BRAIN IMAGING
WITH MRI AND CT

An Image Pattern Approach

BRAIN IMAGING WITH MRI AND CT

An Image Pattern Approach

Edited by

Zoran Rumboldt

Professor of Radiology, Neuroradiology Section Chief and
Fellowship Program Director, Department of Radiology
and Radiological Science, Medical University of
South Carolina, Charleston, South Carolina, USA

Mauricio Castillo

Professor of Radiology and Section Chief of
Neuroradiology, University of North Carolina School of
Medicine, Chapel Hill, North Carolina, USA

Benjamin Huang

Clinical Assistant Professor of Radiology in the
Division of Neuroradiology, University of
North Carolina School of Medicine, Chapel Hill,
North Carolina, USA

Andrea Rossi

Head of the Department of Neuroradiology,
G. Gaslini Children's Research Hospital, Genoa, Italy

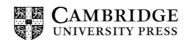

CAMBRIDGE
UNIVERSITY PRESS

CAMBRIDGE UNIVERSITY PRESS

Cambridge, New York, Melbourne, Madrid, Cape Town, Singapore, São Paulo, Delhi, Mexico City

Cambridge University Press

The Edinburgh Building, Cambridge CB2 8RU, UK

Published in the United States of America by Cambridge University Press, New York

www.cambridge.org
Information on this title: www.cambridge.org/9780521119443

First published 2012

Printed and bound in Great Britain by the MPG Books Group

A catalogue record for this publication is available from the British Library

Library of Congress Cataloging-in-Publication Data

Brain imaging with MRI and CT : an image pattern approach / edited by Zoran Rumboldt . . . [et al.].
     p.   cm.
Includes bibliographical references and index.
ISBN 978-0-521-11944-3 (Hardback)
I. Rumboldt, Zoran.
[DNLM: 1. Neuroimaging–methods.   2. Diagnosis, Differential.   3. Magnetic Resonance Imaging–methods.
4.   Tomography, X-Ray Computed–methods. WL 141]
616.8′047548–dc23   2012000482

ISBN 978-0-521-11944-3 Hardback

CONTENTS

Section 1 Bilateral Predominantly Symmetric Abnormalities

Section 2 Sellar, Perisellar and Midline Lesions

Cases

Other Relevant Cases

Section 3 Parenchymal Defects or Abnormal Volume

Cases

Section 4 Abnormalities Without Significant Mass Effect

Cases

A. Primarily Non-Enhancing

Section 5 Primarily Extra-Axial Focal Space-Occupying Lesions

Cases

Section 6 Primarily Intra-Axial Masses

Cases

A. Typically Without Blood Products

Other Relevant Cases

B. Typically With Blood Products

Section 7 Intracranial Calcifications

Cases

CONTRIBUTORS

Mauricio Castillo
Professor of Radiology and Section Chief, Neuroradiology,
University of North Carolina School of Medicine,
Chapel Hill, NC, USA

Alessandro Cianfoni
Associate Professor, Neuroradiology, Image Guided Spinal
Procedures, Department of Radiology and Radiological
Science, Charleston, SC, USA, and
Neuroradiology Section Chief
Neurocenter of Southern Switzerland
Lugano, Switzerland

Chen Hoffmann
Sheba Medical Center, Tel Hashomer, Sakler School of
Medicine, Tel Aviv University, Tel Aviv, Israel

Benjamin Huang
Clinical Assistant Professor of Radiology, Division of
Neuroradiology, University of North Carolina School of
Medicine, Chapel Hill, NC, USA

Maria Gisele Matheus
Assistant Professor, Neuroradiology, Department of
Radiology and Radiological Science, Charleston, SC, USA

Giovanni Morana
Department of Pediatric Neuroradiology, G. Gaslini
Children's Research Hospital, Genoa, Italy

Matthew Omojola
Professor, Section of Neuroradiology, Department of Radiology,
University of Nebraska Medical Center, Omaha, NE, USA

Donna Roberts
Assistant Professor, Neuroradiology, Department of
Radiology and Radiological Science, Charleston,
SC, USA

Andrea Rossi
Head of the Department of Neuroradiology, G. Gaslini
Children's Research Hospital, Genoa, Italy

Zoran Rumboldt
Professor of Radiology, Neuroradiology Section
Chief and Fellowship Program Director, Department
of Radiology and Radiological Science, Medical
University of South Carolina, Charleston,
South Carolina, USA

Mariasavina Severino
Department of Pediatric Neuroradiology, G. Gaslini
Children's Research Hospital, Genoa, Italy

Maria Vittoria Spampinato
Associate Professor, Neuroradiology, Department of
Radiology and Radiological Science, Charleston,
SC, USA

Majda Thurnher
Associate Professor of Radiology, Medical University of
Vienna, Vienna, Austria

Giulio Zuccoli
Section Chief of Neuroradiology, Children's Hospital of
Pittsburgh at the University of Pittsburgh Medical Center,
Pittsburgh, PA, USA

ABBREVIATIONS

αDG	α-dystroglycan	DVST	dural venous sinus thrombosis
AC	arachnoid cyst	DWM	Dandy–Walker malformation
ACE	angiotensin-converting enzyme	EC	ependymal cyst
AD	Alexander disease	ECA	external carotid artery
AD	Alzheimer disease	EDH	epidural (or extradural) hematoma
ADC	apparent diffusion coefficient	EEG	electroencephalography
ADEM	acute disseminated encephalomyelitis	ENB	esthesioneuroblastoma
AESD	acute encephalopathy with biphasic seizures and late reduced diffusion	EPPL	ectopic posterior pituitary lobe
		ESR	erythrocyte sedimentation rate
AG	arachnoid granulation	FA	fractional anisotropy
AGS	Aicardi–Goutières syndrome	FASI	focal areas of signal intensity
ALS	amytrophic lateral sclerosis	FCD	focal cortical dysplasia
AMN	adrenomyeloneuropathy	FCMD	Fukuyama CMD
APD	atypical parkinsonian disorder	FDG	fluorodeoxyglucose
APE	atretic parietal encephalocele	FTD	frontotemporal dementia
AS	aqueductal stenosis	FTLD	frontotemporal lobar degeneration
ATRT	atypical teratoid–rhabdoid tumor	GBM	glioblastoma multiforme
AVM	arteriovenous malformation	GC	gliomatosis cerebri
BBB	blood–brain barrier	GCDH	glutaryl-CoA dehydrogenase
BCAAs	branched-chain amino acids	GCMN	giant cutaneous melanocytic nevi
BCKAs	branched-chain alpha-keto acids	GFAP	glial fibrillary acidic protein
BEH	benign external hydrocephalus	GG	ganglioma
BPP	bilateral perisylvian polymicrogyria	GLHS	Gómez–López–Hernández syndrome
CAA	cerebral amyloid angiopathy	GOM	granular osmiophilic material
CADASIL	cerebral autosomal dominant arteriopathy with subcortical infarcts and leukoencephalopathy	GRE	gradient echo
		HAART	highly active antiretroviral therapy
CAVE	cerebro-acro-visceral early lethality	HCHB	hemichorea–hemiballismus
CBD	cortico-basal degeneration	HD	Huntington disease
CBPS	congenital bilateral perisylvian syndrome	HE	hepatic encephalopathy
CC	corpus callosum	HIE	hypoxic ischemic encephalopathy
CC	cysticercosis	HII	hypoxic–ischemic injury
CCF	carotid-cavernous sinus fistula	HME	hemimegalencephaly
CCM	cerebral cavernous malformations	HOD	hypertrophic olivary degeneration
CD	callosal dysgenesis	HPC	hemangiopericytoma
CDR	clinical dementia rating	HPE	holoprosencephaly
CJD	Creutzfeldt–Jakob disease	HPF	high power field
CMB	classic medulloblastoma	HS	hippocampal sclerosis
CMD	congenital muscular dystrophies	HSAS	hydrocephalus with stenosis of the sylvian aqueduct
CN	cranial nerve		
CNSV	central nervous system vasculitis	HSCT	hematopoietic stem cell transplantation
CPM	central pontine myelinolysis	HSE	herpes simplex encephalitis
CPP	choroid plexus papilloma	IAC	internal auditory canal
CRP	C-reactive protein	ICA	internal carotid artery
CS	cavernous sinus	IHP	idiopathic hypertrophic pachymeningitis
CST	corticospinal tract	iNPH	idiopathic normal pressure hydrocephalus
DAI	diffuse axonal injury	IRIS	immune reconstitution inflammatory syndrome
DAVF	dural arteriovenous fistula		
DCVT	deep cerebral vein thrombosis	JCV	John Cunningham polyomavirus
DI	diabetes insipidus	JS	Joubert syndrome
DIG	desmoplastic infantile gangliogliomas	JSRD	Joubert syndrome related disorders
DIR	double inversion recovery	LA	leukoaraiosis
DMB	desmoplastic/nodular medulloblastoma	LAH	lymphocytic adenohypophysitis
DNET	dysembryoplastic neuroepithelial tumor	LBSL	leukoencephalopathy with brainstem and spinal cord involvement and lactate elevation
DNT	dysembryoplastic neuroepithelial tumor		
DSA	digital subtraction angiography	LCH	Langerhans cell histiocytosis
DVA	developmental venous anomaly	LD	Leigh disease
		LDD	Lhermitte–Duclos disease

LE	limbic encephalitis	PNS	perineural tumor spread
LH	lymphocytic hypophysitis	PRES	posterior reversible encephalopathy syndrome
LIAS	late-onset idiopathic aqueductal stenosis	PSP	progressive supranuclear palsy
LINH	lymphocytic infundibuloneurohypophysitis	PSWCs	periodic sharp and slow wave complexes
LIPH	lymphocytic infundibulopanhypophysitis	PTFE	polytetrafluoroethylene
LM	leptomeningeal melanocytosis	PTH	parathyroid hormone
LN	laminar necrosis	PTPR	papillary tumor of the pineal region
LSV	lenticulo-striate vasculopathy	PVL	periventricular leukomalacia
MA	meningioangiomatosis	PVS	perivascular spaces
MB-EN	medulloblastoma with extensive nodularity	PXA	pleomorphic xanthoastrocytoma
MBS	Marchiafava–Bignami syndrome	rCBV	relative cerebral blood volume
MEB	muscle–eye–brain disease	RCC	Rathke's cleft cyst
MELAS	mitochondrial myopathy, encephalopathy, lactic acidosis, and stroke-like episodes	RCH	remote cerebellar hemorrhage
		RES	rhombencephalosynapsis
MIP	maximum intensity projection	REZ	root entry zone
MLC	megalencephalic leukoencephalopathy with subcortical cysts	SAH	subarachnoid hemorrhage
		SAS	subarachnoid spaces
MLD	metachromatic leukodystrophy	SBH	subcortical band heterotopia
MMC	myelomenigocele	SCC	squamous cell carcinoma
MMSE	mini mental status examination	sCJD	sporadic CJD
MRA	magnetic resonance angiography	SCNSL	secondary CNS lymphoma
MRS	MR spectroscopy	SCP	superior cerebellar peduncles
MS	multiple sclerosis	SD	semantic dementia
MSA	multiple system atrophy	SEGA	subependymal giant cell astrocytoma
MSUD	maple syrup urine disease	SHD	subdural hematoma
MT	magnetization transfer	SIH	spontaneous intracranial hypotension
MTS	mesial temporal sclerosis	SNH	subcortical nodular heterotopia
MVD	microvascular decompression	SOD	septo-optic dysplasia
NASAH	nonaneurysmal SAH	SOV	superior ophthalmic vein
NBIA	neurodegeneration with brain iron accumulation	SS	superficial siderosis
NBO	neurofibromatosis bright objects	SSS	superior sagittal sinus
NCC	neurocysticercosis	SWI	susceptibility-weighted images
NCM	neurocutaneous melanosis	SWS	Sturge–Weber syndrome
ND-LCH	neurodegenerative Langerhans cell histiocytosis	T2WI	T2-weighted imaging
NF1	neurofibromatosis type 1	TCN	therapy-induced (radiation) cerebral necrosis
NH	nodular heterotopia		
NHL	non-Hodgkin lymphoma	TDL	tumefactive demyelinating lesion
NK	nonketotic	TG	tectal glioma
NMO	Neuromyelitis Optica	THS	Tolosa–Hunt syndrome
NPH	normal pressure hydrocephalus	TIA	transient ischemic attack
ONB	olfactory neuroblastoma	TSC	tuberous sclerosis complex
OPG	optic pathway gliomas	UBO	unidentified bright object
PA	pilocytic astrocytomas	vCJD	variant CJD
PACNS	primary angiitis of the CNS	VGAM	vein of Galen aneurysmal malformation
PCNSL	primary CNS lymphoma	VHL	von Hippel–Lindau disease
PCR	polymerase chain reaction	VLCFA	very long chain fatty acids
PD	Parkinson disease	WBRT	whole brain radiation therapy/treatment
PET	positron emission tomography	WBRT	whole-brain radiotherapy
PKAN	pantothenate kinase-associated neurodegeneration	WD	Wallerian degeneration
		WD	Wilson disease
PLIC	posterior limb of the internal capsule	WE	Wernicke encephalopathy
PML	progressive multifocal leukoencephalopathy	WMH	white matter hyperintensities
PNFA	progressive nonfluent aphasia	WWS	Walker–Warburg syndrome
PNH	periventricular nodular heterotopia	X-ALD	X-linked adrenoleukodystrophy

PREFACE

This book was conceived based on the requests and suggestions from radiology residents and neuroradiology fellows (especially once they actually started practicing) and on my own interest in writing a different kind of book. There are already somewhat similar volumes with a differential diagnosis instead of a textbook format; however, the pattern approach, by which the entities are grouped into categories based solely on the imaging findings, represents a novel concept.

The goal of this work is to be useful in real life clinical practice (as well as the board exams) – it is not intended just for neuroradiologists, but probably even more so for practicing general radiologists, neurologists, neurosurgeons, pediatricians and other physicians. The book starts with the bilateral symmetric and midline lesion patterns, as these are the easiest ones to miss, especially by relatively inexperienced readers.

The design has been standardized with images on the left-hand page and the text on the right, and I am personally responsible for the layouts of well over 1500 pictures. Every attempt has been made to include at least two different patients with each entity, and there are only a few with a single one, while frequently the cases comprise images from three or more individuals. The text is concise and broken down into smaller sections, stressing the distinguishing features, both imaging and clinical, with links to other similar cases under the differential diagnosis section.

The book may be used in different ways: by comparing the pattern(s) with an actual clinical case; when looking for characteristics of a certain disease process or a normal variant; for jumping from one case to another through the differential diagnosis sections; as a test (with the right-hand page covered), and even as a regular book from the beginning to the end.

This volume is certainly not aimed at replacing textbooks, but should rather be viewed as a complementary source. It is an attempt at pattern-based approach, not perfect and definitely not all encompassing. There are entities that are not included as separate cases, such as Krabbe disease, neuromyelitis optica, and lacunar infarcts, to name a few, which were for different reasons initially considered. They are, however, listed and briefly described under the differential diagnosis sections. The objective was a book of a reasonable size that would more thoroughly cover the majority of the common and/or radiologically characteristic entities. At some point adding new cases and images, revising text, and updating references had to stop.

I would like to thank all the contributors, especially my co-editors and friends Mauricio, Ben and Andrea. I would also like to acknowledge the colleagues from around the world who have generously provided their excellent cases: Angelika Gutenberg, Chung-Ping Lo, Pranshu Sharma, Se Jeong Jeon, Yasuhiro Nakata and Zoltán Patay. I would like to thank everybody at Cambridge University Press for enabling me to publish the book which I wanted to write for years.

Finally, my special thanks go to my parents, Mirjana and Zvonko, for their continuous support and promotion of academic activity, and to my wife Tihana and daughters Rita, Frida and Zora for their patience and understanding.

Zoran Rumboldt

Bilateral Predominantly Symmetric Abnormalities

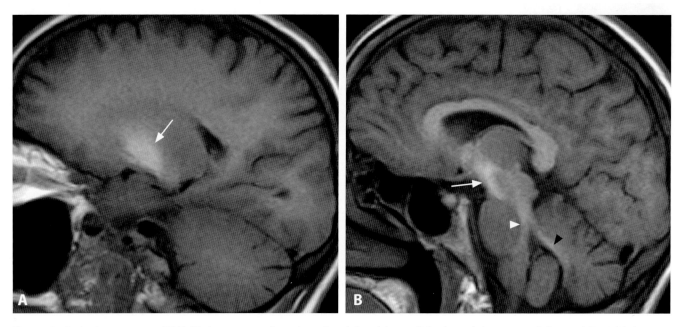

Figure 1. Sagittal non-contrast T1WI (A) demonstrates hyperintensity of the globus pallidus (arrow). A more medial sagittal T1WI (B) shows increased signal in the substantia nigra (arrow), dorsal brainstem (white arrowhead), and cerebellum (black arrowhead).

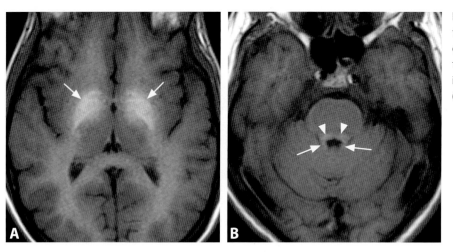

Figure 2. Axial non-contrast T1WI through the basal ganglia (A) shows bilateral bright globus pallidus (arrows). Axial T1WI image through the pons (B) reveals hyperintensity involving superior cerebellar peduncles (arrows) and tectum (arrowheads).

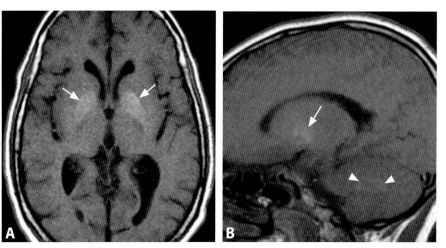

Figure 3. Axial non-contrast T1WI (A) shows a more subtle globus pallidus hyperintensity (arrows). Sagittal T1WI (B) demonstrates high signal in the region of the dentate nucleus (arrowheads) in addition to globus pallidus (arrows).

Hepatic Encephalopathy

MARIA VITTORIA SPAMPINATO

Specific Imaging Findings

Classic brain MR imaging finding in patients with hepatic encephalopathy (HE) is bilateral symmetric globus pallidus hyperintensity on T1-weighted images. When more prominent, high T1 signal is also present in substantia nigra, subthalamic nucleus, tectum, and cerebellar denatate nucleus, with no corresponding findings on T2-weighted images or on CT. Additional MRI findings include diffuse white matter T2 hyperintensity involving predominantly the hemispheric corticospinal tract and focal bright T2 lesions in subcortical hemispheric white matter. MR spectroscopy obtained with short echo time shows depletion of *myo*-inositol. Myo/Cr ratios are decreased not only in cirrhotic patients with clinical or subclinical encephalopathy, but also in individuals without encephalopathy. Increased levels of glutamine/glutamate have also been observed, particularly in severe cases. All these MR imaging findings – bright T1 lesions, white matter T2 hyperintensity, and MRS abnormalities – tend to improve and return to normal with restoration of liver function, such as following a successful liver transplantation. Characteristic MRI appearance of acute hyperammonemic encephalopathy appears to be bilateral symmetric cortical T2 hyperintensity involving the insula and cingulate gyrus, best seen on FLAIR and DWI.

Pertinent Clinical Information

HE includes a spectrum of neuropsychiatric abnormalities occurring in patients with liver dysfunction. Most cases are associated with cirrhosis and portal hypertension or portal-systemic shunts. It is a reversible metabolic encephalopathy, characterized by personality changes and shortened attention span, anxiety and depression, motor incoordination, and flapping tremor of the hands (asterixis). In severe cases, coma and death may occur. Severe forms of hepatic encephalopathy are usually diagnosed clinically; however, mild cases are sometimes difficult to identify even with neuropsychological testing.

Differential Diagnosis

Manganese Intoxication
• indistinguishable T1 hyperintensity (same presumed pathophysiology)

Long-Term Parenteral Nutrition
• indistinguishable T1 hyperintensity (same presumed pathophysiology)
• abnormalities disappear when manganese is excluded from the solution

Physiologic Basal Ganglia Calcifications (187)
• typically punctate to patchy and not diffuse
• calcifications on CT

Neurofibromatosis Type 1 (2)
• typically patchy, not diffuse
• additional areas of involvement

Carbon Monoxide Intoxication (3)
• bright T2 signal and reduced diffusion in bilateral globus pallidus

Hypoxic Ischemic Encephalopathy (7)
• bright T1 signal around the posterior limb of the internal capsule (thalamus, putamen, globus pallidus)
• affects neonates

Kernicterus
• increased T1 and T2 signal of the globus pallidus
• affects neonates

Background

HE (or portal systemic encephalopathy) is caused by inadequate hepatic removal of nitrogenous compounds or other toxins ingested or formed in the gastrointestinal tract. Failure of the hepatic detoxification systems results from compromised hepatic function as well as extensive shunting of splanchnic blood directly into the systemic circulation by porto-systemic collateral vessels. Factors precipitating hepatic encephalopathy in patients with chronic hepatocellular disease include dietary protein load, constipation, and gastrointestinal hemorrhage. As a result, toxic compounds, such as ammonia, manganese, and mercaptans gain access to the central nervous system. These series of events lead to the development of HE. The neurotoxic effects of ammonia are mediated by its effects on several neurotransmitter systems and on brain energetic metabolism. The T1-weighted MRI findings are considered related to the accumulation of manganese, and its serum concentration in cirrhotic patients is tripled compared to normal individuals. Manganese accumulation may lead to parkinsonism, especially with substantia nigra involvement. White matter T2 hyperintensity is thought to be caused by mild brain edema and focal lesions have been linked to spongy degeneration involving the deep layers of the cerebral cortices and the underlying U-fibers.

REFERENCES

1. Rovira A, Alonso J, Córdoba J. MR imaging findings in hepatic encephalopathy. *AJNR* 2008;**29**:1612–21.
2. Spampinato MV, Castillo M, Rojas R, *et al.* Magnetic resonance imaging findings in substance abuse: alcohol and alcoholism and syndromes associated with alcohol abuse. *Top Magn Reson Imaging* 2005;**16**:223–30.
3. Miese F, Kircheis G, Wittsack HJ, *et al.* 1H-MR spectroscopy, magnetization transfer, and diffusion-weighted imaging in alcoholic and nonalcoholic patients with cirrhosis with hepatic encephalopathy. *AJNR* 2006;**27**:1019–26.
4. Matsusue E, Kinoshita T, Ohama E, Ogawa T. Cerebral cortical and white matter lesions in chronic hepatic encephalopathy: MR-pathologic correlations. *AJNR* 2005;**26**:347–51.
5. U-King-Im JM, Yu E, Bartlett E, *et al.* Acute hyperammonemic encephalopathy in adults: imaging findings. *AJNR* 2011;**32**:413–8.

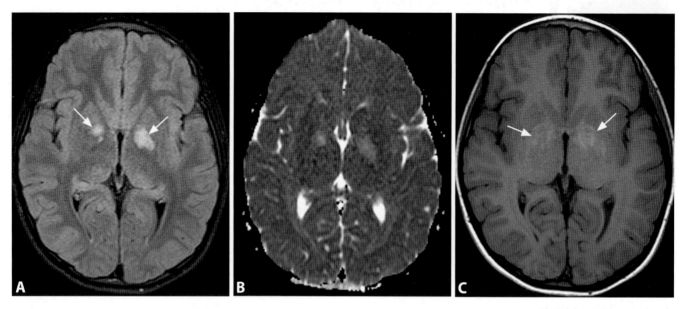

Figure 1. Axial FLAIR image (A) shows bilateral bright signal abnormalities (arrows) in the globi pallidi. There is also increased diffusivity on the ADC map (B) and mild hyperintensity (arrows) on T1WI (C).

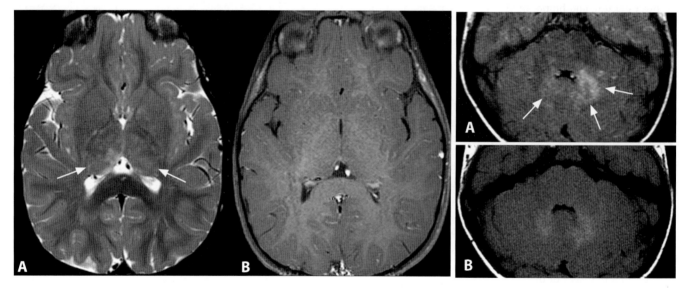

Figure 2. T2WI in another patient (A) depicts multiple hyperintense foci (arrows) predominantly in the thalami without enhancement on post-contrast T1WI (B).

Figure 3. Bright foci in medial cerebellum (arrows) are seen on FLAIR (A) and T1WI (B).

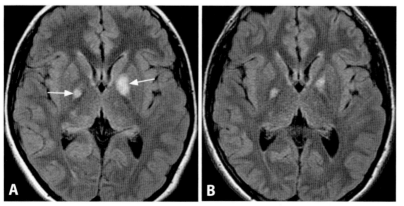

Figure 4. Axial FLAIR image at the basal ganglia level in a 10-year-old patient (A) shows bilateral patchy hyperintense abnormalities primarily involving the globi pallidi (arrows). FLAIR image acquired 3 years later at the same level (B) reveals spontaneous regression of these lesions.

Neurofibromatosis Type 1 – UBOs

ANDREA ROSSI

Specific Imaging Findings

Unidentified bright objects (UBOs) are the most common intra-cranial lesions in patients with neurofibromatosis type 1 (NF1), occurring in about two-thirds of the patients. They typically appear as hyperintense foci on long repetition time (T2-weighted, FLAIR, PD) MR images and iso- to mildly hypointense on T1-weighted images; sometimes they show slight T1 shortening, which has been related to myelin clumping or microcalcification. Mass effect, vasogenic edema, and contrast enhancement are characteristically absent. These lesions typically appear at around 3 years of age, increase in number and size until 10–12 years, and then tend to spontaneously decrease in size and number, or even completely disappear. They are typically multiple and most commonly involve the white matter and basal ganglia (especially the globi pallidi), usually in a bilateral asymmetric fashion. Other common locations include the middle cerebellar peduncles, cerebellar hemispheres, brainstem, internal capsule, splenium of the corpus callosum, and hippocampi. MRS performed within these lesions may be normal or show slightly decreased NAA and increased choline levels.

Pertinent Clinical Information

The correlation between the presence and extent of UBOs and the cognitive deficit or learning disability is still controversial. It has been suggested that the anatomic location of neurofibromatosis bright objects (NBOs) is more important than their presence or number. It seems that thalamic NBOs are in particular significantly associated with neuropsychological impairment. A patient with NF1 may present other CNS lesions (optic pathway tumors and other brain and/or spine low-grade gliomas), skin lesions (café-au-lait spotzs, axillary and inguinal freckling and cutaneous neurofibromas), ocular Lisch nodules and skeletal and skull manifestations (kyphoscoliosis, overgrowth or undergrowth of bone, erosive defects due to neurofibromas, pseudoarthrosis of the tibia and dysplasia of the greater sphenoidal wing).

Differential Diagnosis

Low-Grade Gliomas in NF1
- markedly hypointense on T1-weighted images
- mass effect and possible contrast enhancement
- may also spontaneously regress

Kernicterus
- symmetric bilateral pallidal hyperintensity on T1- and T2-weighted images
- clinical history of neonatal hyperbilirubinemia

PKAN (4)
- symmetric eye-of-the-tiger sign (central hypointensity within hyperintense globi pallidi)

Methylmalonic Aciduria
- symmetric diffuse bilateral pallidal T2 hyperintensity

Hemolytic–Uremic Syndrome
- patients are acutely symptomatic, characteristically with diarrhea and renal failure
- generally symmetric T2 hyperintensity, primarily of the basal ganglia and thalami
- areas of T1 hyperintensity are frequently present, reflecting hemorrhage

Background

UBOs have been described in 60–80% of NF1 cases, but the incidence rises to 90% in patients with concurrent optic glioma. These abnormalities have received numerous designations, among which are "histogenetic foci", focal areas of signal intensity (FASI), non-specific bright foci, and "neurofibromatosis bright objects" (NBOs). The exact nature and significance of UBOs are still unknown. Although they have been related to dysplastic glial proliferation, hamartomatous changes, or heterotopia, no histological evidence has been found to support these hypotheses. Pathological studies, performed in three cases by DiPaolo et al., showed spongiform myelinopathy or vacuolar changes of myelin without frank demyelination, thereby supporting abnormal myelination as a causal factor. Although UBOs are traditionally considered to be transient and benign, proliferative changes (development of tumors from previously recognized UBOs) have been described in children with larger than usual number and volume of NBOs.

REFERENCES

1. Lopes Ferraz Filho JR, Munis MP, Soares Souza A, et al. Unidentified bright objects on brain MRI in children as a diagnostic criterion for neurofibromatosis type 1. Pediatr Radiol 2008; 38:305–10.

2. DiPaolo DP, Zimmerman RA, Rorke LB, et al. Neurofibromatosis type 1: pathologic substrate of high-signal-intensity foci in the brain. Radiology 1995;195:721–4.

3. DeBella K, Poskitt K, Szudek J, Friedman JM. Use of "unidentified bright objects" on MRI for diagnosis of neurofibromatosis 1 in children. Neurology 2000;54:1646–51.

4. Wilkinson ID, Griffiths PD, Wales JK. Proton magnetic resonance spectroscopy of brain lesions in children with neurofibromatosis type 1. Magn Reson Imaging 2001;19:1081–9.

5. Hyman SL, Gill DS, Shores EA, et al. T2 hyperintensities in children with neurofibromatosis type 1 and their relationship to cognitive functioning. J Neurol Neurosurg Psychiatry 2007;78:1088–91.

Brain Imaging with MRI and CT, ed. Zoran Rumboldt et al. Published by Cambridge University Press. © Cambridge University Press 2012.

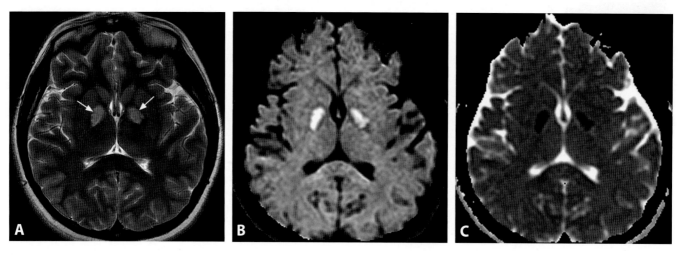

Figure 1. Axial T2WI (A) demonstrates symmetric hyperintense lesions (arrows) in the globi pallidi. Corresponding DWI image (B) shows bright signal of the lesions, which becomes dark on ADC map (C), consistent with reduced diffusivity.

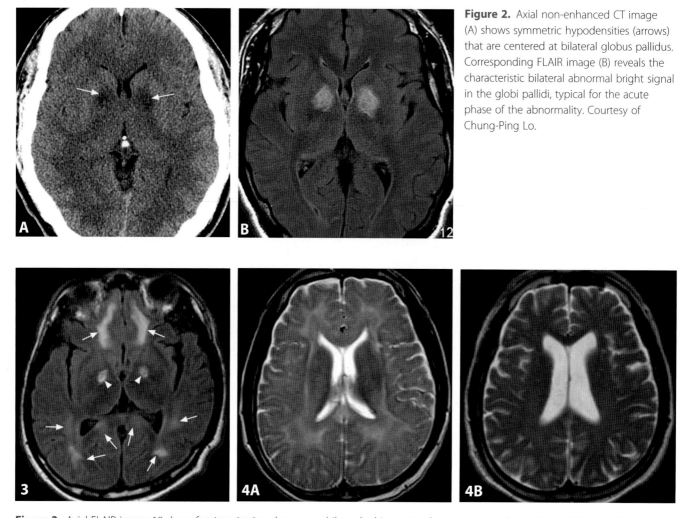

Figure 2. Axial non-enhanced CT image (A) shows symmetric hypodensities (arrows) that are centered at bilateral globus pallidus. Corresponding FLAIR image (B) reveals the characteristic bilateral abnormal bright signal in the globi pallidi, typical for the acute phase of the abnormality. Courtesy of Chung-Ping Lo.

Figure 3. Axial FLAIR image 10 days after intoxication shows new bilateral white matter hyperintensities (arrows), in addition to the initial globi pallidi lesions (arrowheads).

Figure 4. Axial T2WI 1 month later (A) demonstrates diffuse white matter hyperintensity. Corresponding T2WI 19 months later (B) reveals resolution of signal abnormality and progressive brain atrophy. Courtesy of Chung-Ping Lo.

Carbon Monoxide Intoxication

BENJAMIN HUANG

Specific Imaging Findings

The globus pallidus is the most common and characteristic site of brain involvement in acute carbon monoxide (CO) poisoning and CT usually shows symmetric hypodensity. On MRI, the pallidi demonstrate low T1 and high T2 signal with reduced diffusion. T1 hyperintensity and a rim of low T2 signal are sometimes seen, reflecting hemorrhagic necrosis. Patchy or peripheral contrast enhancement may occur in the acute phase. Similar MRI findings are occasionally seen in the substantia nigra, hippocampus and cerebral cortex. In patients who develop a delayed leukoencephalopathy, bilateral symmetric confluent areas of high T2 signal are found in the periventricular white matter and centrum semiovale, along with mildly reduced diffusion. Diffuse white matter involvement may also be present.

Pertinent Clinical Information

Symptoms of mild CO poisoning can include headache, nausea, vomiting, myalgia, dizziness, or neuropsychological impairment. Severe exposures result in confusion, ataxia, seizures, loss of consciousness, or death. Long-term low-level CO poisoning may cause chronic fatigue, affective conditions, memory deficits, sleep disturbances, vertigo, neuropathy, paresthesias, abdominal pain, and diarrhea. On physical examination, patients may demonstrate cherry red lips and mucosa, cyanosis, or retinal hemorrhages. Suspected CO poisoning can be confirmed with blood carboxyhemoglobin levels. Delayed encephalopathy associated with CO toxicity typically occurs 2–3 weeks after recovery from the acute stage of poisoning and is characterized by recurrence of neurologic or psychiatric symptoms. Characteristic symptoms include mental deterioration, urinary incontinence, and gait disturbances. The course of the delayed encephalopathy varies with the severity of intoxication, and symptoms may resolve completely or progress to coma or death.

Differential Diagnosis

Cyanide Intoxication
- may be indistinguishable

PKAN (4)
- symmetric eye-of-the-tiger sign (central hypointensity within hyperintense globi pallidi)

Global Cerebral Anoxia in Mature Brain (13)
- unlikely to preferentially involve globus pallidus
- bilateral deep gray matter and perirolandic cortex involvement

Methanol Intoxication (5)
- characteristic putaminal necrosis
- caudate nucleus may be involved, globus pallidus is typically spared

Leigh Disease (10)
- bilateral brainstem, basal ganglia, and cerebral white matter lesions
- basal ganglia involvement is predominantly in the putamina

Background

CO poisoning is the most frequent cause of accidental poisoning in the US and Europe. Common sources of CO, a by-product of incomplete combustion of carbon-based fuels, include faulty furnaces, inadequately ventilated heating sources, and engine exhaust. CO binds avidly to iron in the hemoglobin molecule, with the affinity 250 times higher than that of oxygen, and forms carboxyhemoglobin. This results in reduction of the oxygen-carrying blood capacity of the subsequent tissue hypoxia. Equally important are the direct cellular effects of CO, primarily inhibition of mitochondrial electron transport enzymes by attaching to their heme-containing proteins. Selective vulnerability of the globus pallidus may be related to its high iron content, as carbon monoxide binds directly to heme iron. Decreased cerebral perfusion from an associated cardiovascular insult contributes to the defect in oxygen transport, and the pathological findings of demyelination, edema, and hemorrhagic necrosis are similar to those of other hypoxic–ischemic lesions. Delayed white matter injury may be the result of polymorphonuclear leukocyte activation, which causes brain lipid peroxidation and myelin breakdown. Low fractional anisotropy (FA) values correlate with damage to the white matter fibers in the subacute phase after CO intoxication in patients with persistent or delayed encephalopathy. Administration of 100% normobaric or hyperbaric oxygen is the mainstay of treatment for acute CO poisoning and may improve long-term neurologic sequelae.

REFERENCES

1. Lo CP, Chen SY, Lee KW, *et al.* Brain injury after acute carbon monoxide poisoning: early and late complications. *AJR* 2007;**189**: W205–11.

2. Kim JH, Chang KH, Song IC, *et al.* Delayed encephalopathy of acute carbon monoxide intoxication: diffusivity of cerebral white matter lesions. *AJNR* 2003;**24**:1592–7.

3. Kinoshita T, Sugihara S, Matsusue E, *et al.* Pallidoreticular damage in acute carbon monoxide poisoning: diffusion-weighted MR imaging findings. *AJNR* 2005;**26**:1845–8.

4. Weaver LK. Clinical practice. Carbon monoxide poisoning. *N Engl J Med* 2009;**360**:1217–25.

5. Beppu T, Nishimoto H, Ishigaki D, *et al.* Assessment of damage to cerebral white matter fiber in the subacute phase after carbon monoxide poisoning using fractional anisotropy in diffusion tensor imaging. *Neuroradiology* 2010;**52**:735–43.

Brain Imaging with MRI and CT, ed. Zoran Rumboldt *et al.* Published by Cambridge University Press. © Cambridge University Press 2012.

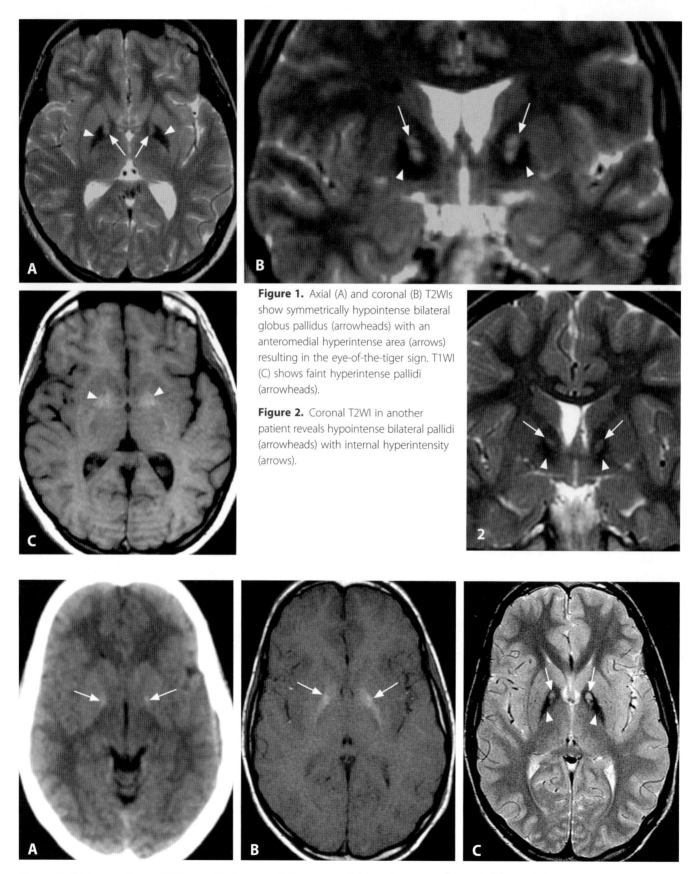

Figure 1. Axial (A) and coronal (B) T2WIs show symmetrically hypointense bilateral globus pallidus (arrowheads) with an anteromedial hyperintense area (arrows) resulting in the eye-of-the-tiger sign. T1WI (C) shows faint hyperintense pallidi (arrowheads).

Figure 2. Coronal T2WI in another patient reveals hypointense bilateral pallidi (arrowheads) with internal hyperintensity (arrows).

Figure 3. Axial non-enhanced CT image (A) shows a subtle anteromedial hyperintensity in bilateral globus pallidus (arrows). Axial T1WI at a similar level shows hyperintensity of the pallidi (arrows), slightly more prominent in the anteromedial aspect. Corresponding T2WI (C) reveals symmetrical bilateral hypointensity of the globus pallidus (arrowheads) containing a focal anteromedial hyperintense area (arrows).

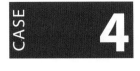

CASE 4

Pantothenate Kinase-Associated Neurodegeneration (Hallervorden–Spatz Syndrome)

ANDREA ROSSI

Specific Imaging Findings

In pantothenate kinase-associated neurodegeneration (PKAN, formerly known as Hallervorden–Spatz syndrome), MRI shows markedly hypointense globi pallidi on T2-weighted images, with a small hyperintense central or anteromedial area. This finding has been labelled the "eye-of-the-tiger" sign and is highly characteristic of PKAN; it is visible on both axial and coronal images. Gradient-echo T2*-weighted images show more profound hypointensity owing to paramagnetic effects. T1-weighted images may show a corresponding high signal intensity of the pallida. There is no contrast enhancement. CT may reveal symmmetrically increased attenuation, primarily in the anteromedial globus pallidus.

Pertinent Clinical Information

This rare autosomal recessive disorder is a part of a group of diseases called "neurodegeneration with brain iron accumulation" (NBIA) which also includes aceruloplasminemia and neuroferritinopathy. PKAN typically presents in older children or adolescents with oromandibular dystonia, mental deterioration, pyramidal signs, and retinal degeneration. Most patients die within 10 years of the clinical onset, although longer survival into early adulthood is possible.

Differential Diagnosis

HARP Syndrome (hypopre-β-lipoproteinemia, acanthocytosis, retinitis pigmentosa, and pallidal degeneration)
• may be indistinguishable

Other Forms of NBIA
• "eye-of-the-tiger" sign absent

Toxic Encephalopathies (CO poisoning) (3)
• globus pallidus T2 hyperintensity without hypointense portion

Kernicterus
• globus pallidus T2 hyperintensity without hypointense portion

Methylmalonic Acidemia
• globus pallidus T2 hyperintensity without hypointense portion

Normal Iron Deposition
• iron starts accumulating in the pallidi during later childhood and adolescence and is usually seen on MRI from approximately 25 years of age onwards

Background

The causal gene, PKAN, is located on the short arm of chromosome 20 and encodes for pantothenate kinase, which regulates the synthesis of coenzyme A from pantothenate, thus participating in fatty acid synthesis and energy metabolism. Defective membrane biosynthesis may result in cysteine increase, which is believed to play a role in the accumulation of iron in the basal ganglia, in turn generating the typical MRI appearance of PKAN. PANK2 mutation analysis confirms the diagnosis, and may be used for prenatal diagnosis in affected families.

Axonal dystrophy with spheroid bodies is found exclusively in the brain, while skin or conjunctival biopsy is typically negative. Abnormal increase of iron deposits within the globus pallidus, with rusty brown discoloration and neuroaxonal swelling, is found on histology. Iron deposits occur either around vessels or as free tissue accumulations and may also involve the substantia nigra and red nuclei. There are associated dystrophic axons and reactive astrocytes in a similar distribution.

REFERENCES

1. Gordon N. Pantothenate kinase-associated neurodegeneration (Hallervorden–Spatz syndrome). *Eur J Pediatr Neurol* 2002;**6**:243–7.
2. Angelini L, Nardocci N, Rumi V. Hallervorden–Spatz disease: clinical and MRI study of 11 cases diagnosed in life. *J Neurol* 1992;**239**:417–25.
3. Zhou B, Westaway SK, Levinson B, *et al.* A novel pantothenate kinase gene (PANK2) is defective in Hallervorden–Spatz syndrome. *Nature Genet* 2001;**28**:345–9.
4. Savoiardo M, Halliday WC, Nardocci N, *et al.* Hallervorden–Spatz disease: MR and pathologic findings. *AJNR* 1993;**14**:155–62.
5. Ching KH, Westaway SK, Gitschier J, *et al.* HARP syndrome is allelic with pantothenate kinase-associated neurodegeneration. *Neurology* 2002;**58**:1673–4.

Brain Imaging with MRI and CT, ed. Zoran Rumboldt *et al.* Published by Cambridge University Press. © Cambridge University Press 2012.

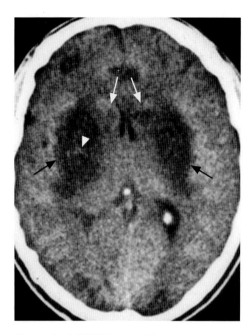

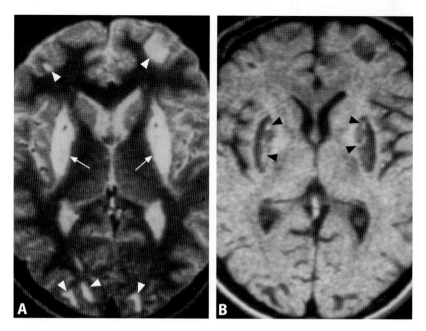

Figure 1. Axial CT image without contrast demonstrates symmetric basal ganglia swelling and hypodensity (arrows). Small hyperdense foci on the right (arrowhead) are consistent with hemorrhage.

Figure 2. Axial T2WI (A) shows symmetric high signal intensity in bilateral putamina (arrows), as well as in subcortical white matter of the left frontal and bilateral occipital lobes (arrowheads). Corresponding T1WI (B) demonstrates predominantly low signal intensity in these regions with a few small foci of higher signal (arrowheads) in the putamina, compatible with small hemorrhages.

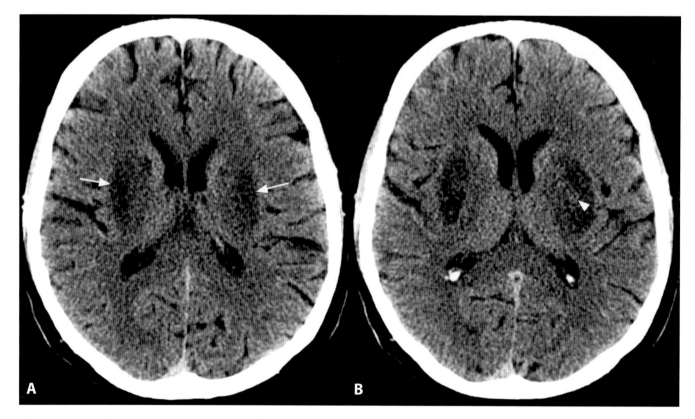

Figure 3. Axial CT images without contrast (A and B) show symmetric bilateral basal ganglia hypodensity (arrows) predominantly involving putamina. Subtle hyperdensity (arrowhead) within the lesions is consistent with hemorrhage. Courtesy of Pranshu Sharma.

Methanol Intoxication

BENJAMIN HUANG

Specific Imaging Findings

Initial CT and MRI studies in patients following methanol ingestion may be normal. CT and MRI performed at least 24 h after ingestion demonstrate characteristic bilateral necrosis of the putamina, which appear hypodense and edematous on CT and hyperintense on T2-weighted MR images. Hemorrhagic foci can also be seen within the putaminal lesions and other basal ganglia may be involved. Contrast-enhanced MR images may demonstrate peripheral enhancement of putaminal and subcortical lesions in the acute phase of injury. Optic nerve MR imaging reveals nonspecific T2 hyperintensity. Other findings seen in patients who survive for several days are non-enhancing areas of necrosis within the peripheral white matter, with sparing of the subcortical white matter U-fibers.

Pertinent Clinical Information

Symptoms of methanol intoxication usually begin after a 12- to 24-h latent period following ingestion. Patients typically experience visual disturbances, including decrease in visual acuity, visual field defects, color blindness, hyperemia of the optic discs, and peripapillary nerve fiber edema, and neurologic symptoms, including weakness, headache, and dizziness. Gastrointestinal complaints (pain, nausea, and vomiting) are also common. With larger consumed doses, seizures, stupor, and coma may occur. Laboratory evaluations will reveal a severe metabolic acidosis. Patients who survive methanol poisoning may have permanent blindness or irreversible neurologic impairments.

Differential Diagnosis

Global Cerebral Anoxia in Mature Brain (13)
- cortical involvement common
- no optic nerve involvement

Creutzfeldt–Jakob Disease (12)
- presence of cortical lesions
- gradual onset of symptoms

Leigh Disease (10)
- brainstem involvement common

Wilson Disease (6)
- brainstem involvement common, "Panda sign"

Carbon Monoxide Intoxication (3)
- globus pallidus lesions, putamen is spared

Background

Methanol is a colorless fluid which smells and tastes similar to ethanol. It is widely used in industry as a denaturant additive to ethanol and is also found in a number of commercially available products including antifreeze, paint removers, windshield washer fluid, and various solvents. Methanol has also been found in bootlegged alcohol and fraudulently adulterated alcoholic beverages. Methanol is metabolized in the liver by the enzyme alcohol dehydrogenase into formaldehyde, which is subsequently metabolized into formic acid, the metabolite which is primarily responsible for methanol's toxicity. Metabolism into formaldehyde is a relatively slow process, which accounts for the latent period observed between ingestion and onset of symptoms. Accumulation of formic acid results in a metabolic acidosis early on. Tissue hypoxia caused by formate inhibition of oxidative metabolism (through effects on cytochrome c oxidase) may explain its toxicity to the brain and optic nerves. Hemorrhagic putaminal necrosis is the pathologic finding that is typical of methanol intoxication, and selective vulnerability of the putamina may be due to their higher oxygen consumption relative to other structures. Acute methanol poisoning is treated with hemodialysis as well as with ethanol or fomepizole, which inhibits metabolism of methanol by alcohol dehydrogenase.

REFERENCES

1. Sefidbakht S, Rasekhi AR, Kamali K, *et al*. Methanol poisoning: acute MR and CT findings in nine patients. *Neuroradiology* 2007;**49**:427–35.
2. Sharma P, Eesa M, Scott JN. Toxic and acquired metabolic encephalopathies: MRI appearance. *AJR* 2009;**193**:879–86.
3. Blanco M, Casado R, Vazquez F, Pumar JM. CT and MR imaging findings in methanol intoxication. *AJNR* 2006;**27**:452–4.
4. Barceloux DG, Bond GR, Krenzelok EP, *et al*. American Academy of Clinical Toxicology practice guidelines on the treatment of methanol poisoning. *Clinical Toxicology* 2002;**40**:415–46.
5. Spampinato MV, Castillo M, Rojas R, *et al*. Magnetic resonance imaging findings in substance abuse. Alcohol and alcoholism and syndromes associated with alcohol abuse. *Top Magn Reson Imaging* 2005;**16**:223–30.

Brain Imaging with MRI and CT, ed. Zoran Rumboldt *et al.* Published by Cambridge University Press. © Cambridge University Press 2012.

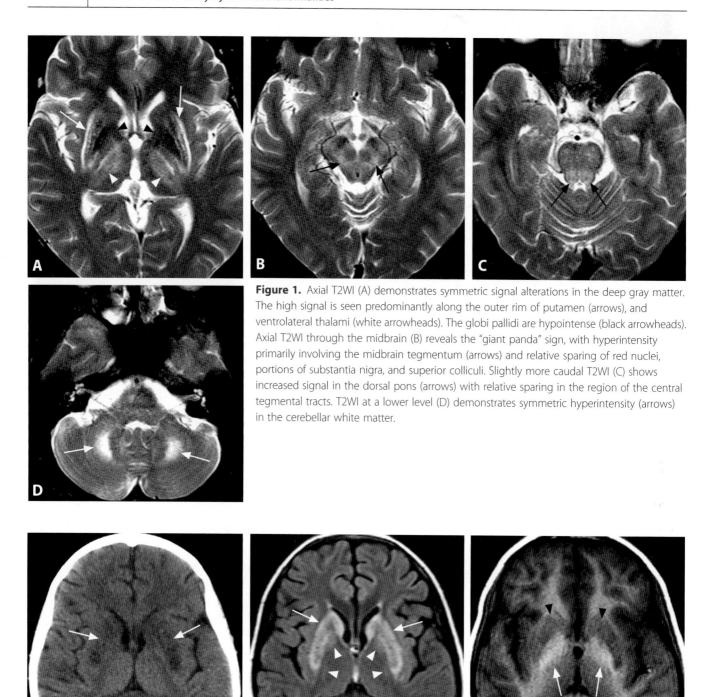

Figure 1. Axial T2WI (A) demonstrates symmetric signal alterations in the deep gray matter. The high signal is seen predominantly along the outer rim of putamen (arrows), and ventrolateral thalami (white arrowheads). The globi pallidi are hypointense (black arrowheads). Axial T2WI through the midbrain (B) reveals the "giant panda" sign, with hyperintensity primarily involving the midbrain tegmentum (arrows) and relative sparing of red nuclei, portions of substantia nigra, and superior colliculi. Slightly more caudal T2WI (C) shows increased signal in the dorsal pons (arrows) with relative sparing in the region of the central tegmental tracts. T2WI at a lower level (D) demonstrates symmetric hyperintensity (arrows) in the cerebellar white matter.

Figure 2. Non-enhanced axial CT (A) in a young girl shows bilateral hypodensity in the basal ganglia (arrows), primarily putamen and caudate head. Axial FLAIR image (B) reveals corresponding hyperintensity (arrows). There is also subtle increase in signal intensity (arrowheads) in bilateral globus pallidus and lateral thalamus. Axial T1WI at a slightly lower level (C) shows bilateral mild decrease in signal intensity of striatum (arrowheads) and hyperintensity of globus pallidus (arrows).

Wilson Disease

BENJAMIN HUANG

Specific Imaging Findings

Symmetric increased T2 signal in the deep gray matter is typical for Wilson disease (WD), primarily involving the putamen, followed by thalami (commonly ventrolateral), caudate, and globus pallidus. Hyperintensity may be characteristically localized to the outer rim of the putamen. Globi pallidi sometimes show very low T2 signal. In some patients the characteristic "giant panda" sign is found in the midbrain: hyperintensity throughout the tegmentum with relative sparing of red nuclei, lateral pars reticulata of the substantia nigra, and superior colliculi. Central and dorsal pons may also be affected. Dorsal pontine involvement with sparing of central tegmental tracts has been described as a second smaller panda face or "panda cub" – relatively low signal of central tegmental tracts represents the eyes and aqueduct represents the mouth. Less frequently affected are claustrum and other gray matter structures, including cortex, as well as the white matter, primarily superior and middle cerebellar peduncles. The lesions are usually of intermediate to low T1 signal intensity and do not enhance with contrast. With severe liver failure, symmetric T1 hyperintensity of globi pallidi may be present, similar to other causes of hepatic dysfunction. Generalized cerebral and cerebellar atrophy are commonly observed with WD. T2 hyperintensities frequently improve with therapy.

Pertinent Clinical Information

WD, also known as hepatolenticular degeneration, affects multiple organ systems and patients can present in strikingly diverse ways. Hepatic dysfunction is the initial manifestation in 40–50% of patients, while 40–60% present with neurologic manifestations. Neurologic symptoms usually start in the late teens, but can occur even earlier. Tremor is most frequent, followed by dysarthria, cerebellar dysfunction, dystonia, gait abnormalities, and autonomic dysfunction. Psychiatric illness is present in up to two-thirds of patients, most commonly personality changes and depression. Kayser–Fleischer rings – brown or green corneal pigmentation caused by sulfur–copper deposition – are the classic WD finding, almost invariably present in individuals with neurologic or psychiatric symptoms. Diagnosis relies on a battery of tests including slit lamp examination, serum ceruloplasmin, bound and unbound serum copper, 24-h urinary copper excretion, and neuroimaging. Liver biopsy for determination of copper content is the single most sensitive and accurate test, usually performed only when noninvasive exams are inconclusive. Patients with WD require lifelong treatment with chelating agents (D-penicillamine) or zinc. Liver transplantation is performed for fulminant hepatic failure.

Differential Diagnosis

Leigh Disease (10)
- T2 hyperintensity may involve subthalamic and cerebellar dentate nucleus
- elevated lactate in basal ganglia and CSF on MRS

Creutzfeldt–Jakob Disease (12)
- lesions are bright on DWI
- prominent cortical involvement
- posteromedial thalamic involvement in variant form

Hypoxic Ischemic Encephalopathy (7)
- lesions have decreased diffusivity in the acute phase
- cortical involvement frequently present
- T1 hyperintensity around the internal capsule
- lactate on MRS

Methanol Intoxication (5)
- putamen primarily affected, frequently with hemorrhage
- possible white matter edema

Background

WD is a rare autosomal-recessive disorder caused by mutations in the *ATP7B* gene located on chromosome 13. ATP7B protein is involved in the process of copper transport by mediating the formation of ceruloplasmin and by transporting excess copper across hepatocyte membranes into the biliary tract. A defect in this protein results in progressive copper accumulation in hepatocytes, ultimately leading to hepatic dysfunction. Once the liver's capacity to store copper is exceeded, unbound copper becomes deposited in other tissues and organs, including the brain. It is assumed that cellular damage is due to direct copper toxicity, but recent evidence suggests that copper elevation induces cell death by reducing levels of XIAP, a protein that inhibits apoptosis. The neuroimaging findings presumably reflect a combination of edema, spongy or cystic gray matter degeneration, gliosis, myelinolysis, and demyelination.

REFERENCES

1. Kim TJ, Kim IO, Kim WS, *et al*. MR imaging of the brain in Wilson disease of childhood: findings before and after treatment with clinical correlation. *AJNR* 2006;**27**:1373–8.

2. Sinha S, Taly AB, Ravishankar S, *et al*. Wilson's disease: cranial MRI observations and clinical correlation. *Neuroradiology* 2006;**48**:613–21.

3. King AD, Walshe JM, Kendall BE, *et al*. Cranial MR imaging in Wilson's disease. *AJR* 1996;**167**:1579–84.

4. van Wassenaer-van Hall HN, van den Heuvel AG, Algra A, *et al*. Wilson disease: findings at MR imaging and CT of the brain with clinical correlation. *Radiology* 1996;**198**:531–6.

Brain Imaging with MRI and CT, ed. Zoran Rumboldt *et al*. Published by Cambridge University Press. © Cambridge University Press 2012.

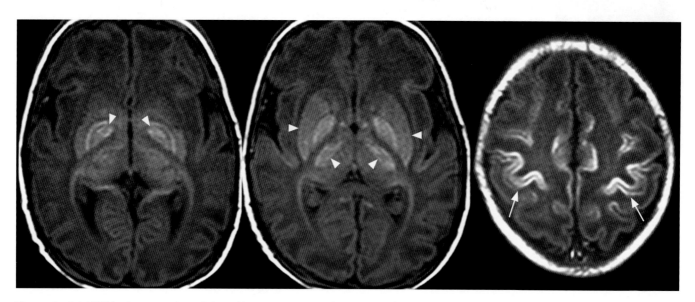

Figure 1. Axial T1WIs show prominent bilateral hyperintensities within putamina, globi pallidi and lateral thalami (arrowheads) around the posterior limb of the internal capsule (PLIC), with relative caudate head sparing. There is also bilateral cortical brightness (arrows) around the precentral sulcus.

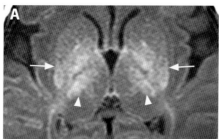

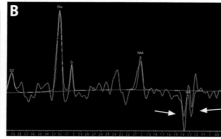

Figure 2. Bilateral bright posterior lentiform nucleus (arrow) and ventrolateral thalamus (arrowhead), surrounding relatively dark PLIC on T1WI (A). Intermediate echo time MRS (B) shows prominent lactate (arrows).

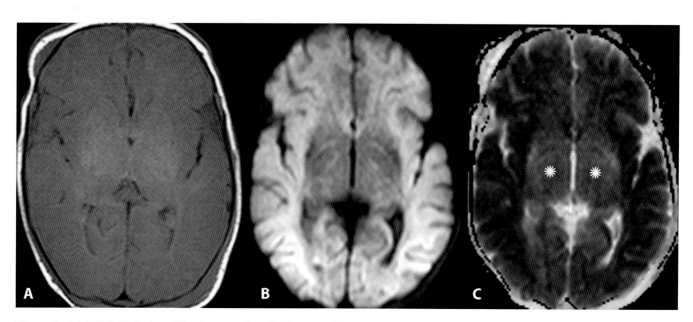

Figure 3. Axial T1WI (A) depicts diffuse brain swelling, PLIC is not visible. Corresponding DWI (B) and ADC maps (C) reveal widespread reduced diffusion with relative sparing of central gray matter (*).

Hypoxic Ischemic Encephalopathy in Term Neonates

MARIASAVINA SEVERINO

Specific Imaging Findings

The findings in Hypoxic Ischemic Encephalopathy (HIE) are variable and depend on brain maturity, severity and duration of insult, and timing of imaging studies. In moderate-to-severe HIE at term, the central gray matter is the most frequently affected with lesions in the lentiform nuclei and thalami, typically adjacent to the posterior limb of the internal capsule (PLIC). Cortical abnormalities are characteristically found in the perirolandic area. These lesions are T1 hypointense and T2 hyperintense in the acute phase (first 2 days), becoming T1 hyperintense after 3–5 days. An early sign is the loss PLIC on conventional MR sequences. The most reliable sign of HIE, which also remains for a long time, is the reversal of normal PLIC T1 hyperintensity compared to the adjacent lentiform nucleus and thalamus.

In severe and prolonged HIE at term, there is diffuse brain swelling and edema, usually sparing the basal ganglia, brainstem, and cerebellum. The lesions rapidly evolve by cavitation, developing into multicystic encephalopathy. In mild HIE, typical MRI features are characterized by parasagittal lesions involving vascular boundary zones (watershed injury pattern). Diffusion imaging shows corresponding bright DWI signal and reduced apparent diffusion coefficient (ADC) values in the first 24 h. These abnormalities peak at 3–5 days and pseudonormalize by about the end of the first week. MR spectroscopy demonstrates lactate peak in the affected regions. A glutamine–glutamate (Glx) peak may also be elevated.

Pertinent Clinical Information

Term neonates with HIE show signs of intrapartum distress, severe functional depression with low Apgar scores and metabolic acidosis documented in the cord blood. They require resuscitation at birth and have neurological abnormalities in the first 24 h (apnea, seizures and hypotonia) with electroencephalographic (EEG) abnormalities. Sarnat and Sarnat classification is based on clinical scoring system for developmental outcome subdividing the infants with HIE into three groups: normal, mildly abnormal, and definitely abnormal.

Differential Diagnosis

Kernicterus
- bilateral increased T1 and T2 signal usually isolated to the globus pallidus

Urea-Cycle Disorders
- bilateral T2 hyperintensities of the lentiform nuclei, insular and perirolandic cortex
- absence of thalamic injury

Manganese Intoxication; Hepatic Encephalopathy (1)
- T1 hyperintensity of the globi pallidi without putaminal or thalamic involvement
- T1 hyperintensity may be present in substantia nigra, tectum, cerebellum

Leigh Disease (10)
- lesions of the putamen, caudate nucleus and globus pallidus with thalamus usually spared
- brainstem and cerebellar dentate nuclei are commonly involved

Non-Ketotic Hyperglycinaemia
- in addition to PLIC, dorsal brain stem and cerebral peduncles are involved
- glycine peak is shown by proton MR spectroscopy at 3.56 ppm

Background

Perinatal HIE occurs in up to 2/1000 live births and is a significant cause of mortality and severe neurological disability, accounting for 15–28% of children with cerebral palsy. The exact pathophysiology of HIE is not completely understood, the lack of sufficient blood flow in conjunction with its decreased oxygen content leads to loss of normal cerebral autoregulation and diffuse brain injury. It may result from fetal cardiac and vascular compromise, either *in utero* (placental abruption, fetomaternal hemorrhage, fetal bradycardia, maternal hypotension or preeclampsia, and tight nuchal cord or cord prolapse) or postnatally (severe hyaline membrane disease, meconium aspiration, or congenital heart anomalies). Treatment consists of supportive care, but new emerging neuroprotective strategies, such as hypothermia and administration of excitatory amino acid antagonists, have been developed to prevent brain injury that occurs immediately following the causative insult. It has been shown that favorable outcome is very likely if the T1 signal intensity in the posterolateral putamen is less than in the PLIC, whereas adverse outcome is very likely if putamen is equal to or brighter than PLIC.

REFERENCES

1. Liauw L, van der Grond J, van den Berg-Huysmans AA, *et al*. Is there a way to predict outcome in (near) term neonates with hypoxic-ischemic encephalopathy based on MR imaging? *AJNR* 2008;**29**:1789–94.
2. Huang BY, Castillo M. Hypoxic–ischemic brain injury: imaging findings from birth to adulthood. *Radiographics* 2008;**28**:417–39.
3. Chao CP, Zaleski CG, Patton AC. Neonatal hypoxic–ischemic encephalopathy: multimodality imaging findings. *Radiographics* 2006;**26**(Suppl 1):S159–72.
4. Triulzi F, Parazzini C, Righini A. Patterns of damage in the mature neonatal brain. *Pediatr Radiol* 2006;**36**:608–20.

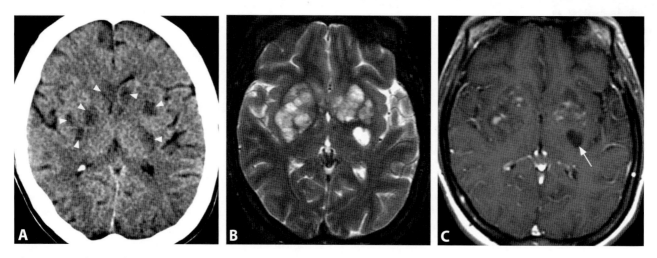

Figure 1. Axial non-enhanced CT image (A) in a patient with AIDS shows multifocal bilateral basal ganglia hypodensities (arrowheads). Corresponding T2WI (B) demonstrates multiple hyperintense lesions in the basal ganglia. On post-contrast T1WI (C) there is enhancement within several but not all of these lesions – note the non-enhancing lesion in the tail of the left putamen (arrow).

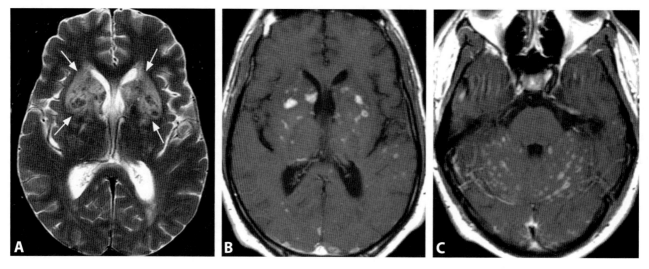

Figure 2. Axial T2WI (A) and post-contrast T1WI (B) in a different patient show multiple lesions, predominantly located in the basal ganglia, but also scattered throughout the cerebral hemispheres. There is marked edema (arrows) associated with the basal ganglia lesions. Innumerable enhancing nodules throughout the cerebellar hemispheres are depicted on post-contrast T1WI (C).

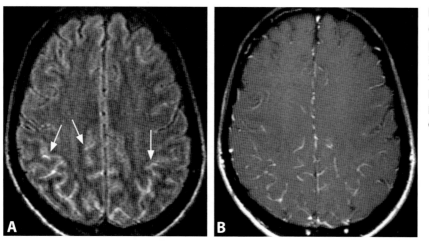

Figure 3. Axial FLAIR image at the level of the centrum semiovale (A) in an immunocompetent patient demonstrates bilateral increased signal intensity (arrows) within the posterior sulcal subarachnoid space, suggesting the presence of proteinaceous material. Corresponding post-contrast T1WI (B) reveals leptomeningeal enhancement within these sulci.

Cryptococcosis

BENJAMIN HUANG

Specific Imaging Findings

Manifestations of cryptococcal CNS infection are varied and include: (1) meningoencephalitis, (2) gelatinous pseudocysts, (3) parenchymal or intraventricular miliary nodules/cryptococcomas, or (4) a combination of these findings. Imaging studies (especially CT) may frequently be normal or show just ventriculomegaly, which is the most common radiologic abnormality. Meningoencephalitis appears as cortical and subcortical hyperintensity on FLAIR images with associated leptomeningeal (often nodular) enhancement. Gelatinous pseudocysts appear as rapidly enlarging, well-demarcated, cystic lesions in the basal ganglia and deep white matter of low density on CT, and signal similar to cerebrospinal fluid (CSF) on T2- and T1-weighted MRI, without contrast enhancement. On FLAIR images, the lesions may be hyperintense to CSF. The finding of multiple cysts/dilated perivascular spaces in an immunosuppressed patient is highly suspicious for cryptococcal infection. Cryptococcomas appear as enhancing nodular intra-axial lesions (usually in the deep gray matter and cerebellum) or as intraventricular lesions with enlarged choroid plexus (choroid plexitis), leading to hydrocephalus. They are T2 hyperintense similar to pseudocysts, range in size from a few millimeters to several centimeters, and may have surrounding edema.

Pertinent Clinical Information

The CNS and the lung are the two primary sites of infection with *Cryptococcus neoformans*. Patients with CNS cryptococcosis typically present with nonspecific signs of subacute or chronic meningitis or meningoencephalitis, including headaches, fever, lethargy, nausea, vomiting, or memory loss over a period of several weeks. The diagnosis is confirmed by encapsulated yeast cells on direct microscopic examination of the CSF with India ink, positive CSF cultures for *C. neoformans*, or detection of the cryptococcal capsular polysaccharide antigen in the CSF. Without appropriate antifungal treatment, cryptococcal meningitis is uniformly fatal.

Differential Diagnosis

Dilated Perivascular Spaces (168)
- absent parenchymal or leptomeningeal enhancement
- no T2 hyperintensity around the fluid-containing spaces

Other Meningoencephalitides
- no perivascular space enlargement

Cerebral Toxoplasmosis (157)
- focal ring enhancing lesions, "eccentric target sign"
- no perivascular space dilatation

Primary CNS Lymphoma (158)
- focal enhancing lesions with low ADC values
- no perivascular space dilatation

Background

Cryptococcus neoformans is a ubiquitous yeast-like fungus found in soil contaminated by bird excreta. It is the most common fungal CNS pathogen and the third most common cause of CNS infection overall (behind HIV and *Toxoplasma*) in AIDS patients. CNS cryptococcosis can also occur in immunocompetent individuals. The organism spreads to the CNS by hematogenous dissemination from a pulmonary focus, and reactivation of a latent infection is also possible. The organisms extend from the basal cisterns into the brain via the perivascular (Virchow–Robin) spaces, resulting in pseudocysts filled with the fungi and their gelatinous capsular material. Cryptococcomas are histologically chronic granulomatous reactions with relatively few organisms or lesions containing numerous organisms with only mild inflammation; the latter form resembles gelatinous pseudocysts both radiographically and histologically. The degree of contrast enhancement in cryptococcomas correlates to an individual's immune status – in severely immunosuppressed patients there is less inflammatory change and less enhancement. Immune reconstitution inflammatory syndrome (IRIS) may be associated with *Cryptococcus* – symptoms of acute cryptococcal meningitis typically occur weeks to months after starting a highly active antiretroviral therapy (HAART) regimen.

REFERENCES

1. Tien RD, Chu PK, Hesselink JR, *et al.* Intracranial cryptococcosis in immunocompromised patients: CT and MR findings in 29 cases. *AJNR* 1991;**12**:283–9.
2. Mathews VP, Alo PL, Glass JD, *et al.* AIDS-related CNS cryptococcosis: radiologic–pathologic correlation. *AJNR* 1992;**13**:1477–86.
3. Smith AB, Smirniotopoulos JG, Rushing EJ. From the archives of the AFIP. Central nervous system infections associated with human immunodeficiency virus infection: radiology–pathologic correlation. *Radiographics* 2008;**28**:2033–58.
4. Haddow LJ, Colebunders R, Meintjes G, *et al.* Cryptococcal immune reconstitution inflammatory syndrome in HIV-1-infected individuals: proposed clinical case definitions. *Lancet Infect Dis* 2010;**10**:791–802.
5. Perfect JR, Casadevall A. Cryptococcosis. *Infect Dis Clin N Am* 2002;**16**:837–74.

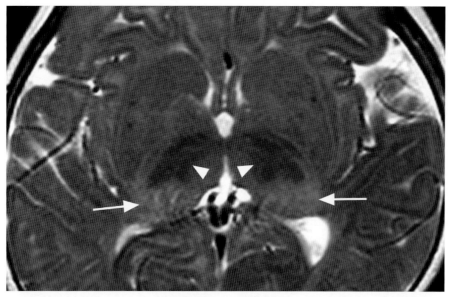

Figure 1. Axial T2WI obtained in a macrocephalic infant with psychomotor retardation and seizures reveals symmetric very low signal intensity of the ventral thalami (arrowheads). There is associated hyperintensity (arrows) of the posterior thalami.

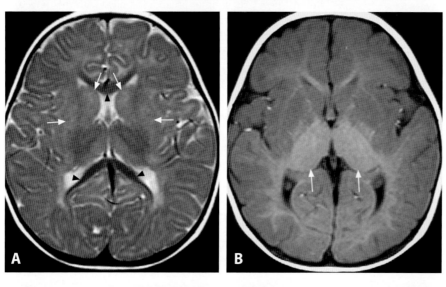

Figure 2. Axial T2WI (A) in a 4-year-old patient shows swelling and increased signal intensity in the basal ganglia (arrows). The cerebral hemispheric white matter shows diffuse abnormal hyperintensity with sparing of the corpus callosum (arrowheads). Axial T1WI (B) shows hyperintensity of the thalámi (arrows).

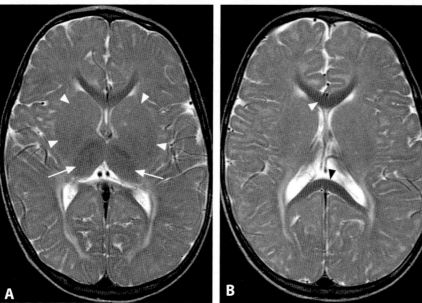

Figure 3. Axial T2WI (A) in a 12-year-old patient with extrapyramidal symptoms and psychosis shows hyperintensity of the cerebral white matter. There is a mild symmetric increased signal intensity with swelling of the basal ganglia (arrowheads), while the thalami are hypointense (arrows). T2WI at a higher level (B) better shows notable sparing of the corpus callosum (arrowheads). Courtesy of Zoltán Patay.

Gangliosidosis GM2

MARIASAVINA SEVERINO

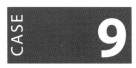

Specific Imaging Findings

Imaging findings in Tay–Sachs (Infantile GM2 Gangliosidosis Type B) and Sandhoff diseases (Infantile GM2 Gangliosidosis Type O) are quite similar. The lesion pattern in a macrocephalic infant is highly suggestive and includes symmetrical hyperdensities within the thalami and/or basal ganglia on brain CT. The thalami are typically hyperintense on T1-weighted images and hypointense on T2-weighted images. In Tay–Sachs disease the posterior part of the thalami may be T2 hyperintense. The putamina, caudate nuclei and globi pallidi are swollen and hyperintense on T2-weighted images. Widespread white matter changes within the cerebral hemispheres are also noted with sparing of corpus callosum, anterior commissure, and posterior limbs of the internal capsules. Brain atrophy appears in the final stages of the disease. Diffusion imaging is usually unremarkable. Brain MRS shows decline in the NAA, increased choline and progressive elevation of *myo*-inositol. In juvenile and adult GM2 gangliosidosis, there is cerebral and cerebellar atrophy, generally in combination with slight white matter signal changes. A decrease in T2 signal intensity of the thalami is also found in a number of other diseases caused by genetic mutations and it seems to be a sign of lysosomal disease.

Pertinent Clinical Information

Patients with infantile GM2 Gangliosidosis forms are macrocephalic and present before 6 months of age with a progressive neurological disease characterized by psychomotor deterioration, pyramidal and later extrapyramidal (choreoathetosis) signs, feeding problems, and generalized tonic–clonic seizures. In the later stages of the disease, patients are usually deaf and blind (with a cherry-red spot in one or both maculae in most cases). Hepatosplenomegaly may be present in Sandhoff disease. Death usually occurs between 2 and 3 years of age. Patients with juvenile (onset at 2–6 years) and adult (onset at 10–40 years) forms usually exhibit a slower progression of the disease with dysarthria, extrapyramidal dysfunction, dementia, psychosis, and depression.

Differential Diagnosis

Krabbe Disease
- dentate nuclei usually involved while signal abnormality in the basal ganglia is lacking
- white matter disease does not spare the corpus callosum
- presence of optic nerve enlargement and cranial nerve/spinal roots enhancement

Fucosidosis
- additional T2 hypointensity and T1 hyperintensity of the globi pallidi

Neuronal Ceroid Lipofuscinosis
- severe cerebral and cerebellar atrophy associated with white matter signal changes
- frequent optic nerve atrophy

Status Marmoratus
- hyperdense thalami on CT
- white matter signal changes associated with global brain atrophy

Toluene Toxicity
- diffuse atrophy
- loss of differentiation between the gray and white matter
- T2 hypointensity may also involve basal ganglia
- older patients (teenagers, adults)

Background

GM2 gangliosidoses are rare lysosomal storage disorders caused by autosomal recessive mutations in the genes encoding β-hexosaminidase A and/or B, and GM2 activator glycoprotein. Deficient activity of these enzymes leads to accumulation of GM2 gangliosides inside neuronal lysosomes, leading to cell death. There are three major, biochemically distinct types: B, O, and AB. Among the B and O types, infantile, juvenile, and adult forms can be distinguished; the AB variant is known only as an infantile form. Tay–Sachs disease (B) is more common in Ashkenazi Jews while Sandhoff disease (O) and AB variant have no ethnic predilection. The treatment is supportive and mainly aimed at seizure control.

REFERENCES

1. Autti T, Joensuu R, Aberg L. Decreased T2 signal in the thalami may be a sign of lysosomal storage disease. *Neuroradiology* 2007;**49**:571–8.
2. Koelfen W, Freund M, Jaschke W, *et al*. GM-2 gangliosidosis (Sandhoff's disease): two year follow-up by MRI. *Neuroradiology* 1994;**36**:152–4.
3. Patay Z. Metabolic disorders. In: Pediatric Neuroradiology Brain. Tortori-Donati P, Rossi A, eds. Springer, New York, NY, 2005.
4. Maegawa GH, Stockley T, Tropak M, *et al*. The natural history of juvenile or subacute GM2 gangliosidosis: 21 new cases and literature review of 134 previously reported. *Pediatrics* 2006;**118**:e1550–62.
5. Steenweg ME, Vanderver A, Blaser S, *et al*. Magnetic resonance imaging pattern recognition in hypomyelinating disorders. *Brain* 2010;**133**:2971–82.

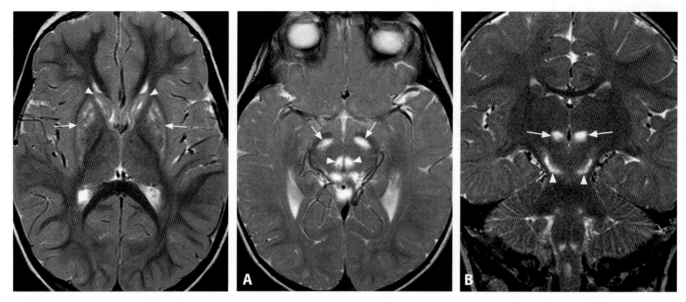

Figure 1. Axial T2WI shows symmetric hyperintensity in caudate (arrowheads) and putamen (arrows).

Figure 2. Axial T2WI (A) shows symmetric midbrain hyperintensities, including substantia nigra (arrows), central tegmental tract (arrowheads) and periaqueductal gray. Coronal T2WI (B) reveals involvement of thalami (arrows), subthalamic nucleus (arrowheads), and medulla.

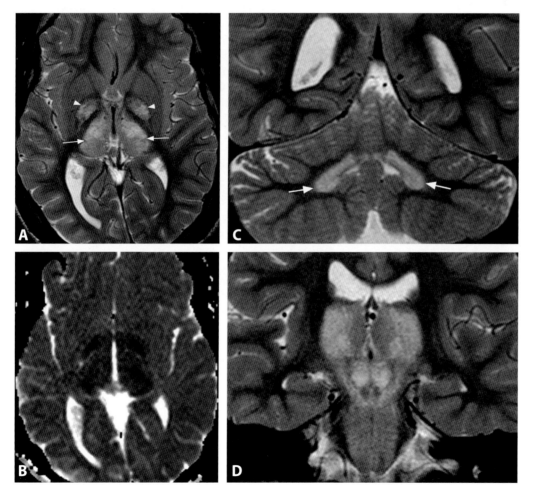

Figure 3. Axial T2WI (A) in a different patient shows bilateral hyperintense involvement of thalamus (arrows) and globus pallidus (arrowheads) along with reduced diffusion on corresponding ADC map (B). Coronal T2WIs (C, D) also demonstrate widespread hyperintense signal changes of the dentate nuclei (arrows) and within the brainstem.

Leigh Disease

MARIASAVINA SEVERINO

Specific Imaging Findings

MR imaging in Leigh disease (LD) usually reveals bilateral symmetrical T2 hyperintense lesions of the deep gray matter and brainstem. Putamen is typically involved, followed by the caudate nuclei. The globi pallidi and thalami area less frequently affected. Brainstem lesions including the subthalamic nuclei, substantia nigra, red nuclei, colliculi, periaqueductal gray matter, and medulla oblongata are commonly present. Cerebellar dentate nuclei are also a frequent location of T2 hyperintensity. Spinal cord, hemispheric white matter and cerebral cortex involvement may occur. Acutely affected areas may show reduced diffusivity on ADC maps. MRS usually reveals elevated lactate, most prominent within the lesions. Normal MRS, however, does not exclude LD.

Pertinent Clinical Information

Leigh disease is a frequently lethal disorder that usually presents during infancy, and rarely during childhood and later in life. Developmental delay, seizures, and altered consciousness are the most common presenting symptoms. Generalized weakness, hypotonia, nystagmus, ataxia, dystonia, lactic acidosis and respiratory failure with apneas are also frequently present. Visceral manifestations comprise failure to thrive, cardiomyopathy, liver function impairment and proximal renal tubulopathy.

Differential Diagnosis

Kernicterus

- bilateral increased T1 and T2 signal intensity in the globus pallidus
- usual sparing of the thalami (the subthalamic nuclei can be involved)

Neonatal Hypoxic Ischemic Encephalopathy (7)

- posterior part of the lentiform nuclei, lateral thalami, dorsal brainstem, perirolandic cortex
- hyperintensities on T1-weighted images surrounding PLIC

Wilson Disease (6)

- globi pallidi hyperintense on T1-weighted images (with liver involvement)

Encephalitis

- brainstem is usually spared
- lesions are usually asymmetrical

Juvenile Huntington Disease (91)

- may be indistinguishable in the early phase
- caudate and putaminal atrophy appears later

Glutaric Aciduria Type 1 (16)

- high T2 signal of the basal ganglia may be associated with leukoencephalopathy
- widening of the sylvian fissures is characteristic

Background

LS, also known as subacute necrotizing encephalopathy, is a genetically heterogeneous mitochondrial disorder embracing a wide spectrum of defects in enzymes involved in cerebral oxidative metabolism. It is caused by mitochondrial DNA mutations (maternally inherited) or nuclear DNA mutations. Accordingly, inheritance may be X-linked recessive (e.g. pyruvate dehydrogenase deficiency), autosomal recessive (e.g. some respiratory chain complex I and COX deficiencies), or maternal (mitochondrial DNA), depending on the underlying mutation. Pathologically, the lesions are consistent with demyelination leading to spongiform necrosis, capillary proliferation, cavitation, and gliosis in the vulnerable structures, which are highly dependent on energy consumption. Although there is no causal treatment of CNS manifestations of LS, various symptomatic therapeutic measures are available, such as dietary modifications with substitution of vitamins, coenzymes and hormones, quinone derivates and dichloroacetate.

REFERENCES

1. Arii J, Tanabe Y. Leigh syndrome: serial MR imaging and clinical follow-up. *AJNR* 2000;**21**:1502–9.

2. Lee H-F, Tsai C-R, Chi C-S, *et al*. Leigh syndrome: clinical and neuroimaging follow-up. *Pediatr Neurol* 2009;**40**:88–93.

3. Rossi A, Biancheri R, Bruno C, *et al*. Leigh Syndrome with COX deficiency and SURF1 gene mutations: MR imaging findings. *AJNR* 2003;**24**:1188–91.

4. Valanne L, Ketonen L, Majander A, *et al*. Neuroradiologic findings in children with mitochondrial disorders. *AJNR* 1998;**19**:369–77.

5. Friedman SD, Shaw DW, Ishak G. The use of neuroimaging in the diagnosis of mitochondrial disease. *Dev Disabil Res Rev* 2010;**16**:129–35.

Brain Imaging with MRI and CT, ed. Zoran Rumboldt *et al*. Published by Cambridge University Press. © Cambridge University Press 2012.

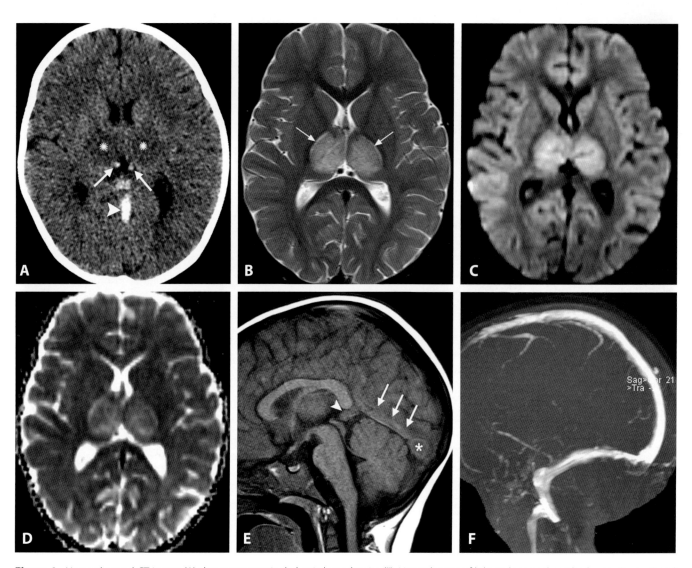

Figure 1. Non-enhanced CT image (A) shows symmetric thalamic hypodensity (*). Hyperdensity of bilateral internal cerebral veins (arrows) and straight sinus (arrowhead) is also present. Axial T2WI (B) reveals symmetric increased signal throughout thalami (arrows). Corresponding DWI (C) and ADC map (D) both show increased signal, indicating vasogenic edema. Sagittal T1WI (E) shows intermediate signal intensity within the straight sinus (arrows), vein of Galen (arrowhead), and torcular herophili (*). Sagittal MIP image from TOF MRV (F) demonstrates complete absence of flow in the deep venous system.

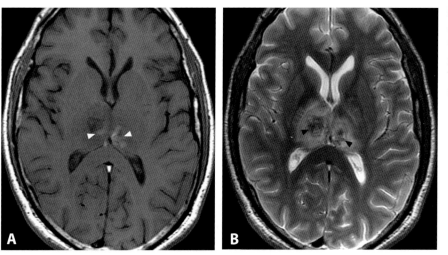

Figure 2. Axial T1WI (A) and T2WI (B) in a different patient demonstrate bilateral thalamic edema (diffusely low T1 and high T2 signal) with hemorrhagic areas, seen as foci of T1 hyperintensity and T2 hypointensity (arrowheads).

Deep Cerebral Vein Thrombosis (DCVT)

BENJAMIN HUANG

Specific Imaging Findings

Symmetric bilateral thalamic edema (hypodense on CT, hypointense on T1, and hyperintense on T2-weighted images), which may extend into the basal ganglia, midbrain, and adjacent deep white matter, is the characteristic imaging finding in DCVT. Unilateral thalamic involvement has also been reported. Thalamic hemorrhage is common, and intraventricular hemorrhage can also be seen. On DWI, the areas of edema will usually demonstrate increased ADC (compatible with vasogenic edema), rather than reduced diffusion typically seen in arterial infarctions.

Thrombus is usually evident within the affected vessels, primarily internal cerebral veins, which appear hyperdense on unenhanced CT, with reported sensitivity and specificity of this "attenuated vein sign" at 99–100%. On MRI, venous thrombus will appear iso- to hyperintense to brain on unenhanced T1-weighted images, with loss of normal flow voids on T2-weighted images. Time-of-flight MR venography (MRV) will demonstrate absence of normal flow-related signal within the thrombosed veins; however, in some cases, time-of-flight MRV may appear falsely negative due to high signal from thrombus simulating normal flow. Contrast-enhanced CT or MRV will demonstrate a filling defect. Thrombosis of the superficial dural sinuses can also be present.

Pertinent Clinical Information

Patients with DCVT tend to present with a short history (usually less than a week), most commonly of headache and reduced consciousness. D-dimer levels have low positive predictive value, but they are useful in ruling out cerebral venous thrombosis, given their high negative predictive value. Predisposing conditions include genetic or acquired prothrombotic disorders, cancer, pregnancy and puerperium, and oral contraceptive use. In contrast to thrombosis of the superficial dural venous sinuses, deep venous system occlusion is more likely to result in death (13–37%) or significant long-term morbidity.

Differential Diagnosis

Encephalitis
- patent veins on MRV
- may involve other areas of cerebrum or cerebellum

Artery of Percheron Infarction
- paramedian thalamic location
- always reduced diffusion on ADC maps

Top of the Basilar Syndrome
- occipital and medial temporal involvement
- shows reduced diffusion

Background

The deep cerebral veins drain the thalami, basal ganglia, and deep white matter. These veins include the thalamic veins, thalamostriate veins, internal cerebral veins, basal veins of Rosenthal, vein of Galen, and the straight sinus. The vein of Galen then joins with the inferior sagittal sinus to form the straight sinus, which communicates with the dural venous sinuses at the torcular herophili. DCVT occurs in roughly 16% of patients with cerebral venous thrombosis, and is associated with poorer outcomes than dural venous thrombosis, due to the lack of a substantial collateral drainage pathway. Signal abnormality observed within the thalami and basal ganglia in deep venous thrombosis is primarily due to venous congestion and resultant vasogenic edema, rather than cytotoxic edema, which is typically seen with arterial ischemic infarction. Even areas of reduced diffusion may be reversible. The mainstay of treatment for DCVT is heparin. In cases of severe neurologic deterioration, endovascular catheter-directed thrombolytic therapy (and possibly open surgical thrombectomy) is required.

REFERENCES
1. Poon CS, Chang JK, Swarnkar A, et al. Radiologic diagnosis of cerebral venous thrombosis: pictorial review. AJR 2007;189:S64–75.
2. Linn J, Pfefferkorn T, Ivanicova K, et al. Noncontrast CT in deep cerebral venous thrombosis and sinus thrombosis: comparison of its diagnostic value for both entities. AJNR 2009;30:728–35.
3. Herrmann KA, Sporer B, Youstry TA. Thrombosis of the internal cerebral vein associated with transient unilateral thalamic edema: a case report and review of the literature. AJNR 2004;25:1351–5.
4. Lovblad KO, Bassetti C, Schneider J, et al. Diffusion-weighted MRI suggests coexistence of cytotoxic and vasogenic oedema in a case of deep cerebral venous thrombosis. Neuroradiology 2000;42:728–31.
5. Pfefferkorn T, Crassard I, Linn J, et al. Clinical features, course and outcome in deep cerebral venous system thrombosis: an analysis of 32 cases. J Neurol 2009;256:1839–45.

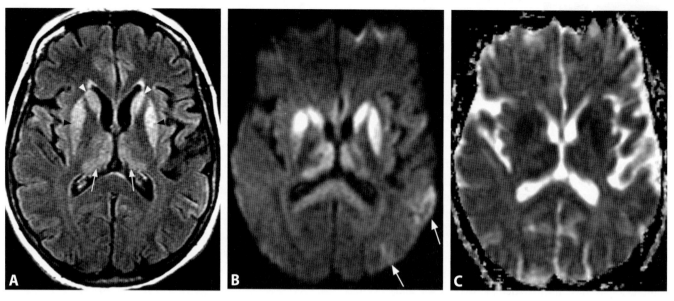

Figure 1. Axial FLAIR image (A) demonstrates symmetric increased signal intensity in the bilateral caudate heads (white arrowheads) and putamina (black arrowheads), as well as in the medial thalami and pulvinar thalami (arrows). Corresponding DWI image (B) and ADC map (C) show reduced diffusion within these affected areas. There is also reduced diffusion in the cortex of the left posterior temporal lobe (arrows), which is more prominent than on the FLAIR image.

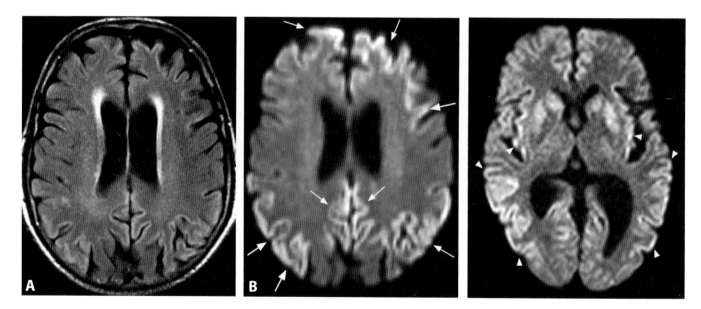

Figure 2. MR imaging in a different patient without any suspicion for the diagnosis on the initial clinical presentation. Axial FLAIR (A) image shows a very subtle increase in cortical signal intensity involving bilateral frontal and parietal lobes. These findings (arrows) are much better appreciated on the corresponding DWI (B).

Figure 3. Axial DWI shows bilateral hyperintensity involving caudate and putamen, as well as cortical gray matter, predominantly of the insula and temporal lobes (arrowheads).

Creutzfeldt–Jakob Disease (CJD)

BENJAMIN HUANG

Specific Imaging Findings

The classic imaging finding is symmetric high signal on DWI and FLAIR images in the corpora striata (caudate and putamen), in the cerebral cortex, and possibly in the thalami. Isolated involvement of the cortex alone or the deep gray matter alone is less common. In the early phase of disease, signal changes may only be detectable on DWI, which is the most sensitive test for diagnosing CJD. There is no contrast enhancement. Diffusion changes persist for weeks to months, and may disappear in the late stages of disease. A prominent symmetrical hyperintense T2 and DWI signal in the pulvinar thalami (the "pulvinar sign") is characteristic of variant CJD (vCJD). Involvement of the medial thalamus is also common, and the combination of both findings has been referred to as the "hockey-stick" sign. Signal changes in the pulvinar with sporadic CJD (sCJD) are less pronounced than changes in the striata.

Pertinent Clinical Information

The most common form of CJD, accounting for 85–90% of cases of human prion disease, is the sCJD. It typically occurs in the seventh decade of life with rapidly progressive dementia, focal neurologic signs and visual disturbances. CSF analysis for the presence of 14-3-3 proteins is 95% sensitive for the diagnosis of sCJD, but has a low specificity. EEG will show periodic sharp and slow wave complexes (PSWCs) in about 60–70% of patients with sCJD. The mean duration of this uniformly fatal disease is 6 months. vCJD has been linked with bovine spongiform encephalopathy (BSE, "mad cow disease"). It predominantly affects young patients (<30 years), has a more prolonged clinical course (median disease duration 14 months), and psychiatric features predominate early in its course. The pathologic protein in vCJD can be readily detected in palatine tonsil biopsy specimen. Only half of patients with vCJD will have elevated 14-3-3 levels in the CSF. PSWCs are not seen in vCJD patients.

In addition to sCJD and vCJD, other forms of human prion disease include hereditary disease (familial CJD and others), iatrogenic CJD (transmitted via contaminated surgical instruments, corneal or dura mater transplants, or after use of contaminated human growth hormone), and kuru. Clinical features of familial and iatrogenic CJD are similar to those of sCJD.

Differential Diagnosis

Global Cerebral Anoxia in Mature Brain (13)
- acute clinical onset (not progressive)

MELAS (164)
- younger patients
- gyriform swelling and enhancement
- deep white matter involvement
- elevated lactate on MRS

Seizure-Related Changes (Peri-Ictal MRI Abnormalities) (104)
- history of seizures
- no basal ganglia involvement
- gyriform swelling, contrast enhancement may be present

Background

Prion diseases are characterized pathologically by spongiform gray matter degeneration, neuronal loss, and astrocytic gliosis. It is hypothesized that the sporadic form of the disease results from transformation of the normal cellular prion protein (PrP^C) into an abnormal, insoluble form (PrP^{Sc}) which accumulates in the brain and induces neuronal death and spongiform change. Antemortem reductions in ADC values are correlated with spongiform changes seen at autopsy. In vCJD, thalamic gliosis, which is most severe in the pulvinar, is believed to account for the pulvinar sign seen on MRI.

Subtypes of CJD have been described based on polymorphisms at codon 129 of the prion protein gene, PRNP, which codes for either methionine or valine. Homozygosity at this site appears to be a predisposing factor for sCJD, while vCJD is associated exclusively with homozygotes for the methionine allele.

REFERENCES

1. Tschampa HJ, Zerr I, Urbach H. Radiologic assessment of Creutzfeldt–Jakob disease. *Eur Radiol* 2007;**17**:1200–11.

2. Ukisu R, Kushihashi T, Tanaka E, *et al.* Diffusion-weighted MR imaging of early stage Creutzfeldt–Jakob disease: typical and atypical manifestations. *Radiographics* 2006;**26**:S191–204.

3. Young GS, Geschwind MD, Fischbein NJ, *et al.* Diffusion-weighted and fluid-attenuated inversion recovery imaging in Creutzfeldt–Jakob disease: high sensitivity and specificity for diagnosis. *AJNR* 2005;**26**:1551–62.

4. Meissner B, Kallenberg K, Sanchez-Juan P, *et al.* Isolated cortical signal increase on MR imaging as a frequent lesion pattern in sporadic Creutzfeldt–Jakob disease. *AJNR* 2008;**29**:1519–24.

5. Manners DN, Parchi P, Tonon C, *et al.* Pathologic correlates of diffusion MRI changes in Creutzfeldt–Jakob disease. *Neurology* 2009;**72**:1425–31.

Brain Imaging with MRI and CT, ed. Zoran Rumboldt *et al.* Published by Cambridge University Press. © Cambridge University Press 2012.

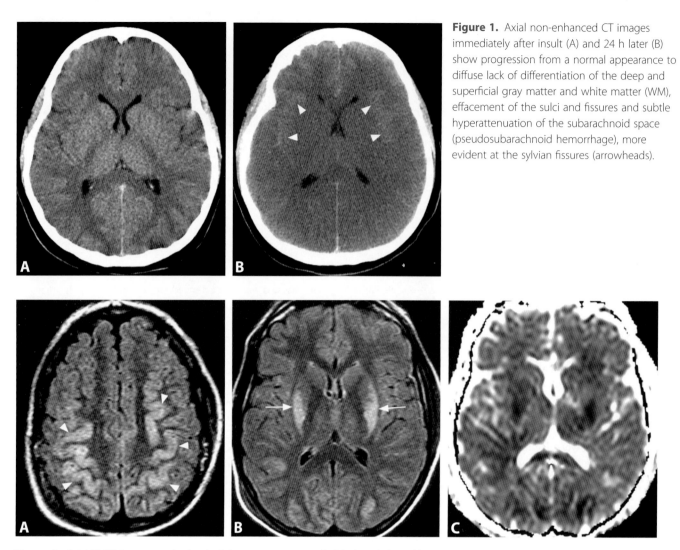

Figure 1. Axial non-enhanced CT images immediately after insult (A) and 24 h later (B) show progression from a normal appearance to diffuse lack of differentiation of the deep and superficial gray matter and white matter (WM), effacement of the sulci and fissures and subtle hyperattenuation of the subarachnoid space (pseudosubarachnoid hemorrhage), more evident at the sylvian fissures (arrowheads).

Figure 2. Axial FLAIR images at the level of the centrum semiovale (A) show bilateral hyperintense signal of the posterior frontal and parietal cortex (arrowheads). FLAIR image at the basal ganglia level (B) in addition to the bilateral cortical hyperintensity reveals high signal in the putamina (arrows). Corresponding ADC map (C) shows symmetrical low signal consistent with reduced diffusion of the affected areas.

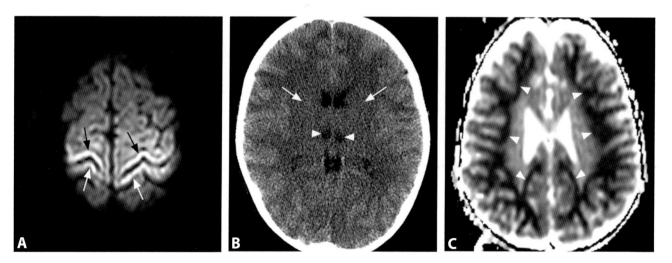

Figure 3. DWI image (B) reveals bilateral symmetric perirolandic cortical hyperintensity (arrows). CT image on the following day (A) shows bilateral loss of differentiation and hypodensity of the deep gray matter (arrows). Additionally, there are focal intrathalamic areas of even lower attenuation (arrowheads). ADC map obtained after 10 days shows atrophy and shifting of the reduced diffusion to the subcortical WM (arrowheads).

Global Cerebral Anoxia in Mature Brain

MARIA VITTORIA SPAMPINATO AND ZORAN RUMBOLDT

Specific Imaging Findings

Global cerebral anoxia (hypoxic–ischemic injury, HII) findings vary depending on the duration and severity of insult, brain maturity, and type and timing of imaging studies with different presentations in premature neonates, full-term neonates, and older children and adults. In all three scenarios the lesions are bilateral and predominantly symmetrical. The spectrum of mild to severe findings in mature brains on non-contrast CT are: (1) poor differentiation of the cortical gray matter from subcortical white matter with sulcal effacement, predominantly affecting the arterial boundary zones; (2) loss of deep gray and white matter definition; (3) relative hyperdensity of the subarachnoid space (pseudosubarachnoid hemorrhage); (4) relatively hyperdense cerebellum (bright cerebellum); (5) hypodense brainstem; and (6) herniations. MRI shows hyperintense T2 (and low T1) signal of the affected areas, especially cortical, when CT findings may be absent. Diffusion MRI is the most sensitive technique with bright lesions on DWI and low ADC values involving deep gray matter, cortex, and cerebellum in the early stages. Perirolandic and deep gray matter involvement is observed in term neonates. Profound HII in older children and adults affects the deep gray matter nuclei, cortices, hippocampi, and cerebellum. Areas of reduced diffusion shift from the gray matter to the white matter in the subacute phase, when laminar enhancement of the cortex and patchy enhancement of the deep gray matter may be present on post-contrast images. This is followed by T1 bright cortical laminar necrosis in the late subacute phase and cortical atrophy and progressive white matter changes in the chronic stage.

When initial anoxia is followed by ischemia the white matter may be preferentially involved, even within the first few days.

Pertinent Clinical Information

The prognosis of HII is poor with death or significant neurological deficits as the most frequent outcomes. Imaging plays an important role in the diagnosis and treatment of HII, helping guide management and providing information about long-term prognosis. Basal ganglia and thalamic involvement on CT and MR imaging has been highly associated with poor outcome.

Differential Diagnosis

Encephalitis
- findings usually not evident on CT images
- deep gray matter involvement may be symmetrical, if cortical lesions are present they are usually asymmetrical
- mild or no mass effect

Creutzfeldt–Jacob Disease (12)
- no significant mass effect
- protracted gradual clinical presentation

PRES (32)
- patchy bilateral involvement with posterior brain predominance
- primarily affecting the subcortical white matter with sparing of the cortex
- rarely shows low ADC values (usually nonreversible lesions)

Background

Anoxic brain injury is a devastating result of prolonged hypoxia progressing to subsequent coma. The causes can be due to direct impairment in oxygen supply (anoxia/hypoxia), exogenous intoxication (histotoxic), hypoglycemia, or circulatory (ischemic/oligemic). The pathophysiology of HII is complex, the pattern of involvement varies with the severity of the insult and the state of brain maturation. Brain tissue damage is related to energy demand and cerebral vasculature autoregulation. In premature neonates HII predominantly affects the periventricular white matter, most likely due to high energy demand of the germinal matrix. Full-term babies show marked damage in areas of high myelination (corticospinal tracts). The mature brain shows preferential tissue damage at the boundary arterial zones and areas of higher energy demand such as the cortex and deep gray matter. The cascade of events that culminates with HII includes cerebral vascular autoregulation, injury mediated by excitotoxicity, apoptosis, inflammatory protease cascades, and free radicals. ASL MR perfusion studies demonstrate cerebral hyperperfusion following global anoxia, probably resulting from loss of cerebral vascular resistance autoregulation. Promising new neuroprotective strategies designed to limit the extent of brain injury caused by HII are currently under investigation.

REFERENCES

1. Takahashi S, Higano S, Ishii K, et al. Hypoxic brain damage: cortical laminar necrosis and delayed changes in white matter at sequential MRI imaging. *Radiology* 1993;**189**:449–56.

2. Arbelaez A, Castillo M, Mukherji SK. Diffusion-weighted MR imaging of global cerebral anoxia. *AJNR* 1999;**20**:999–1007.

3. Chalela JA, Wolf RL, Maldjian JA, Kasner SE. MRI identification of early white matter injury in anoxic-ischemic encephalopathy. *Neurology* 2001;**56**:481–5.

4. Huang BY, Castillo M. Hypoxic–ischemic brain injury: imaging findings from birth to adulthood. *Radiographics* 2008;**28**:417–39.

5. Pollock JM, Whitlow CT, Deibler AR, et al. Anoxic injury-associated cerebral hyperperfusion identified with arterial spin-labeled MR imaging. *AJNR* 2008;**29**:1302–7.

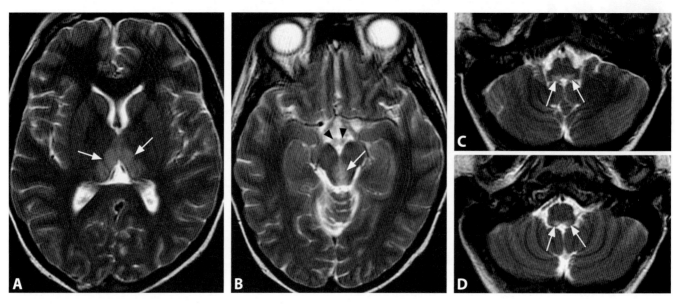

Figure 1. Axial T2WI images show symmetric bilateral hyperintensity in the bilateral medial thalami (arrows in A); the tectum of the midbrain and the periaqueductal gray matter (arrow in B); mammillary bodies (arrowheads in B); the medial vestibular nuclei (arrows in C); and prepositus hypoglossal nuclei (arrows in D).

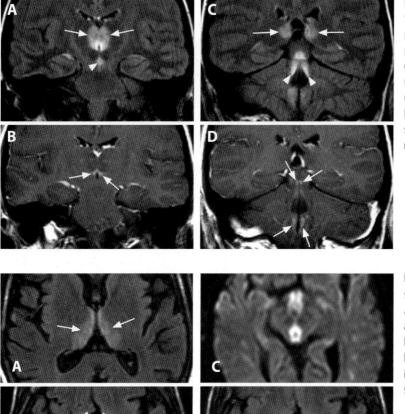

Figure 2. Coronal FLAIR (A) shows hyperintensity in the thalami (arrows), along the third ventricle, and in the periaqueductal gray matter (arrowhead). Corresponding post-contrast T1WI (B) reveals periventricular enhancement (arrows). Hyperintensity in the thalami (arrows), mesencephalon, superior cerebellar peduncles (arrowheads) and along the fourth ventricle on another FLAIR image (C). Post-contrast T1WI (D) shows symmetric enhancement in most of the affected regions (arrows).

Figure 3. Axial FLAIR images show abnormal increased signal along the medial nuclei of the thalami (arrows in A) as well as in the periaqueductal region (arrow in B) and along the third ventricle (arrowheads in B). Hyperintensity is also present on the corresponding DWI (C). Follow-up FLAIR image (D) shows significant improvement of the periaqueductal and periventricular signal abnormalities.

Wernicke Encephalopathy

GIULIO ZUCCOLI

Specific Imaging Findings

In Wernicke encephalopathy (WE, Wernicke–Korsakoff syndrome) symmetric signal intensity alterations in the mammillary bodies, medial thalami, periventricular regions of the third ventricle, tectal plate, and periaqueductal gray matter are typical MRI findings. Selective involvement of the cranial nerve nuclei, cerebellum, dentate nuclei, fornix, splenium of the corpus callosum, cerebral cortex, and basal ganglia characterize nonalcoholic WE. Lesions in the basal ganglia mainly affect the putamen and are most frequently observed in children. The lesions are iso to hypointense to the gray matter on T1-weighted images and T2 hyperintense. DWI also shows high signal intensity in the acute phase with variable ADC values. Enhancement of the mammillary bodies is most frequently observed in the alcholic population and may be the only imaging finding. Degree of enhancement is quite variable. Hemorrhagic transformation is rare.

Brain atrophy develops in chronic WE, in particular of the fornices and mammillary bodies, while T2 hyperintensity becomes less obvious.

Pertinent Clinical Information

WE is an acute neurologic disorder resulting from thiamine (vitamin B1) deficiency and its incidence is underestimated in both adult and pediatric patients. Clinical presentation is characterized by changes in consciousness, ocular dysfunction, and ataxia. However, this triad is not present in many patients. The most common presenting symptom is nonspecific mental status changes. Untreated patients can progress to irreversible brain damage leading to Korsakoff syndrome and, eventually, to death.

Differential Diagnosis

Artery of Percheron Infarction
- bilateral medial thalamic and rostral mesencephalic lesions

Deep Venous Thrombosis (11)
- symmetric thalamic lesions with possible extension and hemorrhage
- high T1 signal of intraluminal clot in the internal cerebral veins
- filling defect on contrast-enhanced images and absence of flow on MRV/CTV

Encephalitis; Acute Disseminated Encephalomyelitis (ADEM) (112)
- usually also multifocal involvement of the gray and white matter
- usually patchy and asymmetric

Extrapontine Osmotic Myelinolysis (66)
- often associated with central pontine involvement (central pontine myelinolysis)
- external capsule, putamen and caudate nucleus often affected
- osmotic myelinolysis and WE may coexist

Variant Creutzfeldt–Jakob Disease (12)
- increased T2 signal in the pulvinar thalami
- involvement of putamen and caudate, cortical gray matter
- extensive areas of reduced diffusion involving cortical and deep gray matter

Primary CNS Lymphoma (158)
- usually low to isointense T2 signal
- mass effect, avid enhancement, surrounding vasogenic edema

Neuromyelitis Optica (NMO)
- spinal cord and optic nerve involvement

Hypoxic Ischemic Encephalopathy (7)
- acutely thalamic increased T2 signal, normal to decreased T1 signal
- usually T2 hyperintensity in (perirolandic) cortical areas
- low ADC in the acute phase
- T1 hyperintensity around the posterior limb of the internal capsule later on

Leigh Disease (10)
- thalamus, basal ganglia and brainstem involved
- low ADC in the acute phase

Krabbe Disease/Lysosomal Genetic Defects (9)
- decreased T2 and increased T1 signal of the thalamus

Background

Although alcoholism is a common predisposing factor for the development of WE, the disease can also be caused by malignancy, total parenteral nutrition, abdominal surgery, prolonged vomiting, hemodialysis, diarrhea, magnesium depletion, unbalanced nutrition, and infections. Glucose load may precipitate the disorder. The frequency of WE in children appears to be similar to that observed in adults. Mortality is estimated at 17%. In a thiamine-deficient state, increased metabolic requirements and inability to regulate the osmotic gradients may result in cytotoxic edema followed by permanent neuronal loss. In the acute phase, petechial hemorrhages, hypertrophic endothelial changes, reactive gliosis, and necrosis are seen on histology. Progression of this disease is preventable with prompt diagnosis and emergent intravenous thiamine administration. The prognosis depends on the time from diagnosis to thiamine supplementation.

REFERENCES

1. Zuccoli G, Siddiqui N, Cravo I, et al. Neuroimaging findings in alcohol-related encephalopathies. AJR 2010;195:1378–84.
2. Zuccoli G, Cravo I, Bailey A, et al. Basal ganglia involvement in Wernicke encephalopathy: report of 2 cases. AJNR 2011;32:E129–31.
3. Zuccoli G, Siddiqui N, Bailey A, Bartoletti SC. Neuroimaging findings in pediatric Wernicke encephalopathy: a review. Neuroradiology 2010;52:523–9.
4. Zuccoli G, Pipitone N. Neuroimaging findings in acute Wernicke's encephalopathy: review of the literature. AJR 2009;192:501–8.
5. Sechi G, Serra A. Wernicke's encephalopathy: new clinical settings and recent advances in diagnosis and management. Lancet Neurol 2007;6:442–55.

Brain Imaging with MRI and CT, ed. Zoran Rumboldt *et al.* Published by Cambridge University Press. © Cambridge University Press 2012.

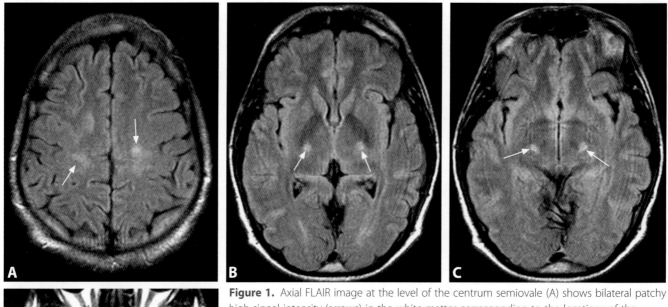

Figure 1. Axial FLAIR image at the level of the centrum semiovale (A) shows bilateral patchy high signal intensity (arrows) in the white matter corresponding to the locations of the corticospinal tracts (CST). Axial FLAIR image at the level of the basal ganglia (B) shows a very high and abnormal signal intensity in the posterior limb of bilateral internal capsules (arrows) corresponding to the location of CST. Axial FLAIR image at a slightly more inferior level (C) shows hyperintensity in both CST (arrows) as they course through the midbrain. FLAIR image (D) shows high signal of the CST (arrows) in the pons.

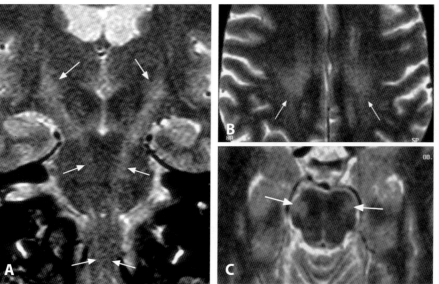

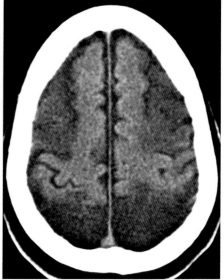

Figure 2. Coronal T2WI (A) in a different patient reveals hyperintensity along bilateral CST (arrows) from the basal ganglia level through the spinal cord. Corresponding axial T2WI images show high signal intensity of bilateral CST at the centrum semiovale (arrows in B) and the brainstem (arrows in C).

Figure 3. Non-enhanced axial CT in a patient with end-stage disease shows marked atrophy in bilateral frontal and parietal regions.

Amyotrophic Lateral Sclerosis

MAURICIO CASTILLO

Specific Imaging Findings

In amyotrophic lateral sclerosis (ALS) T2-weighted MR images, and particularly T2* (gradient echo), may show dark areas of increased iron deposition in the pre- and post-central gyri. This finding needs to be interpreted with caution, because it is also a part of normal aging. Increased T2 signal involving the corticospinal tracts (CSTs) from their subcortical beginning into the brainstem and medulla is characteristic. This finding should also be cautiously interpreted, as the posterior aspect of the CST travelling through the posterior limb of the internal capsule is less myelinated and may be slightly bright on T2-weighted and FLAIR images. These regions are T1 hypointense and this may be accentuated by adding magnetization transfer to the sequence. Faint linear subcortical hyperintensities on T2 sequences have been reported, particularly in the medial temporal lobes. The thickness of the primary motor cortex is reduced. The brain shows diffuse atrophy in the chronic phase, which may be more prominent in the parietal and frontotemporal regions. MRS is nonspecific and shows low NAA, creatine and glutamate; it may be used to follow the effects of treatment. DTI shows increased diffusivity and reduced volumes of the CSTs. CT shows only atrophy. MRI of the spinal cord is usually normal.

Pertinent Clinical Information

Early symptoms may be mild and nonspecific and are commonly overlooked. These include twitching, cramps and muscle stiffness or weakness. Most of the early symptoms affect the extremities, particularly the lower ones. Symptoms progress until patients are unable to walk. About a quarter of patients present with brainstem symptoms including speech and swallowing difficulties; eventually all patients lose speech and are unable to swallow. Progressive muscle weakness and atrophy may be followed by spasticity and hyperreflexia. Additional neuropsychiatric symptoms such as anxiety and depression complicate the clinical state. Some patients develop neurocognitive abnormalities similar to those encountered in frontotemporal dementia. However, in most patients cognition remains intact until death. Eye muscle control is maintained throughout life. All patients experience respiratory difficulties which require assisted ventilation. Superimposed pneumonia is a common cause of death.

Differential Diagnosis

Primary Lateral Sclerosis
- clinically only the upper motor neurons are affected

Wallerian Degeneration (78)
- tends to be unilateral and the causative lesion is almost always evident

Normal
- high signal on T2-weighted and FLAIR images in the corticospinal tracts and low signal in the pericentral gray matter may be more prominent at 3.0 T

Background

This is a rare, progressive neurodegenerative disorder (a.k.a. Lou Gehrig disease) in which a mutation in the gene encoding for superoxide dismutase leads to death of motor neurons. Exactly what sets off this mutation is unclear, but viruses, toxins, heavy metals, immune system abnormalities and hereditary conditions have been implicated (most cases are, however, sporadic). Higher levels of glutamate are also found in the brains of ALS patients. Both upper and lower motor neurons degenerate and this is accompanied by Wallerian degeneration of the corresponding white matter tracts. ALS affects individuals between 40 and 60 years of age, slightly more commonly men. Muscle weakness is progressive, untreatable and ultimately fatal. Most patients die from respiratory insufficiency about 5 years after initial diagnosis. About 10% of patients survive more than 10 years (physicist Stephen Hawking is a famous example). Sensory and autonomic functions are spared.

REFERENCES
1. Matsusue E, Sugihara S, Fujii S, et al. Cerebral cortical and white matter lesions in amyotrophic lateral sclerosis with dementia: correlation with MR and pathologic examinations. *AJNR* 2007;**28**:1505–10.
2. Ngai S, Tang YM, Du L, Stuckey S. Hyperintensity of the precentral gyral subcortical white matter and hypointensity of the precentral gyrus on fluid-attenuated inversion recovery: variations with age and implications for the diagnosis of amyotrophic lateral sclerosis. *AJNR* 2007;**28**:250–4.
3. Da Rocha AJ, Oliveira ASB, Fonseca RB, et al. Detection of corticospinal tract compromise in amyotrophic lateral sclerosis with brain MR imaging: relevance of the T1-weighted spin-echo magnetization transfer contrast sequence. *AJNR* 2004;**25**:1509–15.
4. Mezzapesa DM, Ceccarelli A, Dicuonzo F, et al. Whole-brain and regional brain atrophy in amyotrophic lateral sclerosis. *AJNR* 2007;**28**:255–9.
5. Wang S, Opotani H, Biello M, et al. Diffusion tensor imaging in amyotrophic lateral sclerosis: volumetric analysis of the corticospinal tract. *AJNR* 2006;**27**:1234–8.

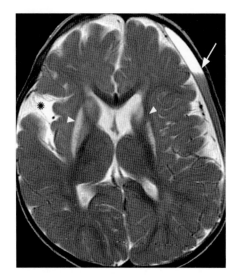

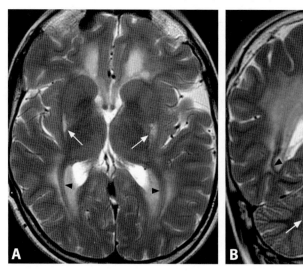

Figure 1. Axial T2WI shows subdural hematoma (arrow) and right sylvian fissure (*) expansion with basal ganglia hyperintensity and atrophy (arrowheads). Courtesy of Zoltán Patay.

Figure 2. Axial T2WI (A) reveals selective involvement of the posterior lentiform nuclei with hyperintense signal (arrows). Note diffuse white matter hyperintensity with spared optic radiations (arrowheads). Coronal T2WI (B) additionally depicts dentate nucleus involvement (arrows). Again note spared optic radiations (arrowheads).

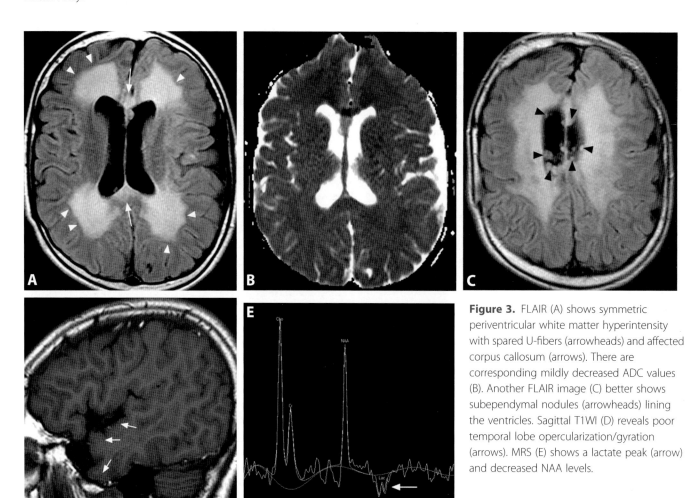

Figure 3. FLAIR (A) shows symmetric periventricular white matter hyperintensity with spared U-fibers (arrowheads) and affected corpus callosum (arrows). There are corresponding mildly decreased ADC values (B). Another FLAIR image (C) better shows subependymal nodules (arrowheads) lining the ventricles. Sagittal T1WI (D) reveals poor temporal lobe opercularization/gyration (arrows). MRS (E) shows a lactate peak (arrow) and decreased NAA levels.

Glutaric Aciduria Type 1

MARIASAVINA SEVERINO

Specific Imaging Findings

MR findings in glutaric aciduria type 1 (GA-1) in addition to macrocephaly include characteristic bilateral small anterior poles of temporal lobes with poor opercularization and widened sylvian fissure, subdural collections, and basal ganglia lesions. Central gray matter abnormalities variably include symmetric T2 hyperintensities and volume loss of the basal ganglia and dentate nucleus, with thalamus occasionally involved. In acutely affected areas there may be reduced diffusivity and MRS reveals elevated lactate with decreased levels of NAA. Abnormalities are often seen within the midbrain with involvement of white matter structures, tegmentum and substantia nigra and sparing of red nuclei, producing the "giant panda face" sign. The white matter may be primarily involved in GA-1, characteristically in the periventricular regions with sparing of the U-fibers and optic radiations. Diffusion may be persistently reduced with decreased ADC values within the lesions. Additional findings include subependymal nodules and pseudocysts.

Pertinent Clinical Information

The disease has a variable clinical presentation and severity. Patients may remain asymptomatic or mildly affected, with macrocephaly only, or they may present with encephalopathic crises in infancy or childhood after an initially normal development. These episodic crises typically occur following a trigger event (infection, immunization, surgery) and are characterized by hypotonia, spasticity, dystonia, rigidity, orofacial dyskinesia, seizures, opisthotonic posturing, decreased consciousness, and coma. Recovery is slow and often incomplete.

Differential Diagnosis

Non-Accidental Trauma

- subdural hematomas may be associated with subarachnoid hemorrhages
- multiple parenchymal lesions without symmetric GM and WM abnormalities
- skull and skeletal fractures

Wilson Disease (6)

- similar basal ganglia and mesencephalic involvement ("giant panda face" sign)
- globi pallidi are T1 hyperintense (with liver involvement)
- absence of subdural collections and widened sylvian fissure

Juvenile Huntington Disease (91)

- symmetric putaminal changes followed by caudate atrophy
- absence of subdural collections and widened sylvian fissure

Leigh Disease (10)

- absence of subdural collections and widened sylvian fissure

Physiologic Subarachnoid Space Enlargement (Benign External Hydrocephalus) (87)

- transient, self-limiting enlargement of the subarachnoid spaces
- absence of associated brain lesions

Tuberous Sclerosis Complex (TSC) (107, 198, 199)

- subependymal nodules are calcified (dark on T2*WI) and may enhance
- presence of cortical tubers
- absence of subdural collections, widened sylvian fissure, and deep gray matter lesions

Background

GA-1 is an autosomal recessive disorder of amino acid metabolism caused by deficiency of glutaryl-CoA dehydrogenase (GCDH), a mitochondrial enzyme necessary for the degradation of lysine, hydroxylysine and tryptophan. The condition has an estimated prevalence of 1 in 30 000 with most children presenting within the first 2 years of life. The *GCDH* gene is located on chromosome 19q13.2 and many different mutations have been described with no apparent correlation between genotype and phenotype. The pathogenesis of CNS lesions in GA-1 is poorly understood, but seems to be related to glutaric and 3-hydroxy-glutaric acid excitotoxicity. Early treatment (low protein diet supplemented with riboflavin and carnitine and aggressive treatment of catabolic states) may prevent or ameliorate crises and imaging features. Inclusion of this rare disease in the newborn screening disease panel significantly improves the neurological outcome of affected individuals.

REFERENCES

1. Desai NK, Runge VM, Crisp DE, *et al.* Magnetic resonance imaging of the brain in glutaric acidemia type I: a review of the literature and a report of four new cases with attention to the basal ganglia and imaging technique. *Invest Radiol* 2003;**38**:489–96.

2. Heringer J, Boy SP, Ensenauer R, *et al.* Use of guidelines improves the neurological outcome in glutaric aciduria type I. *Ann Neurol* 2010;**68**:743–52.

3. Righini A, Fiori L, Parazzini C, *et al.* Early prenatal magnetic resonance imaging of glutaric aciduria type 1: case report. *J Comput Assist Tomogr* 2010;**34**:446–8.

4. Oguz KK, Ozturk A, Cila A. Diffusion-weighted MR imaging and MR spectroscopy in glutaric aciduria type 1. *Neuroradiology* 2005;**47**:229–34.

5. Twomey EL, Naughten ER, Donoghue VB, *et al.* Neuroimaging findings in glutaric aciduria type 1. *Pediatr Radiol* 2003;**33**:823–30.

Brain Imaging with MRI and CT, ed. Zoran Rumboldt *et al.* Published by Cambridge University Press. © Cambridge University Press 2012.

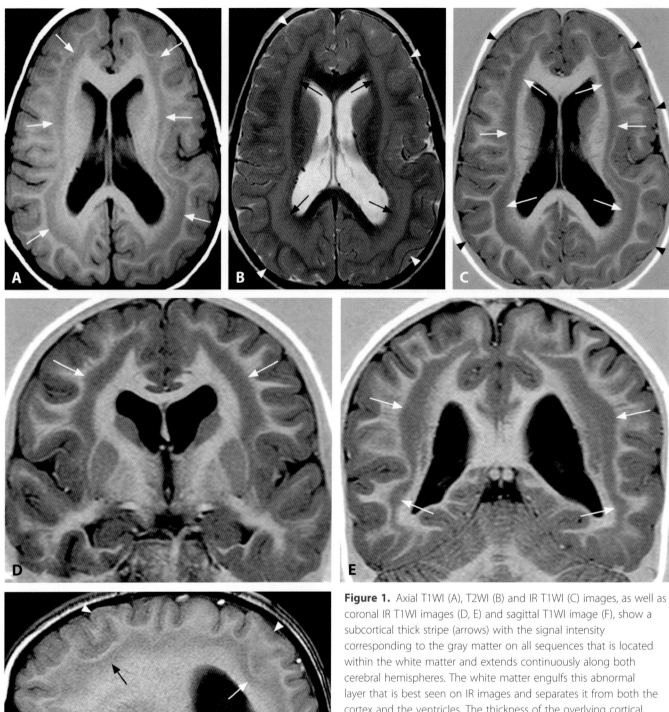

Figure 1. Axial T1WI (A), T2WI (B) and IR T1WI (C) images, as well as coronal IR T1WI images (D, E) and sagittal T1WI image (F), show a subcortical thick stripe (arrows) with the signal intensity corresponding to the gray matter on all sequences that is located within the white matter and extends continuously along both cerebral hemispheres. The white matter engulfs this abnormal layer that is best seen on IR images and separates it from both the cortex and the ventricles. The thickness of the overlying cortical mantle is preserved but the gyral pattern is somewhat rudimentary with decreased sulcation (arrowheads).

Subcortical Band Heterotopia

ANDREA ROSSI

Specific Imaging Findings

Subcortical band heterotopia (SBH) on MR imaging shows a symmetric band of heterotopic gray matter located deep to the cortical mantle and embedded within well-defined, smoothly marginated layers of normal-appearing white matter that separate it from both the overlying cerebral cortex and the underlying lateral ventricle. The heterotopic band is isointense with gray matter on all MR sequences. The cerebral cortex is usually normal; however, it can be thickened with a pachygyric configuration. A more severe malformation that overlaps with classic lissencephaly and band heterotopia is characterized by SBH in the occipital regions and pachygyria in the frontal regions. There is a gross correlation between the thickness of the heterotopic band and of the overlying cortex – patients with pachygyria tend to have thicker heterotopic bands. The hemispheric extent of the heterotopias is variable, ranging from complete to partial (sparing either frontal or posterior regions).

Pertinent Clinical Information

Most patients with subcortical band heterotopia are females who present with seizures and a variable degree of cognitive impairment. However, about 25% of affected children possess normal or near-normal intelligence. The malformation is sometimes discovered in mothers of boys with X-linked lissencephaly when they are investigated after the malformation has been diagnosed in their offspring. There is a gross relationship between the degree of disability and the thickness of the heterotopic band of neurons. Patients with a well-developed cortex may have a better clinical picture, and the onset of epilepsy occurs later. The lifespan is likely to be shortened in patients with severe mental retardation, intractable epilepsy, or both.

Differential Diagnosis

Lissencephaly (19)

- flat brain surface with absence (agyria) or paucity (pachygyria) of convolutions and intervening sulci
- shallow sylvian fissures with figure-of-eight brain configuration
- three-layered cortical mantle (molecular/outer cellular layers, sparse cell layer, and thick inner cellular layer composed of arrested neurons)

Subependymal (Nodular) Heterotopia (117)

- isolated or multiple, uni- or bilateral nodules with gray matter signal intensity immediately adjacent to the ventricular surface

Focal Subcortical Heterotopia

- variably sized nodules of heterotopic gray matter within subcortical brain
- typically asymmetric, continuous with thinned overlying cortex with a swirling appearance
- no intervening white matter layers
- may be giant and simulate neoplasm

Background

SBH, also known as double cortex, is the least severe form within the spectrum of classical lissencephaly, a congenital abnormality of cortical development caused by arrested migration of neurons between the germinative matrix and the cortical mantle. SBH is characterized by a poorly organized band of arrested neurons engulfed within the white matter, typically with a relatively normal overlying cerebral cortex. Both SBH and lissencephaly are caused by mutations of either the *LIS1* gene on chromosome 17 or the *DCX* gene on the X chromosome, which are implicated in the process of neuronal migration. There is a variable degree of severity in the lissencephaly spectrum ranging from complete agyria (grade 1) to SBH (grade 6). While *DCX* mutations cause full-blown lissencephaly in males (who possess only a single gene on the X chromosome), SBH mostly affects females, with roughly half of neurons expressing the mutated allele. SBH has exceptionally also been demonstrated in males as a consequence of minor missense mutations of *DCX* or *LIS1*. Subcortical bands restricted to the frontal lobes are typically associated with mutations of *DCX*, whereas subcortical bands limited to the posterior lobes are usually found with *LIS1* mutations.

REFERENCES

1. Barkovich AJ, Jackson DE Jr, Boyer RS. Band heterotopias: a newly recognized neuronal migration anomaly. *Radiology* 1989;**171**:455–8.
2. Barkovich AJ, Guerrini R, Battaglia G, *et al*. Band heterotopia: correlation of outcome with magnetic resonance imaging parameters. *Ann Neurol* 1994;**36**:609–17.
3. Pilz DT, Kuc J, Matsumoto N, *et al*. Subcortical band heterotopia in rare affected males can be caused by missense mutations in DCX (XLIS) or LIS1. *Hum Mol Genet* 1999;**8**:1757–60.
4. Uyanik G, Aigner L, Couillard-Despres S, *et al*. DCX-related disorders. In: Pagon RA, Bird TC, Dolan CR, Stephens K, eds. *GeneReviews* [Internet]. Seattle (WA): University of Washington, Seattle; 1993–2007 Oct 19.
5. Dobyns WB, Das S. LIS1-Associated lissencephaly/subcortical band heterotopia. In: Pagon RA, Bird TC, Dolan CR, Stephens K, eds. *GeneReviews* [Internet]. Seattle (WA): University of Washington, Seattle; 1993–2009 Mar 03.

Brain Imaging with MRI and CT, ed. Zoran Rumboldt *et al*. Published by Cambridge University Press. © Cambridge University Press 2012.

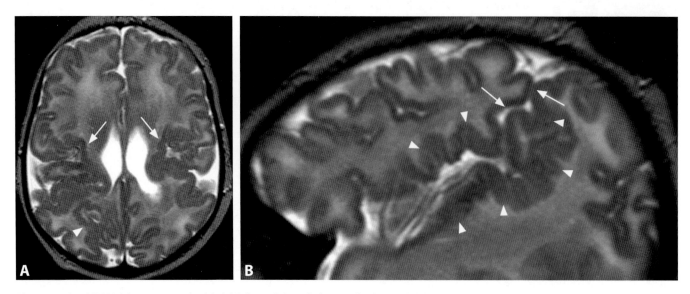

Figure 1. Axial T2WI (A) in a 1-month-old child shows bilateral abnormally thin and delicate cortex (arrows), extending posteriorly to the right parietal lobe (arrowheads). There is a sharp but undulating and irregular interface with the adjacent unmyelinated white matter. Sagittal T2WI (B) shows verticalized elongated sylvian fissure (arrows) festooned by the abnormal cortex (arrowheads).

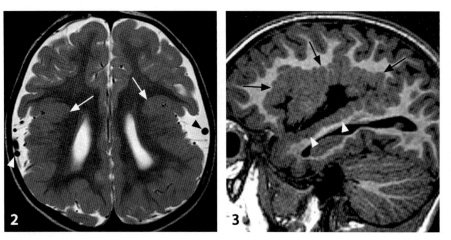

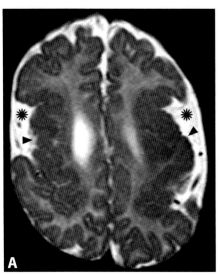

Figure 2. Axial T2WI in a 3-year-old patient reveals thick and coarse appearance of bilateral perisylvian cortex (arrows), extending to parietal regions. Note enlarged overlying veins (arrowheads).

Figure 3. Sagittal T1WI from 3D acquisition in another patient shows irregular and bumpy perisylvian cortex (arrows) extending to the temporal lobe (arrowheads) with irregular corrugated gray–white junction.

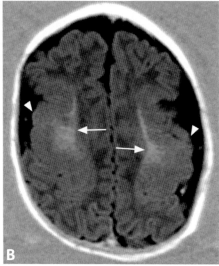

Figure 4. Axial T2WI (A) in a 2-month-old patient with swallowing difficulties and seizures shows bilateral abnormally thick cortex with a bumpy irregular appearance (arrowheads) and adjacent very wide sylvian fissures (*). The abnormal cortical thickening (arrowheads) is even more conspicuous on a slightly more cephalad IR T1WI (B), adjacent to the myelinated white matter (arrows).

Bilateral Perisylvian Polymicrogyria (BPP)

MARIASAVINA SEVERINO

Specific Imaging Findings

In bilateral perisylvian polymicrogyria (BPP), MRI demonstrates an abnormal configuration of the cortical ribbon and irregular gray–white matter junction suggestive of multiple small gyri bilaterally around the sylvian fissures. The mildest forms of perisylvian polymicrogyria involve part of the perisylvian cortex, usually the posterior region, while the most severe forms extend beyond the perisylvian area to the frontal, occipital, and temporal lobes with a perisylvian gradient (i.e. maximal severity in the perisylvian cortex). The spectrum of cortical morphology is wide: the cortex may be normal to thick with a delicate or coarse appearance, and the cortical surface may range from bumpy and irregular to smooth. Moreover, the appearance of BPP depends on the stage of maturity/myelination of the brain: in unmyelinated regions, the inner surface of the polymicrogyric cortex looks thin and finely undulated, while in myelinated areas it looks thicker and relatively smooth. The underlying white matter usually appears decreased in volume. The sylvian fissures have an abnormally verticalized orientation extending far more posteriorly than normal into the parietal regions and may be abnormally forked along their course. The fronto-temporo-parietal opercula present an abnormally open appearance, which is frequently associated with an overlying large anomalous venous structure. CT may show abnormal sylvian fissures and thickened adjacent cortex.

Pertinent Clinical Information

Clinical presentation of BPP (also known as congenital bilateral perisylvian syndrome – CBPS) varies among patients depending on the extent of cortical involvement and includes epilepsy, developmental delay and cognitive impairment, while the most characteristic feature is pseudobulbar palsy (Foix–Chavany–Marie syndrome), which is found in essentially all sporadic cases. Patients usually present with swallowing difficulties and anarthria or severe dysarthria resulting from disturbed voluntary control of the facio-pharyngeo-glosso-masticatory muscles. Arthrogryposis and/or lower motor neuron disease may also be associated. Callosotomy may be effective for patients with intractable seizures.

Differential Diagnosis

Pachygyria
- few sulci are present and the gyri are broad
- cortical thickness usually 6–9 mm

Lissencephaly (19)
- few or no sulci are seen on the cortical surface
- cortical thickness usually at least 1 cm
- brain circumference may be reduced

Glutaric Aciduria Type 1 (16)
- sylvian fissures are wide but without abnormal posterior extension
- no polymicrogyria
- bilateral deep gray and white matter abnormalities
- elevated lactate on MR spectroscopy

Background

Polymicrogyria is one of the most common cortical malformations due to disturbed post-migratory cortical organization and its most common location is around the sylvian fissure. It is characterized histologically by an excessive number of small irregular gyri, with obliterated sulci due to fusion of the molecular layers, and abnormal cortical lamination. BPP is the best-known and most frequent bilateral symmetrical polymicrogyria. Bilateral polymicrogyrias are overall slightly more common than the unilateral forms, and also include frontal, fronto-parietal, parasagittal parieto-occipital, and generalized syndromes. BPP can be graded based on MRI, with grade 1 being the most severe and extensive and grade 4 limited to the posterior perisylvian region. Most BPP cases are sporadic, but genetic heterogeneity is suggested by reports of X-linked, autosomal recessive and autosomal dominant cases. Interestingly, asymmetric BPP with a striking predisposition for the right hemisphere has also been reported in children with the chromosome 22q11.2 deletion. Familial cases tend to be less severe, sometimes presenting with just developmental reading disorder. Agenesis of the arcuate fasciculus, a major language tract in the perisylvian region, is a recently described finding on DTI in BPP patients with severe impairment and no speech development.

REFERENCES

1. Barkovich AJ, Hevner R, Guerrini R. Syndromes of bilateral symmetrical polymicrogyria. *AJNR* 1999;**20**:1814–21.
2. Leventer RJ, Jansen A, Pilz DT, *et al.* Clinical and imaging heterogeneity of polymicrogyria: a study of 328 patients. *Brain* 2010;**133**:1415–27.
3. Barkovich AJ. Current concepts of polymicrogyria. *Neuroradiology* 2010;**52**:479–87.
4. Brandão-Almeida IL, Hage SR, Oliveira EP, *et al.* Congenital bilateral perisylvian syndrome: familial occurrence, clinical and psycholinguistic aspects correlated with MRI. *Neuropediatrics* 2008;**39**:139–45.
5. Hehr U, Schuierer G. Genetic assessment of cortical malformations. *Neuropediatrics* 2011;**42**:43–50.

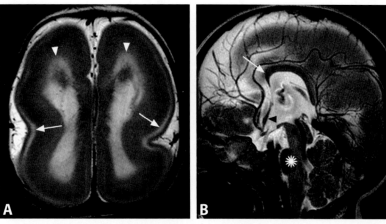

Figure 1. Axial T2WI (A) shows a figure-of-eight cerebral configuration with shallow sylvian fissures. The cortex is very thick and smooth, while the white matter is thin (arrowheads), with lack of the normal gray–white matter interdigitation. Note the bright peripheral circumferential band (arrows). Sagittal T2WI (B) reveals callosal dysgenesis (arrow), thick lamina terminalis (arrowhead) and hypoplastic pons (*).

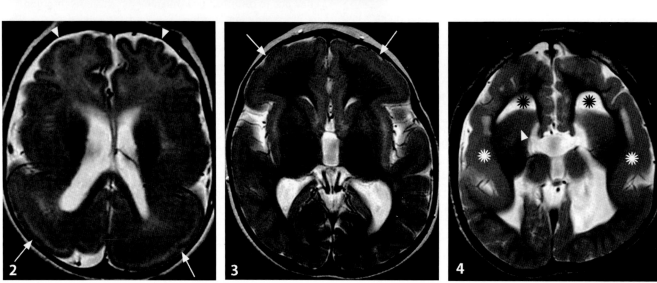

Figure 2. Axial T2WI in a boy with *LIS1* mutation shows predominantly posterior abnormality of thick and smooth cortex (arrows) with posterior to anterior gradient and relatively preserved frontal regions (arrowheads).

Figure 3. Axial T2WI in a girl with *DCX* mutation reveals predominantly frontal abnormally thick and smooth cortical ribbon (arrows) with an anterior to posterior pattern.

Figure 4. Axial T2WI in a girl with *TUBA1A* mutation demonstrates bilateral perisylvian pachygyria (white *), abnormal shape of frontal horns (black *) of the lateral ventricles and absent anterior limb of internal capsules resulting in lack of separation of the caudate nucleus and putamen (arrowhead) and typical basal ganglia dysgenesis.

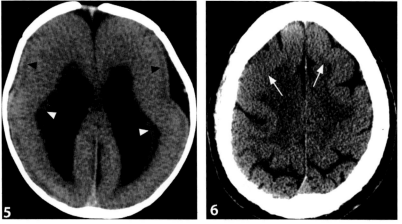

Figure 5. Non-enhanced axial CT shows agyric cerebral hemispheres. Peripheral thin dark line (black arrowhead) within thick cortex corresponds to sparse cell zone. A small amount of white matter is only found in the periventricular area (white arrowhead).

Figure 6. Axial CT in another patient shows pachygyria with thick cortical mantle (arrows).

Lissencephaly

MARIASAVINA SEVERINO

Specific Imaging Findings

Lissencephaly is characterized by absent (agyria) or decreased (pachygyria) cortical convolutions, resulting in a smooth cerebral surface. The affected cortex is abnormally thick, usually measuring 10–15 mm in agyria with almost no visible sulcation, and 6–9 mm in pachygyria (also called "incomplete lissencephaly") with the presence of only a few shallow sulci and broad gyri. Complete agyria or pachygyria are unusual, and most cases are a combination of agyria and pachygyria. The thick, smooth cortex characteristically shows a peripheral stripe of high T2 signal and low CT attenuation, corresponding to sparse cell zone. The white matter is very thin and may be reduced to periventricular areas only. Several different patterns of lissencephaly have been described depending on the severity of the gyral simplification and the gradient along the anterior to posterior axis, with good correlation between the phenotypic spectrum and the underlying genetic abnormality. The most severe pattern is characterized by complete agyria with smooth cerebral surface and absent opercularization ("figure eight" configuration of the brain). Children with *LIS1* and *TUBA1A* mutations have predominant posterior lissencephaly with a posterior to anterior (P>A) gradient. *TUBA1A* mutations may also show perisylvian pachygyria with typical dysgenesis of the anterior limb of the internal capsules. Children with *DCX* mutations have predominant anterior lissencephaly, with anterior to posterior (A>P) gradient. Other lissencephaly-associated abnormalities may include microcephaly, commissural abnormalities (in particular callosal anomalies), brainstem abnormalities (such as severe hypoplasia of the pons and medulla) and abnormalities of the cerebellum (in particular hypo/dysplasia of the vermis).

Pertinent Clinical Information

The clinical manifestations are usually closely dependent on the severity of anatomic malformation. Patients with severe classical lissencephaly have early developmental delay, profound or severe mental retardation, early diffuse hypotonia which may evolve to spastic quadriplegia, and feeding problems. The lifespan is shortened in most cases. Less severe malformations such as pachygyria are accompanied by milder impairment with moderate mental retardation. Seizures occur in over 90% of patients and represent an independent contributor to intellectual disability and developmental delay. The Miller–Dieker syndrome is a contiguous gene deletion syndrome due to deletion of multiple genes at the tip of the short arm of chromosome 17 and characterized by predominantly posterior lissencephaly, facial dysmorphisms and occasionally other congenital abnormalities. Other subtypes of lissencephaly (called "lissencephaly variants") have been described in patients harbouring mutations of *RELN*, *ARX*, and *VLDLR* genes. *RELN*-associated lissencephaly is characterized by severe cerebellar hypoplasia. *ARX* mutations are associated with predominant posterior lissencephaly, abnormal white matter signal, and corpus callosum agenesis; these patients typically present ambiguous genitalia.

Differential Diagnosis

Polymicrogyria (103)
- usually thinner cortical ribbon of bumpy, corrugated appearance
- irregular gray–white matter interface

Congenital Muscular Dystrophies (Cobblestone Complex) (92)
- "pebbly" surface of the brain
- cerebellar and ocular abnormalities
- congenital muscular dystrophy

Lissencephaly Secondary to CMV (184)
- thin cortex
- calcifications

Background

Lissencephaly is a cortical malformation caused by disturbed neuronal migration. In approximately 80% of cases a genetic cause can be found. Six genes have been so far identified (*LIS1*, *DCX*, *ARX*, *RELN*, *YWHAE* and *TUBA1A*). These genes are required for optimal tangential and radial migration of neurons during brain development. Lissencephaly has been subdivided into several types based on both brain imaging and pathology: "classic lissencephaly" due to *LIS1*, *DCX*, and *TUBA1A* mutations, "variant lissencephaly" due to *RELN*, *VLDLR*, and *ARX* mutations, and the cobblestone complex. Lissencephaly is histologically characterized by thick and poorly organized cortex with four primitive layers including an outer marginal zone with increased cellularity (layer 1), a superficial cortical layer with diffusely scattered large pyramidal neurons (layer 2), a relatively neuron-sparse zone (layer 3) and a deep thick cortical gray zone with medium and small neurons often oriented in columns (layer 4).

REFERENCES

1. Jissendi-Tchofo P, Kara S, Barkovich AJ. Midbrain–hindbrain involvement in lissencephalies. *Neurology* 2009;**72**:410–8.
2. Kara S, Jissendi-Tchofo P, Barkovich AJ. Developmental differences of the major forebrain commissures in lissencephalies. *AJNR* 2010;**31**:1602–7.
3. Mochida GH. Genetics and biology of microcephaly and lissencephaly. *Semin Pediatr Neurol* 2009;**16**:120–6.
4. Guerrini R, Parrini E. Neuronal migration disorders. *Neurobiology of Disease* 2010;**38**:154–66.
5. Morris-Rosendahl DJ, Najm J, Lachmeijer AM, *et al.* Refining the phenotype of alpha-1a tubulin (TUBA1A) mutation in patients with classical lissencephaly. *Clin Genet* 2008;**74**:425–33.

Brain Imaging with MRI and CT, ed. Zoran Rumboldt *et al.* Published by Cambridge University Press. © Cambridge University Press 2012.

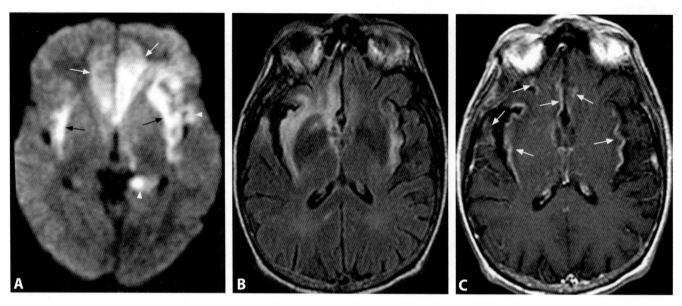

Figure 1. Axial DWI image (A) shows very bright signals in bilateral paramedial basal frontal lobes (white arrows), both insulae (black arrows) and left temporal lobe (arrowheads). FLAIR image at a similar level (B) shows hyperintense signal in bilateral insular and frontal location as well as in the anterior right temporal lobe. Corresponding post-contrast T1WI (C) reveals cortical enhancement (arrows) of these areas.

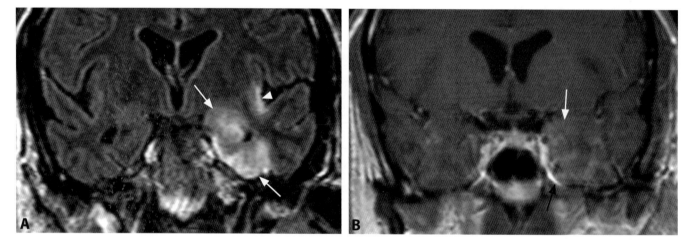

Figure 2. Coronal FLAIR image (A) shows hyperintensity involving the cortex and subcortical white matter of the mesial left temporal lobe (arrows). There is also involvement of the left insula (arrowhead). Postcontrast T1WI image at a similar level (B) shows mild peripheral enhancement (arrows) in the mesial left temporal lobe.

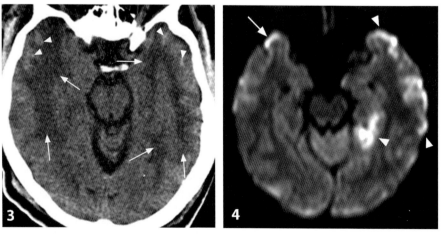

Figure 3. Non-enhanced CT image shows abnormal hypodensity in both temporal lobes (arrows), right greater than left, with small hyperdense areas of hemorrhage (arrowheads).

Figure 4. Axial DWI shows asymmetric hyperintensity in the temporal lobes, left (arrowheads) greater than right (arrow).

Herpes Simplex Encephalitis

MAURICIO CASTILLO AND ZORAN RUMBOLDT

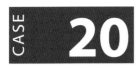

Specific Imaging Findings

As herpes simplex encephalitis (HSE) may clinically simulate stroke or tumor and early treatment is a must, identification by imaging is imperative and MRI is the method of choice. The process usually initially involves the mesial temporal lobes but may quickly extend to the insula (classically skipping the basal ganglia), the frontobasal regions, along the interhemispheric region, and then to the rest of the temporal, frontal and parietal lobes. Areas involved tend to be bilateral with generally asymmetrical degree of involvement. All lesions are of low T1 and high T2 signal, bright on DWI and with reduced diffusion on ADC maps. The advantage of FLAIR and especially DWI sequences is that the abnormalities are much more conspicuous early in the process. Contrast enhancement, particularly of the involved cortex, occurs in the later stages and meningeal enhancement may also be present. Hemorrhage may occur at any time of the infection. Perfusion study shows normal to low relative cerebral blood volume, as in other infectious and inflammatory processes. In addition to high choline and NAA, MR spectroscopy shows lipids and lactate. CT may show edema involving the temporal lobes but usually becomes positive only in advanced disease and should not be used to make the initial diagnosis. The abnormal signal in the mesial temporal lobes in patients with HHV-6 encephalopathy tends to be transient in contrast to persistent abnormality in patients with HSE.

Differential Diagnosis

Limbic Encephalitis (21)
- gradual and not acute onset
- CSF analysis shows different parameters than for HSE

Seizure-Induced Cortical Changes (104)
- generally unilateral
- usually known to have seizures
- on repeated study after seizures are controlled abnormalities generally resolve

Gliomas (165, 166)
- mesial temporal lobe tumors tend to be unilateral
- usually mass-like appearance

Pertinent Clinical Information

HSE is typically characterized by a sudden onset of fever and headaches, rapidly progressing to alterations of consciousness, seizures and coma if not promptly treated. Most patients are young and atypical clinical presentations are commonly seen in the youngest ones. CSF shows high number of lymphocytes and proteins. The diagnosis is established by positive PCR in CSF (sensitivity and specificity of over 95%) which may, however, be negative early on. Early EEG points to abnormalities in the temporal lobes. Among the most common symptoms in survivors are chronic epilepsy, memory and personality changes, and hearing loss.

Background

Unlike the perinatal encephalitis caused by HSV type 2, HSV type 1 has been considered the most common sporadic viral encephalitis in the world and occurs at any age without gender predominance. Most patients are below 30 years of age and believed to have a normal immune system. It is thought that the first infection, generally subclinical or mildly clinically symptomatic, involves the upper respiratory airways. From here the virus infects the cranial nerves, particularly the trigeminal and travels to the Gasserian ganglia where it will remain in a dormant state for variable periods of time. The acute encephalitis is due to either reactivation of this dormant virus or infection by a new one. Reactivation has been linked to any condition that increases stress in humans. The virus then invades the brain, particularly the limbic areas and results in an acute hemorrhagic and necrotizing process. This process is accompanied by severe edema and abundant lymphocytes. Soon after, the infection spreads to the insula, frontal and less commonly parietal regions. Hyperintense lesions involving the cortex and adjacent white matter on DWI in the appropriate clinical setting should be considered HSE until proven otherwise. Once HSE is considered in the differential diagnosis, administration of antiviral antibiotics must be immediately started. Delay in proper therapy leads to mortality rates from 50% to over 80%. Regardless of treatment, nearly 50% of patients will show neurologic sequelae.

REFERENCES
1. Demaerel P, Wilms G, Robberecht W *et al.* MRI of herpes simplex encephalitis. *Neuroradiology* 1992;**34**:490–3.
2. Noguchi T, Yoshiura T, Hiwatashi A, *et al.* CT and MRI findings of human herpesvirus 6-associated encephalopathy: comparison with findings of herpes simplex virus encephalitis. *AJR* 2010;**194**: 754–60.
3. Baskin HJ, Hedlund G. Neuroimaging of herpesvirus infections in children. *Pediatr Radiol* 2007;**37**:949–63.
4. Vossough A, Zimmerman RA, Bilaniuk LT, Schwartz EM. Imaging findings of neonatal herpes simplex virus type 2 encephalitis. *Neuroradiology* 2008;**50**:355–66.

Brain Imaging with MRI and CT, ed. Zoran Rumboldt *et al.* Published by Cambridge University Press. © Cambridge University Press 2012.

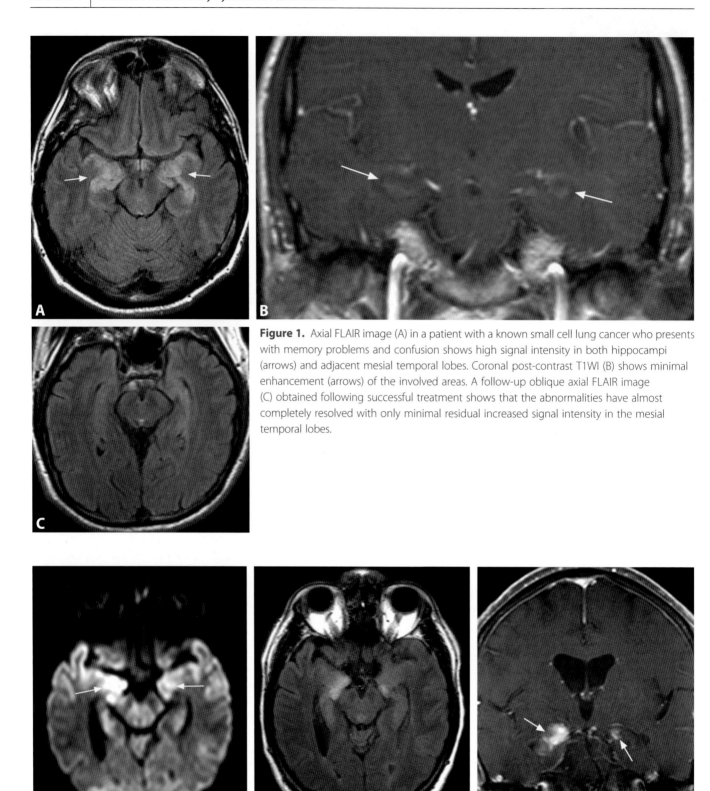

Figure 1. Axial FLAIR image (A) in a patient with a known small cell lung cancer who presents with memory problems and confusion shows high signal intensity in both hippocampi (arrows) and adjacent mesial temporal lobes. Coronal post-contrast T1WI (B) shows minimal enhancement (arrows) of the involved areas. A follow-up oblique axial FLAIR image (C) obtained following successful treatment shows that the abnormalities have almost completely resolved with only minimal residual increased signal intensity in the mesial temporal lobes.

Figure 2. Axial DWI image (A) shows cortical hyperintensity in bilateral anterior temporal lobe, most prominent in the uncus (arrows), right greater than left. This was consistent with T2 shine-through phenomenon as ADC maps were unremarkable. Corresponding FLAIR image (B) also shows hyperintense signal of bilateral uncus and anterior hippocampus. Coronal fat saturated post-contrast T1WI (C) reveals hippocampal enhancement (arrows) bilaterally, right greater than left. In this patient who presented with memory difficulties lymphoma was diagnosed in the work-up following the imaging diagnosis.

Limbic Encephalitis

MAURICIO CASTILLO

Specific Imaging Findings

In limbic encephalitis (LE), the mesial temporal lobes show bright T2 signal and may appear swollen or of normal width. Contrast enhancement is commonly absent, but when present may be patchy or have a bizarre configuration and distribution. About 50% of patients show bilateral involvement, often asymmetrical. The lesion may extend from the amygdala to the tail of the hippocampus. Other areas which are occasionally involved include the parahippocampal gyrus, temporal white matter stem, thalamic pulvinar, dentate nuclei and cerebellar cortex. With the passage of time, the signal abnormality resolves (although not completely in many patients) and the affected area loses volume. ADC measurements have been inconclusive and thus not helpful, while high signal intensity in DWI is thought to be due to shine-through phenomenon. Proton MR spectroscopy may show low n-acetylaspartate, normal choline and occasionally high glutamate/glutamine and lactate. In some patients, all metabolites are low.

Pertinent Clinical Information

Symptoms tend to start relatively acutely and include: cognitive dysfunction, recent memory difficulties, hallucinations, bizarre behavior, seizures, sleep disturbances, and speech disturbances. Symptoms are present in about 80% of patients who have an abnormal MRI study. The symptoms may be similar to those seen in Alzheimer and Creutzfeldt–Jakob diseases but their more acute onset and the presence of underlying neoplasias helps differentiate among them. To make the diagnosis, CSF must be free of malignant cells, viruses and other pathogens.

Differential Diagnosis

Herpes Simplex Encephalitis (20)
* acute onset with fever
* CSF analysis shows different parameters than for LE

Seizure-Induced Cortical Changes (104)
* generally unilateral
* usually known to have seizures
* if study is repeated after seizures are controlled abnormalities generally resolve

Gliomas (165, 166)
* mesial temporal lobe tumors tend to be unilateral
* usually mass-like appearance
* MRS may show elevated choline which is not seen in LE

Background

LE is a rare disorder which is due to a paraneoplastic disorder in over half of patients. It occurs most commonly with small cell carcinoma of the lung, but may be seen in other primary tumors such as lymphoma, thymoma, adenocarcinoma of the colon, renal cell cancer, breast, prostate, ovary and testicular cancers, and neuroblastoma. It is estimated that about 1% of these patients will develop LE. Because patients with LE show abnormal antibodies in CSF it is believed that the disease is immune-mediated (so-called "onconeural" antibodies). The most commonly found antibody is named Hu (rarely, LE can be Hu negative) and multiple others have been implicated. It is thought that these antibodies affect the voltage-gated potassium channels in the cells leading to depolarization and subsequent damage. After the initial insult there is infiltration by T cells. It is this "second hit" that is thought to result in permanent neuronal damage and gliosis. Perivascular and interstitial infiltrates are composed of B lymphocytes and CD4$^+$ and CD8$^+$ T lymphocytes, with microglial proliferation and neuronophagia. FDG-PET usually shows hypermetabolism in one or both temporal lobes and findings rarely correlate with MRI. LE may occur without underlying malignancy (especially in children), most notably following allogeneic hematopoietic stem-cell transplant, which has been associated with human herpesvirus-6 (HHV6) infection. Treatment is geared towards the control of the underlying condition. Otherwise, even if it resolves, LE eventually relapses. Corticosteroids and intravenous immunoglobulin are used for direct treatment of LE, aimed at preventing permanent cognitive and behavioral deficits, along with immunomodulators (such as cyclophosphamide) and plasmapheresis. Paraneoplastic LE has an unpredictable course and death may occur even just a few days after onset of symptoms.

REFERENCES

1. Urbach H, Soeder BM, Jeub M, et al. Serial MRI of limbic encephalitis. *Neuroradiology* 2006;**48**:380–6.

2. Thueri C, Muller K, Laubenberger J, et al. MR imaging of autopsy-proved paraneoplastic limbic encephalitis in non-Hodgkin lymphoma. *AJNR* 2003;**24**:507–11.

3. Gorniak RJ, Young GS, Wiese DE, et al. MR imaging of human herpesvirus-6-associated encephalitis in 4 patients with anterograde amnesia after allogeneic hematopoietic stem-cell transplantation. *AJNR* 2006;**27**:887–91.

4. Anderson NE, Barber PA. Limbic encephalitis – a review. *J Clin Neurosci* 2008;**15**:961–71.

5. Basu S, Alavi A. Role of FDG-PET in the clinical management of paraneoplastic neurological syndrome: detection of the underlying malignancy and the brain PET–MRI correlates. *Mol Imaging Biol* 2008;**10**:131–7.

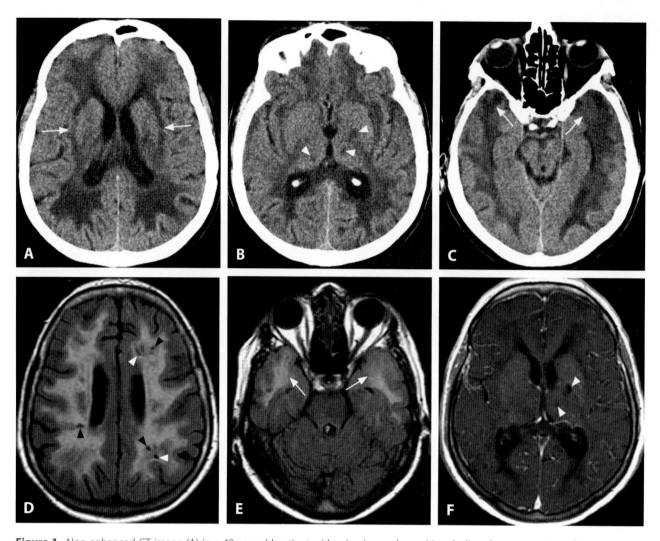

Figure 1. Non-enhanced CT image (A) in a 49-year-old patient with migraine and cognitive decline shows extensive white matter hypodensity, involving bilateral external capsules (arrows). CT image at a lower level (B) better shows lacunar infarcts (arrowheads). CT (C) reveals extension of the hypodensity into bilateral anterior temporal white matter (arrows). FLAIR image (D) shows additional lacunar infarcts (arrowheads) along with extensive diffuse white matter hyperintensity. FLAIR at a lower level (E) shows high signal of bilateral anterior temporal white matter (arrows). Post-contrast T1WI (F) again shows deep lacunar infarcts (arrowheads). The involved white matter is hypointense and there is no abnormal enhancement.

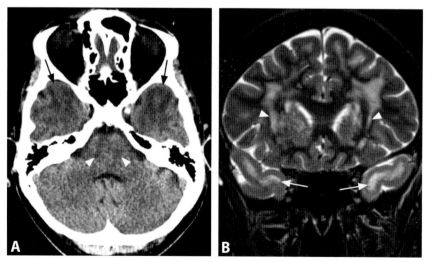

Figure 2. Non-enhanced axial CT image (A) in a 30-year-old patient with migraine with aura shows hypodense subcortical white matter of both anterior temporal lobes (arrows). There is also a vague pontine hypodensity (arrowheads). Coronal STIR image (B) reveals diffusely increased signal of the cerebral white matter, including the external capsules (arrowheads) and anterior temporal lobes (arrows).

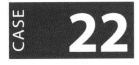

CADASIL (Cerebral Autosomal Dominant Arteriopathy with Subcortical Infarcts and Leukoencephalopathy)

ZORAN RUMBOLDT

Specific Imaging Findings

Cerebral autosomal dominant arteriopathy with subcortical infarcts and leukoencephalopathy (CADASIL) has a characteristic imaging appearance with involvement of the bilateral anterior temporal lobe white matter and the external capsules on both CT and MR imaging. The involved white matter is diffusely hypodense on CT, of low T1 signal and T2 hyperintense. There is no associated mass effect or contrast enhancement and the involved areas have increased diffusivity with increased signal on ADC maps. The lesions start to appear in the subcortical white matter at around 20 years of age and subsequently extend into the deep gray matter and brainstem. Lacunar infarctions are very common and usually appear by 30 years of age in the subcortical white matter, internal capsule, deep gray matter, and brainstem. The number of lacunar infarctions increases with age. Microbleeds, best seen as areas of "blooming" signal loss on T2* imaging, are frequently present. While these findings, primarily in the external capsules and even more so in the anterior temporal white matter, are highly characteristic for CADASIL, none of them are pathognomonic and may be seen with the much more common sporadic microangiopathy. However, the combination of typical findings in a young adult is highly suggestive of this disorder.

Pertinent Clinical Information

The main clinical manifestations are recurrent ischemic stroke, migraine, psychiatric symptoms (mostly mood disorders), and progressive cognitive impairment. Migraine, very commonly with aura, is the most common initial symptom. The long clinical course (several decades) and variable onset of symptoms even within families can result in many CADASIL patients being initially misdiagnosed with multiple sclerosis, dementia, or CNS vasculitis. The diagnosis is confirmed by the presence of granular osmiophilic material (GOM) in skin biopsies, which is 100% specific.

Differential Diagnosis

Sporadic Small Vessel Disease (Leukoaraiosis) (27)
- involvement of the anterior temporal lobe is highly unusual
- external capsule rarely involved
- older patients

Chronic MS
- absence of microbleeds
- focal MS lesions with characteristic location and shape are frequently present

Megalencephalic Leukoencephalopathy with Subcortical Cysts (van der Knapp Disease) (23)
- anterior temporal lobe expansion with cysts

- absence of lacunar infarcts and microbleeds
- most commonly occurs in infants

HIV Encephalopathy (25)
- usually prominent atrophy
- absence of lacunar infarcts

Limbic Encephalitis (21)
- anterior temporal gray matter involvement
- contrast enhancement and reduced diffusion may occur

Background

CADASIL is the most common hereditary cerebral small vessel disease, caused by missense point mutations or small deletions of the *Notch3* gene, which encodes a large single-pass transmembrane receptor. The brain arterioles are the main targets, but extracerebral small blood vessels are also affected. GOM, found in the walls of affected vessels, refers to small or medium-size (20–40 μm) extracellular electron-dense granular deposits observed on electron microscopy. *Notch3* immunostaining of skin biopsy specimens has been recently introduced as a simplified supportive test. Catheter cerebral angiography frequently results in neurological complications and should be avoided in patients suspected of CADASIL. DTI detects ultrastructural tissue damage even in areas that appear normal on conventional MRI and mean diffusivity was found to be a predictor of clinical progression. Cognitive decline, especially executive dysfunction, is strongly associated with increase in lacunar infarcts. The exact prevalence of this disorder is currently unknown, with the number of reported CADASIL families steadily increasing as this entity is becoming more widely known. At present there is no specific treatment.

REFERENCES

1. van den Boom R, Lesnik Oberstein SA, Ferrari MD, et al. Cerebral autosomal dominant arteriopathy with subcortical infarcts and leukoencephalopathy: MR imaging findings at different ages – 3rd–6th decades. *Radiology* 2003;**229**:683–90.

2. O'Sullivan M, Jarosz JM, Martin RJ, et al. MRI hyperintensities of the temporal lobe and external capsule in patients with CADASIL. *Neurology* 2001;**56**:628–34.

3. Chabriat H, Levy C, Taillia H, et al. Patterns of MRI lesions in CADASIL. *Neurology* 1998;**51**:452–7.

4. Choi JC. Cerebral autosomal dominant arteriopathy with subcortical infarcts and leukoencephalopathy: a genetic cause of cerebral small vessel disease. *J Clin Neurol* 2010;**6**:1–9.

5. Liem MK, van der Grond J, Haan J, et al. Lacunar infarcts are the main correlate with cognitive dysfunction in CADASIL. *Stroke* 2007;**38**:923–8.

45

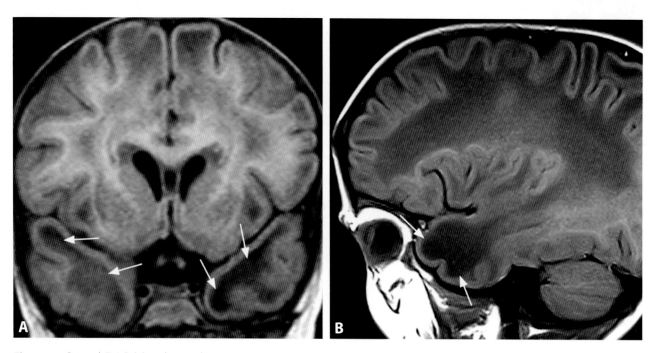

Figure 1. Coronal FLAIR (A) and sagittal T1WI (B) reveal typical subcortical cysts in the temporal poles (arrows). There is also less prominent diffusely abnormal low T1 signal of the white matter.

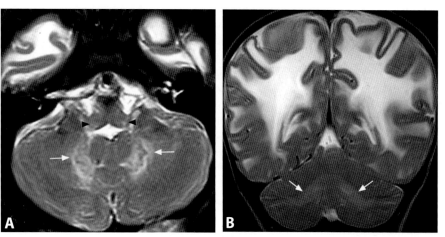

Figure 2. Axial (A) and coronal (B) T2WI depict mild cerebellar white matter hyperintensities with bilateral involvement of the dentate hilus (arrows). There is slight hyperintensity of the bilateral inferior olivary nuclei (arrowheads) and much more prominent diffuse high signal abnormality involving the supratentorial white matter.

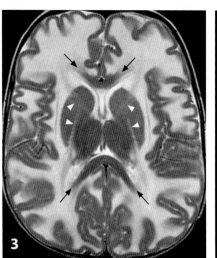

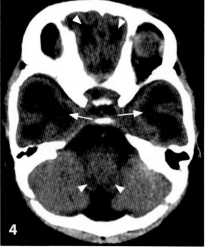

Figure 3. Axial T2WI shows diffuse cerebral swelling and white matter hyperintensity including the U-fibers and external/extreme capsules. Corpus callosum (arrows) and internal capsules (arrowheads) are less affected. Gyri appear swollen but cortex is intact.

Figure 4. CT shows temporal cysts (arrows), along with frontal and brainstem hypodensities (arrowheads).

Megalencephalic Leukoencephalopathy with Subcortical Cysts

MARIASAVINA SEVERINO

Specific Imaging Findings

MRI shows diffuse cerebral white matter swelling and T2 hyperintensity with involvement of U-fibers and early appearance of typical subcortical cysts, particularly in the frontotemporal regions, best shown by FLAIR and T1WI. Over time these cysts may increase in size and number. The corpus callosum and internal capsules are relatively preserved. Subtle signal changes may be present within the brainstem, especially along the pyramidal tracts. Cerebellar white matter is usually of a mildly abnormal signal and not swollen. The deep gray matter structures are intact and there is no abnormal contrast enhancement. Brain atrophy develops on follow-up studies. A more benign variant is characterized by milder initial findings with subcortical cysts limited to the temporal region. In this form, the white matter abnormalities and cysts decrease over time. In adults with the disease, atrophy is present instead of brain swelling, with enlargement of the ventricles and other CSF spaces. On ADC maps there is increased diffusivity of the affected white matter. MRS shows decreased levels of all metabolites in cystic areas and decreased NAA within white matter lesions.

Pertinent Clinical Information

Megalencephalic leukoencephalopathy with subcortical cysts (MLC) is characterized by early macrocephaly (developing during the first year of life) and delayed motor and cognitive deterioration. Mild delay in gross motor milestones is followed by slowly progressive ataxia and spastic paraparesis. Mental deterioration and seizures develop in later stages of the disease. Minor head trauma may induce temporary deterioration. Extrapyramidal disorders (dystonia and athetosis), dysphagia and speech problems can appear in the second and third decades. The clinical features progress very slowly with variable life expectancy (from teens to forties). In the recently described benign variant of MLC, motor functions may improve over time. The disease has also been identified in adults with similar clinical history and neurological findings.

Differential Diagnosis

Canavan Disease (24)
- subcortical cysts are usually absent
- typical involvement of thalamus and globus pallidus
- characteristic increased NAA peak on MRS

Alexander Disease (33)
- leukoencephalopathy with frontal predominance
- contrast enhancement of affected brain structures almost invariably present
- cystic degeneration occurs mainly in the deep frontal white matter
- CT hyperdense and high T1/low T2 periventricular rims

Congenital CMV Infection (184)
- microcephaly
- calcifications
- polymicrogyria
- fixed deficits, without progression

Congenital Muscular Dystrophy (92)
- hypoplastic brainstem and cerebellum
- possible cortical malformations
- characteristic cerebellar subcortical microcysts

GM2 or GM1 Gangliosidosis (9)
- prominent involvement of the deep gray matter
- absence of cysts
- low T2/high T1 signal of the thalami

Background

MLC is a rare autosomal recessive leukoencephalopathy and approximately 80% of MLC patients harbor mutations of the *MLC1* gene on chromosome 22. This gene encodes a membrane protein (MLC1) with unknown function, which is mainly expressed in astrocytes of perivascular, subependymal, and subpial regions. This location suggests a possible role for MLC1 in a transport process across the blood–brain barrier. MLC patients without *MLC1* mutations have also been described and they present with two distinct phenotypes: classic and benign (in which there is no decline of motor functions). Brain biopsy in MLC shows fine uniform vacuolation of white matter with wide separation of myelinated axons. Laboratory investigations are typically normal and there is no other organ involvement. Therapy is strictly supportive.

REFERENCES

1. Miles L, DeGrauw TJ, Dinopoulos A, *et al*. Megalencephalic leukoencephalopathy with subcortical cysts: a third confirmed case with literature review. *Pediatr Dev Pathol* 2009;**12**:180–6.

2. van der Knaap MS, Lai V, Köhler W, *et al*. Megalencephalic leukoencephalopathy with cysts without MLC1 defect. *Ann Neurol* 2010;**67**:834–7.

3. López-Hernández T, Ridder MC, Montolio M, *et al*. Mutant glial CAM causes megalencephalic leukoencephalopathy with subcortical cysts, benign familial macrocephaly, and macrocephaly with retardation and autism. *Am J Hum Genet* 2011;**88**:422–32.

4. Patay Z. Metabolic disorders. In: *Pediatric Neuroradiology Brain*. Tortori-Donati P, Rossi A, eds. Springer, New York NY 2005.

5. Brockmann K, Finsterbusch J, Terwey B, *et al*. Megalencephalic leukoencephalopathy with subcortical cysts in an adult: quantitative proton MR spectroscopy and diffusion tensor MRI. *Neuroradiology* 2003;**45**:137–42.

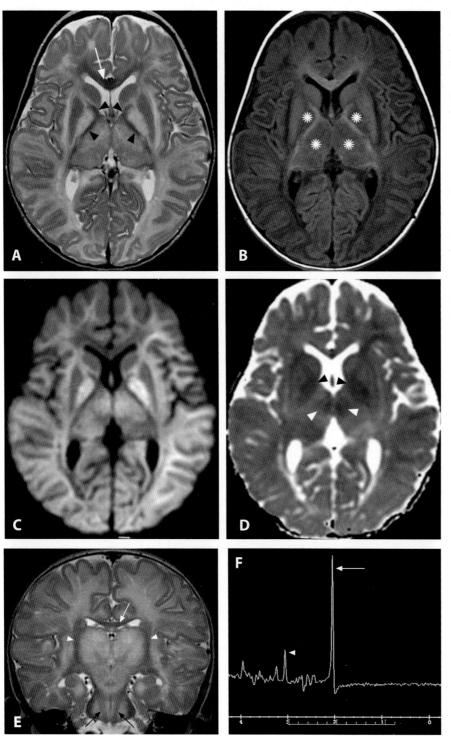

Figure 1. MRI in an 18-month-old boy. Axial T2WI (A) and T1WI (B) show diffusely abnormal signal of supratentorial white matter with involvement of subcortical fibers and relative sparing of corpus callosum (arrow) and genu and posterior limb of the internal capsule (arrowheads), suggesting a centripetal pattern. Note bilateral swelling and abnormal signal of thalami and globi pallidi (*) with sparing of the striatum and claustrum. DWI (C) and ADC map (D) show decreased diffusion throughout the involved white matter, consistent with intramyelin edema. Abnormal diffusivity is also present in both thalami and globi pallidi (arrowheads). Coronal T2WI (E) shows diffuse hyperintensity of the thalami, midbrain, and pons, with relative sparing of the corpus callosum (white arrow), internal capsules (arrowheads), and pyramidal tracts (black arrows). Proton MRS (TE 144 ms; F) shows pathognomonic prominent increase of the NAA peak (arrow). Compare to the creatine peak (arrowhead).

Canavan Disease

ANDREA ROSSI AND CHEN HOFFMAN

Specific Imaging Findings

MRI shows a diffuse leukoencephalopathy with swelling of the white matter, involving both the supratentorial and the infratentorial compartments. There is a centripetal pattern of involvement, with relative sparing of the internal capsules and corpus callosum until later stages of the disease. The affected white matter appears T1 hypointense and hyperintense on T2-weighted images, with signal approaching that of the CSF, due to diffuse spongy degeneration. The same regions are bright on DWI and dark on ADC maps, consistent with reduced diffusivity of water, compatible with intramyelinic edema. The gray matter of the thalami and globi pallidi is also involved, whereas the caudate nuclei, putamina, and claustra are spared. There is no pathological enhancement of affected structures following contrast administration. Canavan disease has a pathognomonic appearance on proton MR spectroscopy with a marked increase of the NAA peak, as a result of its accumulation within the brain tissue. Other possible and nonspecific MR spectroscopy findings include decrease of choline and creatine, increased *myo*-inositol levels, and presence of lactate.

Pertinent Clinical Information

There are three clinical variants of Canavan disease: neonatal, infantile, and juvenile, of which the infantile (presenting by age 3–6 months) is by far the most common. Patients present with macrocrania, hypotonia, lethargy, seizures, spasticity, optic atrophy, and developmental delay. The clinical phenotype is variably severe depending on the degree of enzyme activity in individual cases. The disorder is now considered to be more prevalent than commonly thought, with a range of clinically milder forms that are characterized by later onset and prolonged length of survival. In typical cases, demise occurs after a few years. Lithium administration appears to be beneficial in patients with Canavan disease.

Differential Diagnosis

Pelizaeus–Merzbacher Disease

- diffuse lack of myelination on both T1- and T2-weighted images with white matter showing less profound T2 hyperintensity
- absence of diffusion abnormality
- NAA not elevated on MRS

Alexander Disease (33)

- white matter is involved with an anterior-to-posterior gradient
- subcortical white matter initially spared

- bifrontal periventricular rim is hyperdense on CT and of low T2/high T1 signal
- periventricular contrast enhancement
- brainstem involvement with contrast enhancement

Megalencephalic Leukoencephalopathy with Subcortical Cysts (van der Knaap Disease) (23)

- white matter diffusely swollen and with increased diffusivity
- basal nuclei are spared
- characteristic subcortical cysts at temporal poles and superior frontal lobes

Background

Canavan disease is an autosomal recessive disease caused by mutation of the *ASPA* gene on chromosome 17 encoding for aspartoacylase, an enzyme metabolizing *N*-acetylaspartate (NAA) into acetate and aspartate. This results in brain accumulation of NAA. A proposed role of NAA, which is found only in neurons, is in brain water homeostasis. NAA regulates the molecular efflux water pump system that accounts for fluid balance between intra- and extracellular spaces of the myelinated white matter. Thus, excessive NAA would lead to water accumulation in white matter with resulting intramyelinic edema, spongy degeneration, demyelination, and glial cell loss. The effects of lithium on metabolic and signaling pathways in the brain vary depending on the specific clinical condition – while it increases levels of NAA in patients with bipolar disorder, a drop in NAA is observed in patients with Canavan disease, along with improved myelination on DTI and other MR imaging techniques.

REFERENCES

1. Janson CG, McPhee SW, Francis J, *et al*. Natural history of Canavan disease revealed by proton magnetic resonance spectroscopy (1H-MRS) and diffusion-weighted MRI. *Neuropediatrics* 2006;**37**:209–21.
2. Michel SJ, Given CA 2nd. Case 99: Canavan disease. *Radiology* 2006;**241**:310–4.
3. Patay Z. Diffusion-weighted MR imaging in leukodystrophies. *Eur Radiol* 2005;**15**:2284–303.
4. Yalcinkaya C, Benbir G, Salomons GS, *et al*. Atypical MRI findings in Canavan disease: a patient with a mild course. *Neuropediatrics* 2005;**36**:336–9.
5. Assadi M, Janson C, Wang DJ, *et al*. Lithium citrate reduces excessive intra-cerebral N-acetyl aspartate in Canavan disease. *Eur J Paediatr Neurol* 2010;**14**:354–9.

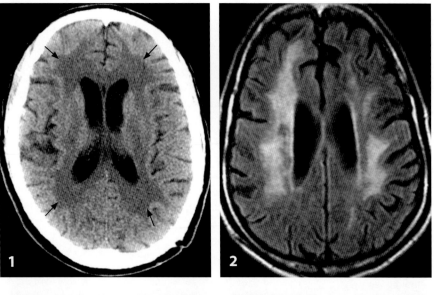

Figure 1. Axial non-enhanced CT image at the level of the lateral ventricles shows diffuse white matter hypodensity (arrows).

Figure 2. Axial FLAIR image in a different patient shows patchy but still confluent periventricular white matter hyperintensities and diffuse brain atrophy.

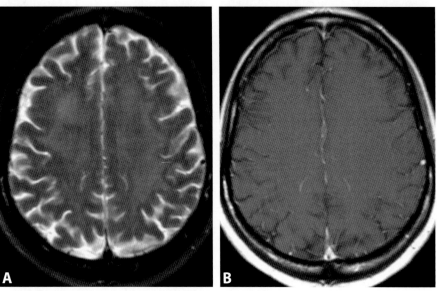

Figure 3. Axial T2WI at the level of centrum semiovale (A) shows bilateral "cloud-like" abnormal high signal intensity involving most of the hemispheric white matter as well as cortical atrophy. Note relative sparing of the subcortical white matter. Post-contrast T1WI (B) at a slightly lower level shows isointensity of the affected white matter and no enhancement.

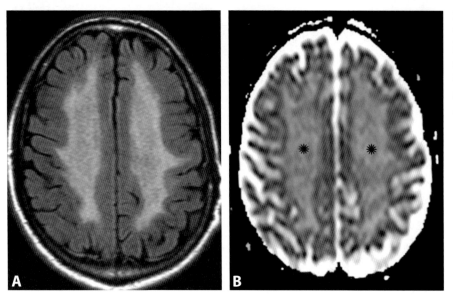

Figure 4. Axial FLAIR image (A) in a patient with severe disease shows a prominent bilateral diffuse hyperintensity of the white matter with relative sparing of the subcortical U-fibers. ADC map at a similar level (B) demonstrates increased diffusion (*) of the abnormal white matter.

HIV Encephalopathy

ZORAN RUMBOLDT AND MAURICIO CASTILLO

Specific Imaging Findings

The most common finding in HIV encephalopathy is diffuse brain atrophy, which is progressive and more prominent in the patients with dementia. White matter lesions which are better seen on MRI are the second most common finding. They are characteristically diffuse; however, patchy, focal or punctate lesions may also be seen. They are of low attenuation on CT and T2 hyperintense, while isointense to minimally hypointense and therefore inconspicuous on T1-weighted images. The abnormalities show increased diffusion and typically spare the subcortical U-fibers. Contrast enhancement and mass effect are absent and the overlying gray matter may appear atrophic. Typically, it has a "cloud-like" appearance which may involve both hemispheres and cross the corpus callosum. These abnormalities may improve with treatment. At the start of the disease, MRS shows low NAA and high choline and *myo*-inositol. In the chronic stages all metabolites are low. Perfusion studies show low relative cerebral blood flow. DTI shows low fractional anisotropy throughout the brain including the normal-appearing white matter.

Pertinent Clinical Information

HIV-related encephalopathy is the most common cause of dementia in younger individuals (20–45 years of age). Its incidence is declining possibly due to the widespread use of highly active anti-retroviral therapy (HAART) given to nearly all infected patients. The most prominent symptoms include cognitive impairment and motor dysfunction. Attention, speed of information processing, and learning efficiency are primarily impaired. Brain involvement is present in over 90% of HIV-infected patients.

Differential Diagnosis

Microangiopathy (Leukoaraiosis) (27)
- usually less confluent and diffuse
- microbleeds and lacunar infarcts may be present

Radiation/Chemotherapy-Induced Leukoencephalopathy (26)
- history of whole-brain radiation and/or intrathecal chemotherapy

Chronic MS
- presence of focal lesions with very low T1 signal/hypodensity ("black holes")
- history of MS usually known

Posterior Reversible Encephalopathy Syndrome (32)
- primarily affects the subcortical white matter, possible cortical involvement
- predominantly posterior location

Progressive Multifocal Leukoencephalopathy (116)
- asymmetrical single or multifocal lesion with low T1 signal
- involvement of subcortical U-fibers
- mild mass effect common
- lower magnetization transfer ratio of PML lesions
- more severe reduction in NAA and increase in choline levels, prominent lactate on MRS

CMV encephalitis
- possible ventriculitis, otherwise indistinguishable

Background

The HIV virus belongs to the retroviral family which integrates itself into the host's DNA. Of the two viruses, HIV-1 is more common with over 35% of infected individuals progressing to full AIDS. Although this virus results in many opportunistic infections and neoplasias, it also directly involves the CNS. The virus enters the brain and resides in microglia and macrophages. Activation of immunity-related cells leads to release of toxins which damage neurons and astrocytes. At autopsy the brain shows atrophy that is predominantly fronto-parietal. There is loss of gray matter volume and pallor of the white matter. There is diffuse microglial reaction and presence of multinucleated giant cells, while lymphocytic infiltration is minimal or absent. Although neuronal loss is prominent, gliosis is not and frank myelin destruction is absent. Mineralization of blood vessels is also present in children. Infection with HIV-2 is less common and has a longer course than that with HIV-1. Clinically and by imaging they are indistinguishable. Generalized atrophy and white matter T2 hyperintensity also occur in patients with CMV encephalitis and cannot be differentiated from HIV encephalopathy. Highly active antiretroviral therapy (HAART) may result in stabilization or even regression of white matter and metabolite abnormalities. Progression of lesions on initial follow-up studies is frequently due to immune reconstitution inflammatory syndrome (IRIS) after the initiation of HAART.

REFERENCES

1. Thurnher MM, Post MJD. Neuroimaging in the brain in HIV-1-infected patients. *Neuroimaging Clinics North Am* 2008;**18**:93–118.
2. Filipi DG, Ulug AM, Ryan E, *et al*. Diffusion tensor imaging of patients with HIV and normal-appearing white matter on MR images of the brain. *AJNR* 2001;**22**:277–83.
3. Dousset V, Armand JP, Lacoste D, *et al*. Magnetization transfer study of HIV encephalitis and progressive multifocal leukoencephalopathy. *AJNR* 1997;**18**:895–901.
4. Smith AB, Smirniotopoulos JG, Rushing EJ. From the archives of the AFIP: central nervous system infections associated with human immunodeficiency virus infection: radiologic-pathologic correlation. *Radiographics* 2008;**28**:2033–58.
5. Rumboldt Z, Thurnher MM, Gupta RK. Central nervous system infections. *Semin Roentgenol* 2007;**42**:62–91.

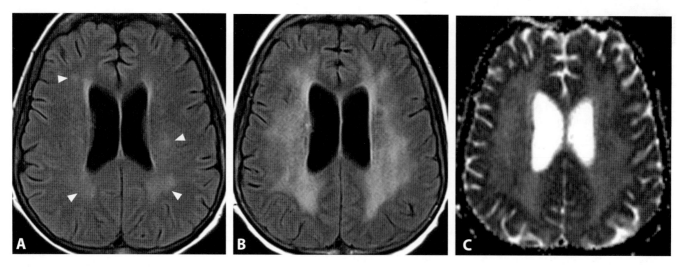

Figure 1. Axial FLAIR image (A) shortly after completion of radiation treatment shows subtle bilateral ill-defined areas of increased signal (arrowheads) in the deep white matter. Corresponding FLAIR image 3 months later (B) shows increase in size and coalescence of the WM hyperintensities, without mass effect and with a somewhat transparent "fluffy" appearance. The abnormalities are also hyperintense on ADC map (C), consistent with increased diffusivity.

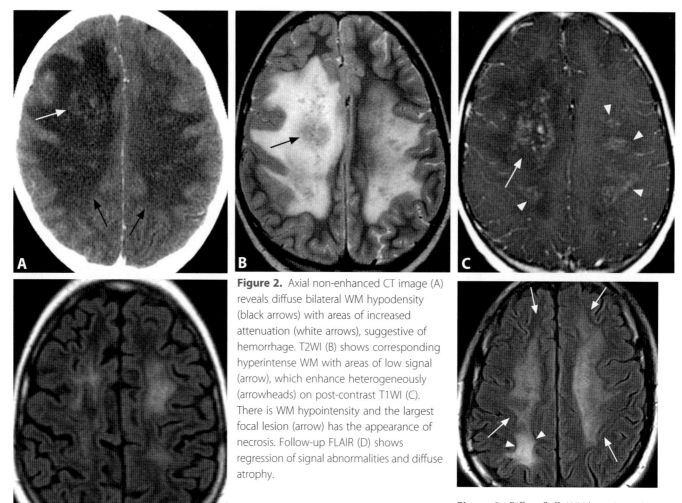

Figure 2. Axial non-enhanced CT image (A) reveals diffuse bilateral WM hypodensity (black arrows) with areas of increased attenuation (white arrows), suggestive of hemorrhage. T2WI (B) shows corresponding hyperintense WM with areas of low signal (arrow), which enhance heterogeneously (arrowheads) on post-contrast T1WI (C). There is WM hypointensity and the largest focal lesion (arrow) has the appearance of necrosis. Follow-up FLAIR (D) shows regression of signal abnormalities and diffuse atrophy.

Figure 3. Diffuse fluffy WM hyperintensity (arrows) and a focal brighter edema (arrowheads) adjacent to a treated metastasis on FLAIR.

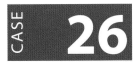

26 Radiation- and Chemotherapy-Induced Leukoencephalopathy

MARIA VITTORIA SPAMPINATO

Specific Imaging Findings

Radiation-induced leukoencephalopathy presents with rapidly progressive, symmetric CT hypodensities and T2 hyperintensities in the periventricular and deep white matter, initially with sparing of the corpus callosum and subcortical arcuate fibers. Over time, lesions increase in size and coalesce leading to a confluent pattern with smooth peripheral margins. Concurrent cerebral atrophy may develop and rapidly progress. The affected white matter is of increased diffusivity on ADC maps and gradual decrease of rCBV on perfusion imaging may be observed. Pediatric patients may develop a mineralizing microangiopathy months or years following radiation or more commonly combined chemoradiation, with large calcifications within the affected white matter. Symptomatic reversible methotrexate toxicity shows T2 hyperintense areas in the supratentorial and cerebellar cortex and subcortical white matter in addition to deep white matter changes. Chemotherapy with or without radiotherapy, typically including intrathecal methotrexate, may lead to disseminated necrotizing leukoencephalopathy, characterized by rapidly progressive confluent white matter T2 hyperintensity and T1 hypointensity with internal hemorrhages and corresponding ill-defined areas of enhancement, which can evolve into circular necrotic lesions.

Pertinent Clinical Information

Radiation-induced delayed encephalopathy is a common and serious irreversible condition characterized by neurocognitive deterioration ranging from mild impairment to dementia. Known risk factors include combined radiation and chemotherapy, diabetes, hypertension, and advanced age. It is particularly common following whole-brain radiotherapy (WBRT), which can induce cognitive dysfunction in up to 50% of long-term survivors. Pre-existing leukoaraiosis appears to be a predisposing factor for developing further leukoencephalopathy after WBRT. The developing nervous system is particularly vulnerable and individuals irradiated during childhood for CNS malignancy have lower IQ scores compared to the general population. Disseminated necrotizing leukoencephalopathy may occur with combined chemoradiation (typically high-dose methotrexate) and is characterized by rapidly progressive dementia, ataxia, psychomotor and psychiatric disturbances. Seizures, coma, and death can occur in the most severe cases.

Differential Diagnosis

Chronic Microangiopathy (Leukoaraiosis) (27)
- typically scattered and asymmetric areas of abnormal signal
- concomitant basal ganglia and deep white matter lacunar infarcts
- usually progresses over the course of years, not months
- possible deep gray and white matter microhemorrhages

CNS Vasculitis (123)
- characteristic scattered areas of leptomeningeal enhancement may be present

- cortical and subcortical infarctions
- intraparenchymal and/or subarachnoid hemorrhage
- beading of the intracranial arterial branches on angiograms

HIV Encephalitis (25)
- diffuse homogenous white matter T2 hyperintensity without associated low T1 signal or enhancement

Chronic Multiple Sclerosis
- at least some characteristic focal lesions are usually present, such as juxtacortical plaques, involvement of middle cerebellar peduncles and calloso-septal interface
- spinal cord and optic nerves are frequently affected

Background

Despite advances in radiation delivery methods, damage to normal structures remains an important issue, especially in light of widespread use of combined chemoradiotherapy, development of radiosurgery, and increasing number of long-term survivors. There are three phases of pathophysiological response to irradiation: acute phase (after the first few fractions) with mostly reversible loosening of microvascular endothelial tight junctions; subacute phase (6–12 weeks after irradiation) with demyelination secondary to death of myelin-producing oligodendrocytes, which can be followed by regrowth and remyelination; irreversible chronic phase with vascular wall thickening, diminished glial cells, and diffuse demyelination. The mechanisms of chemotherapy-induced neurotoxicity are incompletely understood and include direct toxic effects on axons, oligodendrocytes, and progenitor stem cells, as well as secondary immunologic reactions, oxidative stress, and microvascular insult.

Disseminated necrotizing leukoencephalopathy, initially described in children with metastatic meningeal acute lymphoblastic lymphoma treated with methotrexate and whole-brain RT, has been associated with all age groups, various chemotherapeutics, and other neoplasms.

REFERENCES

1. Pruzincova L, Steno J, Srbecky M, *et al*. MR imaging of late radiation therapy- and chemotherapy-induced injury: a pictorial essay. *Eur Radiol* 2009;**19**:2716–27.

2. Oka M, Terae S, Kobayashi R, *et al*. MRI in methotrexate-related leukoencephalopathy: disseminated necrotising leukoencephalopathy in comparison with mild leukoencephalopathy. *Neuroradiology* 2003;**45**:493–7.

3. Ziereisen F, Dan B, Azzi N, *et al*. Reversible acute methotrexate leukoencephalopathy: atypical brain MR imaging features. *Pediatr Radiol* 2006;**36**:205–12.

4. Perry A, Schmidt RE. Cancer therapy-associated CNS neuropathology: an update and review of the literature. *Acta Neuropathol* 2006;**111**:197–212.

5. Soussain C, Ricard D, Fike JR, *et al*. CNS complications of radiotherapy and chemotherapy. *Lancet* 2009;**374**:1639–51.

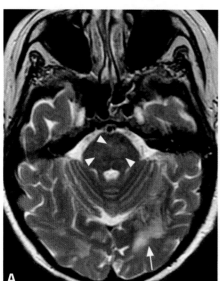
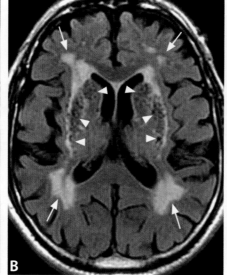
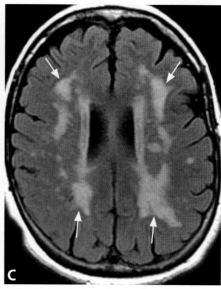

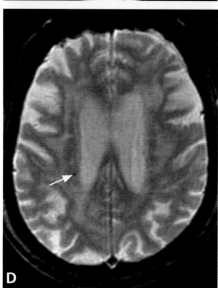

Figure 1. Axial T2WI through the pons and occipital lobes (A) shows patchy confluent hyperintense areas in the pons (arrowheads). A chronic posterior cerebral artery infarct is present in the left temporo-occipital area (arrow). Axial FLAIR images through the basal ganglia (B) and lateral ventricles (C) show innumerable small "holes" (arrowheads) within the basal ganglia (so-called "état criblé") as well as patchy confluent areas of hyperintensity (arrows) throughout the periventricular, deep, and subcortical white matter that are more prominent posteriorly, without associated mass effect. Axial T2*WI through the lateral ventricles (D) again shows the extensive white matter signal abnormalities. Additionally, there is a punctate area of very low signal (arrow) in the right corona radiata, caused by magnetic susceptibility effect and representing a chronic microhemorrhage.

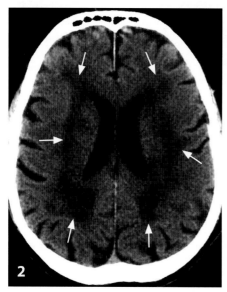
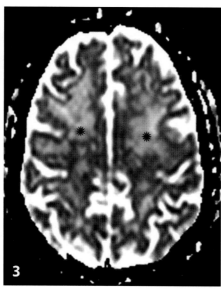

Figure 2. CT shows extensive patchy and confluent periventricular, deep, and subcortical white matter hypodensities (arrows) in the cerebral hemispheres, without mass effect.

Figure 3. ADC map shows high signal intensity (*) in bilateral centrum semiovale, representing increased diffusion of water molecules in the affected white matter, presumably due to gliosis and myelin rarefaction.

Leukoaraiosis (Microangiopathy)

ALESSANDRO CIANFONI

Specific Imaging Findings

Leukoaraiosis (LA) and white matter hyperintensities (WMH) are the interchangeable terms used for bilateral non-enhancing white matter abnormalities without mass effect that are hypodense on CT, of high T2 signal, and with increased diffusion (bright on ADC maps). The abnormalities can be punctate or patchy with irregular borders; they are often confluent and involving large areas of white matter, especially in the periventricular subependymal regions, where they may form "caps" and "rims". The lesions tend to spare the temporal lobes and corpus callosum. T2 hyperintensities frequently also involve the deep gray matter structures. Microangiopathy is considered responsible for these imaging findings. There is a frequent coexistence of dilated perivascular spaces (PVS, Virchow–Robin spaces), lacunar infarcts, chronic microbleeds, and diffuse brain volume loss. Differentiation between PVS and lacunar infarcts is best accomplished with FLAIR images: hypodense areas with gliotic hyperintense borders are present in lacunar infarcts. A number of imaging grading systems have been formulated, but are rarely used in clinical practice.

Pertinent Clinical Information

WMH are almost universal in patients over 65 years of age and are also found in younger individuals. There is therefore a large overlap between asymptomatic aging individuals with LA and patients with vascular risk factors, such as arterial hypertension, hypercholesterolemia, diabetes mellitus, and amyloid angiopathy. LA is associated with lacunar infarcts and cerebral hemorrhages. Periventricular lesions are related to cognitive decline, whereas subcortical ones may be related to late-onset depression. Lesion extension is a predictor for the subsequent rate of progression. Subjects with punctate abnormalities have a low tendency for progression, whereas individuals with confluent changes tend to progress rapidly.

Differential Diagnosis

Normal Aging Brain; Migraine Headaches
- differentiation on imaging studies possible only if infarcts or microbleeds are present

Hepatic Encephalopathy (1)
- T1 bright globi pallidi, otherwise indistinguishable

CADASIL (22)
- younger patients (usually <40 years of age)
- predilection for temporal and subinsular white matter

Multiple Sclerosis (115)
- ovoid morphology, perivenular orientation
- juxta-cortical, corpus callosum, and temporal lesions
- possible contrast enhancement

- deep gray matter involvement is very rare (common in ADEM)

Radiation-/Chemotherapy-Induced Leukoencephalopathy (26)
- abnormalities are extensive, symmetric, typically smooth and not patchy
- appropriate history

HIV encephalopathy (25)
- typically diffuse white matter involvement, without focal lesions

CNS Vasculitis (123)
- acute and chronic lesions often coexist
- common leptomeningeal contrast enhancement
- subarachnoid or parenchymal hemorrhages may be present

Background

On histology, there is decreased afferent vascular density; severe arteriosclerosis and arteriolosclerosis are usually found, while venous collagenosis and obstruction have also been described. Periventricular WMHs correlate with myelin pallor, dilation of perivascular spaces, discontinuity of the ependymal lining, and subependymal gliosis. Deep and subcortical WMHs reflect myelin pallor and widening of perivascular spaces. Clinical correlates are much less clear, with large overlap between normal asymptomatic population, patients with mild cognitive impairment, and patients with vascular dementia. The localization of lesions is important, with a possible greater impact on cognition by the lesions in the basal ganglia and thalami. The final clinical result is probably multifactorial, including lesion burden, localization, pathological substrate, and brain atrophy.

REFERENCES

1. Lövblad KO, Assal F, Pereira VM, et al. Magnetic resonance imaging of vascular diseases of the white matter. Top Magn Reson Imaging 2009;20:343–8.

2. Gouw AA, van der Flier WM, Fazekas F, et al. Progression of white matter hyperintensities and incidence of new lacunes over a 3-year period: the Leukoaraiosis and Disability Study. Stroke 2008;39:1414–20.

3. de Leeuw FE, de Groot JC, Achten E, et al. Prevalence of cerebral white matter lesions in elderly people: a population based magnetic resonance imaging study. The Rotterdam Scan Study. J Neurol Neurosurg Psychiatry 2001;70:9–14.

4. Moody DM, Thore CR, Anstrom JA, et al. Quantification of afferent vessels shows reduced brain vascular density in subjects with leukoaraiosis. Radiology 2004;233:883–90.

5. Jagust WJ, Zheng L, Harvey DJ, et al. Neuropathological basis of magnetic resonance images in aging and dementia. Ann Neurol 2008;63:72–80.

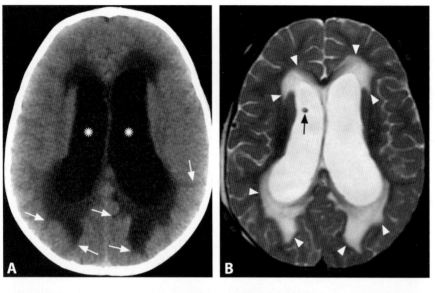

Figure 1. Non-enhanced CT image (A) shows dilation of the lateral ventricles (*) and periventricular hypodensities adjacent to the frontal horns and trigones. Some hypodensities extend into the subcortical white matter (arrows), resembling vasogenic edema. Corresponding T2WI after shunting (B) again shows frontal and parietal "caps" (arrowheads) of periventricular edema with hyperintense signal. Note the drainage catheter (arrow).

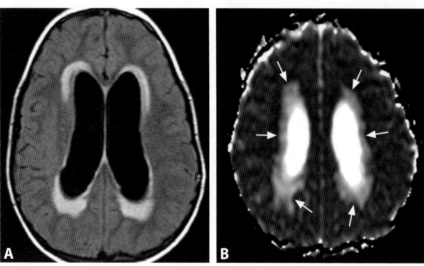

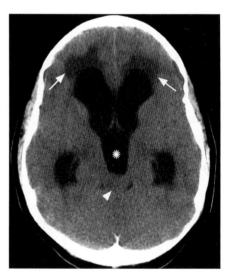

Figure 2. Axial FLAIR image (A) shows smooth hyperintense "caps" adjacent to the lateral ventricles. ADC map at a higher level (B) reveals very high diffusion of periventricular abnormalities (arrows), approaching that of CSF.

Figure 3. CT shows dilated third (*) and lateral ventricles with bifrontal edema (arrows). Tectal mass (arrowhead).

Figure 4. Axial FLAIR image shows temporal horn ectasia (arrowheads) and a thin periventricular hyperintensity (arrows).

Figure 5. FLAIR shows dilated ventricles with slightly undulating borders (arrowheads). Shunt is suggested by the artifact (arrow). Periventricular hyperintensity is due to chronic transependymal CSF resorption and WM damage.

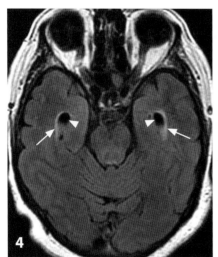

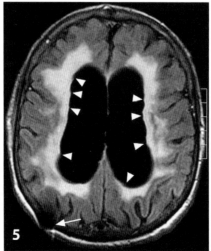

Periventricular Edema in Acute Hydrocephalus

ALESSANDRO CIANFONI

Specific Imaging Findings

Periventricular white matter halo, most commonly around the lateral ventricles, shows low density on CT, increased diffusion and high T2 signal, which is best seen as hyperintensity on FLAIR images. Periventricular edema is invariably associated with ventriculomegaly and signs of high ventricular pressure: dilated temporal horns; rounded frontal horns; bowed, thinned and stretched corpus callosum; ballooned third ventricle; sulcal effacement. There is no contrast enhancement. The periventricular rim has indistinct borders on CT, and smooth, well-delineated margins on FLAIR images. It commonly contours the entire lateral ventricles, extending along the temporal horns. Maximum halo thickness is generally around the frontal horns and the trigones. On sagittal T2-weighted imaging dilated hyperintense perivenular subependymal spaces can be seen, radiating outward with finger-like appearance. In long-standing hydrocephalus, the periventricular halo can show ill-defined margins and white matter thinning due to gliotic scarring. With newly diagnosed acute hydrocephalus, the main distinction is between obstructive and communicating hydrocephalus. If no obvious obstructing masses or subarachnoid hemorrhage are evident to explain the hydrocephalus, cisternographic MR techniques (volumetric high-resolution heavily T2WI), or CT cisternography, can be used to detect thin webs obstructing the CSF outflow.

Pertinent Clinical Information

Obstructive and non-obstructive conditions leading to imbalance between the production and the resorption of CSF, resulting in accumulation of CSF, cause increased intraventricular CSF pressure. Depending on the rate of the ventricular pressure changes, presentations range from signs and symptoms of frank intracranial hypertension (papilledema, headache, worse in the recumbent position and early in the morning, nausea and projecting vomiting, lethargy) to more subtle gait disturbances, headache, ophthalmoplegia, and cognitive decline. Hemorrhage as well as leptomeningeal inflammatory, infectious, or neoplastic disease are possible causes of communicating hydrocephalus.

Differential Diagnosis

Microangiopathy (Leukoaraiosis) (27)
- periventricular bright T2 rim has less well-defined borders, appears to fade outward
- more prominent along the frontal horns and especially trigones ("caps"), rare along the temporal horns
- associated with more diffuse white matter changes, multifocal or confluent
- absence of ventriculomegaly and signs of increased intraventricular pressure

Chronic (Compensated) Hydrocephalus
- periventricular gliosis, with more ill-defined margins
- no signs of increased intracranial pressure, sulci are usually not effaced, ventricular borders are undulating
- signs of parenchymal volume loss, with periventricular white matter thinning

Primary CNS Lymphoma (158)
- the ependyma is thickened, and may protrude inward in the ventricles
- contrast enhancement is invariably present
- T2 signal is usually relatively low, and diffusion is reduced

Ventriculitis/Ependymitis (129)
- typically with linear contrast enhancement along the ependyma
- intraventricular material can be depicted, best seen on FLAIR and DWI

Background

Periventricular edema in acute hydrocephalus reflects in part the attempt of the brain to reabsorb the accumulated intraventricular CSF through the subependymal interstitium, and in part the damage to the ependymal lining caused by the increased intraventricular pressure and ependymal stretching. The ependyma loses its barrier function and CSF invades the subependymal and periventricular white matter interstitium. If not corrected rapidly this ensues in white matter inflammation, ischemia, demyelination, gliosis and scarring. The cause of hydrocephalus needs to be diagnosed, and the most appropriate treatment initiated as early as possible, with ventricular shunting, surgical obstruction removal, or third ventriculostomy, depending on the cause. A rapid decrease in white matter ADC values has been observed after CSF diversion. Lumbar puncture for CSF analysis remains the gold standard for diagnosis of subarachnoid hemorrhage and leptomeningeal disease, when imaging is inconclusive.

REFERENCES

1. Di Chiro G, Arimitsu T, Brooks RA, et al. Computed tomography profiles of periventricular hypodensity in hydrocephalus and leukoencephalopathy. Radiology 1979;130:661–6.
2. Zimmerman RD, Fleming CA, Lee BC, et al. Periventricular hyperintensity as seen by magnetic resonance: prevalence and significance. AJR 1986;146:443–50.
3. Bruni JE, Del Bigio MR, Clattenburg RE. Ependyma: normal and pathological. A review of the literature. Brain Res 1985;356:1–19.
4. James AE Jr, Flor WJ, Novak GR, et al. The ultrastructural basis of periventricular edema: preliminary studies. Radiology 1980;135:747–50.
5. Leliefeld PH, Gooskens RH, Braun KP, et al. Longitudinal diffusion-weighted imaging in infants with hydrocephalus: decrease in tissue water diffusion after cerebrospinal fluid diversion. J Neurosurg Pediatr 2009;4:56–63.

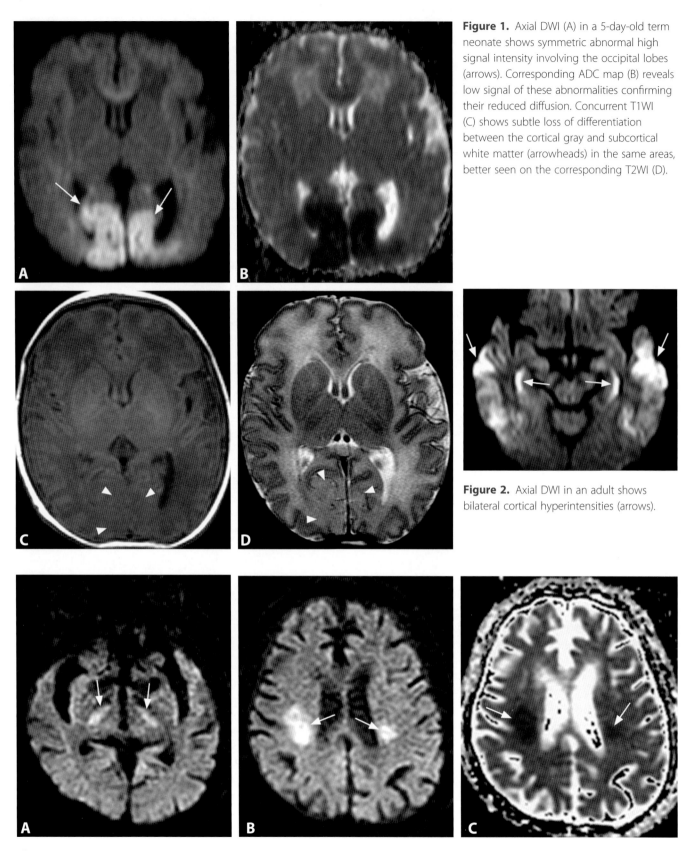

Figure 1. Axial DWI (A) in a 5-day-old term neonate shows symmetric abnormal high signal intensity involving the occipital lobes (arrows). Corresponding ADC map (B) reveals low signal of these abnormalities confirming their reduced diffusion. Concurrent T1WI (C) shows subtle loss of differentiation between the cortical gray and subcortical white matter (arrowheads) in the same areas, better seen on the corresponding T2WI (D).

Figure 2. Axial DWI in an adult shows bilateral cortical hyperintensities (arrows).

Figure 3. Axial DWI (A) in a 75-year-old woman with rapid mental deterioration shows bilateral hyperintensity in the internal capsule (arrows). DWI at a higher level (B) shows hyperintensity involving bilateral corona radiata (arrows). Corresponding ADC map (C) confirms reduced diffusion of these lesions (arrows). The imaging abnormalities disappeared 4 days later following appropriate treatment. Figures 2 and 3 courtesy of Se Jeong Jeon.

Hypoglycemia

BENJAMIN HUANG

Specific Imaging Findings

Hypoglycemia may affect different areas in infants and older patients. In neonates it causes symmetric cortical and subcortical abnormalities, predominantly in the posterior cerebral hemispheres. CT demonstrates edema affecting the parietal and occipital lobes. MRI shows subtle cortical and subjacent white matter T1 hypointensity and T2 hyperintensity. Reduced diffusion is a very sensitive early finding. MRS demonstrates reduced NAA and the presence of lipids and/or lactate. Subacutely, the cortex will develop increased T1 and low T2 signal. Atrophy and gliosis occur in the chronic stage. Diffuse white matter injury may be more common in hypoglycemic neonates than previously believed.

In adults, hypoglycemia can affect either gray matter (primarily cortex) alone, white matter alone, or both. Abnormalities are again typically bilateral and symmetric. White matter T2 hyperintensities with reduced diffusion are found in the centrum semiovale and periventricular area, and, more characteristically in the internal capsule and corpus callosum (typically in the splenium – "boomerang" lesion). The findings may resolve with treatment, especially the white matter lesions.

Pertinent Clinical Information

Symptoms and signs of hypoglycemia in neonates are nonspecific and include cyanotic spells, apnea, refusal to feed, hypothermia, and seizures. Ultimately convulsions or coma may occur. Long-term sequelae include cerebral palsy, epilepsy, developmental delay, and visual impairment. In adults and older children, symptoms of hypoglycemia reflect two major mechanisms. One is related to catecholamine release from activation of the autonomic nervous system, which is the physiologic counterregulatory response to hypoglycemia. These symptoms include tachycardia, anxiety, sweating, and palpitations. The second symptom group reflects the effects of glucose deprivation on the brain and includes progressive neurologic impairment, seizures, and coma.

Differential Diagnosis

Global Anoxic Brain Injury (7, 13)
- characteristically watershed territory involvement in neonates
- perirolandic cortex and deep gray matter selectively affected

Creutzfeldt–Jakob Disease (12)
- very different clinical history with gradual onset of symptoms
- spared white matter

Hyperammonemia
- preferential involvement of the insular cortex and cingulate gyrus

Seizure-Related Changes (104)
- usually unilateral
- usually known seizure history
- isolated lesion in the splenium may be indistinguishable from hypoglycemia by imaging

Susac Syndrome (113)
- more focal and scattered lesions
- gradual onset of symptoms with headaches

Herpes Simplex Encephalitis (20)
- temporal lobes are involved in a characteristically asymmetric bilateral or even unilateral fashion
- laboratory testing does not show hypoglycemia
- fever and headache are typically present

Background

Historically, hypoglycemia has been defined as a serum glucose concentration below 40–45 mg/dl, but differing threshold values have been proposed depending upon the maturational state of the brain and patient's clinical status. Infants can tolerate lower glucose levels than adults, potentially due to decreased glucose requirements of the immature brain and its ability to utilize lactate. In fact, hypoglycemia is common in the newborn period and may be seen in up to 8% of low-risk infants. This is typically transient and responds to glucose administration. Neonatal brain injury due to hypoglycemia is rare and generally requires severe, prolonged, or recurrent episodes. Proposed mechanisms include primary energy failure and excitotoxic edema, but the exact mechanisms and the reasons for selective vulnerability of the parietal and occipital lobes remain unclear. In adults, hypoglycemia may be caused by overdoses of insulin or oral hypoglycemic agents, insulin-producing tumors, or systemic processes. Treatment is based on reversal of acute hypoglycemia either orally or intravenously, and the underlying causes need to be addressed.

REFERENCES
1. Barkovich AJ, Ali FA, Rowley HA, Bass N. Imaging patterns of neonatal hypoglycemia. *AJNR* 1998;**19**:523–8.
2. Kim SY, Goo HW, Lim KH, *et al*. Neonatal hypoglycaemic encephalopathy: diffusion-weighted imaging and proton MR spectroscopy. *Pediatr Radiol* 2006;**36**:144–8.
3. Ma JH, Kim YJ, Yoo WJ, *et al*. MR imaging of hypoglycemic encephalopathy: lesion distribution and prognosis prediction by diffusion-weighted imaging. *Neuroradiology* 2009;**51**:641–9.
4. Kang EG, Jeon SJ, Choi SS, *et al*. Diffusion MR imaging of hypoglycemic encephalopathy. *AJNR* 2010;**31**:559–64.
5. Kim JH, Choi JY, Koh SB, Lee Y. Reversible splenial abnormality in hypoglycemic encephalopathy. *Neuroradiology* 2007;**49**:217–22.

Brain Imaging with MRI and CT, ed. Zoran Rumboldt *et al.* Published by Cambridge University Press. © Cambridge University Press 2012.

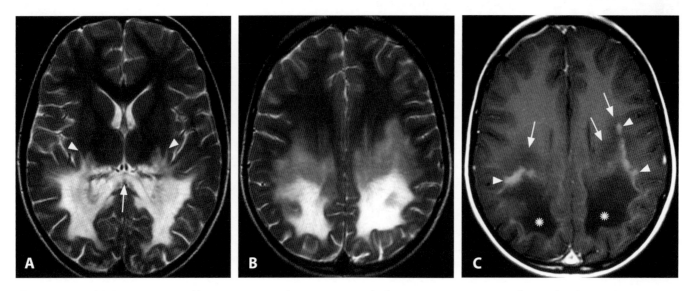

Figure 1. T2WI (A) shows symmetrical hyperintensities in the parieto-occipital white matter, posterior parts of internal and external capsules (arrowheads), as well as the splenium of corpus callosum (arrow) and postero-lateral thalami. T2WI at a higher level (B) reveals different signal intensities of the bilateral symmetric lesions. Corresponding post-contrast T1WI (C) reveals enhancement at the edge of the lesions delineating three distinct zones: the central burned-out zone (prominently T1 hypointense and T2 hyperintense, *), the intermediate inflammatory zone (faintly T2 hyperintense and enhancing, arrowheads) and the most peripheral demyelination zone (T1 hypointense and T2 hyperintense on, arrows).

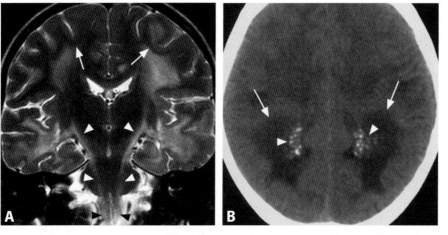

Figure 2. Coronal T2WI (A) in an 8-year-old boy depicts bilateral cerebral white matter hyperintensity as well as the corticospinal tract involvement (arrowheads), with sparing of the subcortical U-fibers (arrows). Non-enhanced CT image (B) demonstrates punctate calcifications (arrowheads) within the bilateral symmetric hypodense lesions (arrows).

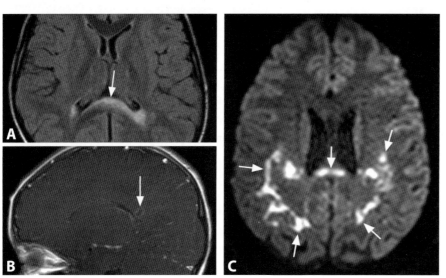

Figure 3. Axial FLAIR image (A) in a 6-year-old boy very early in the course of the disease shows hyperintensity limited to the splenium of the corpus callosum (arrow). Corresponding sagittal post-contrast T1WI (B) reveals rim enhancement (arrow) of the splenium lesion. Axial DWI obtained at a later date (C) demonstrates very high signal intensity (arrows) characteristic for the advancing front of the disease.

X-Linked Adrenoleukodystrophy (X-ALD)

MARIASAVINA SEVERINO

Specific Imaging Findings

The childhood form of X-linked adrenoleukodystrophy (X-ALD) shows the typical parieto-occipital pattern (up to 85% of patients) with symmetric involvement of the white matter, splenium and posterior body of corpus callosum. The progression pattern is centrifugal and postero-anterior starting from the splenium with sparing of subcortical U fibers. Contrast enhancement and reduced diffusion at the advancing lesion margins are characteristic, corresponding to active demyelination, axonal damage and inflammation. CT may show dystrophic calcifications within the affected areas. Brain stem lesions involving the corticospinal, corticobulbar, visual, and auditory tracts are frequently associated. The frontal variant (about 15% of cases) shows involvement of the frontal periventricular white matter, the genu and anterior body of the corpus callosum and the anterior limbs of internal capsules; the outer borders of the lesions may enhance with contrast. The atypical presentation of childhood cerebral X-ALD (2.5% of cases) is characterized by combined but separate involvement of the frontal and parieto-occipital white matter. Central portions of the X-ALD lesions show high ADC and low FA values, correlating with histologic findings. In addition to nonspecific decrease in NAA with increased lactate and choline, MRS shows elevated *myo*-inositol levels, which correlate with disease severity.

Adrenomyeloneuropathy (AMN) in adults is characterized by spinal cord atrophy often with signal changes in the posterior limbs of the internal capsules, brainstem (with relative sparing of tegmental structures), and cerebellar white matter.

Pertinent Clinical Information

X-ALD is a progressive disorder with several clinical phenotypes. In the childhood cerebral form the onset is usually between 4 and 8 years. It initially resembles attention deficit disorder; progressive impairment of cognition, vision, hearing, and motor function follow and often lead to total disability and death within a few years. Adrenomyeloneuropathy (AMN) manifests most commonly in the late twenties with myelopathy and neuropathy (progressive paraparesis, sphincter disturbances, sexual dysfunction) and impaired adrenocortical function; the disease is slowly progressive over decades. The third phenotype, "Addison disease only", presents between 2 years of age and adulthood without neurological dysfunction; some neurologic disability (most commonly AMN) usually develops later. Approximately 20% of female X-ALD carriers develop an AMN-like disorder with later onset and milder course.

Differential Diagnosis

Periventricular Leukomalacia (31)

- signal changes and volume loss in the parieto-occipital periventricular white matter with enlarged "wavy" lateral ventricles
- no contrast enhancement

Alexander Disease (33)

- frontotemporal white matter involvement with anteroposterior progression pattern and periventricular rims
- affected deep gray matter
- contrast enhancement of ventricular ependyma, periventricular rim, deep gray matter, dentate nucleus and brainstem

Metachromatic Leukodystrophy (34)

- periventricular "butterfly-shaped" hemispheric involvement with radial stripes on T2WI
- no contrast enhancement of the affected WM
- descending long tracts in the brainstem are affected
- frequent enhancement of cranial nerves and cauda equina

Background

X-ALD is an X-linked peroxisomal disorder with a prevalence between 1 : 20 000 and 1 : 50 000. It has a wide phenotypical variability ranging from the symptomatic cerebral form to the asymptomatic with biochemical defects only. The deficient gene *ABCD1* codes for a membrane protein (adrenoleukodystrophy protein or ALDP) required for the transport of fatty acids into peroxisomes. The accumulation of very long chain fatty acids (VLCFA) leads to an inflammatory leukodystrophy in children (cerebral X-ALD) or to a non-inflammatory distal axonopathy in adults (AMN). About 93% of the cases have inherited the *ABCD1* mutation; 7% have a de-novo mutation. X-ALD patients benefit from supportive care and dietary treatment (Lorenzo's oil). Allogeneic hematopoietic stem cell transplantation (HSCT) is the only treatment that can arrest cerebral demyelination and result in a long-term good quality of life, if performed at an early stage of X-ALD.

REFERENCES

1. Kim JH, Kim HJ. Childhood X-linked adrenoleukodystrophy: clinical–pathologic overview and MR imaging manifestations at initial evaluation and follow-up. *Radiographics* 2005;**25**: 619–31.

2. Barkovich AJ, Ferriero DM, Bass N, Boyer R. Involvement of the pontomedullary corticospinal tracts: a useful finding in the diagnosis of X-linked adrenoleukodystrophy. *AJNR* 1997;**18**:95–100.

3. van der Voorn JP, Pouwels PJ, Powers JM, *et al.* Correlating quantitative MR imaging with histopathology in X-linked adrenoleukodystrophy. *AJNR* 2011;**32**:481–9.

4. Vijay K, Ouyang T. Anterior pattern disease in adrenoleukodystrophy. *Pediatr Radiol* 2010;**40**(Suppl 1):S157.

5. Cartier N, Aubourg P. Hematopoietic stem cell transplantation and hematopoietic stem cell gene therapy in X-linked adrenoleukodystrophy. *Brain Pathol* 2010;**20**:857–62.

Brain Imaging with MRI and CT, ed. Zoran Rumboldt *et al.* Published by Cambridge University Press. © Cambridge University Press 2012.

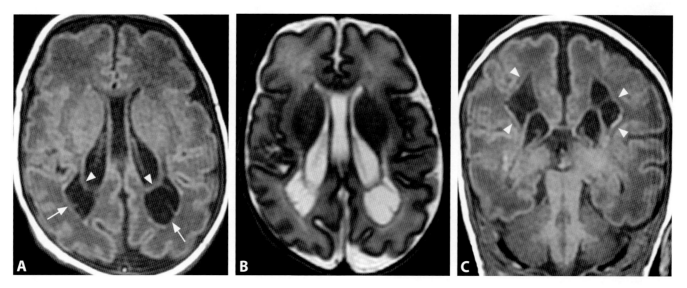

Figure 1. Axial T1WI (A) and T2WI (B) in a pre-term infant show multicystic involution of the bilateral peritrigonal white matter (arrows). The ependymal lining is still visible (arrowheads) and thin sepations separate the cysts. These will be resorbed and incorporated within dilated ventricular trigones. Coronal T1WI again shows the periventricular cysts. The adjacent white matter is notably thinned (arrowheads).

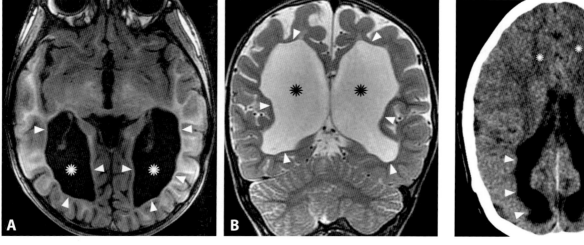 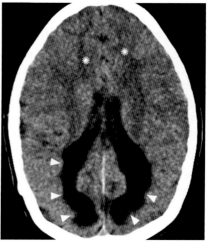

Figure 2. Axial T1WI (A) and coronal T2WI (B) show the chronic stage with irregular contours of dilated ventricular trigones (*) and extreme thinning of the periventricular white matter (WM, arrowheads).

Figure 3. CT shows wavy dilated trigones without visible adjacent WM (arrowheads). Compare to frontal WM (*).

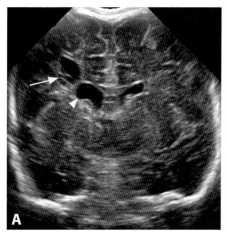 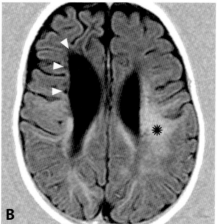

Figure 4. Coronal neonatal head ultrasound image (A) shows periventricular cysts (arrow) and dilated right frontal horn (arrowhead). Follow-up axial IR T1WI (B) shows severe reduction of the right frontal WM, dilated right frontal horn, and small periventricular cysts (arrowheads). Note normal thickness and myelination of the contralateral WM (*).

Periventricular Leukomalacia (PVL)

ALESSANDRO CIANFONI

Specific Imaging Findings

The earliest imaging signs of periventricular leukomalacia (PVL) are periventricular hyperechogenicity on brain ultrasound scans, corresponding to areas of low ADC value on MRI. In the subacute stage, there is cystic cavitation of the most severely affected areas, typically the peritrigonal parietal white matter. These cystic areas tend to coalesce, and are eventually incorporated by the ventricular trigones, that become dilated, characteristically with wavy contours. Depending on the extent of parenchymal damage, variable degrees of peritrigonal white matter thinning and T2 hyperintensity, roughly symmetrical dilatation of the ventricular trigones, and calcarine cortex atrophy are present at later stages. The parenchymal damage can sometimes be associated with micro-hemorrhages, revealed in the chronic stage as hypointense dots in the periventricular areas or hypointense ependymal lining on T2*-weighted MR imaging. There is no intervening normal-appearing parenchyma between the trigonal walls and the periventricular injured white matter. Unilateral and/or frontal PVL is much less common.

Pertinent Clinical Information

Pre-term neonates can present with hemodynamic instability and partial asphyxia. The end result of the related brain insults is most commonly PVL. Term neonates with hypoperfusion or partial asphyxia present brain injuries in different locations due to different topography of watershed areas in the term brain, and different regional brain vulnerability. Patients with PVL are usually affected by variable severity of spastic paraparesis, as well as visual and cognitive impairment.

Differential Diagnosis

Terminal Areas of Myelination

- the peritrigonal white matter is the last to become fully myelinated, relative T2 hyperintensity can be seen in normal individuals at 20 years of age and beyond
- normal-appearing white matter is seen between the ependyma and the areas of terminal myelination
- no white matter thinning

Chronic Hydrocephalus

- more diffuse ventricular enlargement with expanded "ballooned" appearance
- ventricular borders are smooth, not irregular and wavy

X-ALD (30)

- contrast enhancement and low diffusion of the advancing edge
- straight ventricular contours

- initial involvement of the splenium of corpus callosum
- progressive disease

Corpus Callosum Dysgenesis (71)

- partial or complete absence of corpus callosum
- dilation of the ventricular trigones and occipital horns (colpocephaly); however, the contours of the ventricles are not wavy, but straight and parallel
- no periventricular white matter signal abnormality

Background

PVL reflects the final multifactorial injury to the immature brain caused by hemodynamic instability, and/or hypoxia. Infection can be a precipitating factor. The predominant involvement of peritrigonal white matter reflects the location of watershed areas in the pre-term brain, vascular immaturity of the deep periventricular white matter, and most likely a regional selective vulnerability. Particularly vulnerable progenitors of the myelin-forming oligodendrocytes are likely localized in the posterior periventricular white matter in the pre-term stage. DTI and fiber-tracking techniques reveal lesions beyond the areas of T2 signal abnormality and may predict the degree of neurologic impairment. *In utero* transient venous hypertension may be responsible for the atypical frontal PVL. Transient engorgement and/or thrombosis of deep medullary veins may be responsible for white matter damage that can lead to a PVL pattern.

REFERENCES

1. Dyet LE, Kennea N, Counsell SJ, et al. Natural history of brain lesions in extremely preterm infants studied with serial magnetic resonance imaging from birth and neurodevelopmental assessment. *Pediatrics* 2006;**118**:536–48.
2. Deng W, Pleasure J, Pleasure D. Progress in periventricular leukomalacia. *Arch Neurol* 2008;**65**:1291–5.
3. Murakami A, Morimoto M, Yamada K, et al. Fiber-tracking techniques can predict the degree of neurologic impairment for periventricular leukomalacia. *Pediatrics* 2008;**122**:500–6.
4. Nagae LM, Hoon AH Jr, Stashinko E, et al. Diffusion tensor imaging in children with periventricular leukomalacia: variability of injuries to white matter tracts. *AJNR* 2007;**28**:1213–22.
5. Arrigoni F, Parazzini C, Righini A, et al. Deep medullary veins involvement in neonates with brain damage: an MR imaging study. *AJNR* 2011;**32**:2030–6.

Brain Imaging with MRI and CT, ed. Zoran Rumboldt *et al.* Published by Cambridge University Press. © Cambridge University Press 2012.

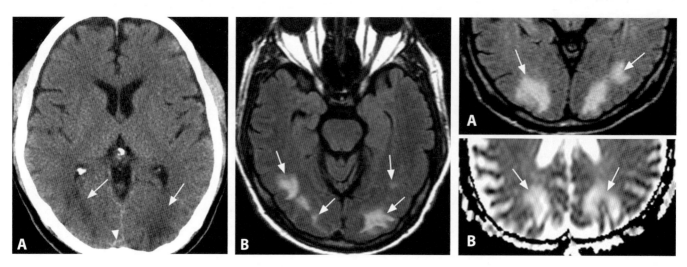

Figure 1. Non-enhanced CT image shows subtle bilateral occipital subcortical hypodensities (arrows). A small focus of hemorrhage (arrowhead) is present. FLAIR image (B) shows subcortical hyperintensities (arrows) in occipital/posterior temporal lobes.

Figure 2. Posterior subcortical hyperintensities on FLAIR (A) and increased diffusion of lesions (arrows) on ADC (B).

Figure 3. Axial T2WI (A) shows multiple patchy areas of hyperintense signal (arrows) predominantly within the subcortical white matter involving frontal and parietal lobes. Coronal FLAIR image (B) shows high signal intensity lesions in bilateral cerebellar white matter (arrowheads), in addition to the scattered supratentorial areas of hyperintensity.

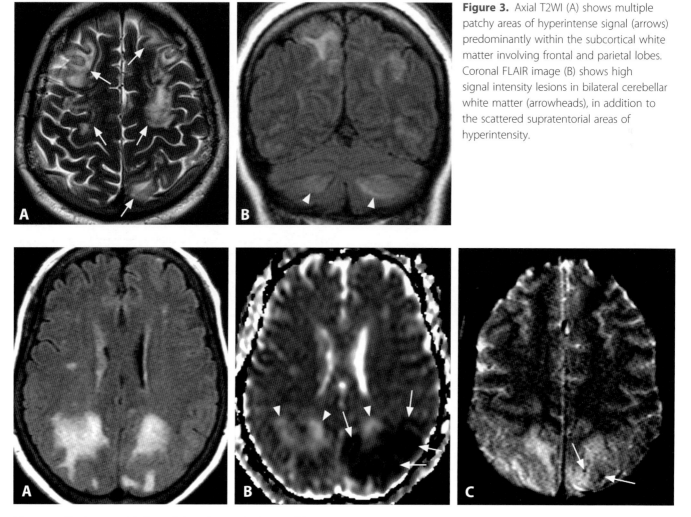

Figure 4. FLAIR image (A) shows bilateral parietal subcortical hyperintensities. ADC map (B) reveals corresponding areas of increased (arrowheads) but also reduced diffusion (arrows). T2*WI at a slightly higher level (C) shows small foci of signal loss (arrows), consistent with hemorrhage.

Posterior Reversible Encephalopathy Syndrome (PRES, Hypertensive Encephalopathy)

MARIA VITTORIA SPAMPINATO AND ZORAN RUMBOLDT

Specific Imaging Findings

Posterior Reversible Encephalopathy Syndrome (PRES) usually shows characteristic bilateral, predominantly symmetric, patchy areas of hyperintense T2 signal in the subcortical regions of the parietal and occipital lobes. Cortex may also be involved, while mass effect is absent to minimal. In addition to the primary parietal–occipital pattern, patchy bilateral T2 hyperintensities are also found in holohemispheric and superior frontal patterns, and may be present in the cerebellum, basal ganglia, and brainstem. There is characteristically increased diffusion on ADC maps corresponding to vasogenic edema, while contrast enhancement is absent to minimal, usually leptomeningeal. Hemorrhage, either subarachnoid or parenchymal, is associated with vasogenic edema in a minority of patients. Areas of reduced diffusion are found in some cases, likely representing infarction. More prominent cases of PRES are visible on CT as ill-defined foci of subcortical low attenuation. Vascular studies commonly show evidence of vasculopathy with irregular and beaded appearance of distal intracranial arteries, which is, similar to other imaging findings, typically reversible. Findings on perfusion studies can span from decreased to increased cerebral blood flow, which may depend on the timing, underlying etiology, and brain area.

Pertinent Clinical Information

The most common presentations include headache, altered mentation, nausea, and visual disturbances. Symptoms may develop acutely or over several days and may lead to generalized seizures and coma. Various conditions place patients at risk of PRES, the most common are pre-eclampsia/eclampsia, hypertensive crisis, following transplantation, autoimmune diseases, infection/sepsis/shock, and after cancer chemotherapy. Hypertension is considered the most frequent predisposing factor; however, it is absent in 20–40% of patients. Discontinuation of the triggering medication or resolution of the predisposing condition usually results in clinical improvement and reversal of PRES imaging findings. PRES is not necessarily reversible and may lead to infarctions, especially if appropriate treatment is delayed.

Differential Diagnosis

Venous Infarcts (181)
- usually asymmetric or unilateral
- associated intraparenchymal hemorrhage is common
- the vasogenic edema may be indistinguishable
- dural sinus or cortical vein thrombosis is usually visible

Parasagittal Arterial Infarcts
- prominent reduced diffusion in acute phase
- gyriform contrast enhancement in subacute phase

Encephalitis
- preferential gray matter involvement

CNS Vasculitis (123)
- patchy and asymmetric acute infarcts
- focal gyriform enhancement
- scattered punctate white matter T2 hyperintensities
- multiple areas of focal narrowing and dilation involving intracranial arteries

Vasogenic Edema Surrounding Expansile Masses (Metastases, Abscesses) (155, 156)
- rarely symmetric
- focal dense contrast enhancement of the lesions within the vasogenic edema

Background

The etiology of PRES remains unclear and controversial. Imaging typically demonstrates symmetric vasogenic edema in a watershed distribution and laboratory studies frequently reveal evidence of endothelial injury. Severe hypertension leading to failed vascular autoregulation and subsequent hyperperfusion with endothelial injury remains a popular explanation for the development of PRES. The alternative and earlier theory proposes that systemic toxicity causes endothelial injury with vasoconstriction and hypoperfusion, which then lead to ischemia and subsequent vasogenic edema. Clinical studies have shown that brain edema is actually lower in severely hypertensive patients and hypertensive animal models have failed to demonstrate systemic toxicity. The conditions associated with PRES have a similar immune challenge present and develop a similar state of T-cell/endothelial cell activation that may be the basis of leukocyte trafficking and vasoconstriction. These systemic features along with current vascular and perfusion imaging findings appear to support the theory of vasoconstriction coupled with hypoperfusion. Considering the fact that PRES is not necessarily posterior in location nor spontaneously reversible, a modification of the acronym into Potentially Reversible Encephalopathy Syndrome has been suggested.

REFERENCES

1. Bartynski WS. Posterior reversible encephalopathy syndrome, part 1: fundamental imaging and clinical features. *AJNR* 2008;**29**:1036–42.
2. Bartynski WS. Posterior reversible encephalopathy syndrome, part 2: controversies surrounding pathophysiology of vasogenic edema. *AJNR* 2008;**29**:1043–9.
3. McKinney AM, Short J, Truwit CL, *et al.* Posterior reversible encephalopathy syndrome: incidence of atypical regions of involvement and imaging findings. *AJR* 2007;**189**:904–12.
4. Sharma A, Whitesell RT, Moran KJ. Imaging pattern of intracranial hemorrhage in the setting of posterior reversible encephalopathy syndrome. *Neuroradiology* 2010;**52**:855–63.
5. Mueller-Mang C, Mang T, Pirker A, *et al.* Posterior reversible encephalopathy syndrome: do predisposing risk factors make a difference in MRI appearance? *Neuroradiology* 2009;**51**:373–83.

Brain Imaging with MRI and CT, ed. Zoran Rumboldt *et al.* Published by Cambridge University Press. © Cambridge University Press 2012.

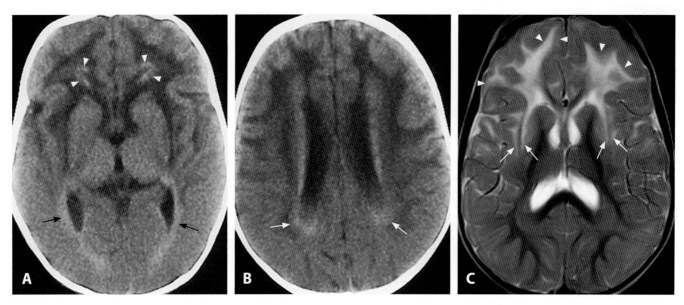

Figure 1. Axial CT images (A, B) in an infant with macrocephaly show diffuse frontal white matter hypodensity with hyperdense bifrontal periventricular rim (arrowheads) and subependymal regions (arrows). T2WI at a similar level (C) shows white matter hyperintensities with involvement of U-fibers (arrowheads) and external/extreme capsule (arrows). Caudate heads and putamina are hyperintense and slightly atrophic.

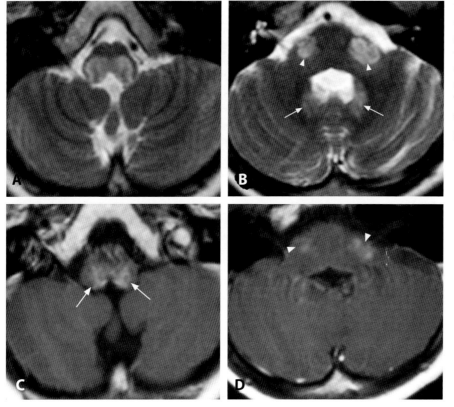

Figure 2. Axial T2WIs (A, B) in an 8-year-old child with developmental regression and spasticity show bilateral hyperintense lesions within the posterior medulla, dentate nuclei (arrows) and middle cerebellar peduncles (arrowheads). Corresponding post-contrast T1WIs (C, D) reveal moderate enhancement in the medulla (arrows) and middle cerebellar peduncles (arrowheads).

Alexander Disease

MARIASAVINA SEVERINO

Specific Imaging Findings

The most common infantile form of Alexander disease (AD) is characterized by frontotemporal white matter abnormalities (CT hypodense, low T1 and high T2 signal) with typical anteroposterior progression pattern, involvement of U-fibers and possible cystic degeneration. The external and extreme capsules are usually involved. There are characteristic T1 hyperintense and T2 hypointense periventricular frontal rims, hyperdense on CT. The deep gray matter may be swollen and T2 hyperintense showing gradual volume loss. Brainstem abnormalities are primarily involving the medulla and midbrain. Contrast enhancement is seen in ventricular ependyma, periventricular rim, frontal white matter, optic chiasm, fornix, basal ganglia, thalamus, dentate nucleus, and brainstem. Hydrocephalus may occcur due to aqueductal stenosis. Atypical MRI findings are more commonly observed in juvenile and adult AD and include: predominant or isolated involvement of posterior fossa, multifocal tumor-like brainstem lesions, signal abnormalities or atrophy of the medulla or spinal cord and garland-like features along the ventricular wall. MRS may show markedly decreased NAA, with increased *myo-*inositol, choline, and lactate.

Pertinent Clinical Information

There are three clinical subgroups of AD: infantile (birth to 2 years), juvenile (2–12 years), and adult forms. Infantile AD presents with increasing macrocephaly, failure of normal development, seizures, serious feeding problems, and rapid neurologic deterioration with average survival of 3 years. In juvenile AD, macrocephaly is less frequent and patients usually suffer from progressive signs of bulbar dysfunction, developmental regression, ataxia and spasticity with average survival of 8 years. The adult form is the most variable, with later onset and slower progression (average survival of 15 years). A neonatal variant has also been reported, characterized by rapid progression leading to severe disability or death within the first 2 years of life.

Differential Diagnosis

Canavan Disease (24)
- no frontal preponderance
- involvement of thalamus and globus pallidus, sparing of caudate nucleus and putamen
- no contrast enhancement
- characteristic increased NAA peak on MRS

Frontal Variant of X-Linked Adrenoleukodystrophy
- absent periventricular rims
- contrast enhancement at the outer border of the white matter lesions
- involvement of geniculate bodies
- brain stem lesions primarily involve corticospinal and other long tracts

Metachromatic Leukodystrophy (34)
- Periventricular "butterfly-shaped" cerebral white matter involvement with radial stripes on T2WI
- no contrast enhancement of the affected WM
- involvement of descending long tracts in the brainstem

Megalencephalic Leukoencephalopathy with Subcortical Cysts (van der Knaap Disease) (23)
- diffuse cerebral white matter changes and swelling
- typical anterior temporal cysts
- no contrast enhancement

Brainstem Glioma (63)
- absence of symmetry
- prominent mass effect
- no associated supratentorial abnormalities

Background

Alexander disease is a rare leukodystrophy caused by dominant mutations in the gene encoding glial fibrillary acidic protein (GFAP) on chromosome 17q.21. GFAP is the main intermediate filament protein expressed in mature astrocytes of the central nervous system. All mutations identified to date appear to exert a dominant toxic effect with accumulation of Rosenthal fibers (abnormal intracellular protein aggregates containing GFAP and small stress proteins) within astrocytes. Prior to the availability of molecular genetic testing the diagnosis was confirmed by the detection of diffuse accumulation of Rosenthal fibers in the brain by biopsy or autopsy. Increased levels of proteins and presence of αβ-crystallin, GFAP and heat shock protein 27 have been observed in the CSF. No specific therapy is currently available for AD and the management is entirely supportive. The classic teaching is that the resulting pathophysiology presumably disturbs the normal interaction between astrocytes and oligodendrocytes, resulting in demyelination. An alternative explanation could be hyperplasia and hypertrophy of astrocytes, as in low-grade gliomas.

REFERENCES

1. van der Knaap MS, Naidu S, Breiter SN, *et al*. Alexander disease: diagnosis with MR imaging. *AJNR* 2001;**22**:541–52.
2. van der Voorn JP, Pouwels PJ, Salomons GS, *et al*. Unraveling pathology in juvenile Alexander disease: serial quantitative MR imaging and spectroscopy of white matter. *Neuroradiology* 2009;**51**:669–75.
3. Farina L, Pareyson D, Minati L, *et al*. Can MR imaging diagnose adult-onset Alexander disease? *AJNR* 2008;**29**:1190–6.
4. Vázquez E, Macaya A, Mayolas N, *et al*. Neonatal Alexander disease: MR imaging prenatal diagnosis. *AJNR* 2008;**29**:1973–5.
5. van der Knaap MS, Salomons GS, Li R, *et al*. Unusual variants of Alexander's disease. *Ann Neurol* 2005;**57**:327–38.

Brain Imaging with MRI and CT, ed. Zoran Rumboldt *et al*. Published by Cambridge University Press. © Cambridge University Press 2012.

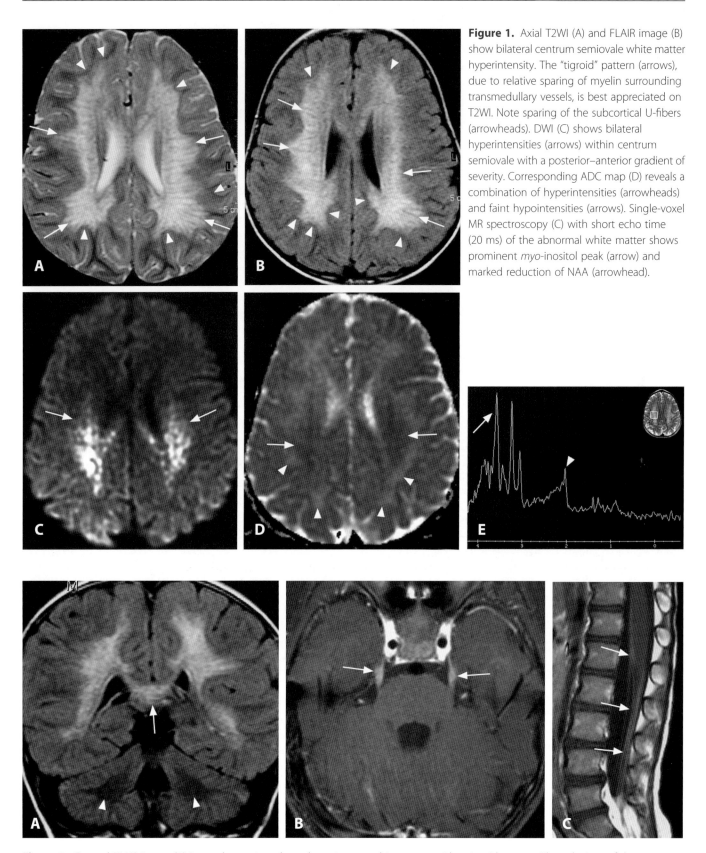

Figure 1. Axial T2WI (A) and FLAIR image (B) show bilateral centrum semiovale white matter hyperintensity. The "tigroid" pattern (arrows), due to relative sparing of myelin surrounding transmedullary vessels, is best appreciated on T2WI. Note sparing of the subcortical U-fibers (arrowheads). DWI (C) shows bilateral hyperintensities (arrows) within centrum semiovale with a posterior–anterior gradient of severity. Corresponding ADC map (D) reveals a combination of hyperintensities (arrowheads) and faint hypointensities (arrows). Single-voxel MR spectroscopy (C) with short echo time (20 ms) of the abnormal white matter shows prominent *myo*-inositol peak (arrow) and marked reduction of NAA (arrowhead).

Figure 2. Coronal FLAIR image (A) in another patient shows hyperintense white matter with a tigroid pattern. The splenium of the corpus callosum is involved (arrow), while the cerebellar white matter is spared (arrowheads). Post-contrast axial fat saturated T1WI through the pons (B) shows bilaterally enhancing trigeminal nerves (arrows). Sagittal post-contrast T1WI of the lumbar spine (C) reveals enhancing cauda equina (arrows).

Metachromatic Leukodystrophy

ANDREA ROSSI AND ZORAN RUMBOLDT

Specific Imaging Findings

Metachromatic leukodystrophy (MLD) is a classical leukodystrophy with initially pure white matter involvement. Hyperintense T2 signal of supratentorial white matter with sparing of the subcortical white matter is typical, at least in the initial stages. The "tigroid" pattern is a peculiar radial stripe appearance within the centrum semiovale due to sparing of perivascular myelin around transmedullary vessels – this finding is strongly suggestive of MLD. The imaging appearance varies over time with a progressive posterior–anterior and centrifugal gradient of white matter involvement. The brainstem and cerebellum are spared until the very late stages. The abnormal white matter does not enhance with contrast; however diffuse enhancement of cranial nerves and cauda equina is typically present. DWI may show a tigroid pattern and more diffuse hyperintense abnormalities, without consistent reduction in ADC values, likely representing a combination of T2-shine through and truly reduced diffusion. Thalamic T2 hypointensity frequently develops over time. MR spectroscopy is nonspecific, with decreased NAA, increased *myo*-inositol, and presence of lactate; NAA levels correlate with motor function.

Pertinent Clinical Information

There are several clinical phenotypes of MLD according to the age of onset, with the late infantile form accounting for 70% of cases. In this form, patients present between 6 months and 3 years of age with hypotonia, dysarthria, ataxia, unsteady gait and progressive loss of motor skills. They develop peripheral neuropathy, which may be painful, optic atrophy, and become paraplegic and later quadriplegic. Decerebration and demise occur between 3 and 6 years of the onset. The juvenile (onset at 4–16 years) and adult (onset at 16–30 years) forms usually have a less aggressive course, and prolonged survival is reported. Clinical signs include spasticity, ataxia, and progressive cognitive decline. Epilepsy and purely psychiatric findings may also be encountered. Diagnosis is based on a combination of increased urinary excretion of sulfatides and arylsulfatase A activity in peripheral leukocytes and cultured fibroblasts. Exceptional cases of activator deficiency (in which patients lack saposin B) show normal arylsulfatase A levels but increased urinary sulfatides. In relatively more frequent instances of so-called pseudodeficiency (genetic polymorphisms with reduced enzyme activity), low arylsulfatase A activity is found without clinical signs of MLD, and normal urinary sulfatides confirm the diagnosis.

Differential Diagnosis

Krabbe Disease
- more prominent posterior–anterior gradient during early course of disease
- tigroid pattern less pronounced if present
- early involvement of cerebellum and brainstem is present
- early increased CT attenuation and decreased T2 signal of the thalami
- thickened optic chiasm may be seen

Pelizaeus–Merzbacher Disease
- diffuse hypomyelination of the whole brain
- earlier clinical onset during infancy
- typical nystagmus

Congenital CMV Infection (184)
- patchy confluent periventricular and centrum semiovale white matter hyperintensities
- asymmetric involvement, no radial tigroid pattern, stable without progression
- cystic cavitations in temporal poles
- frequent calcifications

Periventricular Leukomalacia (31)
- predominantly posterior periventricular white matter gliosis and posterior corpus callosum atrophy
- atrophic white matter with compensatory enlargement of ventricular trigoni
- history of prematurity, possible hypoxic–ischemic distress

Background

Metachromatic leukodystrophy (MLD) is caused by deficiency of cerebroside sulfatase, an enzyme composed of two subunits: arylsulfatase A enzyme (gene located on chromosome 22) and its activator protein, called saposin B (gene located on chromosome 10). Although deficiency of either subunit may cause MLD, arylsulfatase A deficiency is significantly more frequent than activator deficiency. Cerebroside sulfatase deficiency results in accumulation of galactocerebroside sulfate within oligodendrocytes and Schwann cells, causing myelin to become unstable and eventually break down. The disease becomes clinically manifest when arylsulfatase A activity is reduced to less than 10% of normal controls. The different age-related clinical phenotypes are closely correlated to known genotypic variations.

REFERENCES

1. Martin A, Sevin C, Lazarus C, *et al.* Toward a better understanding of brain lesions during metachromatic leukodystrophy evolution. *AJNR* 2012 Apr 26. [Epub ahead of print]

2. van der Voorn JP, Pouwels PJ, Kamphorst W, *et al.* Histopathologic correlates of radial stripes on MR images in lysosomal storage disorders. *AJNR* 2005;**26**:442–6.

3. Polten A, Fluharty AL, Fluharty CB, *et al.* Molecular basis of different forms of metachromatic leukodystrophy. *N Eng J Med* 1991;**324**:18–22.

4. Patay Z. Diffusion-weighted MR imaging in leukodystrophies. *Eur Radiol* 2005;**15**:2284–303.

5. Morana G, Biancheri R, Dirocco M, *et al.* Enhancing cranial nerves and cauda equina: an emerging magnetic resonance imaging pattern in metachromatic leukodystrophy and Krabbe disease. *Neuropediatrics* 2009;**40**:291–4.

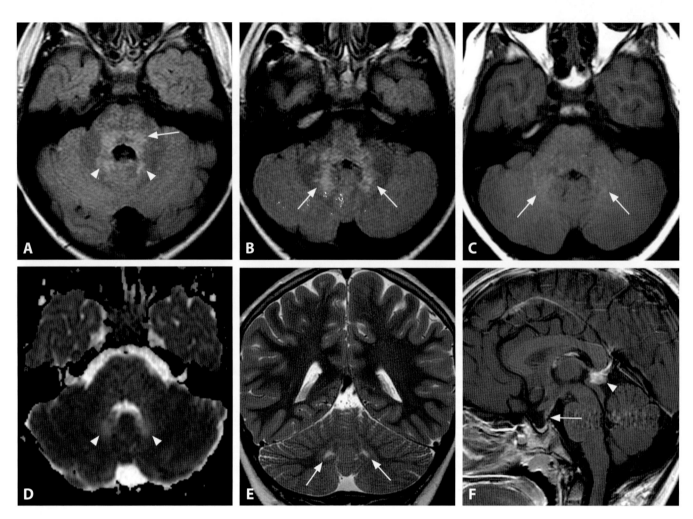

Figure 1. Axial FLAIR image (A) in a teenager with history of osteolytic lesions shows hyperintensity of the dorsal pons (arrow) and adjacent cerebellum (arrowheads). FLAIR at a lower level (B) shows high signal in the dentate nuclei (arrows) and brainstem. T1WI without contrast (C) reveals subtle hyperintense and hypointense signals (arrows) of the affected areas. ADC map (D) shows increased diffusivity of the lesions (arrowheads). Coronal T2WI (E) demonstrates hyperintensity (arrows) of bilateral dentate nucleus. Post-contrast midsagittal T1WI (F) reveals a very thin pituitary infundibulum (arrow) and mildly enlarged enhancing pineal gland (arrowhead). There was no abnormal cerebellar or brainstem enhancement.

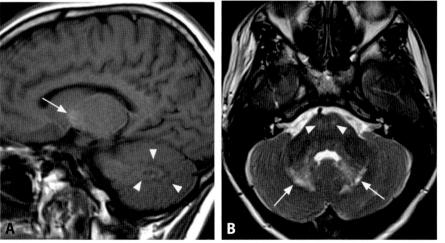

Figure 2. Sagittal T1WI without contrast (A) in a patient with history of diabetes insipidus now presenting with tremor and ataxia shows a hyperintensity in the basal ganglia (arrow) and mixed high and low signals in the dentate nuclei (arrowheads). Axial T2WI (B) reveals bright signal of dentate nuclei (arrows) and the pons. Note high signal of the corticospinal tracts (arrowheads).

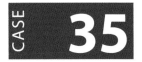
Neurodegenerative Langerhans Cell Histiocytosis (ND-LCH)

ZORAN RUMBOLDT AND ANDREA ROSSI

Specific Imaging Findings

Neurodegenerative Langerhans cell histiocytosis (ND-LCH) develops years after the initial disease presentation and presents on CT as symmetric nonenhancing hypodensities in the dentate nuclei region of the cerebellum, sometimes with calcifications. On MRI, the symmetric cerebellar lesions are T2 hyperintense with hypointense and/or hyperintense signals on T1-weighted images. The abnormalities may be limited to the deep cerebellar gray matter or extend to the surrounding white matter, and can eventually result in CSF-like "holes". T2 hyperintensities may also be found in the pontine tegmentum and/or pontine pyramidal tracts. T1 hyperintensity of the basal ganglia is another characteristic finding, which may be limited to globus pallidus. All of these lesions do not show mass effect or contrast enhancement, and are the second most frequent presentation of CNS LCH, after the extra-axial involvement of the pituitary gland and hypothalamus. Slight hyperintensity of the dentate nucleus on T1WI may be the initial finding, followed by T2 hyperintensity and subsequent slow extension of T2 hyperintensity to the cerebellar white matter. In the cerebral hemispheres, dilated perivascular spaces and white matter T2 hyperintensities may be encountered.

The entire spectrum of intracranial LCH findings can be classified into four groups: (1) osseous lesions in the craniofacial bones and/or skull base with or without soft-tissue extension; (2) intracranial extra-axial disease in the hypothalamic–pituitary region, pineal gland, meninges, choroid plexus, and ependyma; (3) intra-axial degenerative disease in the gray and/or white matter with a striking symmetry of the lesions and a clear predominance in the cerebellum and basal ganglia; (4) localized or diffuse atrophy.

Pertinent Clinical Information

ND-LCH is a slowly progressive process with overt symptoms occuring on average 6 years after the initial LCH diagnosis, with a highly variable severity and course. The MRI signal intensity abnormalities in the cerebellum and basal ganglia do not necessarily correlate with neurologic deterioration. Neurologic symptoms range from subtle tremor to profound ataxia, dysarthria, spastic diparesis, and psychiatric disease. Long-term survivors of multisystem LCH, particularly patients with CNS involvement, may develop significant cognitive deficits.

Differential Diagnosis

Neurofibromatosis Type 1 (2)
- signal abnormalities are more common in the deep gray matter than the cerebellum

- areas of abnormal signal tend to be asymmetric and with a cloudy appearance
- additional NF1 lesions are frequently present

Chronic Liver Failure (1)
- T1 hyperintensity limited to globus pallidus in the basal ganglia
- no history of LCH

Krabbe Disease
- early bilateral involvement of supratentorial white matter
- thalami are hyperdense on CT and of low T2 signal
- usually no signal abnormality in the basal ganglia
- optic nerve enlargement
- contrast enhancement of cranial nerves and spinal roots
- younger age

Background

Three types of LCH lesions can be distinguished on neuropathology: (1) circumscribed granulomas in the meninges or choroid plexus, with variable presence of CD1a$^+$ cells and pronounced CD8$^+$ T-cell infiltration; (2) granulomas within connective tissue with partial infiltration of the adjacent CNS parenchyma by CD1a$^+$ histiocytes, associated with T-cell-dominated inflammation and nearly complete loss of neurons and axons, and gliosis; (3) neurodegenerative lesions mainly affecting the cerebellum and brainstem without CD1a$^+$ cells and with an inflammatory process dominated by CD8$^+$ lymphocytes, tissue degeneration, microglial activation, and gliosis. These neurodegenerative lesions resembling paraneoplastic encephalitis are the found in patients with ND-LCH. Recurrent bilateral FDG-PET abnormalities with hypometabolism in the cerebellum, basal ganglia, and frontal cortex, along with increased metabolism in the amygdala appear to be typical for ND-LCH. Functional changes in these regions may be detected even in the absence of any apparent MRI lesions.

REFERENCES

1. Prosch H, Grois N, Wnorowski M, *et al*. Long-term MR imaging course of neurodegenerative Langerhans cell histiocytosis. *AJNR* 2007;**28**:1022–8.
2. Wnorowski M, Prosch H, Prayer D, *et al*. Pattern and course of neurodegeneration in Langerhans cell histiocytosis. *J Pediatr* 2008;**153**:127–32.
3. Demaerel P, Van Gool S. Paediatric neuroradiological aspects of Langerhans cell histiocytosis. *Neuroradiology* 2008;**50**:85–92.
4. Ribeiro MJ, Idbaih A, Thomas C, et al. 18F-FDG PET in neurodegenerative Langerhans cell histiocytosis: results and potential interest for an early diagnosis of the disease. *J Neurol* 2008;**255**:575–80.
5. Grois N, Prayer D, Prosch H, *et al*. Neuropathology of CNS disease in Langerhans cell histiocytosis. *Brain* 2005;**128**:829–38.

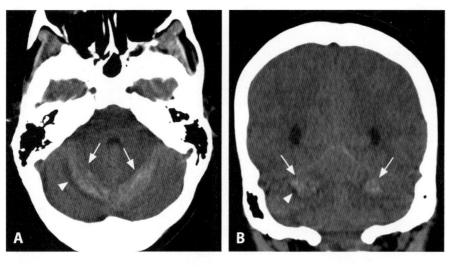

Figure 1. Non-enhanced CT images in axial (A) and coronal (B) planes following frontal craniotomy show hyperdense material consistent with hemorrhage within the lateral superior portion of the bilateral cerebellar hemispheres (arrows). There is a small amount of surrounding hypodensity (arrowheads) corresponding to extruded serum and edema. The axial image (A) shows a streaky linear pattern of the hemorrhage that follows the folia.

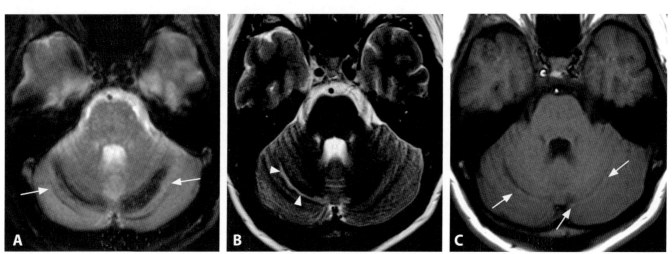

Figure 2. Axial T2* MR image (A) in another patient shows linear bilateral very low signal (arrows) in the superior cerebellum, suggestive of hemorrhage. Corresponding T2WI (B) shows a rim of hypointensity with linear distribution and subtle central hyperintensity (arrowheads) on the right. T1WI (C) shows very faint linear hyperintensities (arrows). The findings are consistent with blood products.

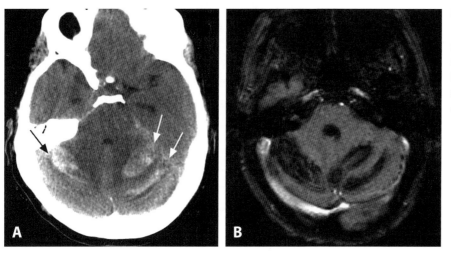

Figure 3. Non-enhanced axial CT image (A) in a patient with headache following lumbar spine surgery shows striped hyperdense material (arrows) in the cephalad portion of both cerebellar hemispheres. T2* MR image at a similar level (B) reveals prominent signal loss of the lesions, consistent with hemorrhage.

Remote Cerebellar Hemorrhage

MARIA GISELE MATHEUS

Specific Imaging Findings

Remote cerebellar hemorrhage (RCH) typically occurs bilaterally along the superior aspect of the cerebellum following the cerebellar folia in a linear arched pattern that has been termed "zebra sign". A recent RCH is seen as multiple linear hyperdensities on non-enhanced CT images. The same striped pattern is found on MRI, and it follows the signal intensity characteristics that vary according to the age of hemorrhage. The susceptibility effect from blood products is seen as signal loss on T2* MR sequences, gradient echo (GRE) or susceptibility-weighted images (SWI). Unilateral RCH is infrequent. Vascular studies, CTA, MRA, or DSA, reveal intact appearance of the venous sinuses and other vascular structures, without signs of thrombosis.

Pertinent Clinical Information

RCH is a rare complication of cranial and spinal surgeries that include opening of the dura. It has been reported following a wide range of procedures, from laminectomies and lumbar CSF drainages to temporal lobectomies, vascular neurosurgery, supratentorial tumor resections, and even single burr hole drainages. The most common symptoms are decreased level of consciousness, headache, nausea, and dizziness. The onset of symptoms is in the range from a few hours to a number of days after the surgical procedure. RCH is frequently benign and self-limited, but it may entail significant morbidity and result in death.

Differential Diagnosis

Hemorrhagic Venous Thrombosis (181)

- presence of thrombus in intracranial venous structures
- "zebra sign" with bilateral striped pattern is highly unusual

Hypertensive Hematoma (177)

- characteristically located deep in the cerebellar white matter (dentate nucleus)
- round or oval and unilateral

AVM-related Hemorrhage (182)

- usually unilateral
- hemorrhage is adjacent to abnormal vascular structures – flow voids, best seen on T2WI
- enlarged feeding and draining vessels may be present

Background

The pathophysiological mechanism of RCH is disputed, but it is probably venous bleeding secondary to significant intraoperative or postoperative loss of CSF. Multiple risk factors have been described, such as systemic hypertension and antiplatelet agents, but postsurgical negative pressure drainage of CSF is the only clear predisposing factor. The most accepted explanation is the development of CSF leak following a dural tear with excessive CSF drainage and consequent sagging of the cerebellum, which in turn leads to stretching of the infratentorial bridging veins. The bleeding occurs in the areas of the cerebellum where most of the draining veins are located. The presence of a downward or upward pressure gradient stretches the cerebellar veins with subsequent hemorrhage, while venous infarction may occur in some cases. RCH typically presents following supratentorial and spinal surgery; however, it has also been described with infratentorial procedures, such as following foramen magnum decompression. RCH is poorly known and hence probably underdiagnosed. The incidence of symptomatic RCH is estimated to range from 0.08 to 0.3%, while the incidence of asymptomatic cases is not known and may be susbstantially higher. Early detection and correct interpretation of the typical imaging findings may help to avoid further aggravation of symptoms. Prognosis significantly depends on severity of hemorrhage and patient age. Outcome in more than 50% of all cases is good with only mild residual neurological symptoms or complete recovery, while death occurs in approximately 10–15% of patients.

REFERENCES

1. Amini A, Osborn AG, McCall TD, Couldwell WT. Remote cerebellar hemorrhage. *AJNR* 2006;**27**:387–90.
2. Cevik B, Kirbas I, Cakir B, *et al.* Remote cerebellar hemorrhage after lumbar spine surgery. *Eur J Radiol* 2009;**70**:7–9.
3. Chalela JA, Timothy M, Kelley M, *et al.* Cerebellar hemorrhage caused by remote neurological surgery. *Neurocrit Care* 2006;**5**:30–4.
4. Brockmann M, Groden C. Remote cerebellar hemorrhage: a review. *Cerebellum* 2006;**5**:64–8.
5. Park JS, Hwang JH, Park J, *et al.* Remote cerebellar hemorrhage complicated after supratentorial surgery: retrospective study with review of articles. *J Korean Neurosurg Soc* 2009;**46**:136–43.

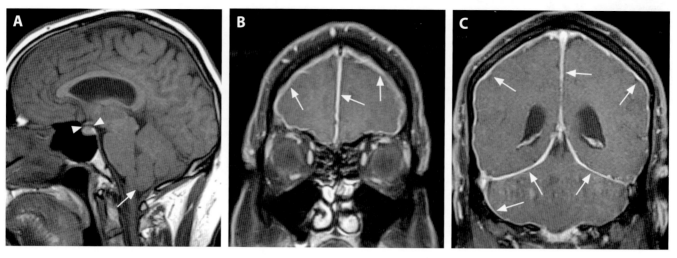

Figure 1. Midsagittal T1WI without contrast (A) shows the "sagging brain" appearance with effaced suprasellar cisterns (arrowheads) and slightly low lying cerebellar tonsils (arrow). Coronal post-contrast T1WIs with fat saturation (B, C) reveal diffuse dural enhancement (arrows).

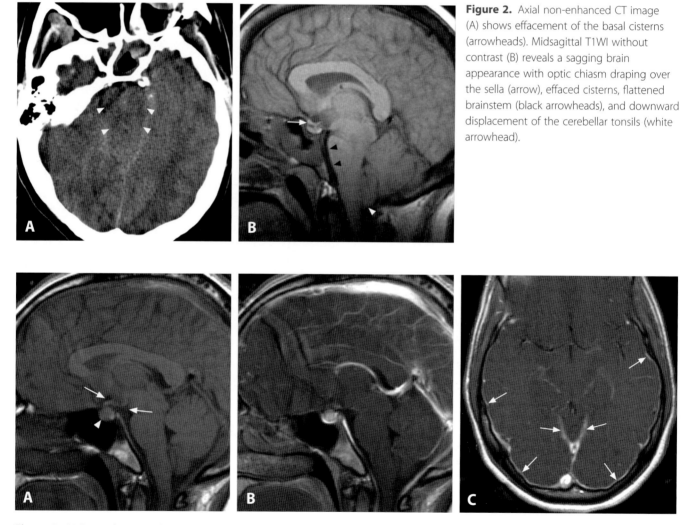

Figure 2. Axial non-enhanced CT image (A) shows effacement of the basal cisterns (arrowheads). Midsagittal T1WI without contrast (B) reveals a sagging brain appearance with optic chiasm draping over the sella (arrow), effaced cisterns, flattened brainstem (black arrowheads), and downward displacement of the cerebellar tonsils (white arrowhead).

Figure 3. Midsagittal T1WI without contrast (A) shows narrowing of the basal cisterns (arrows) and pituitary enlargement (arrowhead). Corresponding post-contrast image (B) shows pituitary hyperemia. Axial post-contrast T1WI (C) demonstrates engorgement of the dural sinuses and thickened enhancing pachymeninges (arrows).

Spontaneous Intracranial Hypotension

MARIA VITTORIA SPAMPINATO

Specific Imaging Findings

Spontaneous Intracranial Hypotension (SIH) typically presents with a "sagging brain" imaging appearance with downward displacement of the brain stem and cerebellar tonsils, loss of the basal cisterns, flattened brainstem, bowing of the optic chiasm over the sella, pituitary hyperemia, and effacement of the ventricles and sulci. Diffuse pachymeningeal thickening is bright on FLAIR images with characteristic contrast enhancement, although absent in some cases. Subdural hygromas or less commonly hematomas can also be found. Clinical improvement is not always accompanied by prompt resolution of the MRI findings. Spinal MRI and CT myelography can demonstrate extra-dural fluid collections indicating the location of the CSF leak. MRI may also show meningeal enhancement and dilation of the internal vertebral venous plexi, especially at C1–C2 level. High T2 signal intensity between the spinous processes of C1 and C2 is highly characteristic for SIH.

Pertinent Clinical Information

SIH is a clinical syndrome in which low CSF volume results in orthostatic headache, occurring within 15 min after a change from supine to standing position, and improvement or resolution after lying down. The headache may be diffuse or localized, most commonly to the occipital and suboccipital regions. Associated symptoms in severe cases include nausea, vomiting, photophobia, vertigo, tinnitus, visual loss, diplopia, and even coma. It can occur following a minor trauma, strenuous exercise, sexual activity, or a bout of sneezing or coughing. A low opening pressure (less than 6 cm H_2O) is usually found on lumbar puncture; however, it may be within normal limits. Imaging tests therefore play a key role in the diagnosis.

Differential Diagnosis

Chiari 1 Malformation
- low-lying cerebellar tonsils with normal appearance of the brainstem and cisterns, without brain "sagging"

Chronic Subdural Hematoma (133)
- enhancing meninges are enclosing blood products
- normal appearance of the brainstem and cisterns

Neoplastic Dural Involvement
- dural thickening is usually irregular and nodular
- usually normal appearance of the brainstem and cisterns

Idiopathic Hypertrophic Pachymeningitis (136)
- "split dura" sign – enhancement along the inner and outer surfaces with central non-enhancing dura
- normal appearance of the brainstem and cisterns

Postoperative Changes
- evidence of/known craniotomy
- usually normal appearance of the brainstem and cisterns

Background

SIH syndrome is characterized by low CSF pressure without any history of trauma. SIH is an important cause of new persistent headaches with a peak incidence around 40 years of age. The estimated prevalence is 2–5 per 100 000 individuals with a female-to-male ratio of 2:1. SIH is often associated with connective tissue disorders such as Marfan syndrome or Ehlers–Danlos syndrome. The spine is the common source of spontaneous CSF leak, typically from meningeal diverticula and tears in nerve root sleeves. The majority of leaks occur along the cervico-thoracic junction. Radioisotope cisternography, CT myelography, and MRI have been used to identify the etiology of SIH. According to the Monro–Kellie rule, the intracranial volume is always constant and represents the sum of the volumes of blood, brain, and CSF. With the brain volume being constant, the volumes of blood and CSF vary reciprocally. When loss of CSF and CSF hypotension occur, a compensatory increase in intracranial blood volume leads to pachymeningeal venous hyperemia, giving the appearance of thickened dura. Downward brain displacement causes headache by traction on pain-sensitive structures, particularly the dura. Conservative treatment includes bed rest, hydration, and analgesics. If the symptoms persist, epidural blood patches are usually effective, while surgical duraplasty is occasionally necessary.

REFERENCES
1. Tosaka M, Sato N, Fujimaki H, et al. Diffuse pachymeningeal hyperintensity and subdural effusion/hematoma detected by fluid-attenuated inversion recovery MR imaging in patients with spontaneous intracranial hypotension. AJNR 2008;29:1164–70.
2. Yuh EL, Dillon WP. Intracranial hypotension and intracranial hypertension. Neuroimaging Clin N Am 2010;20:597–617.
3. Medina JH, Abrams K, Falcone S, Bhatia RG. Spinal imaging findings in spontaneous intracranial hypotension. AJR 2010;195:459–64.
4. Watanabe A, Horikoshi T, Uchida M, et al. Diagnostic value of spinal MR imaging in spontaneous intracranial hypotension syndrome. AJNR 2009;30:147–51.
5. George U, Rathore S, Pandian JD, Singh Y. Diffuse pachymeningeal enhancement and subdural and subarachnoid space opacification on delayed postcontrast fluid-attenuated inversion recovery imaging in spontaneous intracranial hypotension: visualizing the Monro–Kellie hypothesis. AJNR 2011;32:E16.

SECTION 2

Sellar, Perisellar and Midline Lesions

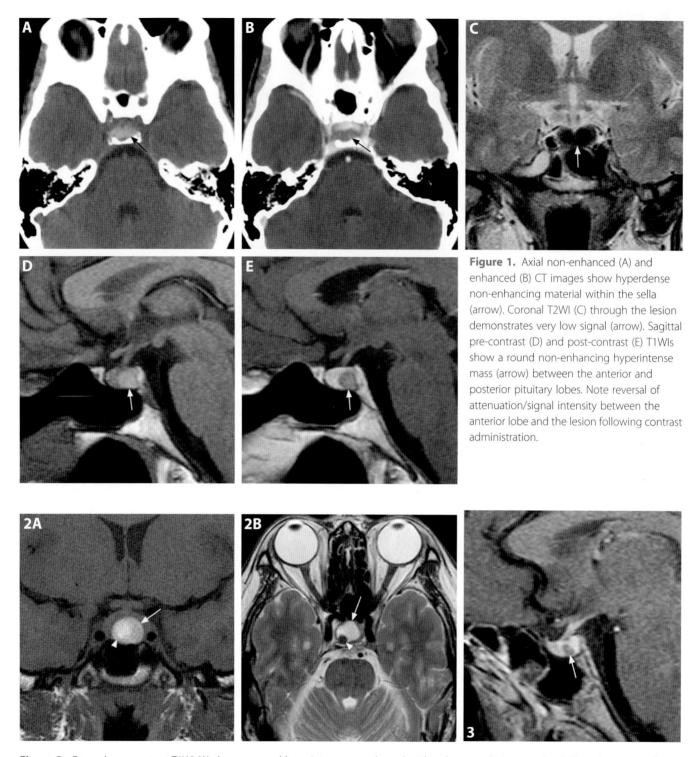

Figure 1. Axial non-enhanced (A) and enhanced (B) CT images show hyperdense non-enhancing material within the sella (arrow). Coronal T2WI (C) through the lesion demonstrates very low signal (arrow). Sagittal pre-contrast (D) and post-contrast (E) T1WIs show a round non-enhancing hyperintense mass (arrow) between the anterior and posterior pituitary lobes. Note reversal of attenuation/signal intensity between the anterior lobe and the lesion following contrast administration.

Figure 2. Coronal non-contrast T1WI (A) shows a round hyperintense mass (arrow) within the central pituitary gland. There is an area of even higher intensity (arrowhead) within the right side of the lesion. Axial T2WI (B) demonstrates overall hyperintensity of the sellar mass with a hypointense nodule (arrowhead) in its right posterior aspect.

Figure 3. Sagittal post-contrast T1WI shows a non-enhancing area (arrow) between the anterior and posterior pituitary lobes. This may represent a pars intermedia cyst or Rathke's cleft cyst.

Specific Imaging Findings

Rathke's cleft cyst (RCC) is located at the central portion of the pituitary gland, in the midline between the anterior and posterior lobes, and is typically bright on CT and T1-weighted MR images. T1 signal, however, varies and can be as low as that of the CSF. The size ranges from a few millimeters to 4 cm. The cyst frequently includes a suprasellar component, while in some cases the gland may be displaced inferiorly leading to "an egg in a cup" appearance. On T2-weighted images, RCC may range from hypointense to hyperintense. A helpful sign is the presence of one of more internal nodules of high T1 and low T2 signal, reflecting cholesterol and protein clusters. RCCs are not calcified and do not enhance with contrast media. A thin rim of enhancement may be present within the adjacent glandular tissue, presumably due to compression and/or inflammatory changes. Characteristic reversal of signal intensities between the anterior lobe and the RCC may be seen when comparing pre- and post-contrast MR or CT images. Single-shot fast spin-echo diffusion MR imaging may be helpful as it shows high ADC values of the RCC contents.

Pertinent Clinical Information

RCC is frequently an incidental imaging finding. Headache, hyperprolactinemia, menstrual irregularities and sexual dysfunction are common presenting symptoms. Hypopituitarism and diabetes insipidus are less frequent. When large enough, compression on the optic chiasm leads to visual field defects. Cyst removal via a transsphenoidal surgical approach is a safe and effective treatment. Re-accumulation occurs in a minority of patients, more commonly in cysts with CSF-like signal intensities on MRI.

Differential Diagnosis

Pituitary Adenoma (39, 41)
- characteristic eccentric lateral location (except for ACTH-secreting tumors)
- contrast enhancement (although usually delayed)

Craniopharyngioma (44, 202)
- calcifications (around 90% of cases)
- contrast enhancement (at least along the periphery, outside the gland)

- suprasellar location is typical
- characteristic multicystic appearance is common

Pars Intermedia Cyst
- may be indistinguishable from a small RCC with low T1 and high T2 signal

Background

RCCs are benign, sellar and/or suprasellar lesions originating from the remnants of Rathke's pouch. They are found in 12–33% of normal pituitary glands on routine autopsies, while symptomatic cases are rare. RCC and craniopharyngioma are thought to have the common embryological origin from remnants of the Rathke's pouch, and even lesions with combined features of both Rathke's cleft cyst and craniopharyngioma have been described. The main distinguishing characteristic on histology is the structure of the wall: Rathke's cleft cyst is lined with a single cell layer, while craniopharyngioma contains thicker multilayered membrane. The imaging features of the Rathke's cleft cyst are thought to relate to its contents: the thicker the fluid is the higher the CT density and T1 signal intensity. Hyperintensity on T1-weighted images may be associated with chronic inflammation that can potentially cause irreversible endocrine dysfunction. Cases of lymphocytic hypophysitis related to a ruptured Rathke's cleft cyst have also been described.

REFERENCES

1. Byun WM, Kim OL, Kim D. MR imaging findings of Rathke's cleft cysts: significance of intracystic nodules. *AJNR* 2000;**21**:485–8.
2. Nishioka H, Haraoka J, Izawa H, Ikeda Y. Magnetic resonance imaging, clinical manifestations, and management of Rathke's cleft cyst. *Clin Endocrinol (Oxf)* 2006;**64**:184–8.
3. Wen L, Hu LB, Feng XY, *et al.* Rathke's cleft cyst: clinicopathological and MRI findings in 22 patients. *Clin Radiol* 2010;**65**:47–55.
4. Kunii N, Abe T, Kawamo M, *et al.* Rathke's cleft cysts: differentiation from other cystic lesions in the pituitary fossa by use of single-shot fast spin-echo diffusion-weighted MR imaging. *Acta Neurochir (Wien)* 2007;**149**:759–69.
5. Rumboldt Z. Pituitary lesions. In: *Neuroradiology (Third Series) Test and Syllabus.* Castillo M, ed. American College of Radiology, Reston VA 2006;37–59.

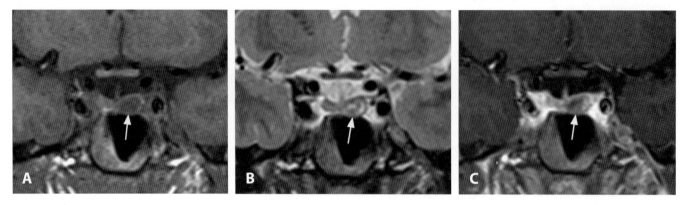

Figure 1. Coronal T1WI (A) through the sella turcica in a patient with hyperprolactinemia shows a left-sided hypointense pituitary lesion (arrow). The lesion is of heterogenous predominantly high signal (arrow) on corresponding T2WI (B). Post-contrast T1WI (C) reveals hypoenhancement of the small mass (arrow).

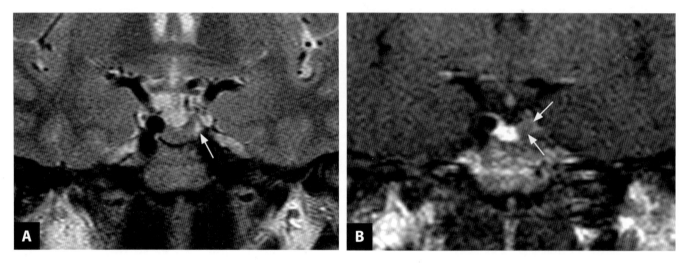

Figure 2. Coronal T2WI (A) reveals a subtle hyperintensity (arrow) in the left lateral aspect of the pituitary (arrow) in another patient. Corresponding early dynamic post-contrast image (B) reveals a larger area of delayed enhancement (arrows). Dynamic images frequently increase the confidence in lesion detection.

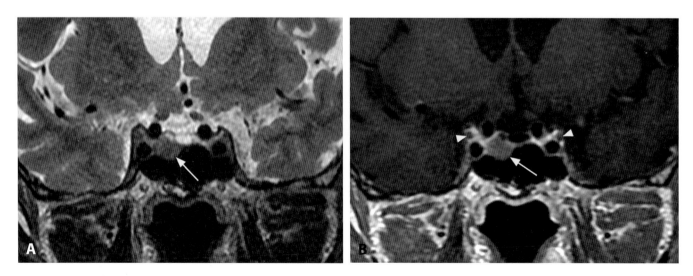

Figure 3. Coronal T2WI (A) shows a 6 mm isointense lesion extending through the sellar floor (arrow). Corresponding post-contrast T1WI (B) shows a relatively mild lesion enhancement (arrow). Note normal oculomotor nerves (arrowheads) within brightly enhancing cavernous sinuses.

Pituitary Microadenoma

MATTHEW OMOJOLA AND ZORAN RUMBOLDT

Specific Imaging Findings

Pituitary adenoma under 1 cm in size is by convention referred to as microadenoma. Most microadenomas are located laterally within the anterior lobe and may not cause any notable change in the size or contour of the gland. The majority are seen on pre-contrast T1WI as a round or oval, sometimes triangular hypointensity. Some microadenomas may be T1 bright, presumably due to hemorrhagic transformation. T2 hyperintensity is found in the majority of microprolactinomas. Most growth hormone-secreting adenomas are, however, T2 iso to hypointense. Some microadenomas are depicted on T2WI only and some exclusively on post-contrast images. Dynamic imaging detects an additional 10% of lesions. The tumors typically show a different dynamic pattern, usually of delayed or complete lack of enhancement. In rare cases adenomas accumulate contrast medium earlier than the normal gland, reflecting a direct arterial supply due to dural invasion. Delayed imaging may show prominent adenoma enhancement within relatively dark normal gland. Dedicated pituitary imaging, including dynamic post-contrast scans, may also be performed with CT. Adenomas in Cushing disease tend to be located around the midline and are frequently not visualized on imaging studies. Presence of fluid levels is highly indicative of adenomas, representing degeneration and hemorrhage.

Pertinent Clinical Information

Microadenomas may be asymptomatic and discovered in patients investigated for unrelated reasons. Symptomatic microadenomas are usually prolactin-secreting and are more common in women presenting with infertility, amenorrhea and galactorrhea. In men, microadenomas usually present with impotence, prolactin levels are higher, tumors larger and more invasive, and the outcome is worse. There is a solid correlation between the prolactin blood levels and MRI: concentration over 200 ng/ml practically guarantees tumor detection, while imaging is positive in less than half of cases below 50 ng/ml. T2 hypointense prolactinomas tend to have higher prolactin secretion. Microadenomas may also lead to Cushing disease with ACTH-producing tumors, or acromegaly with GH-secreting adenomas. Endovascular venous sampling (from inferior petrosal and/or cavernous sinus) may be necessary for diagnosis in patients with Cushing disease.

Differential Diagnosis

Rathke's Cleft Cyst (38)
- typically T1 hyperintense with low T2 signal intensity
- does not enhance with contrast
- located centrally between the anterior and posterior lobes

Pars Intermedia Cyst
- no contrast enhancement
- central location

Lymphocytic Hypophysitis (40)
- diffuse gland enlargement
- delayed dynamic contrast enhancement of the entire gland
- peripheral low T2 signal may be present
- absence of focal lesions

Arachnoid Cyst (142)
- CSF intensity on all MR sequences
- at least in part suprasellar
- no contrast enhancement

Epidermoid (143)
- at least in part suprasellar
- characteristically very bright on DWI
- no contrast enhancement

Background

Incidental pituitary adenomas are found in about 10% of autopsies. A focal 2–3 mm pituitary lesion on MRI has an approximately 50% chance of representing an incidental insignificant finding. The gland enlarges during puberty, especially in girls, when it may have a convex superior contour and reach 10 mm in height. Such appearance is also common during mid-menstrual cycle in fertile women and during pregnancy, while in the first postpartum week the gland may reach 12 mm in height. The adenohypophysis has a portal rather than a direct arterial blood supply, which enables dynamic MR (or CT) imaging. The normal gland enhances after the infundibulum and cavernous sinuses have already opacified, in a characteristic centrifugal pattern. The tumors that are iso to hypointense to the normal gland on T2WI tend to be fibrotic and indurated (especially if not associated with very high prolactin levels), indicating increased difficulty of surgical resection.

REFERENCES

1. Rumboldt Z. Pituitary adenomas. *Top Magn Reson Imaging* 2006;**16**:277–88.

2. Abe T, Izumiyama H, Fujisawa I. Evaluation of pituitary adenomas by multidirectional multislice dynamic CT. *Acta Radiol* 2002;**43**:556–9.

3. Friedman TC, Zuckerbraun E, Lee ML, *et al.* Dynamic pituitary MRI has high sensitivity and specificity for the diagnosis of mild Cushing's syndrome and should be part of the initial workup. *Horm Metab Res* 2007;**39**:451–6.

4. Patronas N, Bulakbasi N, Stratakis CA, *et al.* Spoiled gradient recalled acquisition in the steady state technique is superior to conventional postcontrast spin echo technique for magnetic resonance imaging detection of adrenocorticotropin-secreting pituitary tumors. *J Clin Endocrinol Metab* 2003;**88**:1565–9.

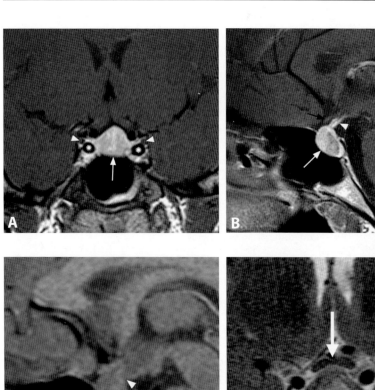

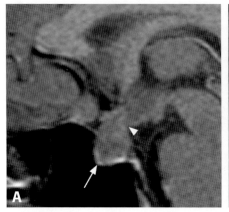

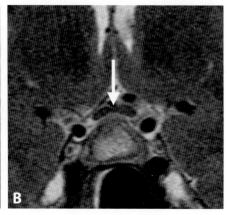

Figure 1. Coronal post-contrast T1WI (A) shows a homogenously enhancing diffusely enlarged pituitary gland (arrow). Normal flow-void in the cavernous internal carotid arteries (*) is surrounded by normal homogenously enhancing cavernous sinus, which cannot be clearly distinguished from the gland. Note non-enhancing oculomotor nerves (arrowhead). Midsagittal post-contrast T1WI (B) shows the enlarged gland (white arrow) with an area of lower signal. Pituitary stalk (arrowhead) is mildly thickened. The optic chiasm (black arrow) is not compressed. Courtesy of Angelika Gutenberg.

Figure 2. Sagittal non-contrast T1WI (A) shows diffuse enlargement of the pituitary infundibulum (arrowhead) and gland (arrow) and absence of the normal posterior pituitary bright spot. The optic chiasm cannot be clearly identified. Coronal T2WI (B) shows enlarged gland with centrally increased and peripherally decreased signal. There is mild mass effect on the optic chiasm (arrow).

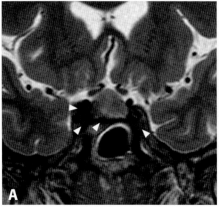

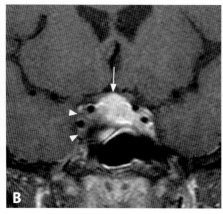

Figure 3. Enlarged pituitary gland is shown on coronal T2WI (A) in a woman with a history of partial hypopituitarism and diabetes insipidus. A very dark area (arrowheads) is present in cavernous sinuses and the sellar floor. Post-contrast T1WI (B) shows homogenous enhancement of the enlarged gland (arrow). The cavernous sinuses are swollen and with poor enhancement, more prominent on the right (arrowheads). Courtesy of Yasuhiro Nakata.

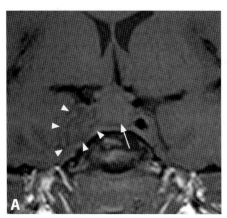

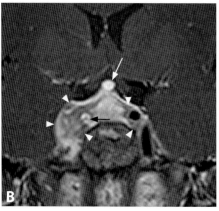

Figure 4. Pre-contrast coronal T1WI (A) in a pregnant patient with headache, right abducens palsy, and diabetes insipidus shows enlarged pituitary gland (arrow). There is absence of normal ICA flow void in the swollen right cavernous sinus (arrowheads). Post-contrast image (B) reveals enhancement of the gland and thickened infundibulum (white arrow). There is only mild enhancement of the cavernous sinuses (arrowheads), less than in the occluded right ICA (black arrow). Courtesy of Angelika Gutenberg.

Lymphocytic Hypophysitis

ZORAN RUMBOLDT AND BENJAMIN HUANG

Specific Imaging Findings

On MRI, lymphocytic hypophysitis (LH) will show symmetric enlargement of the pituitary gland with a homogeneous appearance both on pre- and post-contrast images, an intense gadolinium enhancement, as well as thickened pituitary stalk and loss of the posterior pituitary bright spot. Only some of these features may be present in individual patients. On dynamic contrast-enhanced study there is a prominent delay in pituitary enhancement compared to the normal gland (<60 s). A dark rim at the margins of the gland and in the cavernous sinuses may be seen on T2-weighted images, and this feature may progress over time. Ring-like enhancement, thought to be consistent with central necrosis and enhancement of the diaphragm is occasionally observed.

Pertinent Clinical Information

LH is a rare disease, estimated to be the cause of hypopituitarism in 0.5% of cases and to represent less than 1% of pituitary masses. It is much more common in women and has a striking association with late pregnancy or early postpartum. Patients present with a constellation of symptoms including headache, anterior pituitary dysfunction and hyperprolactinemia. Diabetes insipidus (DI) may be present, and it is the most prominent symptom in some cases. Approximately 40% of patients are misdiagnosed as having pituitary macroadenoma and undergo unnecessary surgery. It has been shown that with the appropriate integration of the MRI and clinical findings 97% of the patients can be correctly diagnosed. The disease may be self-limited, show a relapsing and remitting course, or progress to permanent hypopituitarism.

Differential Diagnosis

Pituitary Macroadenoma (41)
- focal lesions, not diffuse enlargement
- heterogeneous enhancement, lower gadolinium uptake than the normal gland
- normal pituitary stalk and posterior bright spot
- not associated with pregnancy, DI very uncommon

Langerhans Cell Histiocytosis (LCH) (43)
- usually limited to pituitary infundibulum thickening, may involve hypothalamus
- absence of pituitary T2 dark rim
- pineal gland may be enlarged
- lytic osseus lesions are frequently present

Metastasis
- invasion of the bone marrow and optic chiasm may be present

Pituitary Hyperplasia; Hypothyroidism
- normal pituitary stalk and posterior bright spot
- normal rate of enhancement on dynamic post-contrast scans

Normal Pituitary Gland
- normal pituitary signal and enhancement pattern
- normal gland height: ≤ 8 mm in males; ≤ 10 mm in girls and young women; ≤ 12 mm in pregnant or lactating women (loss of posterior lobe bright spot in the third trimester)

Background

Hypophysitis comprises two main histologic forms: lymphocytic and granulomatous. LH is much more common, has a well-established autoimmune pathogenesis, predominantly affects women, frequently presenting in the peripartal period. Granulomatous hypophysitis lacks the female bias and association with pregnancy and has a more aggressive clinical course. They may actually represent different stages of the same disease. Concurrent autoimmune conditions are seen in up to 50% of cases of LH, and cases associated with Rathke's cleft cyst have been described, suggesting cyst rupture as the possible etiology. Depending on the involved portion of the gland, LH can be subdivided into lymphocytic adenohypophysitis (LAH), lymphocytic infundibuloneurohypophysitis (LINH), and lymphocytic infundibulopanhypophysitis (LIPH). Histologic and clinical overlap among different types, however, suggest that these entities have similar etiology and/or represent different stages of the same lesion. LH is histologically characterized by diffuse polyclonal lymphocytic infiltration of the gland. Absence of multinucleated giant cells, histiocytes and granulomas distinguishes LH from granulomatous hypophysitis, which may also occur in sarcoidosis. Steroids and other forms of immunosuppression have been effective in some patients with hypophysitis.

REFERENCES

1. Gutenberg A, Larsen J, Lupi I, et al. A radiologic score to distinguish autoimmune hypophysitis from nonsecreting pituitary adenoma preoperatively. AJNR 2009;3:1766–72.
2. Nakata Y, Sato N, Masumoto T, et al. Parasellar T2 dark sign on MR imaging in patients with lymphocytic hypophysitis. AJNR 2010;31:1944–50.
3. Sato N, Sze G, Endo K. Hypophysitis: endocrinologic and dynamic MR findings. AJNR 1998;19:439–44.
4. Howlett TA, Levy MJ, Robertson IJ. How reliably can autoimmune hypophysitis be diagnosed without pituitary biopsy. Clin Endocrinol (Oxf) 2010;73:18–21.
5. Gutenberg A, Hans V, Puchner MJ, et al. Primary hypophysitis: clinical-pathological correlations. Eur J Endocrinol 2006;155:101–7.

Brain Imaging with MRI and CT, ed. Zoran Rumboldt *et al.* Published by Cambridge University Press. © Cambridge University Press 2012.

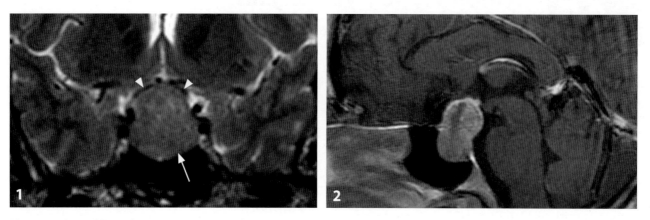

Figure 1. Coronal T2WI shows isointense intrasellar mass (arrow) with suprasellar extension and compression on the optic chiasm and optic nerves (arrowheads). Bilateral cavernous sinuses are intact.

Figure 2. Midsagittal T1WI post-contrast image in a different patient shows mildly heterogeneous sellar and suprasellar mass with a characteristic "snowman" appearance.

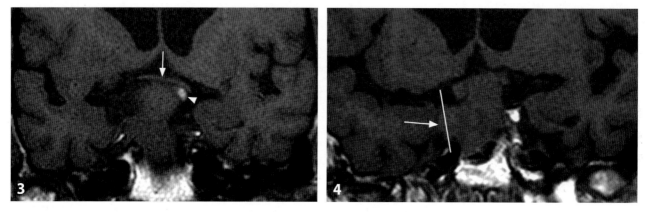

Figure 3. Coronal T1WI without contrast shows displacement of the optic chiasm (arrow) by the sellar mass. The location of the posterior pituitary lobe "bright spot" (arrowhead) is also depicted.

Figure 4. Coronal T1WI shows a sellar mass with right cavernous sinus invasion (arrow). The lesion extends past the lateral intercarotid line (white line; connects the cavernous and supracavernous ICA segments). Compression of the optic chiasm cannot be identified. Unrelated ventriculomegaly.

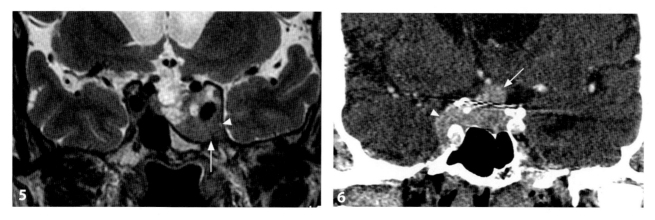

Figure 5. Coronal T2WI shows a left-sided sellar mass extending lateral to the inferior aspect of the cavernous ICA (arrow), invading the cavernous sinus (arrowhead) through the median venous compartment. Incidental prominent ventriculomegaly.

Figure 6. Post-contrast reformatted coronal CT shows an enhancing sellar mass with suprasellar extension (arrow). Invasion of the right cavernous sinus (arrowhead) with the lesion crossing the lateral intercarotid line (bright wall calcifications define the internal carotid arteries).

Pituitary Macroadenoma

MATTHEW OMOJOLA AND ZORAN RUMBOLDT

Specific Imaging Findings

Macroadenomas are frequently of heterogeneous appearance, reflecting cystic, necrotic, or hemorrhagic portions of the neoplasm. Contrast enhancement of the tumors is usually not prominent; the post-contrast images are used to visualize the normal avidly enhancing pituitary tissue. The location of the bright posterior lobe should be established on precontrast T1WI, to minimize chances of permanent postoperative diabetes insipidus. The frequent suprasellar tumor spread leads to the characteristic "figure of 8" or "snowman" appearance. The relationship with the optic chiasm is best evaluated on coronal T2WI, since the chiasm (composed of white matter tracts) is clearly hypointense. Cavernous sinus invasion is assessed on coronal images using virtual intercarotid lines that connect the cavernous and supracavernous ICA segments. Signs of cavernous sinus invasion are: tumor surrounding more than 66% of the cavernous ICA circumference, crossing the lateral intercarotid line, and extending into the medial venous compartment (the portion of the cavernous sinus immediately inferior to the ICA). DWI may show high signal intensity in infarcts and acute hemorrhages of acute pituitary apoplexy. Modern CT scanners can be effectively used when MR imaging is contraindicated.

Pertinent Clinical Information

Pituitary adenomas are more commonly diagnosed in women than in men and nonspecific symptoms, such as headache, are common. By convention 10 mm is used as the size threshold to separate macroadenomas from microadenomas. Non-functional pituitary adenomas present with symptoms associated with compression on the adjacent structures, most notably bitemporal hemianopsia, and are usually diagnosed late when they have reached macroadenoma size. However, hormonally active adenomas may also present as large masses, which is almost a rule for GH-secreting and thyrotropin-secreting tumors. Pituitary apoplexy typically presents with headache, visual impairment and ophthalmoplegia.

Differential Diagnosis

Craniopharyngioma (44, 202)
- typically suprasellar epicenter
- frequent multicystic appearance
- calcifications very common

Rathke's Cleft Cyst (38)
- usually intrasellar in location, suprasellar extension if very large
- typically bright T1 and low T2 signal

Perisellar Aneurysm (51)
- flow void within and/or adjacent to the lesion
- layered appearance ("onion skin") is common

Perisellar Meningioma (47)
- typically arises from the cavernous sinus region
- homogeneous contrast enhancement with dural tail

Arachnoid Cyst (142)
- CSF-like intensity on all MR sequences

Epidermoid (143)
- bright "light bulb" on DWI, may be heterogeneous on FLAIR
- CSF-like intensity on T1 and T2WI

Pituicytoma
- purely suprasellar lesion with avid contrast enhancement resembling meningioma
- uncommon neoplasm, may be indistinguishable from macroadenoma

Background

Pituitary adenomas are by far the most common sellar tumor encountered on imaging, representing about 10–15% of all surgically treated intracranial neoplasms. Estimated overall prevalence is over 10%, however, most of these are asymptomatic, incidentally found in autopsy or radiological studies. Pituitary adenomas produce symptoms by secreting hormones, depressing the secretion of hormones, and/or by mass effect from compression of the adjacent structures. Pituitary adenomas are prone to infarcts and hemorrhages, especially with medical treatment, which are generally subclinical rather than giving rise to life-threatening pituitary apoplexy. Various tumors and other disease processes may occur within the sella simulating the imaging appearance of adenoma; however, their incidence in comparison with adenomas is negligible. Surgical resection is the first-line modality of treatment for macroadenomas, secreting and non-secreting. It seems that transsphenoidal resection of solid tumors with reduced diffusion on ADC maps is more likely to fail. Significant reduction of growth hormone (GH)-secreting tumors may be achieved by somatostatin analogs, preoperatively or when surgery is contraindicated. Radiation therapy, including radiosurgery, is used following incomplete surgical resection, particularly for tumors that are invading the cavernous sinus and are not in contact with the optic chiasm.

REFERENCES

1. Boxerman JL, Rogg JM, Donahue JE, *et al*. Preoperative MRI evaluation of pituitary macroadenoma: imaging features predictive of successful transphenoidal surgery. *AJR* 2010;**195**:720–8.

2. Rumboldt Z. Pituitary adenomas. *Top Magn Reson Imaging* 2006;**16**:277–88.

3. Cottier J-P, Destrieux C, Brunereau L, *et al*. Cavernous sinus invasion by pituitary adenoma: MR imaging. *Radiology* 2000;**215**:463–9.

4. Rogg JM, Tung GA, Anderson G, Cortez S. Pituitary apoplexy: early detection with diffusion-weighted MR imaging. *AJNR* 2002;**23**:1240–5.

5. Hammoud DA, Munter FM, Brat DJ, Pomper MG. Magnetic resonance imaging features of pituicytoma: analysis of 10 cases. *J Comput Assist Tomogr* 2010;**35**:757–61.

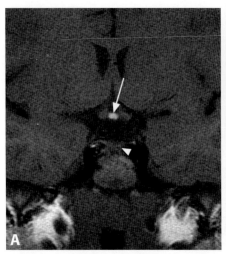
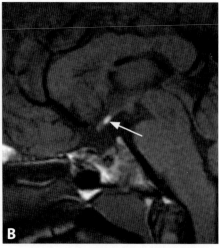

Figure 1. Coronal non-contrast T1WI through the sella (A) in a baby shows a bright spot (arrow) under the midline optic chiasm. The anterior pituitary lobe is present but small (arrowhead). Midsagittal T1WI (B) shows the bright spot (arrow) at the expected superior insertion of the pituitary stalk, which is absent. No other abnormalities were identified in this patient.

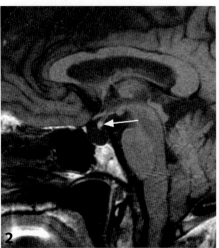
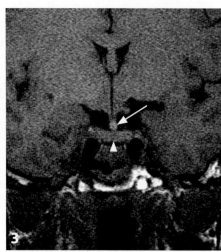

Figure 2. Midsagittal T1WI (A) in an adult shows absent intrasellar gland and a bright spot in the mid pituitary infundibulum (arrow). The inferior portion of the pituitary stalk is absent.

Figure 3. Coronal T1WI in a different patient also shows a bright spot (arrow) in the mid stalk but the anterior lobe (arrowhead) is clearly identified inside the sella.

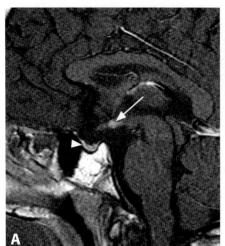
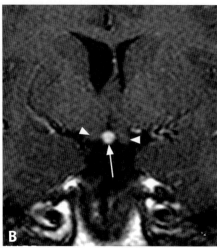

Figure 4. Midsagittal post-contrast T1WI (A) in another young adult shows hyperintense bright spot (arrow) in the hypothalamus at the expected insertion of the pituitary infundibulum, which is absent. The anterior pituitary lobe is small (arrowhead). Coronal post-contrast T1WI (B) shows the bright spot (arrow) between the optic radiations (arrowheads).

Ectopic Posterior Pituitary Lobe

MAURICIO CASTILLO

Specific Imaging Findings

CT is incapable of showing this abnormality and thus MR is the imaging method of choice. The pituitary stalk may be absent, truncated or very thin. The adenohypophysis (anterior pituitary lobe) is generally small but may be absent. The ectopic posterior pituitary lobe (EPPL) is bright on T1-weighted images and may be located anywhere along the expected stalk or in the hypothalamus at the stalk insertion. The EPPL is generally small, 1–3 mm in diameter and does not suppress with fat saturation techniques nor does it change significantly in size and signal intensity after administration of contrast. The intrasellar posterior lobe is absent in all cases. MRI is also the best modality to show the associated brain anomalies.

Pertinent Clinical Information

EPPL is more common in males and may be associated with midline defects (holoprosencephaly, septo-optic dysplasia, Joubert syndrome, midline facial dysraphisms, cleft palate and lip, central megaincisor, Dandy–Walker type malformations, and abnormalities of the olfactory nerves – Kallmann syndrome). This condition occurs in 1 : 5000–20 000 live births. It has been associated with difficult deliveries, and shearing of the stalk during head manipulation may account for it. Children are generally of short stature and delayed physical maturation. Hormones produced by the anterior pituitary gland are of low levels or absent, while those produced by the ectopic posterior lobe are normal or of near-normal levels. Treatment is geared towards replacement of hormones and other associated anomalies.

Differential Diagnosis

Lipoma (76)
- generally larger and more irregular in shape, suppresses with fat saturation
- posterior pituitary lobe in normal position

Dermoid Cyst (75)
- generally larger and more irregular in shape, suppresses with fat saturation
- posterior pituitary lobe in normal position

Craniopharyngioma (44)
- generally larger at diagnosis and with more complex signal intensities
- posterior pituitary lobe in normal position

Rathke's Cleft Cyst (38)
- generally intrasellar, when it involves the stalk it is larger
- posterior pituitary lobe in normal position

Pituitary Stalk Pseudoduplication
- enlarged infundibular recess of the third ventricle

Background

EPPL is also known as a translocated posterior pituitary. Hormones produced in the hypothalamus travel through axonal transport into a reservoir located in the posterior pituitary lobe and from there to the general circulation via the pituitary portal system. These hormones (mainly antidiuretic hormone and oxytocin) travel wrapped in neurosecretory granules, which account for their brightness once they become concentrated within the posterior lobe. Any situation in which the normal anatomic pathway from the hypothalamus to the posterior pituitary becomes interrupted impedes hormonal transport and results in their accumulation in the distal most aspect of the residual path. Thus, when the posterior lobe is ectopic, the normal bright posterior pituitary is not identifiable. The cause of this interruption may be genetic (several gene abnormalities have been found to be associated), vascular (infarction) or traumatic (shearing of the stalk). The posterior lobe may become ectopic when the gland is destroyed by tumor or surgery. EPPL may also be seen with midline anomalies.

REFERENCES

1. Mitchell LA, Thoams PQ, Zacharin MR, Scheffer IE. Ectopic posterior pituitary lobe and periventricular heterotopias: cerebral malformations with the same underlying mechanism? *AJNR* 2002;**23**:1475–81.

2. Kuroiwa T, Okabe Y, Hasuo K, *et al*. MR imaging of pituitary dwarfism. *AJNR* 1991;**21**:161–4.

3. Maintz D, Benz-Bohm G, Gindele A, *et al*. Posterior pituitary ectopia: another hint toward a genetic etiology. *AJNR* 2000;**21**: 1116–8.

4. di Iorgi N, Secco A, Napoli F, *et al*. Developmental abnormalities of the posterior pituitary gland. *Endocr Dev* 2009;**14**:83–94.

5. Rumboldt Z. Pituitary lesions. In: *Neuroradiology (Third Series) Test and Syllabus*. Castillo M, ed. American College of Radiology, Reston VA 2006;37–59.

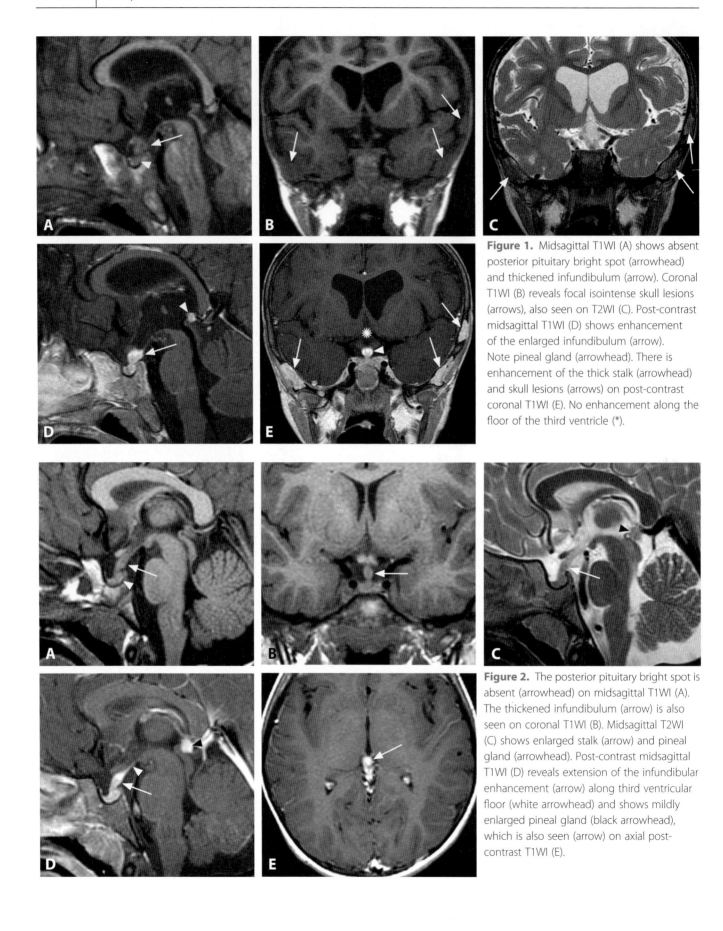

Figure 1. Midsagittal T1WI (A) shows absent posterior pituitary bright spot (arrowhead) and thickened infundibulum (arrow). Coronal T1WI (B) reveals focal isointense skull lesions (arrows), also seen on T2WI (C). Post-contrast midsagittal T1WI (D) shows enhancement of the enlarged infundibulum (arrow). Note pineal gland (arrowhead). There is enhancement of the thick stalk (arrowhead) and skull lesions (arrows) on post-contrast coronal T1WI (E). No enhancement along the floor of the third ventricle (*).

Figure 2. The posterior pituitary bright spot is absent (arrowhead) on midsagittal T1WI (A). The thickened infundibulum (arrow) is also seen on coronal T1WI (B). Midsagittal T2WI (C) shows enlarged stalk (arrow) and pineal gland (arrowhead). Post-contrast midsagittal T1WI (D) reveals extension of the infundibular enhancement (arrow) along third ventricular floor (white arrowhead) and shows mildly enlarged pineal gland (black arrowhead), which is also seen (arrow) on axial post-contrast T1WI (E).

Langerhans Cell Histiocytosis

ZORAN RUMBOLDT AND ANDREA ROSSI

Specific Imaging Findings

Cranial MRI findings in Langerhans cell histiocytosis (LCH) include: (1) lesions of the facial bones, skull base, and calvarium; (2) intracranial extra-axial lesions (hypothalamic–pituitary region, meninges, circumventricular organs); (3) intra-axial changes; and (4) cerebral atrophy. Intracranial findings are typically associated with central diabetes insipidus (DI) and characterized by lack of high signal intensity of the posterior pituitary gland on T1-weighted images (from loss of ADH storage granules) and thickened enhancing pituitary stalk, which measures over 3 and even 7 mm in diameter. However, the posterior pituitary bright spot may persist in DI patients; on the other hand, other disease processes may present in a similar fashion. Hypothalamic (along the floor of the third ventricle) involvement with contrast enhancement can be seen, while pituitary and optic chiasm infiltration are found in some cases. In a minority of patients the infundibulum may be very thin and thread-like, under 1 mm in diameter; it can even be normal on MRI. The pineal gland may also show mild enlargement and contrast enhancement. Progressive reduction in size of the anterior pituitary on MRI is associated with a higher risk of additional endocrine defects. Repeated MRI studies in DI patients are of limited value for assessing a response to therapy, but are important for monitoring bone lesions and possible parenchymal CNS disease.

Pertinent Clinical Information

LCH mainly affects children between 2 and 5 years of age with widely varying clinical manifestations and it may also occur in adults. CNS is affected in around 16% of patients, and DI is the most common manifestation (in 25%), followed by GH deficiency (in 10%) – usually diagnosed years after DI. However, a number of other diseases can cause DI and 30–50% of cases are considered idiopathic. LCH is usually self-limited in the absence of organ dysfunction. Brain involvement appears to be the single most important factor in determining quality of life.

Differential Diagnosis

Germinoma (67)
* frequent increase in the size of the anterior pituitary with thickening of the stalk
* isointense to dark on ADC maps
* increase in size on follow-up studies

Sarcoidosis, TB and Other Granulomatous Diseases (118, 160)
* rarely limited to the sellar region
* parenchymal granulomas may be present
* infiltration into the adjacent brain parenchyma is frequently observed with sarcoidosis

Lymphoma (135)
* rarely limited to the sellar region
* characteristically dark on ADC maps

Craniopharyngioma (44)
* cysts and/or calcifications are almost always present

Pituitary Adenoma (39, 41)
* a focal nodular lesion, typically enhancing less than the pituitary gland

Hypophysitis (40)
* characteristic dark cavernous sinuses and sellar diaphragm on T2WI
* the anterior lobe is very frequently involved and enlarged
* may be indistinguishable

Idiopathic Diabetes Insipidus
* may be indistinguishable

Background

LCH (formerly known as histiocytosis X) is a rare clonal proliferative disorder of a specific dendritic (Langerhans) cell belonging to the monocyte–macrophage system that often presents in childhood and ranges from a solitary lytic bone lesion to a potentially lethal widespread multisystem involvement. The exact pathophysiology is unknown.

The proliferating dendritic cells are S-100 and CD1a positive, and cytoplasmic rod-shaped Birbeck granules on electron microscopy are pathognomonic. Another striking feature is the presence of eosinophils, T cells and multinucleated giant cells. Infiltration of the hypothalamo-pituitary axis has been reported in between 5 and 50% of autopsies in patients with LCH.

REFERENCES

1. Prayer D, Grois N, Prosch H, *et al.* MR imaging presentation of intracranial disease associated with Langerhans cell histiocytosis. *AJNR* 2004;**25**:880–91.

2. Makras P, Samara C, Antoniou M, *et al.* Evolving radiological features of hypothalamo-pituitary lesions in adult patients with Langerhans cell histiocytosis (LCH). *Neuroradiology* 2006;**48**:37–44.

3. D'Ambrosio N, Soohoo S, Warshall C, *et al.* Craniofacial and intracranial manifestations of Langerhans cell histiocytosis: report of findings in 100 patients. *AJR* 2008;**191**:589–97.

4. Marchand I, Barkaoui MA, Garel C, *et al.* Central diabetes insipidus as the inaugural manifestation of Langerhans cell histiocytosis: natural history and medical evaluation of 26 children and adolescents. *J Clin Endocrinol Metab* 2011;**96**:E1352–60.

5. Maghnie M, Cosi G, Genovese E, *et al.* Central diabetes insipidus in children and young adults. *N Engl J Med* 2000;**343**:998–1007.

Brain Imaging with MRI and CT, ed. Zoran Rumboldt *et al.* Published by Cambridge University Press. © Cambridge University Press 2012.

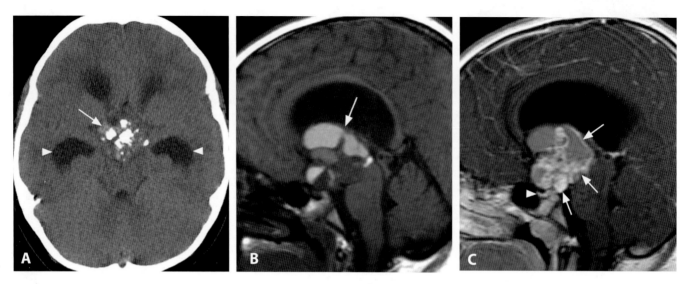

Figure 1. CT image (A) demonstrates suprasellar mass with calcifications (arrow). Hydrocephalus is also present (arrowheads). Midsagittal non-contrast T1WI (B) shows a multiloculated suprasellar mass (arrow) of varying predominantly bright signal intensities. Corresponding post-contrast image (C) shows enhancement of the walls and solid components (arrows). There is a normal pituitary gland in the sella (arrowhead).

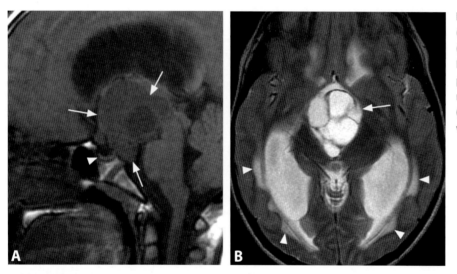

Figure 2. Midsagittal T1WI without contrast (A) shows a lobulated suprasellar mass (arrows) with slightly varying signal intensities. Note retrosellar extension behind a normal pituitary gland (arrowhead). Axial T2WI (B) reveals multicystic structure of the lesion (arrow). There is obstructive hydrocephalus with periventricular edema (arrowheads).

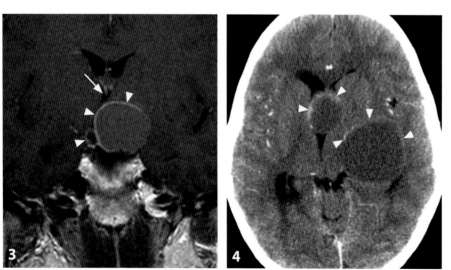

Figure 3. Coronal post-contrast T1WI shows a polycystic mass with thin wall enhancement (arrowheads) and compression on the third ventricle (arrow).

Figure 4. Enhanced axial CT image in another patient shows two oval cystic masses with thin peripheral enhancement (arrowheads).

Craniopharyngioma

MARIA VITTORIA SPAMPINATO

Specific Imaging Findings

The appearance of pediatric craniopharyngiomas is typical: they occupy the suprasellar cistern, have a cystic component and are partially calcified in 90% of cases. Multiple cysts with varying signal intensities are characteristic. Cystic components are typically hyperintense and less commonly isointense to the CSF on T1-weighted images. Fluid-debris levels may be present within the cysts. Solid components have variable signal intensities and they usually enhance with contrast. Enhancement may be minimal and limited to the cyst wall. Compression on the third ventricle is a common feature, which may be accompanied by obstructive hydrocephalus. Optic tract edema is commonly seen in craniopharyngiomas; however, it may occasionally be present in other parasellar tumors. Solid craniopharyngiomas are more common in adults and less frequently contain calcifications.

Pertinent Clinical Information

Patients commonly present with symptoms of increased intracranial pressure, including headache, nausea, vomiting, and symptoms of optic chiasm compression. The most common endocrine abnormality in children consists of growth disturbance, in about 80% of cases. Patients may also present with global hypopituitarism, hyperprolactinemia, or diabetes insipidus.

Differential Diagnosis

Pituitary Macroadenoma (41)
- originates from the sella
- usually isointense with brain and shows solid, frequently delayed, enhancement
- calcifications are rare

Rathke's cleft cyst (38)
- a single ovoid cyst without enhancing nodules, wall enhancement absent to minimal
- calcifications are uncommon, thin and peripheral
- intracystic nodules of low T2 signal may be present

Dermoid (75)
- homogeneous bright T1 signal similar to fat
- absence of enhancement

Epidermoid (143)
- signal similar to CSF on T1WI and T2WI
- heterogeneous signal on FLAIR and characteristically very bright on DWI
- absence of enhancement

Teratoma
- midline mass containing fat, cysts, soft tissue, and calcifications

Background

Craniopharyngiomas are common neoplasms, accounting for 2–5% of all intracranial tumors. They have a bimodal age distribution with a main peak between 5 and 14 years of age and a second smaller peak between the fifth and seventh decades of life. Craniopharyngiomas are thought to originate from remnants of the Rathke's pouch and can occur anywhere along the course of the craniopharyngeal duct, from the nasopharynx to the third ventricle. Most craniopharyngiomas have a suprasellar component, with only 4–25% being entirely intrasellar. Two subtypes of craniopharyngioma have been described: the adamantinomatous (cystic) type, which is more common in children and adolescents although it can be seen at any age, and the papillary (predominantly solid) type, which is seen almost exclusively in adults. Neoplastic cysts contain variable amounts of cholesterol, keratin, protein, methemoglobin, and necrotic debris, which account for their variable appearance on MRI. Treatment usually consists of surgical resection with or without adjuvant radiation therapy, based on whether gross total resection is achieved. Recurrence is infrequent after gross total resection. With subtotal resection, only 47% of patients are disease-free at 5 years, and only 38% are disease-free at 10 years.

REFERENCES

1. Choi SH, Kwon BJ, Na DG, et al. Pituitary adenoma, craniopharyngioma, and Rathke cleft cyst involving both intrasellar and suprasellar regions: differentiation using MRI. Clin Radiol 2007;62(5):453–62.

2. Huang BY, Castillo M. Nonadenomatous tumors of the pituitary and sella turcica. Top Magn Reson Imaging 2005;16:289–99.

3. Curran JG, O'Connor E. Imaging of craniopharyngioma. Childs Nervous System 2005;21:635–9.

4. Karavitaki N, Brufani C, Warner JT, et al. Craniopharyngiomas in children and adults: systematic analysis of 121 cases with long-term follow-up. Clin Endocrinol (Oxf) 2005;62:397–409.

5. Hirunpat S, Tanomkiat W, Sriprung H, Chetpaophan J. Optic tract edema: a highly specific magnetic resonance imaging finding for the diagnosis of craniopharyngiomas. Acta Radiol 2005;46:419–23.

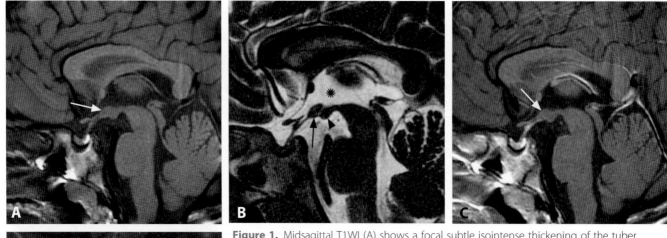

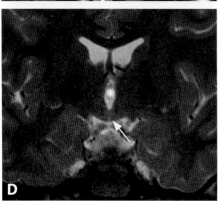

Figure 1. Midsagittal T1WI (A) shows a focal subtle isointense thickening of the tuber cinereum (arrow). Corresponding high resolution 3D T2WI (B) more clearly depicts the small hypothalamic mass (arrow), which is located just anterior to the mammillary body (arrowhead) and bulging upward into the third ventricle (*). The lesion (arrow) does not enhance on corresponding post-contrast T1WI (C). Coronal T2WI (D) shows midline hypothalamic fusion (arrow) at the floor of the third ventricle (*).

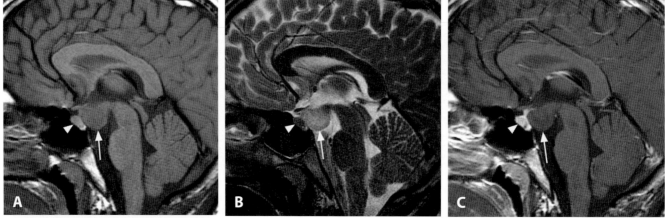

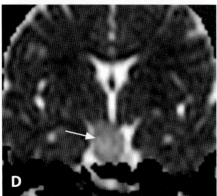

Figure 2. Midsagittal T1WI (A) and T2WI (B) images show a large mass (arrow) that is mildly T1 hypointense and T2 hyperintense with respect to the gray matter. The lesion is originating with a wide sessile base from the inferior surface of the hypothalamus and extends inferiorly, just behind the pituitary gland (arrowhead). There is no enhancement of the mass (arrow) on corresponding post-contrast T1WI (C), in contrast to the pituitary gland (arrowhead). Coronal ADC map (D) demonstrates hyperintensity of the lesion (arrow) compared to the brain parenchyma, consistent with increased diffusivity.

Hypothalamic Hamartoma

ANDREA ROSSI

Specific Imaging Findings

Owing to their isodensity with brain, hypothalamic hamartomas may be difficult to identify on CT scan when their size is small. On MRI, they appear as round to oval solid masses located within or attached to the tuber cinereum, interposed between the pituitary infundibulum anteriorly and the mammillary bodies posteriorly. They are attached with a sessile or pedunculated base to the floor of the third ventricle and typically project caudally into the interpeduncular cistern or, rarely, bulge upward into the third ventricle. The lesions vary in size from a few millimeters up to 4 centimeters. Smaller hamartomas are both T1 and T2 isointense with gray matter, while larger ones tend to be of lower T1 and higher T2 signal, probably because of a larger glial component. The lesions do not enhance with contrast material. Diffusion imaging shows normal to increased ADC values, MR spectroscopy primarily reveals increased *myo*-inositol levels, which correlate with glial component. In rare cases, a large cystic component is associated, extending uni- or bilaterally into the middle cranial fossa.

Pertinent Clinical Information

Patients with hypothalamic hamartomas may be asymptomatic with the lesion found incidentally. However, most patients typically present with either isosexual precocious puberty, caused by overproduction of luteinizing hormone-releasing hormone, or with a peculiar form of partial complex epilepsy called gelastic seizures, manifesting with clonic movements of the chest and diaphragm that simulate laughing. There is no clear-cut correlation between lesion size and clinical presentation, although there is a tendency for larger lesions to present with gelastic epilepsy. In rare instances, patients may have pituitary hormone deficiency ranging from isolated growth hormone deficit to panhypopituitarism, or present with cognitive/behavioural problems.

Differential Diagnosis

Craniopharyngioma (44, 202)
- partly solid, partly cystic suprasellar mass
- calcifications, cysts (at least in part) hyperintense on T1
- solid part enhances

Chiasmatic–Hypothalamic Astrocytoma (46, 173)
- extension to optic nerves and/or tracts may be present
- usually at least partly enhancing, often markedly
- possible association with NF1

Suprasellar Germinoma (67)
- patients present with diabetes insipidus
- enhancing thickening of infundibulum, pituitary stalk
- absent posterior pituitary "bright spot" on T1WI

Pituitary Duplication
- tubomammillary midline fusion produces thickening of third ventricular floor simulating hamartoma
- duplicated pituitary gland and stalk clearly shown on coronal images
- pituitary duplication and hypothalamic hamartoma might represent two parts of a developmental anomaly spectrum

Septo-Preoptic Holoprosencephaly
- minimal form of holoprosencephaly
- lack of midline cleavage in the septal, preoptic, and subcallosal telencephalic regions
- difficult to separate from small intrahypothalamic hamartomas, which are diencephalic in location

Background

Hypothalamic hamartomas are relatively rare congenital malformations that grow at the rate of, or slower than, the surrounding brain tissue. Histologically, they are composed of normal, albeit heterotopic, ganglionic cells, myelinated and unmyelinated fibers, and glial cells. Hypothalamic hamartomas are found in patients with the Pallister–Hall syndrome, an autosomal dominant disease consisting of the variable association of hypothalamic hamartoma, central and postaxial polydactyly, bifid epiglottis, imperforate anus, and renal abnormalities for which molecular genetic testing of *GLI3*, the only gene known to be associated with it, is available clinically. Other syndromes presenting with hamartoma of the hypothalamus include holoprosencephaly polydactyly syndrome (pseudotrisomy 13), Smith–Lemli–Opitz type 2, hydrolethalus syndrome, orofaciodigital type VI syndrome (Varadi–Papp syndrome), and the Cerebro-Acro-Visceral Early lethality (CAVE) syndrome. Treatment is effective in the majority of patients with hypothalamic hamartoma, and may be performed with microsurgery, stereotactic radiosurgery, or radiofrequency ablation.

REFERENCES

1. Booth TN, Timmons C, Shapiro K, Rollins NK. Pre- and postnatal MR imaging of hypothalamic hamartomas associated with arachnoid cysts. *AJNR* 2004;**25**:1283–5.

2. Amstutz DR, Coons SW, Kerrigan JF, *et al*. Hypothalamic hamartomas: correlation of MR imaging and spectroscopic findings with tumor glial content. *AJNR* 2006;**27**:794–8.

3. Freeman JL, Coleman LT, Wellard RM, *et al*. MR imaging and spectroscopic study of epileptogenic hypothalamic hamartomas: analysis of 72 cases. *AJNR* 2004;**25**:450–62.

4. Boudreau EA, Liow K, Frattali CM, *et al*. Hypothalamic hamartomas and seizures: distinct natural history of isolated and Pallister–Hall syndrome cases. *Epilepsia* 2005;**46**:42–7.

5. Rosenfeld JV. The evolution of treatment for hypothalamic hamartoma: a personal odyssey. *Neurosurg Focus* 2011;**30**:E1.

Brain Imaging with MRI and CT, ed. Zoran Rumboldt *et al*. Published by Cambridge University Press. © Cambridge University Press 2012.

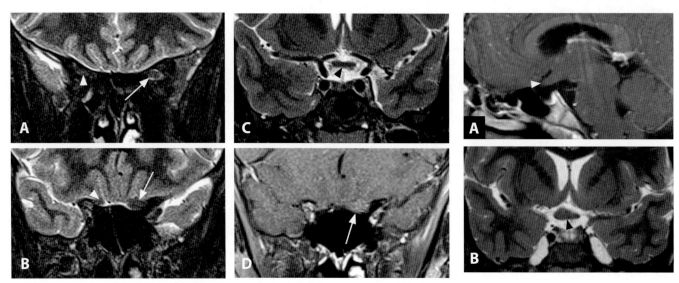

Figure 1. Coronal T2WIs (A–C) show that the left optic nerve is thickened (arrows) compared to the normal nerve on the right (white arrowheads). The optic chiasm is normal (black arrowhead). There is no enhancement of the involved nerve (arrow) on post-contrast T1WI with fat saturation (D).

Figure 2. Sagittal post-contrast T1WI (A) and coronal T2WI (B) show a non-enhancing fusiform enlargement of the right optic nerve and chiasm (arrowheads).

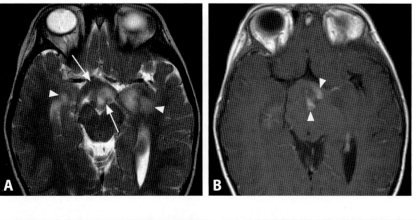

Figure 3. Axial T2WI (A) in a 9-year-old patient with progressive vision loss shows thickening and hyperintensity of the optic chiasm (arrow). The abnormal signal is extending beyond the optic tract into the temporal lobes (arrowheads). Post-contrast T1WI (B) reveals patchy areas of enhancement (arrowheads) within the lesion.

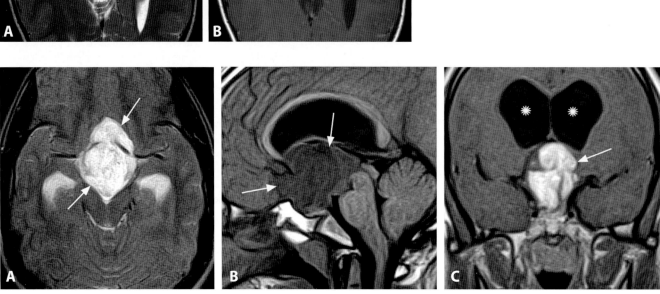

Figure 4. Axial T2WI (A) shows a markedly hyperintense mass (arrow) centered at the optic chiasm. Sagittal pre-contrast T1WI (A) and coronal post-contrast T1WI (B) show dense enhancement of this hypointense mass (arrows). The lesion is involving the hypothalamus and causing hydrocephalus (*).

Optic Glioma

MARIA GISELE MATHEUS

Specific Imaging Findings

Optic pathway gliomas (OPG) are found in the optic nerve, optic chiasm and optic tracts, with unilateral (most common) or bilateral distribution. They typically show fusiform enlargement of the optic pathway, which is iso- to hypodense on non-enhanced CT, T1 iso- to hypointense, and T2 iso- to hyperintense. Post-contrast enhancement varies from completely absent to intense. Kinking of the affected nerve and enlargement of the optic canal are frequently associated findings. OPG may show extension of neoplastic glial cells into the subarachnoid spaces with thickening and enhancement of the perioptic meninges, called "arachnoidal hyperplasia" or "arachnoidal gliomatosis". This finding is almost exclusively seen in patients with neurofibromatosis type-1 (NF-1). On the other hand, cystic components seen as focal well-demarcated areas of hypointense T1 and hyperintense T2 signal are much more common in the sporadic OPG. Sporadic OPGs also tend to be larger, extend beyond the optic pathways, and progress over time. Extension of hyperintense T2 signal into adjacent tissue, especially hypothalamus, is suggestive of invasion. The majority of the OPG are relatively benign tumors and spontaneous regression may occur, especially in association with NF-1. The enhancement pattern may change over time, appear and disappear, which is without clear clinical implications in NF-1 patients. Findings of relatively low *myo*-inositol levels on MR spectroscopy and of increased permeability on perfusion imaging are suggestive of more aggressive neoplasms.

Pertinent Clinical Information

OPG are often asymptomatic, while symptoms are based on the tumor location. Intraorbital OPG may lead to proptosis, strabismus or visual loss, whereas patients with intracranial lesions can present with visual loss, endocrine/hypothalamic disturbance and obstructive hydrocephalus. Overall, the most frequent clinical presentation is diminished vision. OPG associated with NF-1 has a classically indolent course. Management includes observation, surgical excision, chemotherapy, and irradiation.

Differential Diagnosis

Optic Neuritis
- dense contrast enhancement in the acute phase
- only mild thickening of the optic nerve
- typical T2 hyperintensity of the nerve
- typically acute loss of vision, eye tenderness or pain with movement
- may be indistinguishable

Optic Nerve Sheath Meningioma
- avidly enhancing mass encasing the optic nerve
- often shows calcifications and associated hyperostosis of the optic canal
- "dural tail" with intracranial involvement

Hypothalamic Astrocytoma
- arises from the hypothalamus displacing the optic chiasm
- may be indistinguishable as it may be very difficult to establish the site of origin

Hypothalamic Hamartoma (45)
- characteristically arises at the tuber cinereum
- absence of contrast enhancement

Background

OPGs account for approximately 5% of all brain tumors and 10–15% of supratentorial tumors in children, arising anywhere along the optic pathway, from just behind the globe to the occipital cortex. OPG are typically low-grade gliomas, usually pilocytic (PA) and less commonly fibrillary astrocytomas. About 20–30% of patients experience visual impairment, neurologic deficits, and even death. A majority of these tumors are diagnosed during the first decade of life, primarily in the setting of NF-1. Of individuals with NF1, 15–20% will develop an optic nerve PA, which typically shows benign behavior and most commonly arises along the optic nerves. Sporadic OPGs generally tend to be more aggressive and usually originate at the optic chiasm. Pilomyxoid astrocytomas have been recently added as a histological subgroup of OPG with aggressive growth and CSF dissemination. Even large, clinically symptomatic OPGs in non-NF1 patients may undergo spontaneous regression and this possibility should be considered in the planning of treatment.

REFERENCES

1. Kornreich L, Blaser S, Schwarz M, *et al*. Optic pathway glioma: correlation of imaging findings with the presence of neurofibromatosis. *AJNR* 2001;**22**:1963–9.

2. Jost SC, Ackerman JW, Garbow JR, *et al*. Diffusion-weighted and dynamic contrast-enhanced imaging as markers of clinical behavior in children with optic pathway glioma. *Pediatr Radiol* 2008;**38**:1293–9.

3. Harris LM, Davies NP, MacPherson L, *et al*. Magnetic resonance spectroscopy in the assessment of pilocytic astrocytomas. *Eur J Cancer* 2008;**44**:2640–7.

4. Nicolin G, Parkin P, Mabbott D, *et al*. Natural history and outcome of optic pathway gliomas in children. *Pediatr Blood Cancer* 2009;**53**:1231–7.

5. Parsa CF, Hoyt CS, Lesser RL, *et al*. Spontaneous regression of optic gliomas: thirteen cases documented by serial neuroimaging. *Arch Ophthalmol* 2001;**119**:516–29.

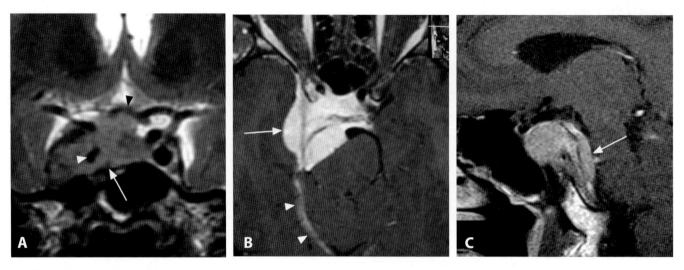

Figure 1. Coronal T2WI (A) shows a right parasellar mass (arrow) centered at the cavernous sinus that encases and narrows the cavernous internal carotid artery (white arrowhead). The optic chiasm is compressed (black arrowhead). Axial post-contrast T1WI with fat saturation (B) shows marked homogenous enhancement of the mass (arrow) with a broad dural base that extends along the tentorium forming a "dural tail" (arrowhead). Sagittal post-contrast T1WI shows extension along the clivus (arrow).

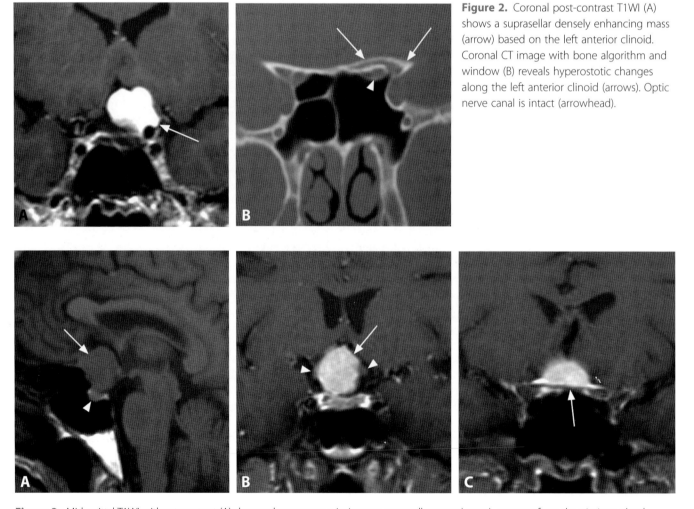

Figure 2. Coronal post-contrast T1WI (A) shows a suprasellar densely enhancing mass (arrow) based on the left anterior clinoid. Coronal CT image with bone algorithm and window (B) reveals hyperostotic changes along the left anterior clinoid (arrows). Optic nerve canal is intact (arrowhead).

Figure 3. Midsagittal T1WI without contrast (A) shows a homogenous isointense suprasellar mass (arrow), separate from the pituitary gland (arrowhead). Coronal post-contrast T1WI (B) reveals marked enhancement of the lesion (arrow), which laterally displaces the optic nerves (arrowheads). A more anterior image (C) of the homogenously enhancing mass shows its broad dural base (arrow) along the planum sphenoidale.

Perisellar Meningioma

ALESSANDRO CIANFONI

Specific Imaging Findings

Perisellar meningiomas originate from the dural walls of the cavernous sinus, the sellar diaphragm, or within the Meckel's cave, with the epicenter characteristically at the edge or outside the sella turcica, commonly suprasellar. The mass is typically hyperdense on CT and the tumor enhances avidly and homogeneously with contrast on CT and MRI. Similar to meningiomas in other locations, they are usually T1 isointense and slightly T2 hypointense to the cortex, of homogenous appearance. Sclerotic hyperostotic changes of the adjacent bone may be present. Like in other intracranial locations, they frequently demonstrate a tapered dural extension, known as the "dural tail" sign. Within the cavernous sinus meningiomas encase the internal carotid artery, typically significantly narrowing its lumen. Bilateral cavernous sinus involvement is occasionally found.

Pertinent Clinical Information

Meningiomas may be clinically silent and represent incidental findings, or can be the cause of different signs and symptoms depending on their size and location, due to compression of adjacent structures. The common presenting symptoms are ophthalmoplegia, visual disturbances, and trigeminal neuralgia. Hormonal disbalances, either increased (usually prolactin) or decreased pituitary hormone levels may also be encountered. The clinical and laboratory findings may simulate those of primary pituitary pathological processes, and imaging plays an essential role in the characterization of these lesions. Suprasellar meningiomas can cause visual field defects and obstructive hydrocephalus; retroclival meningiomas can cause dysfunction of the cranial nerves and brainstem compression; cavernous sinus invasion usually presents with ophthalmoplegia.

Differential Diagnosis

Pituitary Adenoma (41)
- the origin is usually clearly intrasellar, within the gland
- dural thickening is less prominent and only along the tentorium
- internal carotid artery narrowing is extremely rare with cavernous sinus invasion

Nerve Sheath Tumors (141)
- usually heterogenous high T2 signal
- no clear dural base
- grow along the cranial nerves, frequently with a "dumbbell" appearance with trigeminal nerve tumor present both in the basal cistern and Meckel's cave

Cavernous Sinus Hemangioma (48)
- very bright T2 signal, similar to CSF
- extremely avid and early enhancement

Perineural Tumor Spread (121)
- contrast enhancement extends extracranially along trigeminal nerve branches
- no dural base, no dural tail
- other cranial nerves may also be involved
- usually known head and neck cancer

Lymphoma/Inflammatory Masses (Tolosa–Hunt Syndrome, Sarcoidosis) (49, 118, 135)
- may be indistinguishable
- usually more infiltrating and less mass-like
- prompt response to corticosteroid treatment

Metastatic Neoplasm
- may be indistinguishable
- adjacent bone erosion (CT) and marrow infiltration (low T1 on MRI) may be present

Background

The most common mass lesions in the sellar region, following pituitary adenomas, cysts, and craniopharyngiomas, are meningiomas and aneurysms. About 10% of meningiomas occur in this location, where they usually arise at the junction of the clinoid processes and the sellar diphragm (known as tuberculum sella meningiomas), followed by the cavernous sinus and Meckel's cave. Vascularization is through the meningeal external carotid artery branches. Dural origin, extra-axial location, high vascularity and external carotid artery vascularization account for absence of the blood–brain barrier and therefore rapid and dense enhancement. Radiotherapy, including radiosurgery may be the treatment of choice, alone or in combination with microsurgical techniques, as it has a high control rate with few and mild complications.

REFERENCES

1. Cappabianca P, Cirillo S, Alfieri A, et al. Pituitary macroadenoma and diaphragma sellae meningioma: differential diagnosis on MRI. Neuroradiology 1999;41:22–6.
2. Rumboldt Z. Pituitary lesions. In: Neuroradiology (Third Series) Test and Syllabus. Castillo M, ed. American College of Radiology, Reston VA 2006;37–59.
3. Zee CS, Go JL, Kim PE, et al. Imaging of the pituitary and parasellar region. Neurosurg Clin N Am 2003;14:55–80.
4. Litré CF, Colin P, Noudel R, et al. Fractionated stereotactic radiotherapy treatment of cavernous sinus meningiomas: a study of 100 cases. Int J Radiat Oncol Biol Phys 2009;74:1012–7.
5. Spiegelmann R, Cohen ZR, Nissim O, et al. Cavernous sinus meningiomas: a large LINAC radiosurgery series. J Neurooncol 2010;98:195–202.

Brain Imaging with MRI and CT, ed. Zoran Rumboldt et al. Published by Cambridge University Press. © Cambridge University Press 2012.

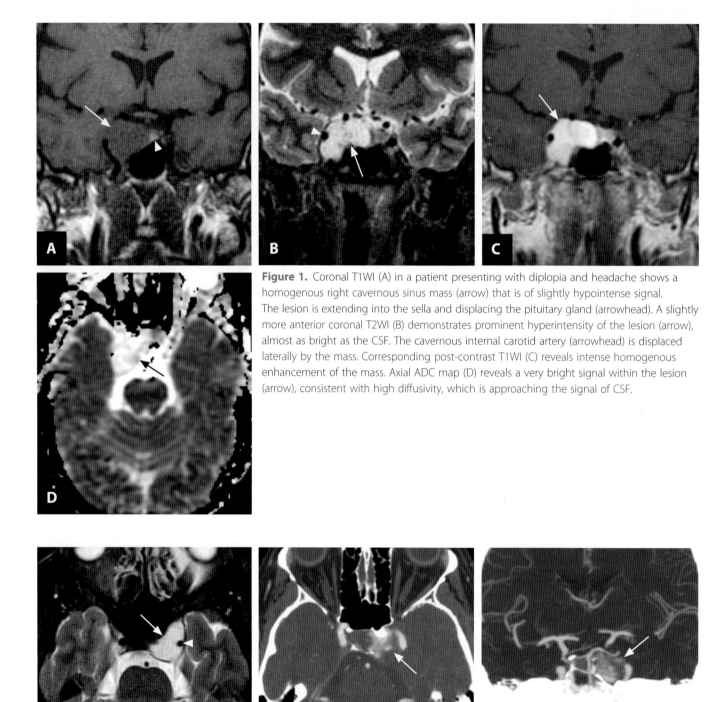

Figure 1. Coronal T1WI (A) in a patient presenting with diplopia and headache shows a homogenous right cavernous sinus mass (arrow) that is of slightly hypointense signal. The lesion is extending into the sella and displacing the pituitary gland (arrowhead). A slightly more anterior coronal T2WI (B) demonstrates prominent hyperintensity of the lesion (arrow), almost as bright as the CSF. The cavernous internal carotid artery (arrowhead) is displaced laterally by the mass. Corresponding post-contrast T1WI (C) reveals intense homogenous enhancement of the mass. Axial ADC map (D) reveals a very bright signal within the lesion (arrow), consistent with high diffusivity, which is approaching the signal of CSF.

Figure 2. Axial T2WI (A) shows a homogenous mass of very high signal (arrow) in the left cavernous sinus. The internal carotid artery (arrowhead) is displaced laterally. Axial source CTA image (B) shows prominent blush (arrow) within the mass following contrast bolus, which is perhaps even better demonstrated on a thick slab coronal reformatted image (C).

Hemangioma of the Cavernous Sinus

ZORAN RUMBOLDT

Specific Imaging Findings

Hemangioma (cavernous hemangioma, cavernous malformation) of the cavernous sinus shows characteristically marked T2 hyperintensity, approaching that of CSF. The tumors are typically homogenous and well-delineated, hypointense on T1-weighted images and with avid post-contrast enhancement. Enhancement may be homogenous or heterogenous, depending on the histologic type. Reflecting their large extracellular spaces, these benign neoplasms also show very high diffusion of water molecules, being almost as bright as CSF on ADC maps. Hemangiomas are hypodense on CT, remodeling of the adjacent bone may be present, without destruction or invasion. Similar to hemangiomas in other parts of the body, these vascular tumors demonstrate progressive filling in with contrast on dynamic and delayed MRI and CT images. Their very early enhancement following contrast bolus has a prominent tumor blush appearance, which may be appreciated on cranial CTA studies.

Pertinent Clinical Information

Cavernous sinus hemangioma may possibly be an incidental finding; however, they usually present with diplopia (extraocular muscle palsy, primarily oculomotor nerve), facial numbness, visual loss and headache. Optimal management is not clear at this time – total microsurgical removal is effective but may be extremely difficult and carries the risk of cranial nerve deficits; low-dose radiosurgery appears to lead to significant tumor shrinkage and clinical improvement. While radiosurgery may also be used following incomplete tumor excision, it is likely to become the treatment modality of choice.

Differential Diagnosis

Meningioma (47)
- usually low T2 signal, dural-based mass, frequently with a dural tail

Schwannoma (141)
- heterogenous with cystic areas, except when very small
- solid portions commonly of increased T2 signal, but not close to CSF
- common dumbbell shape, usually growing along the trigeminal nerve

Chondrosarcoma (53)
- arises from petro-clival junction
- bone destruction, common chondroid calcifications
- heterogenous T2 signal and contrast enhancement

Tolosa–Hunt Syndrome (orbital pseudotumor, idiopathic pachymeningitis) (49)
- not a well-delineated mass
- usually extends into the orbital apex
- not hyperintense on T2-weighted images

Perineural Tumor Spread (121)
- not so bright on T2-weighted images
- contrast enhancement extends extracranially along trigeminal nerve branches
- other cranial nerves may also be involved
- usually known head and neck cancer

Pituitary Adenoma (41)
- arises from the sella, not the cavernous sinus
- homogenous T2 hyperintensity is unusual

Background

Cavernous sinus hemangiomas represent only a small percentage (1–3%) of cavernous sinus masses and they may be of three histologic types: type A is sponge-like with intact pseudocapsule, type B is mulberry-like with incomplete or absent pseudocapsule, and type C consists of both type A and type B components. Tumors with homogeneous contrast enhancement on MRI correspond to histologic type A, whereas types B and C show heterogeneous enhancement. They arise within the cavernous sinus extending laterally by dissecting between the two layers of dura along the floor of the middle cranial fossa. These hemangiomas have rich vascularization, which is reflected in contrast staining on catheter angiograms and CTA studies. They may be dangerous for surgical treatment with the risk of excessive bleeding, but type A is easy to dissect from surrounding structures due to the presence of a pseudocapsule. Total or near-total resection is less common with types B and C. Given the accuracy of imaging and the potentially serious bleeding associated with biopsy sampling or attempted surgical removal, gamma knife radiosurgery may be the primary treatment in patients with a clear neuroimaging diagnosis of cavernous sinus hemangioma.

REFERENCES

1. Yao Z, Feng X, Chen X, Zee C. Magnetic resonance imaging characteristics with pathological correlation of cavernous malformation in cavernous sinus. *J Comput Assist Tomogr* 2006;**30**:975–9.

2. Sohn CH, Kim SP, Kim IM, *et al*. Characteristic MR imaging findings of cavernous hemangiomas in the cavernous sinus. *AJNR* 2003;**24**:1148–51.

3. Jinhu Y, Jianping D, Xin L, Yuanli Z. Dynamic enhancement features of cavernous sinus cavernous hemangiomas on conventional contrast-enhanced MR imaging. *AJNR* 2008;**29**:577–81.

4. Lombardi D, Giovanelli M, de Tribolet N. Sellar and parasellar extra-axial cavernous hemangiomas. *Acta Neurochir (Wien)* 1994;**130**:47–54.

5. Yamamoto M, Kida Y, Fukuoka S, *et al*. Gamma knife radiosurgery for hemangiomas of the cavernous sinus: a seven-institute study in Japan. *J Neurosurg* 2010;**112**:772–9.

Brain Imaging with MRI and CT, ed. Zoran Rumboldt *et al*. Published by Cambridge University Press. © Cambridge University Press 2012.

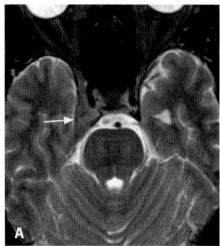
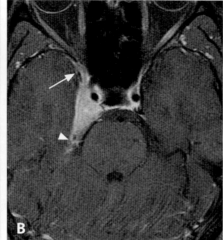
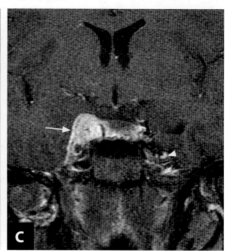
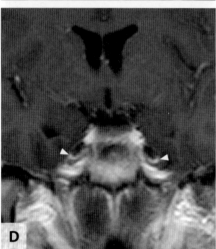

Figure 1. Axial T2WI at the level of the pons (A) shows abnormal intermediate to low signal intensity and expansion of the right cavernous sinus. The lateral dural margin is slightly convex and partially effaced (arrow). Corresponding post-contrast fat-saturated T1WI (B) demonstrates uniform contrast enhancement of the lesion. The process extends anteriorly into the adjacent superior orbital fissure (arrow) and posteriorly toward the tentorium (arrowhead). Note normal left cavernous sinus. Coronal post-contrast fat-saturated T1WI (C) shows enlarged enhancing right cavernous sinus (arrow) with a slightly convex lateral contour. Normal enhancing semilunar ganglion (arrowhead) is seen in the left Meckel's cave. Following treatment with corticosteroids, a coronal post-contrast T1WI 7 months later (D) shows complete resolution of the lesion. Note normal enhancement of bilateral semilunar ganglia (arrowheads).

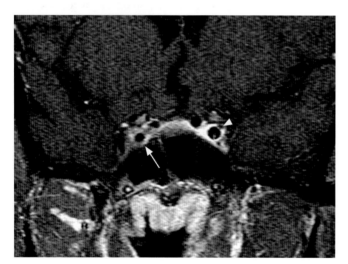

Figure 2. Coronal post-contrast T1WI with fat saturation shows minimal enlargement of the right cavernous sinus (arrow), which enhances less than the normal left cavernous sinus. Normal non-enhancing oculomotor nerve (arrowhead) is clearly depicted on the left, but not on the right, and the caliber of the cavernous internal carotid artery is smaller on the right.

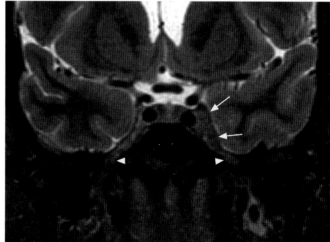

Figure 3. Coronal fat-saturated T2WI in a patient with left-sided painful ophthalmoplegia demonstrates slightly hypointense and enlarged left cavernous sinus (arrows). Note that the affected sinus also has a slightly convex lateral margin, compared to the slightly concave normal side. Bilateral mandibular nerves (arrowheads) at the foramen ovale are also seen.

Tolosa–Hunt Syndrome

BENJAMIN HUANG

Specific Imaging Findings

A unilateral, poorly defined cavernous sinus lesion is characteristic for Tolosa–Hunt syndrome (THS). The lesions are usually slightly dark on T2-weighted images, hypointense to gray matter, and cause increase in size of the sinus with convex bulging of the dural contour. Blurring or complete effacement of the normally hypointense lateral dura may also be present on T2-weighted images. Uniform enhancement is typical, but the degree of enhancement is usually less compared to the unaffected contralateral sinus. Dynamic post-contrast imaging may show small areas of delayed enhancement which gradually fill in on the delayed images. The ipsilateral internal carotid artery will be narrowed in almost one half of patients. In over a third of cases, the process extends anteriorly into the orbital apex via the superior orbital fissure, with abnormal enhancement best seen on fat-saturated post-contrast images. Optic nerve sheath may also be involved.

Pertinent Clinical Information

Painful ophthalmoplegia is the clinical hallmark of THS. Patients classically present with acute, severe periorbital or retroorbital pain followed within days by the onset of diplopia. Visual loss can occur if there is optic nerve involvement. The process is usually unilateral and the diagnosis is based on criteria established by the International Headache Society: (1) one or more episodes of unilateral orbital pain persisting for weeks if untreated; (2) paresis of one or more of the cranial nerves III, IV, or VI and/or demonstration of a granuloma by MRI or biopsy; (3) paresis coinciding with the onset of pain or following it within 2 weeks; (4) resolution of pain and paresis within 72 h of adequate treatment with corticosteroids; and (5) exclusion of other causes with appropriate investigations. Although symptoms are rapidly relieved by steroids, approximately 40% of patients will experience a relapse on either the ipsilateral or, less commonly, contralateral side.

Differential Diagnosis

Meningioma; Sarcoidosis; Lymphoma; Metastasis (47, 118, 135)
- intense contrast enhancement
- may demonstrate dural tail

Carotid–Cavernous Fistula (50)
- proptosis common
- enlarged superior ophthalmic vein
- may see flow voids in the cavernous sinus

Infectious Thrombophlebitis
- usually associated with paranasal sinus disease
- filling defect in cavernous sinus on contrast enhanced imaging

Perineural Spread of Tumor (121)
- extracranial spread along a branch of trigeminal nerve
- other cranial nerves may be affected
- primary head and neck tumor is usually evident

Normal Cavernous Sinus Asymmetry
- no evidence of superior orbital fissure or orbital apex involvement
- signal and enhancement similar to the contralateral cavernous sinus
- normal homogeneous dynamic contrast enhancement

Background

It has been suggested that THS represents a variant of idiopathic inflammatory orbital pseudotumor, and that both of these processes may be within the spectrum of idiopathic inflammatory pachymeningitis. Histologically, THS shows nonspecific inflammation with proliferation of fibroblasts and infiltration of the septa and wall of the cavernous sinus with lymphocytes and plasma cells. Symptoms are likely due to compression of the cranial nerves as they travel through the cavernous sinus. The process may involve the walls of the internal carotid artery, leading to wall thickening and luminal narrowing. The etiology of THS remains unknown, and it is unclear what triggers the inflammatory process which characterizes the syndrome. MR imaging is considered the initial screening study in patients with suspected THS. MRI findings before and after corticosteroid therapy are important diagnostic criteria for the definitive diagnosis of THS and for distinction from other cavernous sinus lesions.

REFERENCES

1. Schuknecht B, Sturm V, Huisman TA, Landau K. Tolosa–Hunt syndrome: MR imaging features in 15 patients with 20 episodes of painful ophthalmoplegia. *Eur J Radiol* 2009;**69**:445–53.
2. Haque TL, Miki Y, Kashii S, *et al*. Dynamic MR imaging in Tolosa–Hunt syndrome. *Eur J Radiol* 2004;**51**:209–17.
3. Yousem DM, Atlas SW, Grossman RI, *et al*. MR imaging of Tolosa–Hunt syndrome. *AJNR* 1989;**10**:1181–4.
4. Colnaghi S, Versino M, Marchioni E, *et al*. ICHD-II diagnostic criteria for Tolosa–Hunt syndrome in idiopathic inflammatory syndromes of the orbit and/or the cavernous sinus. *Cephalalgia* 2008;**28**:577–84.
5. Kline LB, Hoyt WF. The Tolosa–Hunt syndrome. *J Neurol Neurosurg Psychiatry* 2001;**71**:577–82.

Brain Imaging with MRI and CT, ed. Zoran Rumboldt *et al*. Published by Cambridge University Press. © Cambridge University Press 2012.

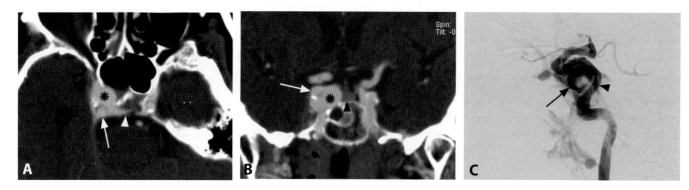

Figure 1. Axial source CTA image (A) shows enlarged enhancing right cavernous sinus (*) and a venous channel connecting the two cavernous sinuses (arrowhead). Right internal carotid artery (ICA; arrow) is seen without presence of direct communication with the sinuses on this image. A coronal CT image reconstructed from the CTA (B) shows the right ICA cavernous segment (white arrow) with associated wall calcification adjacent to the enlarged cavernous sinus (*), from which it cannot be separated. Pituitary gland (black arrow) is mildly displaced. Lateral DSA image following right ICA injection (C) reveals filling of the cavernous sinus (arrow) in the early arterial phase from the ICA (arrowhead).

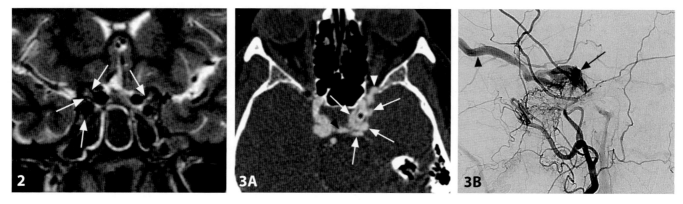

Figure 2. Coronal T2WI through the sella shows multiple linear flow-voids (arrows) that are continuous with cavernous segments of bilateral ICAs.

Figure 3. Axial source CTA image (A) demonstrates contrast filling different compartments (arrows) of an enlarged left cavernous sinus. There is also filling of an enlarged left superior ophthalmic vein (SOV; arrowhead). Left ICA (*) appears separated from the sinus on this image. Right cavernous sinus may also be enlarged. Lateral DSA image following left external carotid artery injection (B) demonstrates early opacification of the cavernous sinus (arrow) and SOV (arrowhead).

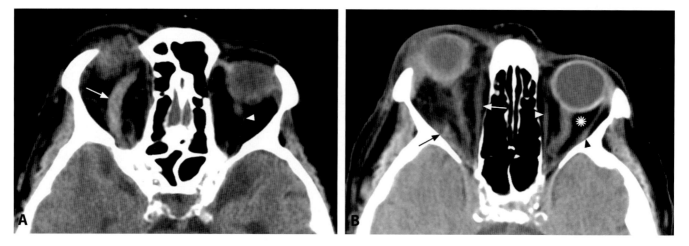

Figure 4. Axial non-enhanced CT image through the superior aspect of the orbits (A) shows a dilated right SOV (arrow). Note normal caliber of the contralateral vein (arrowhead). There is also proptosis. CT through the mid-orbit (B) shows thickening of the right-sided extraocular muscles (arrows) and extensive intraconal edema, seen as overall increased attenuation with fat stranding. Compare to the contralateral normal dark intraconal fat (*) and thin extraocular muscles (arrowheads).

Carotid-Cavernous Sinus Fistula

ZORAN RUMBOLDT

Specific Imaging Findings

The cavernous sinus (CS) ipsilateral to the side of the carotid-cavernous sinus fistula (CCF) is typically enlarged with prominent contrast enhancement, and bilateral CS enlargement may be seen. T2-weighted MR images usually show abnormal flow voids within the CS, which may communicate with the cavernous internal carotid artery (ICA). Abnormal hyperintense flow is also present adjacent to the cavernous ICA on TOF MRA and the fistula site may be observed with other high resolution 3D MRI techniques and, usually to a better advantage, with CTA. Asymmetric and/or diminished pituitary gland enhancement may sometimes be observed. Additional imaging findings are primarily intraorbital: enlarged superior ophthalmic vein (SOV), thickened bulky extraocular muscles, proptosis, and intraorbital edema. Signs of intracranial venous congestion with engorged vessels and cerebral venous hypertension with white matter T2 hyperintensity may be present. Definite diagnosis is with cerebral DSA.

Pertinent Clinical Information

Most cases of CCF are post-traumatic, including rare iatrogenic causes (such as trans-sphenoidal surgery and Gasserian ganglion ablation). Based on the nature of the fistula, CCF is divided into direct and indirect types. Direct CCF is a high-flow lesion and the typical clinical presentation includes the triad of exophthalmos, bruit, and conjunctival chemosis. Diplopia (caused by ophthalmoplegia from compression of the cranial nerves), headache, retroorbital pain, development of glaucoma and decreasing visual acuity may be present in advanced cases. Indirect CCF is a dural arteriovenous fistula (DAVF) and may be of a low-flow or a high-flow variety. It is spontaneous in about 20% of patients, relatively common in postmenopausal women, and may be congenital. Indirect CCF may improve or even heal spontaneously. The treatment of high flow CCF is endovascular embolization, using transvenous or/and transarterial routes. Low flow indirect fistulas may be treated conservatively, including repetitive manual carotid compression by the patient.

Differential Diagnosis

Tolosa–Hunt Syndrome (49)
- absence of flow-voids within the sinus, which is of homogenous low T2 signal
- absence of associated intraorbital findings
- rapid response to corticosteroid treatment

Meningioma (47)
- mass of usually low T2 signal, without flow-voids
- enhancing dural tail may be present

SOV/Cavernous Sinus Thrombosis
- presence of CT hyperdense/T1 hyperintense clot

Thyroid Ophthalmopathy
- thickened bulky extraocular muscles without extraorbital findings
- normal SOV

Orbital Pseudotumor
- intraorbital involvement usually without extraorbital findings
- absence of pathologic flow-voids, normal SOV

Background

Direct CCF is simply described as a single hole connecting ICA with CS and also classified as Type A according to the Barrow's classification. Indirect CCFs are DAVFs and are classified according to the arterial feeders: type B is supplied by ICA branches; external carotid artery (ECA) dural branches are responsible for type C; type D is the most common with contributions from both ICA and ECA. The proximal horizontal segment of the ICA is particularly vulnerable and exposed to traumatic injury. In addition to traumatic causes, pre-existing cavernous ICA aneurysm, weakened vessel wall from inflammatory vascular diseases, and venous thrombosis may be responsible for the fistula. CCFs lead to increased CS pressure with subsequent orbital venous congestion, cranial neuropathies, and glaucoma. MRA and, especially, CTA offer valuable information and may identify the site of the fistula, which is likely to further improve with developing rapid time-resolved (4D) techniques. At the present time, DSA remains the diagnostic modality of choice as it also identifies important associated abnormalities, such as pseudoaneurysms, sinus varices, and cortical venous reflux.

REFERENCES

1. Chen CC, Chang PC, Shy CG, et al. CT angiography and MR angiography in the evaluation of carotid cavernous sinus fistula prior to embolization: a comparison of techniques. AJNR 2005;26:2349–56.

2. Hirai T, Korogi Y, Hamatake S, et al. Three-dimensional FISP imaging in the evaluation of carotid cavernous fistula: comparison with contrast-enhanced CT and spin-echo MR. AJNR 1998;19:253–9.

3. Marques MC, Pereira Caldas JG, Nalli DR, et al. Follow-up of endovascular treatment of direct carotid-cavernous fistulas. Neuroradiology 2010;52:1127–33.

4. Tsai YF, Chen LK, Su CT, et al. Utility of source images of three-dimensional time-of-flight magnetic resonance angiography in the diagnosis of indirect carotid-cavernous sinus fistulas. J Neuroophthalmol 2004;24:285–9.

5. Nishimura S, Hirai T, Sasao A, et al. Evaluation of dural arteriovenous fistulas with 4D contrast-enhanced MR angiography at 3T. AJNR 2010;31:80–5.

Brain Imaging with MRI and CT, ed. Zoran Rumboldt *et al.* Published by Cambridge University Press. © Cambridge University Press 2012.

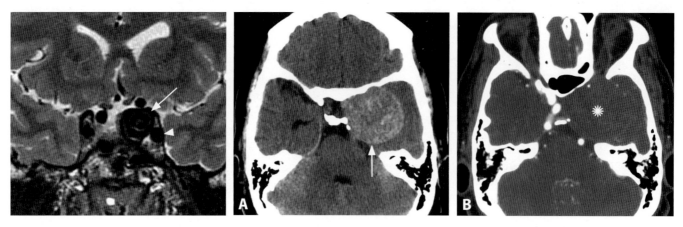

Figure 1. Coronal T2WI shows a round, laminated "onion skin" dark sellar mass (arrow) adjacent to the left internal carotid artery (ICA; arrowhead).

Figure 2. Axial non-enhanced CT image (A) in a patient with left-sided ophthalmoplegia shows a hyperdense round left parasellar mass (arrow). A source axial CTA image (B) shows absence of contrast enhancement within the completely thrombosed mass (*).

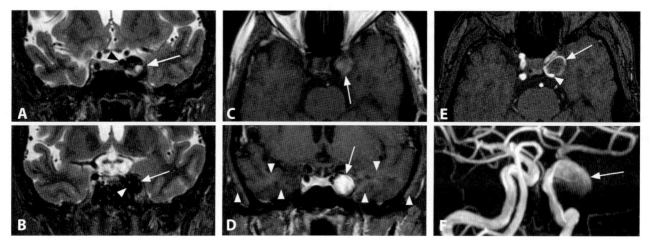

Figure 3. Coronal T2WI (A) shows a round left cavernous sinus mass (arrow) with dark and bright layers, just lateral to the ICA (arrowhead). The lesion (arrow) is inseparable from the ICA (arrowhead) on another T2WI (B). Axial T1WI (C) reveals increased signal of the mass (arrow) and mild pulsatility artifact, which is better seen (arrowheads) on post-contrast coronal T1WI (D) also showing dense lesion enhancement (arrow). Axial 3D TOF magnetic resonance angiography (MRA) source image (E) shows peripheral hyperintensity of the mass, inseparable from the ICA (arrowhead). On MRA maximum intensity projection (MIP; F) the lesion is relatively faint, with ill-defined inferior margin.

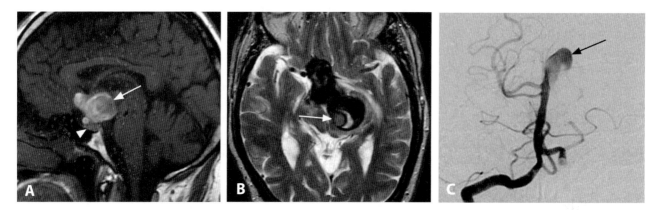

Figure 4. Sagittal T1WI without contrast (A) shows a lobulated bright mass (arrow) just above the pituitary gland (arrowhead). Axial T2WI (B) reveals very low signal of the lesion with an area of layered appearance (arrow) compressing the midbrain (arrowhead). Frontal view of DSA following right vertebral artery injection (C) shows that a small portion of the mass is filling with contrast (arrow) from the basilar artery.

Perisellar Aneurysm

ALESSANDRO CIANFONI

Specific Imaging Findings

Perisellar aneurysms are rarely visible on non-enhanced CT if not calcified or large, when isodense outpouching or lobulation may be present along the course of the vessels, usually cavernous or paraclinoid internal carotid artery (ICA) segments. Sometimes very large aneurysms from other intracranial vessels, primarily the basilar or the anterior communicating arteries, may present as perisellar masses. A small aneurysm in a perisellar location can manifest as a cavernous sinus asymmetry, while large ones may erode into the sphenoid sinus and sella turcica. The aneurysm wall may be calcified, and intraluminal thrombus is hyperdense. Patent aneurysmal lumen enhances the same as the other vessels on post-contrast CT. On T2WI a flow-void outpouching may be seen adjacent to the parent vessel, while the presence of a thrombus leads to T1 hyperintensity. In larger aneurysms a laminated "onion skin" appearance may be seen, due to clot apposition within the lumen, and a pulsatility artifact can be noted along the phase-encoding direction. Post-contrast MRI findings are variable and unpredictable – from flow-void to hyperintensity, due to thrombosis and turbulent flow. CTA, 3D TOF MRA, and contrast-enhanced MRA have very high sensitivity and accuracy for aneurysms. CTA may be limited for aneurysms within the enhancing cavernous sinus and at the skull base. Large aneurysms may be underestimated or even completely absent on TOF MRA due to saturation artifacts caused by turbulent flow. Important diagnostic questions in intracranial aneurysms are patency versus thrombosis, and extra- versus intra-dural location. On CTA the inferior margin of the optic strut marks the likely transition between extra- and intra-dural ICA portions. Direct visualization of the dural ring, as a thin hypointense line, may be achievable on high-resolution volumetric T2WI.

Pertinent Clinical Information

Unruptured aneurysms may clinically present due to compression of the adjacent structures, such as with opthalmoplegia and pituitary dysfunction, or due to embolic events. Misdiagnosis of a neoplasm is rare but can have disastrous consequences and a high level of diagnostic suspicion is necessary in this region. The extra- versus intra-dural location defines prognosis and guides treatment of perisellar aneuryms. The extra-dural ICA aneurysms, confined within the dural reflections of the cavernous sinus, have no potential for subarachnoid hemorrhage, their rupture is not life-threatening, and are usually not treated prophylactically.

Differential Diagnosis

Cavernous Sinus Hemangioma (48)

- avid vascular enhancement is usually slightly delayed on CTA
- extremely T2 bright and homogenous

Craniopharyngioma (and other sellar/perisellar tumors) (44)

- absence of flow-void and continuity with arterial structures
- "onion skin" appearance is highly unusual

Pneumatized Anterior Clinoid

- absence of MR signal caused by the air may mimic flow-void on T1WI and T2WI
- CT is diagnostic demonstrating bone pneumatization

Background

Intracranial ICA aneurysms can be named following the al-Rodhan topographic classification (from proximal to distal: cavernous, transitional, carotid cave, and then the intra-dural ophthalmic, ventral paraclinoid, and superior hypophyseal). If there is partial thrombosis within the aneurysm lumen, which is common in large aneurysms, catheter angiography may significantly underestimate the aneurysm size. In 1–2% of the population the ICA is tortuous, and sometimes has intrasellar extension. This medial deviation may be bilateral, and is known as "kissing carotids". These variations may cause apparent enlargement of a displaced pituitary gland, which should not be confused with an adenoma. It is important to recognize these variations in patients in whom transsphenoidal surgery is planned in order to avoid inadvertent ICA injuries.

REFERENCES

1. Watanabe Y, Nakazawa T, Yamada N, *et al.* Identification of the distal dural ring with use of fusion images with 3D-MR cisternography and MR angiography: application to paraclinoid aneurysms. *AJNR* 2009;**30**:845–50.
2. Gonzalez LF, Walker MT, Zabramski JM, *et al.* Distinction between paraclinoid and cavernous sinus aneurysms with computed tomographic angiography. *Neurosurgery* 2003;**52**:1131–7.
3. Lee N, Jung JY, Huh SK, *et al.* Distinction between intradural and extradural aneurysms involving the paraclinoid internal carotid artery with T2-weighted three-dimensional fast spin-echo magnetic resonance imaging. *J Korean Neurosurg Soc* 2010;**47**:437–41.
4. al-Rodhan NR, Piepgras DG, Sundt TM Jr. Transitional cavernous aneurysms of the internal carotid artery. *Neurosurgery* 1993;**33**:993–6.
5. Jäger HR, Ellamushi H, Moore EA, *et al.* Contrast-enhanced MR angiography of intracranial giant aneurysms. *AJNR* 2000;**21**:1900–7.

Brain Imaging with MRI and CT, ed. Zoran Rumboldt *et al.* Published by Cambridge University Press. © Cambridge University Press 2012.

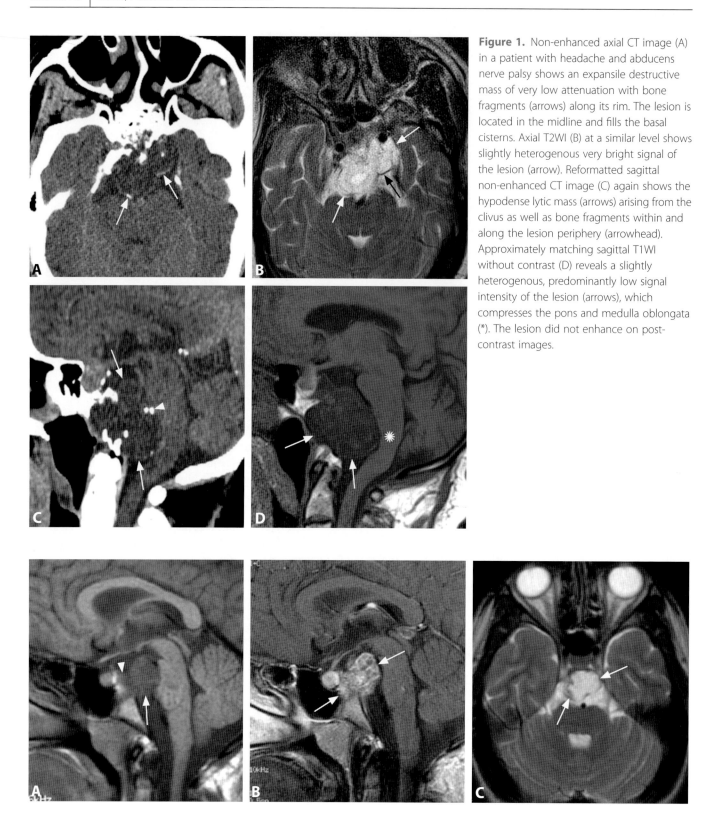

Figure 1. Non-enhanced axial CT image (A) in a patient with headache and abducens nerve palsy shows an expansile destructive mass of very low attenuation with bone fragments (arrows) along its rim. The lesion is located in the midline and fills the basal cisterns. Axial T2WI (B) at a similar level shows slightly heterogenous very bright signal of the lesion (arrow). Reformatted sagittal non-enhanced CT image (C) again shows the hypodense lytic mass (arrows) arising from the clivus as well as bone fragments within and along the lesion periphery (arrowhead). Approximately matching sagittal T1WI without contrast (D) reveals a slightly heterogenous, predominantly low signal intensity of the lesion (arrows), which compresses the pons and medulla oblongata (*). The lesion did not enhance on post-contrast images.

Figure 2. Midsagittal T1WI without contrast (A) shows a hypodense mass (arrow) filling the prepontine cistern and compressing the pons. The lesion is also involving the bone of the dorsum sellae (arrowhead) just behind the pituitary gland. Matching post-contrast T1WI (B) shows heterogenous enhancement of the mass (arrows) that extends from the sphenoid sinus to the brainstem. Axial T2WI (C) shows a very high signal of the midline mass (arrows), similar to the CSF.

Chordoma

ALESSANDRO CIANFONI AND ZORAN RUMBOLDT

Specific Imaging Findings

Chordoma is typically an exophytic mass centered in or around the clivus, characteristically at the midline. It is usually hypodense on CT, iso- to hypointense on T1WI, while predominantly and distinctively of high T2 signal. Chordomas often show septations and lobulations, giving a typical "honeycomb" heterogeneous appearance, with possible round areas of high T1 and low T2 signal. In rare cases they may be predominantly T2 hypointense. Areas of necrosis, hemorrhage, and sequestered bone fragments can cause signal heterogeneity. Chordomas show high diffusion with bright appearance on ADC maps. Post-contrast enhancement is usually heterogeneous and mild, and may be completely absent. CT shows to a better advantage the lytic nature of the lesion, with possible but rare areas of calcification and bone sequestra. Around 15% of these tumors originate off the midline.

Pertinent Clinical Information

The growth of chordomas is usually slow, which accounts for their insidious clinical presentation, often with headache, and/or cranial nerve deficits, most commonly abducens nerve palsy. Both CT and MRI are usually necessary for complete evaluation due to the involvement of soft tissue and bony structures at the skull base.

Differential Diagnosis

Chondrosarcoma (53)
- may be indistinguishable
- characteristically centered off midline, originating from the petro-clival junction
- chondroid matrix calcification (linear, globular, arc-like) is diagnostic, when present

Meningioma (47)
- absence of bone destruction
- isointense to low T2 signal, low ADC values
- intense and homogeneous contrast enhancement

Plasmocytoma/Metastasis
- typically pure lytic bone lesions, prominent exophytic component is rare
- usually darker T2 signal and lower ADC values
- usually more homogeneous pre- and post-contrast appearance

Nasopharyngeal Cancer
- mucosal/submucosal nasopharyngeal origin
- frequent neck lymphadenopathy
- lower T2 signal and ADC values

Pituitary Macroadenoma and Craniopharyngioma (41, 43)
- intrasellar or suprasellar epicenter
- remodeling without bone invasion

Background

Chordomas can be encountered in all age groups, with a peak in the fourth decade of life. They are locally invasive neoplasms originating from notochord remnants. Chordomas of the spheno-occipital synchondrosis represent 35% of chordomas in the adult population, 4% of primary bone tumors, and 1% of all intracranial tumors. They are soft masses at surgery, with gelatinous mucinous components, likely responsible for the high T2 signal and heterogeneous enhancement. In the chondroid variant (1/3 in this location) cartilaginous matrix is found in place of the mucinous component, resulting in generalized lower T2 signal, and more frequent intratumoral calcifications visible on CT. Both chordoma types demonstrate an aggressive clinical course and poor outcome after disease recurrence. The optimal treatment involves radical or near-total surgical resection followed by high-dose radiotherapy. These tumors are locally invasive and frequently recur, but metastases are very rare. Dedifferentiation and sarcomatous degeneration occurs in a few percent of cases. The prognosis is worse compared to chondrosarcomas in the similar location with the 5-year recurrence-free survival in the range of 50–60% and 5-year overall survival around 80%.

REFERENCES

1. Erdem E, Angtuaco EC, Van Hemert R, et al.
Comprehensive review of intracranial chordoma. *Radiographics* 2003;**23**:995–1009.
2. Weber AL, Liebsch NJ, Sanchez R, Sweriduk ST Jr. Chordomas of the skull base. Radiologic and clinical evaluation. *Neuroimaging Clin N Am* 1994;**4**:515–27.
3. Pamir MN, Ozduman K. Analysis of radiological features relative to histopathology in 42 skull-base chordomas and chondrosarcomas. *Eur J Radiol* 2006;**58**:461–70.
4. Almefty K, Pravdenkova S, Colli BO, et al. Chordoma and chondrosarcoma: similar, but quite different, skull base tumors. *Cancer* 2007;**110**:2457–67.
5. Yoneoka Y, Tsumanuma I, Fukuda M, et al. Cranial base chordoma – long term outcome and review of the literature. *Acta Neurochir (Wien)* 2008;**150**:773–8.

Brain Imaging with MRI and CT, ed. Zoran Rumboldt *et al.* Published by Cambridge University Press. © Cambridge University Press 2012.

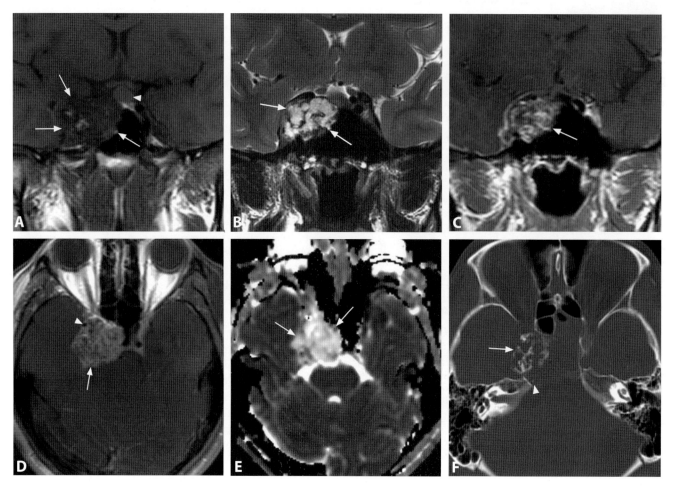

Figure 1. Coronal T1WI (A) shows a predominantly hypointense mass (arrows) with a few small bright areas, lateral and inferior to the pituitary gland (arrowhead). A more anterior coronal T2WI (B) reveals a bright signal of the mass (arrows) with linear areas of very low signal. Post-contrast coronal T1WI (C) shows a multi-septated enhancement of the lesion (arrow). Axial post-contrast image (D) again shows the heterogenous enhancement (arrow). The right internal carotid artery (white arrowhead) is displaced and surrounded by the lesion. ADC map (E) shows very high diffusion of the mass (arrows). Axial CT image with bone algorithm and window (F) reveals septated calcifications within the mass (arrow), corresponding to the T2 hypointense linear areas in B. The lesion has eroded the right petro-clival junction (white arrowhead).

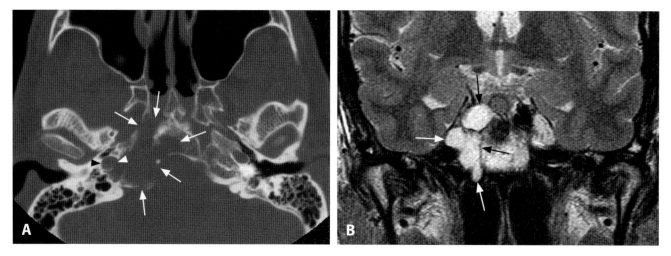

Figure 2. Axial CT image in bone algorithm and window (A) in a different patient shows a lytic expansile lesion (arrows) centered at the right petro-clival junction. Ipsilateral carotid canal (black arrowhead) is well seen, with the mass eroding its medial wall (white arrowhead). No intralesional calcifications are present. Coronal T2WI (B) shows a striking hyperintensity of the right skull base mass (arrows).

Specific Imaging Findings

The characteristic appearance of chondrosarcoma is a mass eroding the petro-clival junction. These tumors show low to intermediate T1 signal and predominantly very bright T2 signal. Heterogenous appearance is frequent with areas of signal loss on T2-weighted images (sometimes along with T1 hyperintensity), caused by matrix mineralization and/or fibrocartilaginous elements. The matrix mineralization with whirls of calcifications represents a very characteristic CT finding, but this is present in less than half of the cases. These tumors are also bright on ADC maps, reflecting very high diffusion. Chondrosarcomas show variable intensity of post-contrast enhancement, usually in a heterogeneous fashion with linear and nodular areas. Distinction from chordomas is not reliable. In rare cases chondrosarcomas may arise at unusual locations, such as the jugular foramen or from the dura of the falx.

Pertinent Clinical Information

Chondrosarcomas are uncommon locally aggressive skull base tumors, which most commonly occur in young patients (on average in the third decade of life) with diplopia (commonly caused by the abducens nerve palsy) and headaches being the most common presenting symptoms. These are generally low-grade tumors, with gradual and slow onset of symptoms, usually with a protracted course before the diagnosis is made. Both CT and MRI are usually necessary for complete evaluation due to the involvement of both soft tissue and bony structures at the skull base. Chondrosarcomas occur at a higher frequency in patients with Ollier's disease and Maffucci's syndrome.

Differential Diagnosis

Chordoma (52)

- arise from the clivus and therefore are typically located more centrally
- whirls of calcifications are usually absent
- may not be distinguishable from chondrosarcoma

Metastasis

- usually not of very high T2 signal
- dark on ADC maps, except for necrotic portions
- enhancement dense and/or with necrotic non-enhancing portions

Schwannoma (141)

- remodeling and not erosion of the bone

- typically along CN V, common "dumbbell" appearance with the lesion involving the subarachnoid trigeminal nerve and the Meckel's cave

Aneurysm (51)

- round to oval shape, continuous with a major vessel, usually ICA
- internal flow-void, flow confirmed on CTA/MRA
- intraluminal clot, frequently with onion-skin appearance

Background

Chondrosarcomas are rare malignant tumors constituting less than 0.16% of all intracranial neoplasms and originating from cartilaginous tissue. The prevailing hypothesis is that they arise from cartilaginous remnants at the skull base, primarily in the petro-clival synchondrosis (also referred to as petro-occipital fissure and petro-clival junction). The majority of chondrosarcomas occur more laterally than chordomas, which arise from the clivus, although overlap occurs in about one-third of cases. The distinction is of clinical importance because chondrosarcomas have a higher local control rate and overall better prognosis than chordomas. Histology with immunohistochemical methods allows reliable differentiation of these tumors. The optimal treatment involves gross total removal, followed by radiotherapy, which reduces the chance of tumor recurrence. Given the frequent involvement of cranial nerves and major vessels by chondrosarcoma, and, on the other hand, a good long-term prognosis, radical surgical resection is rarely attempted, as it could substantially deteriorate patients' quality of life. Treated skull base chondrosarcomas have a 10-year survival rate in the range of 80%.

REFERENCES

1. Meyers SP, Hirsch WL Jr, Curtin HD, *et al.* Chondrosarcomas of the skull base: MR imaging features. *Radiology* 1992;**184**:103–8.
2. Bourgouin PM, Tampieri D, Robitaille Y, *et al.* Low-grade myxoid chondrosarcoma of the base of the skull: CT, MR, and histopathology. *J Comput Assist Tomogr* 1992;**16**:268–73.
3. Brown E, Hug EB, Weber AL. Chondrosarcoma of the skull base. *Neuroimaging Clin N Am* 1994;**4**:529–41.
4. Pamir MN, Ozduman K. Analysis of radiological features relative to histopathology in 42 skull-base chordomas and chondrosarcomas. *Eur J Radiol* 2006;**58**:461–70.
5. Almefty K, Pravdenkova S, Colli BO, *et al.* Chordoma and chondrosarcoma: similar, but quite different, skull base tumors. *Cancer* 2007;**110**:2457–67.

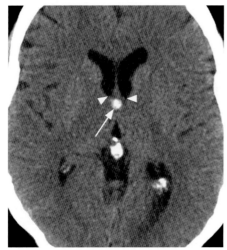

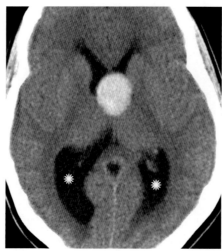

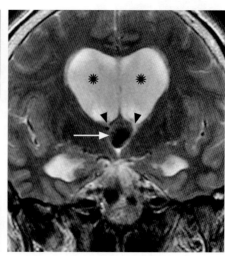

Figure 1. Axial non-enhanced CT image shows a round very bright midline lesion (arrow) at the level of foramina of Monro (arrowheads).

Figure 2. Non-enhanced CT shows a large round hyperdense mass centered in the region of the foramina of Monro, causing obstruction and dilation of lateral ventricles (*).

Figure 3. Coronal T2WI shows markedly hypointense oval third ventricle mass (arrow) obstructing the foramina of Monro (arrowheads) and causing hydrocephalus (*).

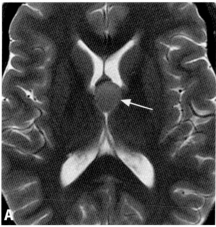

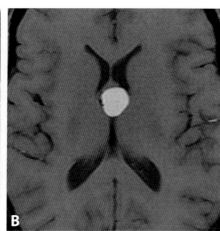

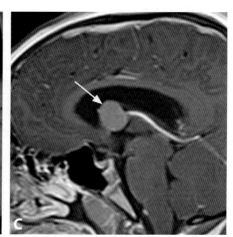

Figure 4. Axial T2WI (A) reveals a non-obstructing rounded structure in the anterior third ventricle (arrow), isointense to the gray matter. Corresponding T1WI (B) shows hyperintensity of the lesion. There is no enhancement of the mass (arrow) at its typical location on sagittal post-contrast T1WI (C).

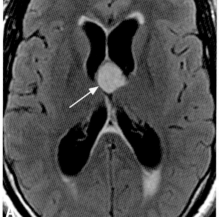

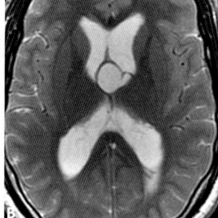

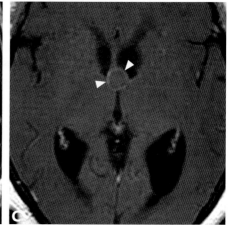

Figure 5. Axial FLAIR image (A) shows an obstructing rounded hyperintense mass (arrow) causing hydrocephalus. The lesion has CSF-like signal on T2WI (B) and post-contrast T1WI (C). There is a very thin linear enhancement of the cyst capsule (arrowheads).

Colloid Cyst

ALESSANDRO CIANFONI

Specific Imaging Findings

Colloid cyst is a round to oval midline intraventricular mass with sharp borders, with origin in the superior and anterior portion of the third ventricle at the foramina of Monro. The fornix columns appear splayed and wrapped around the anterior aspect of larger colloid cysts. The cyst is typically homogeneously hyperdense on CT (in about two-thirds of cases), while it can be isodense and very rarely hypodense. Wall calcifications are extremely rare. The mass is commonly T1 hyperintense, while the T2 signal ranges from low to high, and it can be iso to hypointense to brain on DWI with increased diffusion on ADC maps. Concentric layers or fluid–fluid levels of different signal may be present. Typically there is no contrast enhancement, although occasionally the capsule may enhance. The size of the cyst varies from a few millimeters to several centimeters, and it can be accompanied by obstructive hydrocephalus of the lateral ventricles.

Pertinent Clinical Information

Colloid cysts may be an incidental finding. When symptomatic, they present with headache, classically intermittent and positional, while nausea, vomiting, signs of intracranial hypertension, gait disturbance, visual deficits, memory loss, and altered personality may also occur. Symptoms are believed to be attributable to intermittent ventricular obstruction and hydrocephalus. There are several reported cases of sudden death in patients with non-specific headache, supposedly due to acute hydrocephalus and consequent brain herniation.

Differential Diagnosis

CSF Jet Flow Artifacts at the Foramen of Monro
- usually only on FLAIR and T2WI
- not midline but in the frontal horns of lateral ventricles
- not present in all imaging planes

Intraventricular and Suprasellar Neoplasms (central neurocytoma, subependymal giant cell astrocytoma, subependymoma, craniopharyngioma, hypothalamic gliomas) (44, 150, 170, 171)
- off midline, pure midline presentation is rare
- solid components and/or polycystic, not a single cyst
- contrast enhancement may be present

Choroid Plexus Cyst (147)
- extremely rare in the third ventricle
- calcifications very common

Ependymal Cyst (146)
- extremely rare in the third ventricle
- follows density/signal intensity of CSF

Basilar Tip Aneurysm (51)
- misdiagnosis more common on non-enhanced CT
- sagittal images show the extraventricular origin and continuity with the parent artery
- pulsatility artifacts
- MRA and CTA for confirmation

Background

Colloid cysts represent 1% of all brain masses and 20% of all intraventricular ones. In 99% of cases they arise from the third ventricle and are lined by endoderm. Colloid cysts have a fibrous capsule and contain viscous fluid with variable amounts of gelatinous material, cholesterol, blood, and cell debris. Small, non-obstructing cysts may be followed with serial imaging, while the symptomatic obstructive cysts can be aspirated with intraoperative imaging guidance, resected endoscopically, or removed with microsurgical techniques in open surgery. Spontaneous resolution of the cysts has also been described. Complete or near-complete resection of the entire capsule significantly reduces the rate of recurrence. CT hyperdensity and T2 hypointensity of the cyst suggest very viscous contents. Such findings seem to be predictive of unsuccessful cyst aspiration and surgical resection may be preferred in these cases. On the other hand, the cysts with high viscosity are less likely to grow at serial follow-up imaging studies. One single report on the use of MRS noted a pseudo-NAA peak at 2 ppm, likely representing glycoproteins. Atrophy of the mammillary bodies has been found following surgical removal of colloid cysts, which is likely a consequence of injury to the fornices and may explain occasional difficulties with memory in these patients.

REFERENCES
1. Armao D, Castillo M, Chen H, Kwock L. Colloid cyst of the third ventricle: imaging-pathologic correlation. *AJNR* 2000;**21**:1470–7.
2. Horn EM, Feiz-Erfan I, Bristol RE, *et al*. Treatment options for third ventricular colloid cysts: comparison of open microsurgical versus endoscopic resection. *Neurosurgery* 2007;**60**:613–8.
3. Periakaruppan A, Kesavadas C, Radhakrishnan VV, *et al*. Unique MR spectroscopic finding in colloid-like cyst. *Neuroradiology* 2008;**50**:137–44.
4. Annamalai G, Lindsay KW, Bhattacharya JJ. Spontaneous resolution of a colloid cyst of the third ventricle. *Br J Radiol* 2008;**81**: e20–2.
5. Denby CE, Vann SD, Tsivilis D, *et al*. The frequency and extent of mammillary body atrophy associated with surgical removal of a colloid cyst. *AJNR* 2009;**30**:736–43.

Brain Imaging with MRI and CT, ed. Zoran Rumboldt *et al.* Published by Cambridge University Press. © Cambridge University Press 2012.

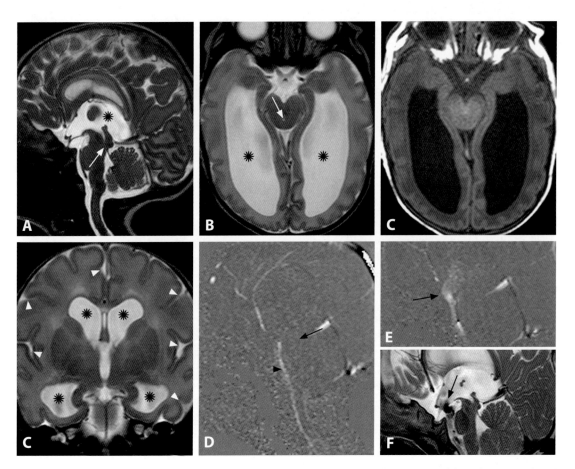

Figure 1. Midsagittal high-resolution 3D T2WI (A) in a newborn shows marked narrowing of the inferior aqueduct (arrow) and third ventricle enlargement (*). Axial T2WI (B) shows absence of normal flow void (arrow). Aqueduct is narrowed but midline. Dilated lateral ventricles (*). T1WI (C) shows no aqueductal hyperintensity ruling out clot, while coronal T2WI (D) reveals commensurate dilation of temporal and frontal horns (*). Despite marked ventricular dilation, patency of subarachnoid spaces is preserved (arrowheads). Sagittal phase-contrast image (E) shows no detectable CSF flow at the aqueduct (arrow) and normal flow ventral to the brainstem (arrowhead). Following third ventriculostomy turbulent flow through the third ventricle floor (arrows) is seen on both phase-contrast (F) and T2WI (G).

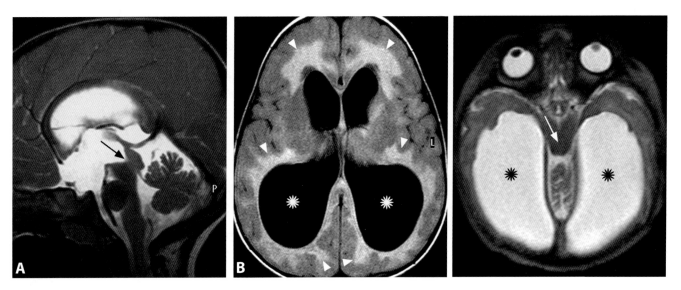

Figure 2. Midsagittal T2WI (A) in a 3-year-old shows obstructed aqueduct (arrow). Axial FLAIR image (B) shows severe ventricular enlargement (*), effaced cortical sulci and extensive periventricular edema (arrowheads), indicating uncompensated hydrocephalus.

Figure 3. Axial T2WI in an infant shows the absence of aqueductal flow-void (arrow) and marked hydrocephalus (*).

Aqueductal Stenosis

ANDREA ROSSI

Specific Imaging Findings

Neuroimaging of aqueductal stenosis (AS) is characterized by a variable, often severe dilation of the supratentorial ventricles and a normal fourth ventricle. Enlargement of the frontal and temporal horns is commensurate; this is an important differential sign from ex-vacuo ventriculomegaly, especially in newborns in whom, owing to compensatory macrocrania, the subarachnoid spaces may remain prominent or even frankly enlarged even with hydrocephalus. The site of stenosis or complete obstruction (either proximal or distal) is best depicted with high-resolution 3D heavily T2WI. Absence of normal aqueductal flow-void on T2WI can be confirmed with flow-sensitive MR techniques (phase-contrast). Periventricular edema is not usually prominent in infants, but becomes more frequent once the cranial sutures have closed, and indicates uncompensated hydrocephalus requiring surgical attention. Septum pellucidum may become fenestrated or even undiscernible with severe long-standing hydrocephalus. Following successful endoscopic third ventriculostomy, T2-weighted and flow-sensitive images will show turbulent CSF flow through the floor of the third ventricle.

Pertinent Clinical Information

Clinical manifestations of AS vary depending on patient age and duration of raised intracranial pressure. Patients with prenatal diagnosis of ventriculomegaly are seen immediately after birth before significant symptoms ensue. During the first two years, presentation is with abnormally accelerated head growth: disproportionately large forehead, wide sutures, tense fontanel, and engorged scalp veins. At this age, neurological signs are insidious including difficulty feeding and laryngeal stridor. Downward gaze deviation ("setting-sun sign") occurs in the most severe cases. Older children present with signs of raised intracranial pressure, including papilledema, strabismus, morning headache, and vomiting. Hormonal deficiencies may result from hypothalamic-pituitary dysfunction. Late-onset idiopathic aqueductal stenosis (LIAS) presents in adults with headaches and normal pressure hydrocephalus symptoms. Endoscopic third ventriculostomy is the preferred treatment for AS with shunting as an alternative.

Differential Diagnosis

Tectal Glioma (62)

- ill-defined T2 hyperintense thickening of the quadrigeminal plate and/or midbrain tegmentum, often asymmetric
- aqueduct is present and displaced off midline on axial images

Aqueductal Clot

- hyperintense aqueduct on T1-weighted images
- evidence of peri- or intraventricular bleed

Hydranencephaly (95)

- fluid cavities fill most of the supratentorial compartment
- scattered brain remnants overlie the cavities without continuity
- thalami are present, but basal nuclei are not

Holoprosencephaly (73)

- absence of midline structures, including interhemispheric fissure and falx
- in alobar form, rudimentary brain surrounds a single ventricle that communicates posteriorly with dorsal sac

Background

AS is typically a malformation with reduced lumen or complete obstruction of the sylvian aqueduct, in the absence of gliosis or extrinsic compression. Ventricular dilation is usually more severe with proximal obstruction. Obstructed CSF flow leads to distension of the supratentorial ventricles and stretching of corpus callosum. In newborns and infants, incompletely ossified skull and unmyelinated brain offer little resistance to progressive ventricular enlargement. Disjunction of intercellular connections causes ependymal cellular loss and diffuse microlacerations with glial proliferation, heterotopias, or diverticular extroversions that damage the periventricular white matter. Subependymal veins may become compressed and cause leakage of fluid in the interstitium. In untreated cases, white matter gliosis and atrophy with relative sparing of both superficial and deep gray matter structures eventually occurs. Aqueductal stenosis occurs in congenital X-linked hydrocephalus with stenosis of the sylvian aqueduct (HSAS), the most common genetic form of congenital hydrocephalus, caused by mutations in the gene for neural cell adhesion molecule L1 (L1CAM) on Xq28. Adducted thumbs are present in about 50% of neonates with HSAS. The clinical picture is variable, ranging from early death to survival with mental retardation and spastic paraplegia. Other structures, such as anomalous veins, may rarely compress the aqueduct.

REFERENCES

1. Stoquart-El Sankari S, Lehmann P, Gondry-Jouet C, et al. Phase-contrast MR imaging support for the diagnosis of aqueductal stenosis. AJNR 2009;30:209–14.
2. Fukuhara T, Vorster SJ, Ruggieri P, Luciano MG. Third ventriculostomy patency: comparison of findings at cinephase-contrast MR imaging and at direct exploration. AJNR 1999;20:1560–6.
3. McAllister JP, Chovan P. Neonatal hydrocephalus. Mechanisms and consequences. Neurosurg Clin North Am 1998;9:73–93.
4. Graf WD, Born DE, Shaw DW, et al. Diffusion-weighted magnetic resonance imaging in boys with neural cell adhesion molecule L1 mutations and congenital hydrocephalus. Ann Neurol 2000;47:113–7.
5. Fukuhara T, Luciano MG. Clinical features of late-onset idiopathic aqueductal stenosis. Surg Neurol 2001;55:132–6.

Brain Imaging with MRI and CT, ed. Zoran Rumboldt et al. Published by Cambridge University Press. © Cambridge University Press 2012.

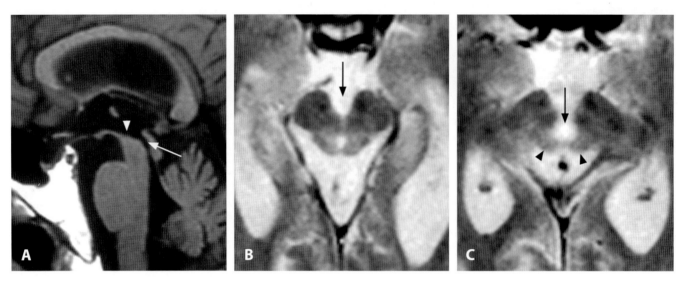

Figure 1. Midsagittal T1WI without contrast (A) shows volume loss of the midbrain with abnormal flattening of its superior contour (arrowhead) along with "funnel-shaped" posterior third ventricle and sylvian aqueduct (arrow). The midbrain resembles the shape of a penguin's head. Axial T2WI through the midbrain (B) reveals widening of the interpeduncular cistern (arrows). A slightly more cephalad T2WI (C) shows widened superior portion of the cerebral aqueduct (arrow) along with mild hyperintensity of the superior colliculi (arrowheads).

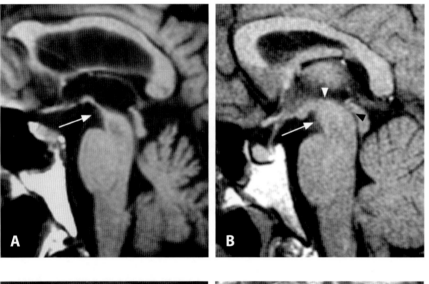

Figure 2. Midsagittal T1WI (A) in another patient shows the characteristic "hummingbird" or "penguin" sign (arrow) due to volume loss of the midbrain tegmentum. Compare to a normal midsagittal T1WI from another individual (B) demonstrating an expected appearance of the midbrain (arrow) with a normal convex superior contour (white arrowhead) and narrow aqueduct (black arrowhead) without cephalad funneling.

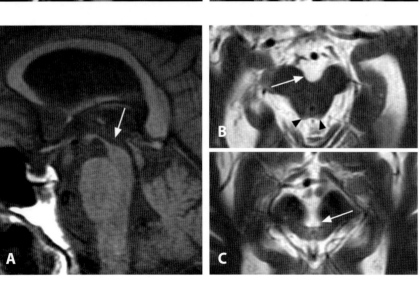

Figure 3. Midsagittal T1WI (A) in a patient with parkinsonism, ophthalmoplegia, and dementia shows the hummingbird sign (arrow). Axial T2WI at the level of cerebral peduncles (B) reveals widened interpeduncular cistern (arrow) and hyperintensity of the superior colliculi (arrowheads). A slightly more cephalad T2WI (C) shows widened inferior aspect of the third ventricle (arrow).

Progressive Supranuclear Palsy (PSP)

ALESSANDRO CIANFONI AND ZORAN RUMBOLDT

Specific Imaging Findings

Progressive supranuclear palsy (PSP) causes a selective atrophy of the rostral midbrain (tegmentum and superior colliculi), with characteristic imaging findings: flattening and concavity of the normally convex superior midbrain contour and a "funnel-shaped" inferior third ventricle on sagittal images; relative increase in the length of the interpeduncular fossa with decreased anteroposterior midbrain diameter on axial images. These changes are responsible for the typical appearance on midsagittal MR images that has been called the "penguin" and "hummingbird" sign, because the shape of the atrophic midbrain resembles the bill of a hummingbird or a penguin's head, and it is a distinguishing feature of PSP. Increased T2 signal of the superior colliculi and periaqueductal gray matter may also be present. A less specific high T2 signal can be observed in the lenticular nuclei, along with T2 hypointensity and increased ADC values of the putamen as well as atrophy of the insular and fronto-temporal cortex.

Pertinent Clinical Information

PSP is a clinical syndrome comprising supranuclear ophthalmoplegia (impaired downward gaze), postural instability, and mild dementia. It is seen mainly in late adult life with a peak during the sixth decade. Clinical presentation includes parkinsonism, axial rigidity, contracture of neck and facial muscles (neck hyperextension and "surprised look"), and disautonomy. ADC measurements, MRI morphometry, DTI and MRS all show abnormal findings at the level of the fronto-temporal cortex, basal ganglia, and midbrain, with limited specificity and sensitivity. PET and SPECT show pre-frontal hypometabolism.

Differential Diagnosis

Parkinson Disease
- absent "penguin/hummingbird" sign, selective atrophy of the substantia nigra
- ADC in the putamina is not increased

Multiple System Atrophy (59)
- in MSA-p there is high T2 signal rim along the dorso-lateral putamen and putaminal T1 hyperintensity
- in MSA-c typical "hot cross bun" T2 bright sign in the pons
- absent "penguin/hummingbird" sign

Cortico-Basal Degeneration
- typical marked fronto-parietal, perirolandic and parasagittal atrophy ("knife blade" atrophy)

Background

PSP is a neurodegenerative disease, neuropathologically defined by the accumulation of neurofibrillary tangles, similar to Alzheimer's dementia and a number of other diseases. These disorders are summarized as tauopathies, because neurofibrillary tangles are composed of intracellular collections of the microtubule-associated protein tau. New insights emphasize that the pathological events that lead to the hyperphosphorylation and aggregation of tau protein in the brain are best considered as dynamic processes that can develop at different rates, leading to different clinical phenomena. PSP is also characterized by neuronal loss, atrophy and gliosis, and ferromagnetic substances accumulation. PSP and multiple system atrophy (MSA) are the most common cause of parkinsonism, after Parkinson's disease (PD), and are grouped, together with cortico-basal degeneration (CBD), into atypical parkinsonian disorders (APDs). In the early disease stages the clinical separation of APDs from PD carries a high rate of misdiagnosis. However, APD and PD are characterized by different natural histories, and require different treatment strategies. Conventional MRI plays an important role in the exclusion of symptomatic parkinsonism due to other pathologies, such as multi-infarct encephalopathy and normal pressure hydrocephalus. While conventional MRI offers specific findings to differentiate PD and APDs in the advanced stages, it is not very reliable in the early phases of the diseases, having several overlapping features. There is ongoing investigation of the advanced MRI techniques in differentiation of PD and individual APDs.

REFERENCES

1. Seppi K, Poewe W. Brain magnetic resonance imaging techniques in the diagnosis of parkinsonian syndromes. *Neuroimaging Clin N Am* 2010;**20**:29–55.
2. Righini A, Antonini A, De Notaris R, *et al*. MR imaging of the superior profile of the midbrain: differential diagnosis between progressive supranuclear palsy and Parkinson disease. *AJNR* 2004;**25**:927–32.
3. Kato N, Arai K, Hattori T. Study of the rostral midbrain atrophy in progressive supranuclear palsy. *J Neurol Sci* 2003;**210**:57–60.
4. Rizzo G, Martinelli P, Manners D, *et al*. Diffusion-weighted brain imaging study of patients with clinical diagnosis of corticobasal degeneration, progressive supranuclear palsy and Parkinson's disease. *Brain* 2008;**131**:2690–700.
5. Williams DR, Lees AJ. Progressive supranuclear palsy: clinicopathological concepts and diagnostic challenges. *Lancet Neurol* 2009;**8**:270–9.

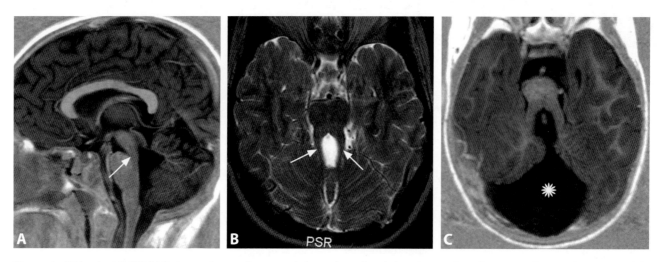

Figure 1. Midsagittal IR T1WI (A) shows abnormally narrow isthmus (arrow) and deep interpeduncular cistern. There is dysgenesis of the cerebellum. Axial T2WI (B) shows very thick superior cerebellar peduncles (SCPs, arrows), giving the brainstem a molar tooth appearance. IR T1WI at a lower level (C) again shows the molar tooth sign and reveals severe hypoplasia of the vermis with large fourth ventricle (*).

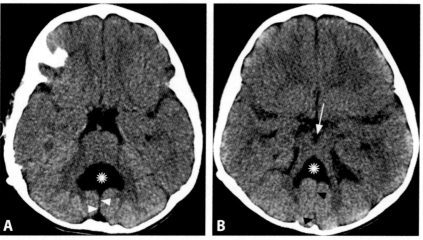

Figure 2. Axial non-enhanced CT images (A, B) in a 3-year-old child show abnormal dilation of the mid fourth ventricle taking the shape of an umbrella (*) and a molar tooth appearance of the brainstem (arrow) with thick horizontal SCPs. There is vermian hypoplasia with a cleft between the cerebellar hemispheres (arrowheads) corresponding to the handle of the umbrella.

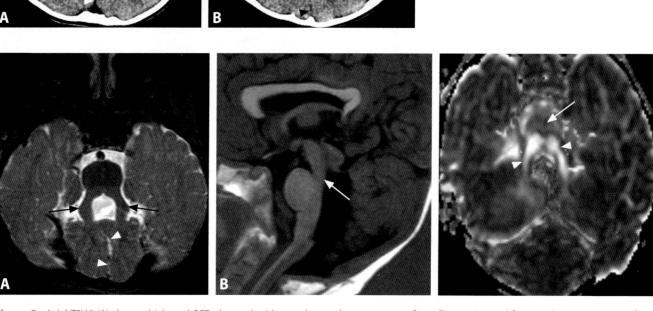

Figure 3. Axial T2WI (A) shows thickened SCPs (arrows) with a molar tooth appearance of the brainstem. There is cerebellar dysgenesis with a cleft separating the superior aspect of the hemispheres (arrowheads). Midsagittal IR T1WI (B) shows a very narrow isthmus (arrow) without the normal hypointense spot and a deep interpeduncular cistern.

Figure 4. Axial fractional anisotropy map from DTI MR scan reveals thickening and horizontal course of the SCPs (arrowheads). The bright SCP commissure is absent (arrow).

Joubert Syndrome

MARIA VITTORIA SPAMPINATO

Specific Imaging Findings

The molar tooth sign on axial brain MRI or CT images is pathognomonic of Joubert syndrome (JS). This sign results from the combination of marked hypoplasia or aplasia of the cerebellar vermis, a narrow isthmus (the area of the midbrain caudal to the inferior colliculi and immediately above the pons), a triangular shaped or "umbrella-shaped" mid-fourth ventricle and a "batwing" appearance of the superior fourth ventricle. The key finding are thickened, elongated and horizontally oriented superior cerebellar peduncles (SCP) with a very deep interpeduncular fossa. In JS patients older than 30 months the absence of SCP decussation can be identified on a mid-sagittal T1WI as a lack of the rounded low signal-intensity area at the level of the ponto-mesencephalic junction, representing the SCP decussation. Diffusion-tensor MR imaging and fiber tractography have been employed to demonstrate the abnormal morphology and aberrant course of the SCP and corticospinal tract. Associated abnormalities may include migration disorders (such as heterotopia), callosal dysgenesis, ventriculomegaly, and cephaloceles.

Pertinent Clinical Information

JS is a rare, autosomal recessive disorder with a distinctive hindbrain malformation. The molar tooth sign was first described in JS; however, it is present in numerous other rare syndromes that are partially overlapping with JS and characterized by abnormalities outside of the CNS in addition to the brainstem and cerebellar findings [e.g. Joubert–polymicrogyria syndrome, Dekaban–Arima syndrome, COACH (Cerebellar vermis hypoplasia, Oligophrenia, Ataxia, Coloboma, and Hepatic fibrosis) syndrome, Varadi–Papp syndrome, Senior–Löchen syndrome]. As a result, it has been suggested to reclassify the syndromes characterized by the molar tooth sign and to describe them collectively as Joubert Syndrome Related Disorders (JSRD). Patients with classic JS present with hypotonia early in life, followed by marked ataxia, neonatal breathing pattern characterized by hyperpnea and apnea, neuro-ophthalmologic abnormalities (including nystagmus and retinal abnormalities), and mental retardation. Facial and cranial features include a large head, broad nasal bridge, high rounded eyebrows, and mild epicanthus. The molar tooth sign is essential for the diagnosis, given the great heterogeneity of clinical presentations, and it may be identified in fetuses on prenatal MRI.

Differential Diagnosis

Dandy–Walker Malformation (93)
- abnormally large posterior fossa
- open fourth ventricle communicating with a dorsal posterior fossa cyst
- absence of the molar-tooth appearance

Cerebellar Vermian Hypoplasia
- vermis is small; however, the brain stem, SCP, and cerebellum are well formed

Rhombencephalosynapis (58)
- fused cerebellar hemispheres, absent vermis
- absence of the molar-tooth appearance

Chiari 2 Malformation (61)
- small posterior fossa, small fourth ventricle, and herniated cerebellar tonsils
- beaked tectum and heart-shaped vermis, absence of the molar-tooth sign
- myelomeningocele

Background

The prevalence of JSRD has been estimated at approximately 1 : 100 000 in the US. Currently eight genes have been implicated in JSRD, accounting for about 50% of causative mutations in JSRD. The genes associated with JSRD synthesize proteins known to be localized in the primary cilium, basal body and centrosome. It has been proposed that the abnormal morphology and function of the ciliary apparatus cause abnormal development of decussating fibers. The absence of crossing of commissural fibers is considered a pathologic hallmark of JSRD, and the abnormality appears to involve the SCP, corticospinal tracts, central pontine tracts and some paramedian nuclei in the vermis and brain stem, while sparing the optic chiasm and corpus callosum. Another key feature of JS is the abnormal development of the structures deriving from the primitive isthmus, including the isthmic segment of the brain stem and vermis. Although essential for the diagnosis, the neuroimaging findings are of limited value in classifying patients with JSRD due to the absence of a correlation with genotype.

REFERENCES

1. Poretti A, Huisman TA, Scheer I, Boltshauser E. Joubert syndrome and related disorders: spectrum of neuroimaging findings in 75 patients. *AJNR* 2011;**32**:1459–63.

2. Maria BL, Quisling RG, Rosainz LC, *et al.* Molar tooth sign in Joubert syndrome: clinical, radiologic, and pathologic significance. *J Child Neurol* 1999;**14**:368–76.

3. Poretti A, Boltshauser E, Loenneker T, *et al.* Diffusion tensor imaging in Joubert syndrome. *AJNR* 2007;**28**:1929–33.

4. Spampinato MV, Kraas J, Maria BL, *et al.* Absence of decussation of the superior cerebellar peduncles in patients with Joubert syndrome. *Am J Med Genet A* 2008;**146A**:1389–94.

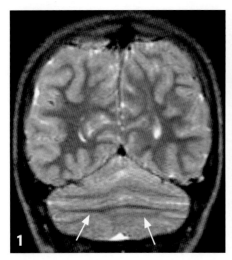
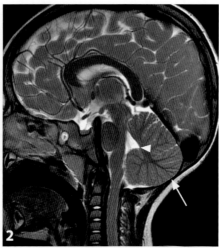

Figure 1. Coronal T2WI shows horizontal cerebellar folia (arrows) with uninterrupted extension from side to side of the cerebellum. The vermis is missing.

Figure 2. Midsagittal T2WI demonstrates absent primary suture (arrow) and rounded posterior margin of the fourth ventricle (arrowhead).

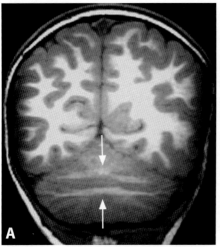
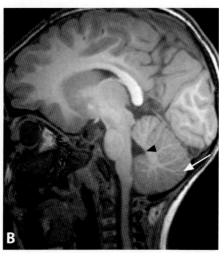

Figure 3. Coronal T1WI reconstructed from a volume GRE acquisition (A) in a child with ataxia and abnormal eye movements shows horizontal cerebellar folia (arrows) with continuous extension across the midline. Sagittal T1WI (B) reveals absence of the primary suture (arrow) with a rounded posterior border of the fourth ventricle (arrowhead).

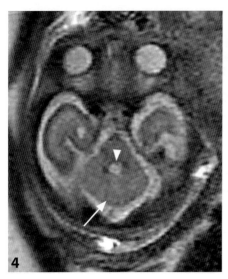
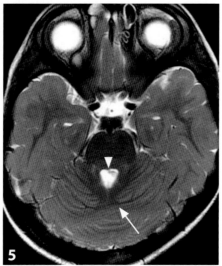

Figure 4. Axial single shot T2WI in a fetus reveals a small "keyhole-shaped" fourth ventricle (arrowhead) and lack of separation between cerebellar hemispheres (arrow).

Figure 5. Axial T2WI shows the characteristic keyhole shape of the narrowed fourth ventricle (arrowhead). Also note fused cerebellar hemispheres with folia extending across the midline (arrow).

Rhombencephalosynapsis

CHEN HOFFMAN

Specific Imaging Findings

MR imaging in rhombencephalosynapsis (RES) shows a characteristic fusion of the cerebellar hemispheres, without separation by a cleft or the vermis. The vermis is absent while the cerebellar dentate nuclei, as well as the middle and superior cerebellar peduncles are fused. The coronal view is most helpful, showing abnormal horizontal orientation of the cerebellar folia that are continuous across the midline, while the typical vermian folial pattern is missing in the midline. The single lobed cerebellum is small, with decreased transverse diameter. In the sagittal plane, the primary fissure is missing and the festigial process of the fourth ventricle is rounded. In the axial plane, the fused structures arch in a horseshoe shape across the midline, resulting in a narrowed and posteriorly pointing fourth ventricle, described as a keyhole, diamond, tear drop, or square. This appearance may suggest RES on CT images; however, the diagnosis is made with MRI. DTI depicts vertically oriented fibers in the midportion of the cerebellum. RES should be considered whenever fetal MRI is performed for the most common indication – ventricular enlargement on prenatal ultrasound.

Pertinent Clinical Information

The clinical presentation of RES is variable, usually including ataxia, hypotonia, involuntary head movements, abnormal eye movements, and/or seizures, and the symptoms may range from mild to debilitating. In a majority of cases, cognitive development is impaired, but this is also markedly variable and ranging from severely handicapped to normal. Obsessive–compulsive disorder, self-mutilation and depression have been observed, while attention deficit and hyperactivity disorders are frequent behavioral problems. The outcome of RES is accordingly unpredictable – some patients die in childhood due to severe disabilities, while others have either subtle or nonexistent clinical signs and the diagnosis is made incidentally in adulthood. The prognosis may depend on the associated abnormalities, particularly supratentorial anomalies and hydrocephalus.

Differential Diagnosis

Chiari II with Chronic Shunting

- cerebellar folia are not horizontal and contiguous across the midline
- may be rarely associated with RES

Congenital Vermian Hypoplasia

- cerebellar hemispheres are not fused but separated by a cleft

Background

RES is a rare congenital malformation with the estimated frequency at 0.13%. It is a sporadic disorder in a majority of cases, thought to result from a disturbed cerebellar development between 28 and 41 days of gestation. The causative factors remain controversial. In the traditional view, the cerebellum arises from two distinct embryonic primordia, followed by development of the vermis. According to this concept, RES would be a consequence of abnormal vermian development with subsequent fusion of the hemispheres. A more recent theory proposes an unpaired cerebellar primordium, so that RES would be caused by a failure in differentiation, leaving the cerebellar hemispheres fused. Experimental studies have identified the "isthmic organizer", a band of neuroepithelium between metencephalon (from which the cerebellar hemispheres derive) and mesencephalon (from which a part of vermis develops) that appears crucial for cerebellar development, and RES may be caused by a genetic defect in this structure. Additional supratentorial midline abnormalities are commonly present with RES, the most frequent being ventriculomegaly secondary to aqueductal stenosis, dysgenesis of the corpus callosum, agenesis of the septum pellucidum, and holoprosencephaly. Fetal MR imaging allows prenatal diagnosis in most cases. RES may also occur as part of a Gómez–López–Hernández syndrome (GLHS), a very rare entity characterized by RES and bilateral parietal alopecia, while trigeminal anesthesia, dysmorphic features, and ataxia are inconsistent findings. Partial rhombencephalosynapsis may be associated with Chiari II malformation.

REFERENCES

1. Toelle SP, Yalcinkaya C, Kocer N, et al. Rhombencephalosynapsis: clinical findings and neuroimaging in 9 children. *Neuropediatrics* 2002;**33**:209–14.
2. Napolitano M, Righini A, Zirpoli S, et al. Prenatal magnetic resonance imaging of rhombencephalosynapsis and associated brain anomalies: report of 3 cases. *J Comput Assist Tomogr* 2004;**28**:762- 5.
3. McAuliffe F, Chitayat D, Halliday W, et al. Rhombencephalosynapsis: prenatal imaging and autopsy findings. *Ultrasound Obstet Gynecol* 2008;**31**:542–8.
4. Poretti A, Alber FD, Bürki S, et al. Cognitive outcome in children with rhombencephalosynapsis. *Eur J Paediatr Neurol* 2009;**13**:28–33.
5. Widjaja E, Blaser S, Raybaud C. Diffusion tensor imaging of midline posterior fossa malformations. *Pediatr Radiol* 2006;**36**:510–7.
6. Utsunomiya H, Takano K, Ogasawara T, et al. Rhombencephalosynapsis: cerebellar embryogenesis. *AJNR* 1998;**19**:547–9.

Brain Imaging with MRI and CT, ed. Zoran Rumboldt *et al.* Published by Cambridge University Press. © Cambridge University Press 2012.

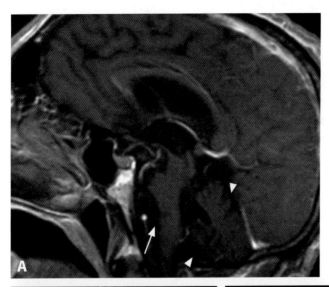

Figure 1. Midsagittal post-contrast T1WI (A) shows significant and disproportionate atrophy of the brainstem (arrow) and cerebellum (arrowheads). Axial FLAIR image (B) shows high signal intensity in the middle cerebellar peduncles (arrows) in a nearly symmetrical fashion with brainstem and cerebellar atrophy. There is a faint suggestion of the hot cross bun sign (arrowhead) in the pons. Axial T2WI (C) shows marked atrophy of the midbrain (arrow) and superior vermis (arrowhead). Axial T1WI (D) shows some dilation of the ventricles, but the degree of atrophy of the cerebral hemispheres is mild compared to the infratentorial structures.

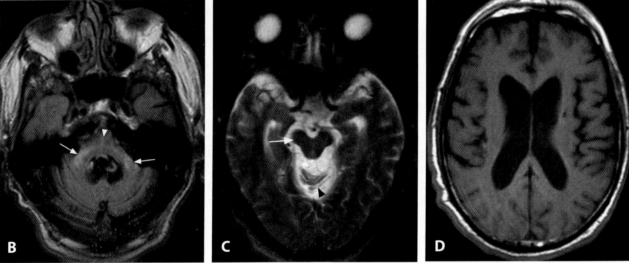

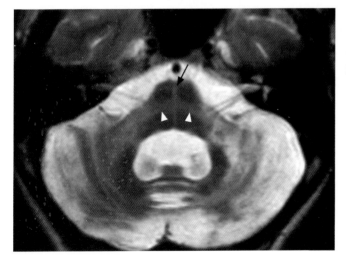

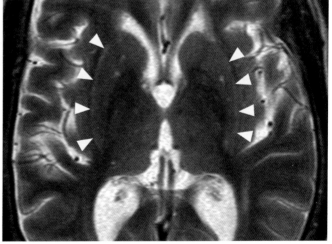

Figure 2. Axial T2WI in a different patient shows marked infratentorial atrophy. Characteristic high signal intensity in the transverse pontine fibers (arrowheads) with the central vertical linear hyperintensity (arrow) produces the hot cross bun sign.

Figure 3. Axial T2WI in a patient with parkinsonian-dominant symptoms shows hyperintense lateral putaminal rim (arrowheads), slightly more prominent on the right side. The image was acquired on a 1.5 T scanner.

Multiple System Atrophy (MSA)

ZORAN RUMBOLDT AND MAURICIO CASTILLO

Specific Imaging Findings

MRI is the imaging method of choice. In MSA-p the putamina may show a T2 hyperintense lateral rim, central low T2 signal and atrophy. On T1WI, the posterior putamen may be slightly bright, which is suggestive of MSA but not pathognomonic. Central T2 hypointensity is accentuated on T2*WI, such as SWI. In MSA-c, FLAIR images may show bilateral symmetric hyperintensity in the middle cerebellar peduncles. This finding, however, may also be found in normal aging individuals. The entire brain shows atrophy, but it tends to be more prominent in the brainstem, cerebellum, and spinal cord. In patients with MSA-c increased T2 signal of the transverse white matter fibers in the lower pons may produce the "hot cross bun" sign. MRI features such as the "hot cross bun" sign have very high specificity and positive predictive value (up to 100%) but low sensitivity (in the range of 60%). Differentiation of MSA from Parkinson disease (PD) and progressive supranuclear palsy (PSP) is challenging and not always possible on standard MR imaging. Putaminal T2 hyperintense lateral rim is a frequent normal finding on 3.0 T scanners.

Pertinent Clinical Information

The most common presentation (> 60% of cases) of MSA is Parkinson-like symptoms. Balance abnormalities are seen in about 20% of patients at presentation and urinary incontinence or retention in about 10%. In males, erectile dysfunction may be an early sign. Due to the lack of balance, falls are quite common early in the disease. MSA progresses rapidly with no periods of remission and patients generally live less than 10 years after the diagnosis is first made. Respiratory problems become prominent as the disease progresses. Vocal cord paralysis may lead to death. No curative treatment exists and management is geared towards control of hypotension and Parkinson-related symptoms.

Differential Diagnosis

Parkinson Disease
- hyperintense lateral putaminal rim and putaminal atrophy are very rare
- absence of infratentorial findings

Progressive Supranuclear Palsy (56)
- characteristic "hummingbird sign" – marked midbrain atrophy on midsagittal images
- absence of "hot cross bun sign"

Chronic Liver Disease (1)
- T1 hyperintensity of the globus pallidus, not putamen

Background

MSA is a sporadic, rare (about 1–3 : 100 000), progressive disorder characterized by autonomic dysfunction, Parkinson-like symptoms, pyramidal tract signs, orthostatic hypotension, impotence, urinary incontinence or retention that are not related to ingestions of medicine or other drugs. It usually affects males over 60 years of age. When MSA has prominent Parkinson symptoms it is called MSA-p (or striatonigral degeneration). When cerebellar signs are predominant it is defined as MSA-c (or olivopontocerebellar atrophy), and Shy–Drager syndrome was previously used in patients with predominant autonomic symptoms. Because the presentation may encompass symptoms of all three diseases, the denomination of MSA was created. The pathologic substrate of MSA is neuronal loss and gliosis involving the basal ganglia, substantia nigra, olivopontocerebellar pathways, intermediolateral columns of the spinal cord, and cerebellar white matter. The hallmarks of the disease are glial cytoplasmic inclusions containing synuclein. T2 hyperintensity of the lateral putaminal rim reflects degeneration of the putaminal lateral margin and/or external capsule. Definite MSA requires neuropathologic confirmation. Probable MSA requires a sporadic, progressive adult-onset disorder including rigorously defined autonomic failure and poorly levodopa-responsive parkinsonism or cerebellar ataxia. Possible MSA requires a sporadic, progressive adult-onset disease including parkinsonism or cerebellar ataxia and at least one feature suggesting autonomic dysfunction plus one other feature that may be a clinical or a neuroimaging abnormality.

REFERENCES
1. Gilman S, Wenning GK, Low PA, et al. Second consensus statement on the diagnosis of multiple system atrophy. *Neurology* 2008;**71**:670–6.
2. Ito S, Shirai W, Hattori T. Putaminal hyperintensity on T1-weighted imaging in patients with the Parkinson variant of multiple system atrophy. *AJNR* 2009;**30**:689–92.
3. Nicoletti G, Fera F, Condino F, et al. MR imaging of middle cerebellar peduncle width: differentiation of multiple system atrophy from Parkinson disease. *Radiology* 2006;**239**:825–30.
4. Ngai, S, Tang YM, Du L, Stuckey S. Hyperintensity of the middle cerebellar peduncles on fluid-attenuated inversion recovery imaging: variation with age and implications for the diagnosis of multiple system atrophy. *AJNR* 2006;**27**:2146–8.
5. Lee WH, Lee CC, Shyu WC, et al. Hyperintense putaminal rim sign is not a hallmark of multiple system atrophy at 3T. *AJNR* 2005;**26**:2238–42.

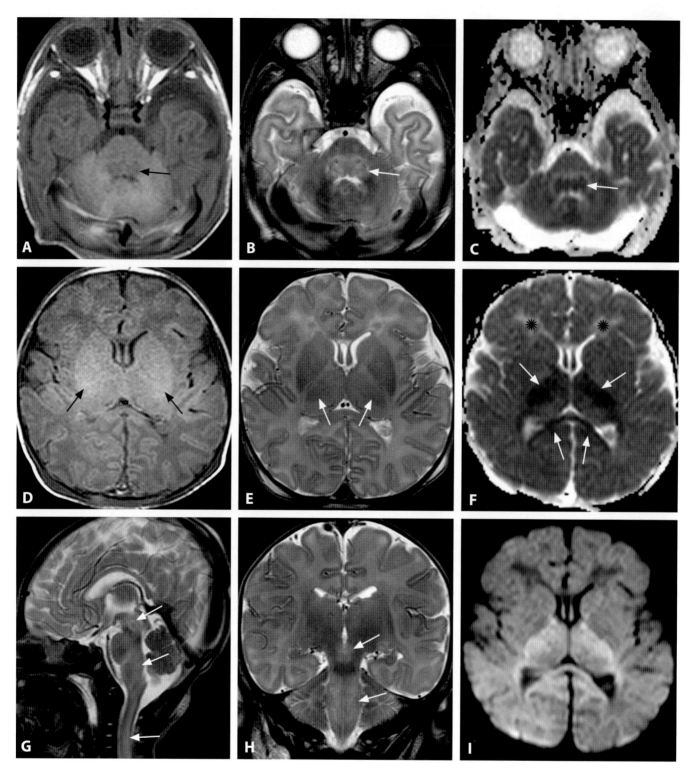

Figure 1. MRI in an 11-day-old newborn. T1WI (A) and T2WI (B) images show a swollen brainstem with abnormal low T1 and high T2 signal intensity of the brainstem tegmentum (arrows). The corresponding ADC map (C) reveals low signal in the tegmentum (arrow). There is absence of the physiological hyperintensity in the posterior limb of the internal capsules (arrows) on T1WI (D), and swollen thalami with hypointensity of their lateral portions (arrows) on T2WI (E). There is mild degree of T1 hypointensity and T2 hyperintensity in bilateral deep frontal white matter. The corresponding ADC map (F) shows decreased diffusivity in the posterior limbs of the internal capsules, lateral thalami, and callosal splenium (arrows), consistent with myelin edema. On the other hand, the deep frontal matter shows increased diffusion (*) consistent with vasogenic edema. On sagittal (G) and coronal (H) T2WIs, swelling and abnormal hyperintensity of the dorsal brainstem and spinal cord (arrows) is depicted. The white matter sein the temporal lobes is mildly hyperintense compared to the frontal white matter. DWI (I) shows the opposite signal intensities compared to the corresponding ADC map (F).

Specific Imaging Findings

The hallmark of MSUD on both CT and MRI is diffuse brain edema and dysmyelination; this results in swelling of the brain with diffuse white matter hypodensity on CT, T1 hypointensity, and hyperintensity on T2-weighted images. Diffusion imaging discriminates between two distinct appearances, depending on the state of myelination of the various brain structures. Abnormalities within myelinated areas show up as low diffusivity (bright on DWI and dark on ADC maps), corresponding to myelin edema – these typically include the dorsal brainstem, deep cerebellar white matter, posterior limbs of the internal capsules, and corticospinal tracts within the cerebral hemispheres. Conversely, the affected nonmyelinated areas appear as increased diffusion (dark on DWI and bright on ADC maps), reflecting vasogenic edema. Proton MR spectroscopy may show an abnormal peak at 0.9–1.0 ppm on both short and long echo-time spectra, produced by the methyl groups of branched-chain amino acids (BCAAs) and branched-chain alpha-keto acids (BCKAs); lactate may be present during metabolic crises. Ultrasound may show echogenic changes at the dorsal part of the pons and medulla, providing a noninvasive imaging method in critically ill newborns.

Pertinent Clinical Information

MSUD presents with four possible variants (classical, intermediate, intermittent, and thiamine-responsive), of which the classical form is the most common and severe. In this variant, typically a few days after an uneventful birth, the affected neonates present with a severe compromise of vital functions, ranging from difficult feeding and vomiting to lethargy and coma. Patients may die from brain edema if untreated. On the other hand, early diagnosis, lifelong dietary restriction, and monitoring of BCAAs may improve the prognosis. However, long-term outcome is usually characterized by some degree of neurological impairment, and episodes of metabolic decompensation in the context of catabolic stress, often associated with intercurrent non-specific illness, commonly recur. Other clinical variants are more uncommon and difficult to diagnose owing to a more insidious presentation and course.

Differential Diagnosis

Hypoxic Ischemic Encephalopathy (7)
• brainstem and cerebellum are spared
• MRS typically shows lactate but not an abnormal peak at 0.9–1.0 ppm
• positive clinical history

Mitochondrial Encephalopathy (Leigh Disease) (10)
• brainstem tegmentum may show reduced diffusivity during metabolic crises

• typically involves gray matter, primarily putamen and caudate with sparing of the white matter
• MRS may show lactate, but not the 0.9–1.0 ppm abnormal peak in older children

Leukoencephalopathy with Brainstem and Spinal Cord Involvement and Lactate Elevation (LBSL)
• cerebral WM affected with relative sparing of the subcortical fibers, dorsal columns and lateral corticospinal tracts of the spinal cord and pyramids in the medulla
• lactate on MRS, but no abnormal peak at 0.9–1.0 ppm
• slowly progressive ataxia, spasticity and dorsal column dysfunction usually starts in childhood or adolescence

Background

MSUD was first recognized as an inherited lethal encephalopathy in the first week of life associated with an unusual odor in the urine of affected children. It is an autosomal recessive disorder in which the breakdown pathway of leucine, isoleucine, and valine (BCAAs) is impaired due to deficiency of the branched-chain α-keto acid dehydrogenase (BCKAD) enzyme. This deficit may be caused by mutations of three genes encoding for the three enzyme subunits E1, E2, and E3, located on chromosomes 19q13.1 and 6p21–p22 (E1 α and β), 1p31 (E2) and 7q31–q32 (E3). Increased concentrations of BCAAs and BCKAs interfere with energy metabolism and myelin synthesis and maintenance through two proposed mechanisms: branched-chain amino acid accumulation causes neurotransmitter deficiencies and growth restriction, while branched-chain ketoacid accumulation results in energy deprivation through Krebs cycle disruption.

REFERENCES

1. Bindu PS, Kovoor JM, Christopher R. Teaching NeuroImages: MRI in maple syrup urine disease. *Neurology* 2010;74:e12.

2. Jan W, Zimmerman RA, Wang ZJ, *et al.* MR diffusion imaging and MR spectroscopy of maple syrup urine disease during acute metabolic decompensation. *Neuroradiology* 2003; 45:393–9.

3. Patay Z. Diffusion-weighted MR imaging in leukodystrophies. *Eur Radiol* 2005;15:2284–303.

4. Tu YF, Chen CY, Lin YJ, *et al.* Neonatal neurological disorders involving the brainstem: neurosonographic approaches through the squamous suture and the foramen magnum. *Eur Radiol* 2005;15:1927–33.

5. Zinnanti WJ, Lazovic J, Griffin K, *et al.* Dual mechanism of brain injury and novel treatment strategy in maple syrup urine disease. *Brain* 2009;132:903–18.

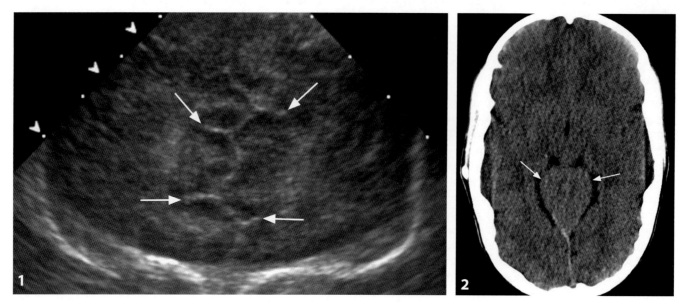

Figure 1. Coronal transcranial sonogram shows absence of the anterior falx cerebri allowing for interdigitation of gyri (arrows).

Figure 2. Axial CT shows an incomplete tentorium resulting in a large incisura through which the cerebellum towers superiorly in the shape of a heart (arrows). The skull is dolicocephalic in shape.

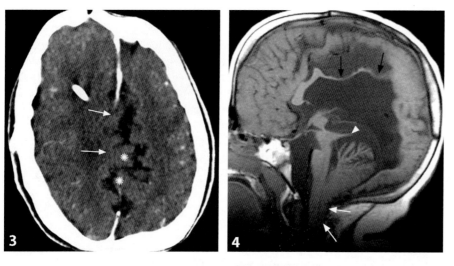

Figure 3. On CT in a different patient post ventricular shunting for hydrocephalus the absent mid falx (arrows) is clearly seen and there is gyral interdigitation (*) across the midline.

Figure 4. Midsagittal T1WI in another patient shows small posterior fossa with prominent herniation of the vermis below the foramen magnum into the spinal canal (white arrows), small brainstem, beaked tectum (arrowhead), increased volume of CSF, and callosal dysgenesis (black arrows).

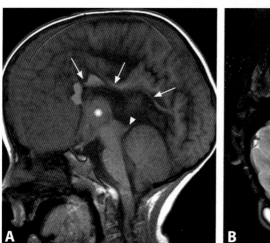
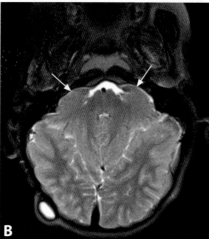

Figure 5. Midsagittal T1WI (A) shows a low-lying cerebellar vermis, posterior medullary kinking, smooth vermis, small brainstem, beaked tectum (arrowhead), large massa intermedia (*) and callosal dysgenesis (arrows). B. Axial T2WI (B) shows anterior extension of the cerebellar hemispheres (arrows) which begin to wrap themselves around the brainstem. Status post-shunting.

Chiari 2 Malformation

MAURICIO CASTILLO

Specific Imaging Findings

Most Chiari 2 malformations are today diagnosed by sonography before birth and encountered abnormalities include: the lemon sign which is due to concavities involving the frontal bones, the banana sign which is due to an abnormal shape of the cerebellar hemispheres with effacement of the cisterna magna, lacunar skull and myelomeningocele (MMC). CT and MR are the imaging methods of choice, but MRI shows the abnormalities to a better extent. On sagittal images the main findings are: herniation of the vermis through the foramen magnum which is large or normal in size, a smooth cerebellar vermis, absent fourth ventricle, small brainstem, beaked tectal plate, large massa intermedia, small third ventricle, variable dilation of the lateral ventricles and dysgenesis of the corpus callosum and stenogyria involving predominantly the occipital lobes. Hippocampi are commonly abnormal, with atypical sulcation of the adjacent mesial temporal cortex. Infratentorially axial images show that the cerebellar hemispheres wrap around the brainstem and that the tentorium is incompletely formed allowing superior protrusion of the cerebellum in the shape of a heart. Axial supratentorial images show an absent falx cerebri with variable interdigitation of the cortical gyri across the midline. Other findings include hydrocephalus, as well as a variety of neuronal migration anomalies.

Pertinent Clinical Information

Chiari 2 and MMC are more common in third-world countries and its overall incidence is about 1 : 1000 live newborns. All patients with an MMC have, by definition, a Chiari 2 malformation. Apart from the obvious MMC the head may be large; they may show lower extremity weakness or paralysis, urinary and anal sphincter dysfunction and multiple cranial neuropathies. Hydrocephalus is the most important issue early on and needs to be treated at the time of MMC closure, and thus all patients with MMC need at least a head ultrasound to exclude it. Later on these patients may develop seizures due to neuronal migration abnormalities and decreased mentation. Chronic abnormalities are generally due to the primary spinal defect (not addressed here), along with spinal cord abnormalities such as hydromyelia, and spasticity.

Differential Diagnosis

Chiari 1 Malformation
- herniation of cerebellar tonsils through a small foramen magnum, a variable degree of hydrocephalus may be present
- absence of additional Chiari 2 findings

Chiari 3 Malformation
- a Chiari 2 plus a parietal and/or occipital MMC

Background

The Chiari 2 malformation represents a group of intracranial anomalies that is typically seen in patients with open spinal dysraphism, generally of the MMC type. Although it is mostly a hindbrain malformation, it is the supratentorial anomalies that have an immediate impact on treatment and prognosis of the patients. Folate is involved in the closure of the neural tube and migration of ectodermal cells over it so that in its absence the neural placode does not fold and remains exposed and uncovered by skin. Chronic CSF leak leads to intracranial hypotension which is believed to cause the caudal displacement of intracranial structures typically seen with Chiari 2 malformation. The abnormality is generally found *in utero* by sonography and/or MRI, or suspected by the increased alfa-fetoprotein in amniotic fluid, as seen in all neural tube defects. Repair of the MMC *in utero* may lead to absence of hindbrain deformities and decreased need for ventricular shunting (which is nearly 100% in patients born untreated).

REFERENCES

1. Hunter JV, Youl BD, Mosely IF. MRI demonstration of midbrain deformity in association with Chiari malformation. *Neuroradiology* 1992;**34**:399–401.
2. Naidich TP, Pudlowski RM, Naidich JB. Computed tomographic signs of Chiari II malformation. II. Midbrain and cerebellum. *Radiology* 1980;**134**:391–8.
3. Ando K, Ishikura R, Ogawa M, *et al.* MRI tight posterior fossa sign for prenatal diagnosis of Chiari type II malformation. *Neuroradiology* 2007;**49**:1033–9.
4. Fujisawa H, Kitawaki J, Iwasa K, Honjo H. New ultrasonographic criteria for the prenatal diagnosis of Chiari type 2 malformation. *Acta Obstet Gynecol Scand* 2006;**85**:1426–9.
5. Miller E, Widjaja E, Blaser S, *et al.* The old and the new: supratentorial MR findings in Chiari II malformation. *Childs Nerv Syst* 2008;**24**:563–75.

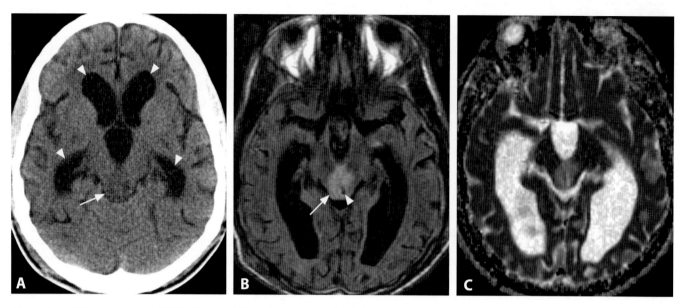

Figure 1. Axial non-enhanced CT (A) shows a thick and expanded slightly hypodense tectum (arrow). There is also ventriculomegaly (arrowheads). Corresponding FLAIR image (B) and ADC map (C) reveal increased signal and diffusion of the mass (arrow). There is mild displacement of the aqueduct (arrowhead).

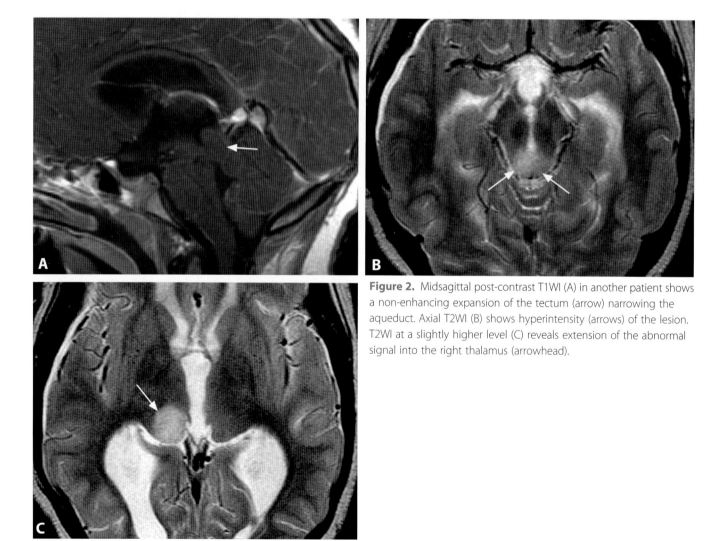

Figure 2. Midsagittal post-contrast T1WI (A) in another patient shows a non-enhancing expansion of the tectum (arrow) narrowing the aqueduct. Axial T2WI (B) shows hyperintensity (arrows) of the lesion. T2WI at a slightly higher level (C) reveals extension of the abnormal signal into the right thalamus (arrowhead).

Specific Imaging Findings

Tectal gliomas (TGs) are located in the tectum of the midbrain, which includes superior and inferior colliculi as well as periaqueductal gray matter. TGs expand the tectum and typically show iso- to low density and signal intensity when compared to the gray matter on non-contrast head CT and T1-weighted MR images. They are usually of increased T2 signal and diffusion. Post-contrast enhancement may be present, but this is not a common finding. The expansion of the tectum can be associated with stenosis or obstruction of the aqueduct and consequent hydrocephalus. Cystic component, calcifications, exophytic growth and tumor extension in the adjacent structures, primarily thalamus, may also occur. Displacement of the aqueduct is a common feature. Tumor size has been reported as a prognostic factor and should be assessed.

Pertinent Clinical Information

TGs are indolent tumors that usually become symptomatic in childhood. The most common presentation is headache and papilledema, which is related to hydrocephalus and resolves after ventricular shunting or ventriculostomy, the most common and essential clinical intervention. Other possible symptoms are Parinaud syndrome, nystagmus, sixth nerve palsy and dysmetria. The large majority of the TGs are low-grade and indolent, while a few show more aggressive growth and an infiltrating pattern, and high-grade gliomas are rare.

Differential Diagnosis

Tectal Hamartoma
- may be indistinguishable from small low-grade glioma
- remains stable over time

Neurofibromatosis Type 1 (NF-1) UBOs (2)
- focal areas of hyperintensity typically in the globus pallidus, thalamus, cerebellum and brainstem with no significant mass effect
- usually disappear in late childhood, may reappear in adolescence

Aqueductal Stenosis (55)
- may show deformity of the tectum; however, without expansion
- funnel-shaped aqueduct above the level of the stenosis
- the aqueduct is not displaced

Background

Tectal glioma is a topographical diagnosis including tumors of different histology. The overwhelming majority are astrocytomas with pilocytic astrocytomas being more common; gangliogliomas and other gliomas are occasionally found. TGs are a peculiar subset of indolent brainstem gliomas with a fairly benign course, generally irrespective of their histology. However, disease progression can be observed and tumor size is, at the present time, the only predictor of a more aggressive behavior with a less-favorable outcome. Management of tumor progression is controversial – the options include resection, biopsy with adjuvant therapy, and conservative management; all with similar outcomes. Endoscopic third ventriculostomy appears to be superior to ventricular shunt placement in the management of hydrocephalus associated with tectal gliomas. Biopsy is generally considered warranted in cases of tumor progression.

REFERENCES

1. Poussaint TY, Kowal JR, Barnes PD, et al. Tectal tumors of childhood: clinical and imaging follow-up. AJNR 1998;**19**:977–83.

2. Friedman DP. Extrapineal abnormalities of the tectal region: MR imaging findings. AJR 1992;**159**:859–66.

3. Ternier J, Wray A, Puget S, et al. Tectal plate lesions in children. J Neurosurg 2006;**104**:369–76.

4. Stark AM, Fritsch MJ, Claviez A, et al. Management of tectal gliomas in childhood. Pediatr Neurol 2005;**33**:33–8.

5. Li KW, Roonprapunt C, Lawson HC, et al. Endoscopic third ventriculostomy for hydrocephalus associated with tectal gliomas. Neurosurg Focus 2005;**18**(6A):E2.

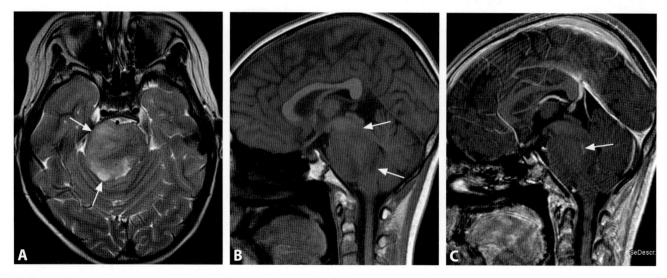

Figure 1. There is an ill-defined mass (arrows) involving over 50% of the cross-sectional diameter of the pons on axial T2WI (A). Pre-contrast T1WI (B) reveals extension into the midbrain and medulla (arrows). Corresponding post-contrast T1WI (C) shows a small focal enhancement (arrow) within the lesion.

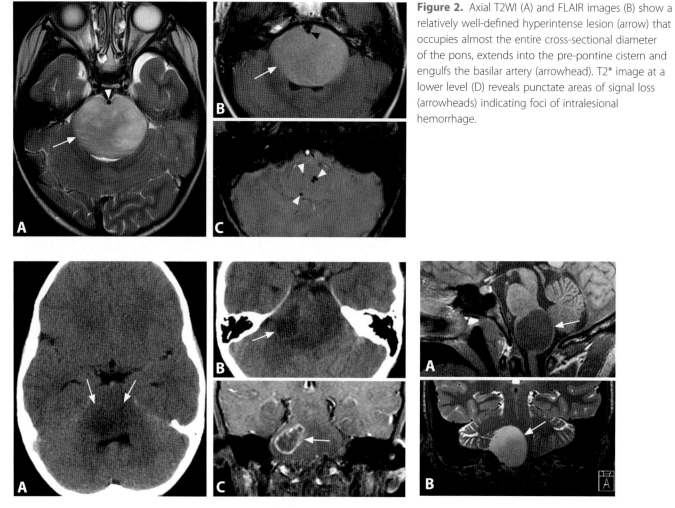

Figure 2. Axial T2WI (A) and FLAIR images (B) show a relatively well-defined hyperintense lesion (arrow) that occupies almost the entire cross-sectional diameter of the pons, extends into the pre-pontine cistern and engulfs the basilar artery (arrowhead). T2* image at a lower level (D) reveals punctate areas of signal loss (arrowheads) indicating foci of intralesional hemorrhage.

Figure 3. Non-enhanced CT (A) shows a hypodensity (arrows) with expansion of the pons. CT at a lower level reveals an area of even lower attenuation (arrow). Coronal fat saturation post-contrast T1WI (C) shows primarily peripheral enhancement (arrow) of that area.

Figure 4. Sagittal T1WI (A) and coronal T2WI (B) show a well-defined lesion (arrows) centered within the medulla.

Imaging Findings

Diffuse brainstem gliomas infiltrate and occupy large portions of the brainstem, best seen as expansile hyperintense lesions on T2WI. They are hypodense on CT, of low T1 signal, and usually with minimal or no enhancement. Areas of necrosis, cystic change, hemorrhage, and focal enhancement may be present. Tumors most commonly arise in the pons and can infiltrate into the mesencephalon, medulla, or cerebellar peduncles. Exophytic growth with effacement of the basilar cisterns and engulfing of the basilar artery is frequently present. Appearance on diffusion imaging varies, usually from slightly brighter to slightly darker compared to the normal brain. MR spectroscopy shows nonspecific elevated choline and decreased NAA; increased lactate appears to be a poor prognostic sign. Focal brain stem tumors occupy less than 50% of the axial diameter of the brainstem, have well-defined margins and frequently an exophytic component.

Pertinent Clinical Information

The mean age at diagnosis is around 8 years, brainstem gliomas rarely occur in adults. Clinical presentation includes multiple cranial neuropathies, long tract signs, and ataxia. Diffuse pontine tumors are the most common and have the worst prognosis with a median survival of 9–18 months. A short duration of symptoms appears to be associated with worse prognosis. MRI is the main diagnostic modality, while biopsy is usually not performed because of the associated risks.

Differential Diagnosis

Pilocytic Astrocytoma (173)
- usually well-defined margins
- usually homogenous contrast enhancement
- very high ADC values

Demyelinating Diseases (112, 115, 125)
- usually multiple lesions with supratentorial involvement
- enhancement is commonly in a shape of an incomplete ring and/or with a fading edge
- truncation rather than deflection of pyramidal tracts on DTI

Encephalitis
- multiple lesions involving supratentorial deep gray matter, frequent cortical involvement
- serology may be positive

Alexander Disease (33)
- symmetric brainstem involvement, minimal mass effect
- usually prominent supratentorial abnormalities

Osmotic Myelinolysis (66)
- typical "trident" appearance with sparing of the corticospinal tracts
- absent to minimal mass effect/brainstem expansion

Background

Brainstem gliomas comprise approximately 10–20% of all pediatric brain tumors. Several classification schemes for brainstem gliomas have been developed, first based on CT and more recently on MRI findings. Tumors are classified based on location (mesencephalon, pons, or medulla), whether the tumor is diffuse or focal, and whether or not the patient has neurofibromatosis type I. Diffuse pontine tumors are the most common and have the worst prognosis, typically being grade III and IV malignant fibrillary astrocytomas on histology. Focal tumors tend to be low-grade astrocytomas and have a better prognosis. Brainstem tumors that occur in the setting of neurofibromatosis type I tend to have a much more indolent course with reports of spontaneous regression. It is therefore recommended to follow neurofibromatosis patients with brainstem tumors with serial imaging unless the tumor demonstrates progressive growth, rapid growth, or the patient becomes symptomatic. Surgery is an option for focal lesions, while treatment for diffuse brainstem gliomas is usually radiation and chemotherapy. Patients with larger diffuse brainstem gliomas, as well as with prominent decrease in tumor volume and diffusion values following treatment have been found to have longer survival intervals, while contrast enhancement is associated with shorter survival. Recently, a subset of children treated with gefitinib and irradiation experienced long-term progression-free survival.

REFERENCES

1. Poussaint TY, Kocak M, Vajapeyam S, *et al.* MRI as a central component of clinical trials analysis in brainstem glioma: a report from the Pediatric Brain Tumor Consortium (PBTC). *Neuro Oncol* 2011;**13**:417–27.

2. Fischbein NJ, Prados MD, Wara W, *et al.* Radiologic classification of brain stem tumors: correlation of magnetic resonance imaging appearance with clinical outcome. *Pediatr Neurosurg* 1996;**24**:9–23.

3. Pollack IF, Stewart CF, Kocak M, *et al.* A phase II study of gefitinib and irradiation in children with newly diagnosed brainstem gliomas: a report from the Pediatric Brain Tumor Consortium. *Neuro Oncol* 2011;**13**:290–7.

4. Giussani C, Poliakov A, Ferri RT, *et al.* DTI fiber tracking to differentiate demyelinating diseases from diffuse brain stem glioma. *Neuroimage* 2010;**52**:217–23.

5. Ueoka DI, Nogueira J, Campos JC, *et al.* Brainstem gliomas – retrospective analysis of 86 patients. *J Neurol Sci* 2009;**281**:20–3.

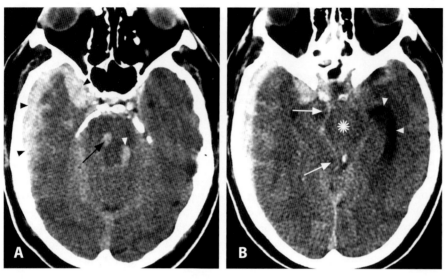

Figure 1. Non-enhanced axial CT image (A) shows a round hemorrhage (arrow) in the upper pons and a second one in its left dorsolateral aspect (white arrowhead). The brainstem is hypodense due to edema. There is subarachnoid hemorrhage and a right subdural hematoma (black arrowheads). A more cephalad CT (B) shows transtentorial herniation of the right uncus (arrows) with compression of the brainstem (*) and dilation of the left lateral ventricle (arrowheads) indicating entrapment.

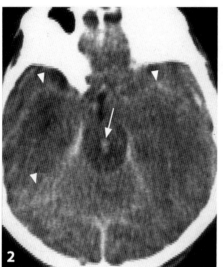
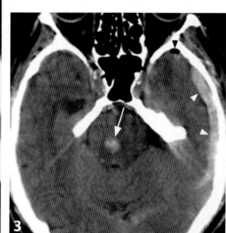

Figure 2. CT image shows a central upper pontine hemorrhage (arrow). There is also diffuse subarachnoid hemorrhage (arrowheads).

Figure 3. CT image in another patient demonstrates a rounded central hemorrhage (arrow) within the upper pons. Also note a left extra-axial hematoma (white arrowheads) and a small amount of pneumocephalus (black arrowhead) indicating skull fracture.

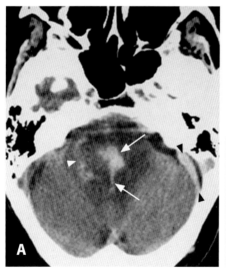
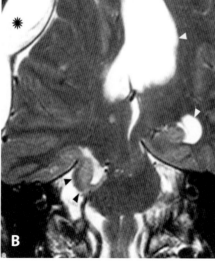

Figure 4. Predominantly linear hemorrhage (arrows) within the mid to lower pons is shown on CT (A). The brainstem is hypodense and swollen from edema. Subarachnoid blood (white arrowhead) and left posterior fossa extra-axial hematoma (black arrowheads) are present. Coronal T2WI (B) reveals right uncal herniation (arrowhead) with contralateral and inferior displacement of the pons. Also note a right epidural hematoma (*), leftward midline shift and enlarged trapped left lateral ventricle (white arrowheads).

Duret Hemorrhage

MAURICIO CASTILLO

Specific Imaging Findings

The imaging method of choice is CT, as these patients tend to be in very poor clinical condition. CT shows low-density edema in the brainstem and generally uncal transtentorial herniation with obliteration of the cisterns. Downward herniation is more difficult to identify, but inferior displacement of the cerebellar tonsils without a clear posterior fossa space-occupying lesion suggests it. Within the hypodense brainstem the acute hemorrhages are seen as focal areas of high density. They tend to be of a linear configuration, extending in from ventral to dorsal, but may have any shape. Hemorrhages are generally found in the pons, but may be located in the medulla and/or midbrain. Duret hemorrhage may be accompanied with other lesions in the brainstem such as shear injuries. MRI with its inherent increased sensitivity to subacute blood products may help to identify them later.

Pertinent Clinical Information

Duret hemorrhages are considered secondary brain injuries and in most patients there is a significant supratentorial abnormality leading to transtentorial herniations. Because intracranial trauma is strongly associated with these hemorrhages, they tend to be found in younger patients. Most patients are obtunded or comatose and show significant brainstem-associated findings (decerebration) which depend also upon the severity of the herniation and extent of the hemorrhages.

Differential Diagnosis

Shearing Injuries (DAI) (114)
- generally affect the dorsolateral aspect of the brainstem
- accompanied by supratentorial axonal injuries, generally not hemorrhagic and bright on DWI

Hypertensive Hematoma (177)
- generally larger
- possible history of uncontrolled hypertension
- no supratentorial acute abnormalities, no transtentorial herniations
- typically spontaneous, non-traumatic

Background

Increased supratentorial pressure leading to transtentorial herniation is the main cause of Duret hemorrhages. These findings were first described in 1955. Regardless of the cause of the herniation, the results are the same. The term Kernohan notch refers to an indentation in the lateral aspect of the upper brainstem contralateral to the herniation, which accompanies Duret hemorrhages. Not only is side-to-side herniation responsible, many think that cranio-caudad herniation must also be present for these bleeds to occur. As the brainstem is displaced there is traction on the perforating arteries, stretching them and tearing them, resulting in bleeding inside the brainstem. It is also possible that veins are stretched, occluded and that the hemorrhages are the result of venous infarctions. Duret hemorrhages may occur after craniotomy and their etiology in this setting is uncertain. Duret hemorrhages generally portray a poor prognosis although patients with a good recovery have been reported.

REFERENCES

1. Parizel PM, Makkat S, Jorens PG, et al. Brainstem hemorrhage in descending transtentorial herniation (Duret hemorrhage). *Intensive Care Med* 2002;**28**:85–8.
2. Stiver SI, Gean AD, Manley GT. Survival with good outcome after cerebral herniation and Duret hemorrhage caused by traumatic brain injury. *J Neurosurg* 2009;**110**:1242–6.
3. Kamijo Y, Soma K, Kishita R, Hamanaka S. Duret hemorrhage is not always suggestive of poor prognosis: a case of severe hyponatremia. *Am J Emerg Med* 2005;**23**:908–10.
4. Duret RL. A rare and little known hemorrhagic syndrome. [In French.] *Brux Med* 1955;**16**:797–800.
5. Chew KL, Baber Y, Iles L, O'Donnell C. Duret hemorrhage: demonstration of ruptured paramedian pontine branches of the basilar artery on minimally invasive, whole body postmortem CT angiography. *Forensic Sci Med Pathol* 2012 Apr 7. [Epub ahead of print]

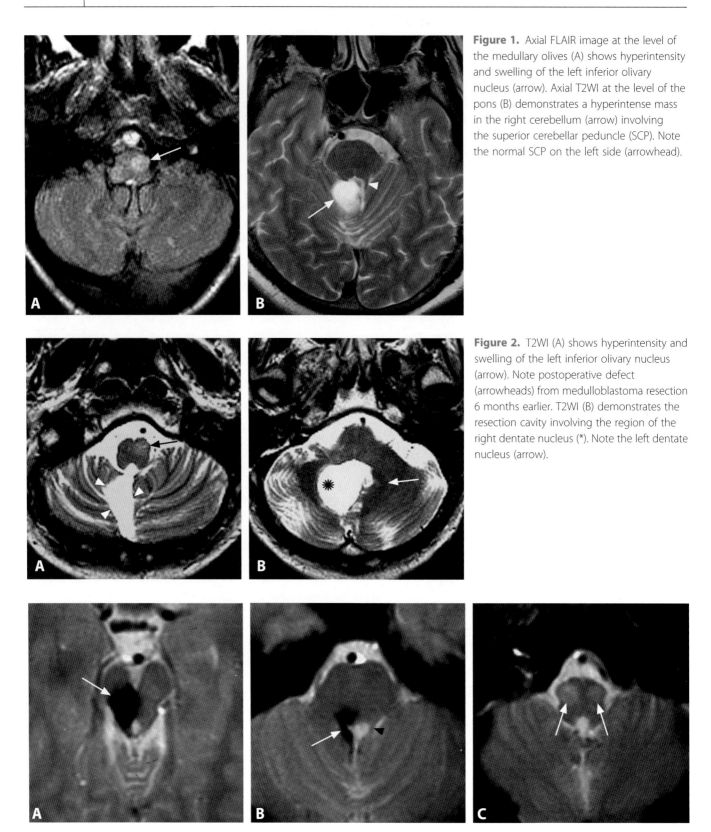

Figure 1. Axial FLAIR image at the level of the medullary olives (A) shows hyperintensity and swelling of the left inferior olivary nucleus (arrow). Axial T2WI at the level of the pons (B) demonstrates a hyperintense mass in the right cerebellum (arrow) involving the superior cerebellar peduncle (SCP). Note the normal SCP on the left side (arrowhead).

Figure 2. T2WI (A) shows hyperintensity and swelling of the left inferior olivary nucleus (arrow). Note postoperative defect (arrowheads) from medulloblastoma resection 6 months earlier. T2WI (B) demonstrates the resection cavity involving the region of the right dentate nucleus (*). Note the left dentate nucleus (arrow).

Figure 3. Axial T2*WI at the level of the midbrain (A) shows an area of signal loss (arrow) in the region of the right red nucleus, consistent with hemosiderin. The patient had hemorrhaged from a cavernoma 8 months earlier. T2*WI at the level of the pons (B) reveals extension of the hemosiderin into the right SCP (arrow). Normal SCP is seen on the left (arrowhead). T2*WI at the level of the medulla (C) shows swollen hyperintense inferior olivary nuclei bilaterally (arrows), right greater than left. Involvement of the red nucleus is responsible for the ipsilateral and of the SCP for the contralateral lesion.

Hypertrophic Olivary Degeneration

ZORAN RUMBOLDT AND BENJAMIN HUANG

Specific Imaging Findings

The finding of an olivary lesion with presence of another abnormality in the contralateral cerebellar dentate nucleus, contralateral superior cerebellar peduncle, ipsilateral red nucleus, or the ipsilateral pontine tegmentum strongly suggests the diagnosis of hypertrophic olivary degeneration (HOD). The earliest finding in HOD is high T2 signal intensity in the inferior olivary nucleus, located anteriorly within the medulla oblongata, which appears within the first month after the symptom onset. This hyperintensity can persist for years and even become permanent. Hyperintensity is followed by hypertrophy, which typically appears 10–18 months after onset, but may be observed by as early as 6 months. Hypertrophy of the inferior olive resolves by 4 years. There is no associated post-contrast enhancement. When the primary lesion is limited to the central tegmental tract, olivary hypertrophy is ipsilateral; when the primary lesion is in the dentate nucleus or in the superior cerebellar peduncle, olivary degeneration is contralateral (the most common and characteristic pattern); when the lesion involves both the central tegmental tract and the superior cerebellar peduncle, HOD is bilateral. Diffusion tensor imaging shows decreased fiber volume and reduced fractional anisotropy in the involved tracts.

Pertinent Clinical Information

Patients with HOD classically present with a palatal tremor or myoclonus, which is characterized by rhythmic involuntary movement of the soft palate, uvula, pharynx, and larynx at one to three cycles per second. Other clinical signs can include dentatorubral tremor, myoclonus of the cervical muscles and diaphragm, and symptoms of cerebellar or brainstem dysfunction. Causes of HOD include infarct, hemorrhage, trauma, demyelinating disease, neoplasm, and it may also be iatrogenic following posterior fossa surgery.

Differential Diagnosis

Infarct (152)
- reduced diffusion in the acute setting
- may enhance, usually in the subacute phase
- edema that may mimic hypertrophy occurs much earlier than hypertrophy of HOD

Neoplasms (Astrocytoma, Lymphoma, Metastases) (63, 135, 155, 173)
- rarely located precisely at the inferior olivary nucleus
- may enhance with contrast
- no additional lesion along the dentato-rubro-olivary pathway (ipsilateral red nucleus, contralateral dentate nucleus)

Multiple Sclerosis (115)
- additional demyelinating lesions are usually present
- active plaques enhance
- rarely located precisely at the inferior olivary nucleus

Background

HOD is a form of trans-synaptic degeneration which occurs in response to a lesion involving the dentato-rubro-olivary pathway (the triangle of Guillain and Mollaret). It is a unique type of degeneration because it is associated with initial enlargement of the affected structure. The triangle of Guillain and Mollaret is defined by the tracts connecting three anatomic structures – the inferior olivary nucleus, the red nucleus, and the contralateral dentate nucleus. Efferents from the dentate nucleus ascend through the superior cerebellar peduncle, cross the decussation of the brachium conjunctivum (located inferior to the red nucleus), and then descend along the central tegmental tract to the inferior olivary nucleus. The circuit is completed by efferent fiber tracts coursing from the inferior olive across the midline and through the inferior cerebellar peduncle to terminate in the original dentate nucleus. Disruption of this pathway affects the reflex arc controlling fine voluntary movements, resulting in symptoms such as palatal myoclonus. HOD is associated with lesions in the first two limbs of the triangle (the dentatorubral tract and central tegmental tract), but not with lesions involving the olivo-dentate fibers. This is because the degenerative changes of HOD are most likely due to olivary deafferentiation. Histologically, the initial olivary signal changes in HOD may be due to neuronal hypertrophy and gliosis associated with demyelination and vacuolization. Delayed development of hypertrophy is most likely a consequence of neuronal and astrocytic hypertrophy, while the subsequent olivary shrinkage likely relates to disappearance of neuronal cells.

REFERENCES

1. Goyal M, Versnick E, Tuite P, et al. Hypertrophic olivary degeneration: metaanalysis of the temporal evolution of MR findings. AJNR 2000;21:1073–7.
2. Birbamer G, Buchberger W, Felber S, et al. MR appearance of hypertrophic olivary degeneration: temporal relationships. AJNR 1992;13:1501–3.
3. Hornyak M, Osborn AG, Couldwell WT. Hypertrophic olivary degeneration after surgical removal of cavernous malformations of the brain stem: report of four cases and review of the literature. Acta Neurochir (Wien) 2008;150:149–56.
4. Shah R, Markert J, Bag AK, et al. Diffusion tensor imaging in hypertrophic olivary degeneration. AJNR 2010;31:1729–31.

Brain Imaging with MRI and CT, ed. Zoran Rumboldt *et al.* Published by Cambridge University Press. © Cambridge University Press 2012.

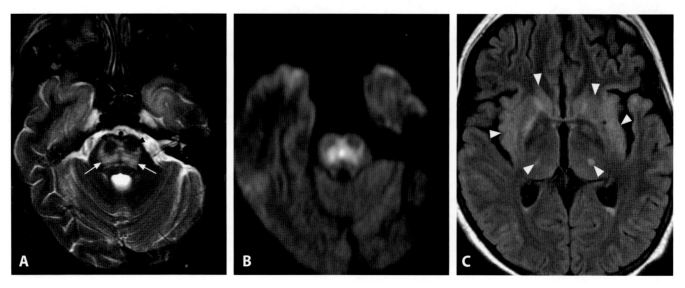

Figure 1. Axial T2WI (A) shows a somewhat trident-shaped area of high signal in the mid pons (arrows) predominantly affecting the regions of the transverse fibers. Note spared corticospinal tracts (arrowheads). Corresponding DWI (B) shows high signal in the lesion. FLAIR image (C) shows additional lesions in the basal ganglia, thalami and the insular cortex bilaterally (arrowheads).

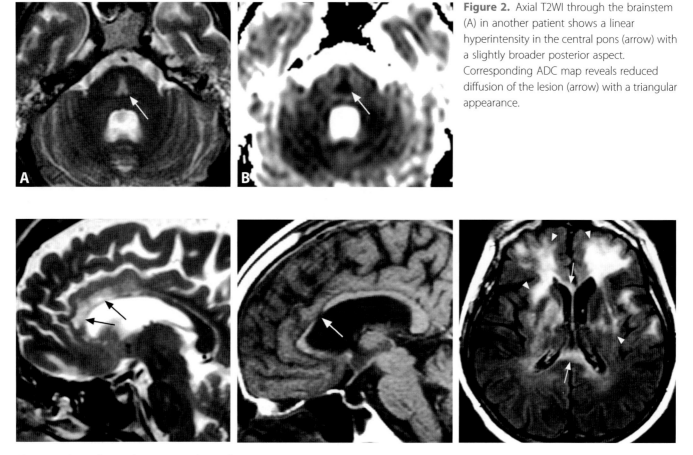

Figure 2. Axial T2WI through the brainstem (A) in another patient shows a linear hyperintensity in the central pons (arrow) with a slightly broader posterior aspect. Corresponding ADC map reveals reduced diffusion of the lesion (arrow) with a triangular appearance.

Figure 3. Sagittal T2WI during acute phase of the disease shows high signal intensity in the anterior body and genu of the corpus callosum (arrows).

Figure 4. Midsagittal T1WI in chronic phase of the disease shows thinning of the corpus callosum with a focal lesion in the anterior body (arrow).

Figure 5. FLAIR image shows involvement of the anterior and posterior callosum (arrows) with extensive abnormalities primarily in the frontal WM and deep GM (arrowheads).

Osmotic Myelinolysis

MAURICIO CASTILLO

Specific Imaging Findings

In central pontine myelinolysis (CPM) CT shows hypodensity in the central mid to lower pons, typically of a somewhat triangular shape with its base located posteriorly and resembling a trident, due to sparing of the corticospinal tracts. The brainstem is not expanded and the abnormality tends to regress and even disappear with time. The lesions are T2 hyperintense with usually less prominent T1 hypointensity. Hemorrhage is not present and contrast enhancement is absent or minimal. DWI shows the lesion to be bright and ADC maps reveal reduced diffusion. Diffusion changes may precede T2 findings by up to 24 hours. MRS may in the acute period show elevated choline, probably due to breakdown of myelin. NAA is decreased and lactate may occasionally be present. DTI may show swelling and displacement of white matter tracts but no frank destruction.

Extrapontine myelinolysis presents as areas of high T2 signal and reduced diffusion involving the supratentorial deep gray matter and/or the corpus callosum. Involvement of the deep gray matter occurs in 10% of patients with CPM. Involvement of the corpus callosum, primarily the body, is generally known as the Marchiafava–Bignami syndrome (MBS). The entire thickness of the callosum is affected, the anterior and posterior commissures as well as the subcortical U-fibers may be involved. The lesions are T1 hypointense and bright on T2 sequences. Peripheral contrast enhancement may occur during the acute to subacute periods. Reduced diffusion correlates with a worse prognosis. DTI shows disruption of axon bundles most marked in the callosal body. If the patients survive, the lesions may resolve completely or diminish in size.

Pertinent Clinical Information

CPM most commonly occurs in chronic alcoholics, but also with debilitating illnesses, in transplant recipients, and others. CPM tends to be associated with hyponatremia and other metabolic disturbances particularly when these are rapidly corrected. Symptoms include tetraplegia, bulbar and pseudobulbar palsies, altered mental status, and rapidly progressive coma. Symptoms may be biphasic with an initial nonspecific acute period followed by mild improvement and then quadraparesis and bulbar palsy.

MBS also typically occurs in alcoholics. Although initially thought to be caused by Chianti wines from Italy, all alcoholic beverages have been implicated. It may be related to a deficiency in vitamin B complex. Symptoms include acute confusion, disorientation, neurocognitive deficits, and seizures. Coma and death may ensue if not promptly treated.

Differential Diagnosis

CPM

Pontine Infarction
- typically unilateral paramedian and not central

Multiple Sclerosis (115)
- usually additional involvement of cerebellar peduncles and supratentorial white matter, particularly in the periventricular regions

Glioma (63)
- presence of mass effect

MBS

Infarction (152)
- frequently unilateral, corresponding to anterior cerebral artery territory

Demyelinating Processes (112, 115)
- usually more focal multiple lesions

Susac Syndrome (113)
- rounded cystic-appearing lesions in corpus callosum

Background

CPM is probably caused by the inability of brain cells to respond to rapid changes in osmolality of the extracellular compartment. This osmotic imbalance affects oligodendrocytes located in the pons, thalami, basal ganglia, and other extrapontine sites. In the pons there is preferential involvement of the transverse fibers. The neurons and axons are preserved and there is little or no inflammation. In MBS, abnormal levels of vitamin B complex may also lead to abnormal function and integrity of oligodendrocytes. However, in MBS the axons may also be affected, leading to frank necrosis. This necrosis in the callosum occurs in a layered fashion, splitting it into three distinct segments – the histological hallmark of the disease. The middle layer is most affected with cystic degeneration. There is only a mild inflammatory reaction, differentiating it from multiple sclerosis and other inflammatory demyelinating processes.

REFERENCES

1. Ruzek KA, Campeau NG, Miller GM. Early diagnosis of central pontine myelinolysis with diffusion-weighted imaging. *AJNR* 2004;**25**:210–3.
2. Liberatore M, Denier C, Filliard P, *et al.* Diffusion tensor imaging and tractography of central pontine myelinolysis. *J Neuroradiol* 2006;**33**:189–93.
3. Arbelaez A, Pajon A, Castillo M. Acute Marchiafava–Bignami disease: MR findings in two patients. *AJNR* 2003;**24**:1955–7.
4. Kallakatta RN, Radhakrishnan A, Fayaz RK, *et al.* Clinical and functional outcome and factors predicting prognosis in osmotic demyelination syndrome (central pontine and/or extrapontine myelinolysis) in 25 patients. *J Neurol Neurosurg Psychiatry* 2011;**82**:326–31.

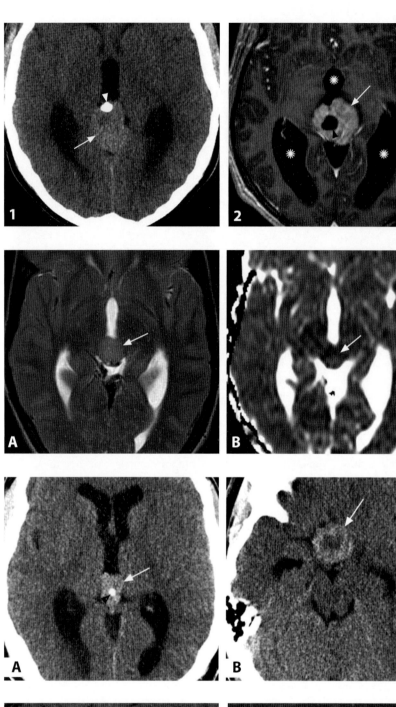

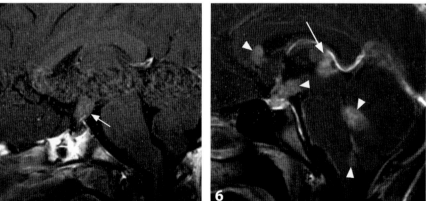

Figure 1. Axial non-enhanced CT shows hyperdense pineal gland mass (arrow) with intact single calcification (arrowhead) anteriorly. There is mild hydrocephalus.

Figure 2. Axial post-contrast T1WI shows enhancing pineal mass (arrow) containing a cyst (arrowhead). Hydrocephalus (*) is present.

Figure 3. Axial T2WI (A) shows relatively isointense solid portions of a pineal mass (arrow), similar to the gray matter. There is no hydrocephalus. The corresponding ADC map (B) shows low diffusion within the lesion (arrow), which is similar to the brain.

Figure 4. Axial CT image (A) shows a slightly hyperdense mass (arrow) that surrounds an intact pineal calcification (arrowhead). A more inferior CT image in this 20-year-old man (B) reveals an additional suprasellar mass (arrow), which is also mildly hyperdense with a central area of lower attenuation.

Figure 5. Midsagittal post-contrast T1WI shows a nonspecific enhancing lesion infiltrating the pituitary infundibulum (arrow).

Figure 6. Midsagittal post-contrast T1WI shows an enhancing pineal gland mass (arrow) as well as enhancing ventricular and suprasellar masses (arrowheads).

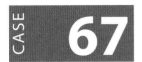

Germinoma

MAURICIO CASTILLO AND ZORAN RUMBOLDT

Specific Imaging Findings

CT of pineal germinomas shows the masses centered at the pineal gland to be slightly hyperdense without contrast, contain a central or peripheral characteristically intact calcification (so-called "engulfed" pineal calcification) and show dense contrast enhancement. Cysts are not uncommon, particularly if the tumor is big, while hemorrhage is rare. The tumors are isointense to brain on T1-weighted images, of isointense to low T2 signal and with ADC values similar to the brain on diffusion imaging. After gadolinium, these tumors show marked enhancement. Another common location for germinomas is the suprasellar region, where they exhibit the same imaging features. It is important to evaluate the entire craniospinal axis after contrast has been given to look for CSF tumor spread. MR spectroscopy shows high choline, low NAA and lactate.

Pertinent Clinical Information

Over 90% of germinomas are found in patients aged under 20 years (peak ages: 12–20 years). Those in the pineal gland are more common in males and the usual clinical findings include: Parinaud syndrome and signs of increased intracranial pressure. Those arising in the suprasellar region produce diabetes insipidus, vision abnormalities and precocious puberty. There is an increased incidence of germinomas in the following syndromes: Down, Klinefelter and neurofibromatosis type 1. Neuroendoscopic procedures are used for both lesion biopsy and management of hydrocephalus associated with these tumors. The risk of tumor dissemination following surgery is minimal when appropriate chemotherapy and radiotherapy are provided postoperatively. The tumors are very radiosensitive, a fact that contributes to a relatively good prognosis, with 10-year overall and progression-free survival in the range of 80–90%. The recurrences are typically located outside the radiation field.

Differential Diagnosis

Pineal

Pineoblastoma (68)
- "exploding" calcifications on CT
- younger patients
- presence of hemorrhage
- typically very dark on ADC maps

Metastasis
- the mass is frequently heterogenous and irregular
- additional lesions are commonly present

Pineocytoma
- older patients (adults)
- well-defined mass

Suprasellar

Chiasmatic/Hypothalamic Astrocytoma (46)
- rarely diffusely enhancing
- relatively bright on T2WI and ADC maps

Langerhans Cell Histiocytosis (43)
- may have additional lesions (skull)
- may be indistinguishable from germinoma

Granulomatous Processes (Sarcoidosis, Tuberculosis) (118, 170)
- usually additional leptomeningeal enhancement

Background

The broader and more encompassing term is germ cell tumors, as not all of these neoplasms are pure germinomas. Pure germinomas have a similar histology to seminomas and are also called dysgerminomas. Germinomas are considered malignant and have variable WHO grades. Although they may contain cysts, the presence of necrosis, calcifications and hemorrhage are less common. They presumably arise from primordial pineal gland cells. They represent about 1% of all intracranial malignancies and about 5% of intracranial tumors in children. In the pediatric population it accounts for over 50% of all tumors arising in the pineal gland. Germinomas are common in male adolescents and have a high prevalence in Japan. Unlike pineal germinomas, those arising in the suprasellar region have no age predominance and are perhaps more common in females. At the time of diagnosis, CSF tumor spread is common. Germinomas in unusual locations (basal ganglia and thalami) are predominantly found in Southeast Asia.

REFERENCES

1. Chang T, Teng MM, Guo WY, Sheng WC. CT of pineal tumors and intracranial germ-cell tumors. *AJNR* 1989;**10**:1039–44.
2. Wang Y, Zou L, Gao B. Intracranial germinoma: clinical and MRI findings in 56 patients. *Childs Nerv Syst* 2010;**26**:1773–7.
3. Dumrongpisutikul N, Intrapiromkul J, Yousem DM. Distinguishing between germinomas and pineal cell tumors on MR imaging. *AJNR* 2012;**33**:550–5.
4. Kawabata Y, Takahashi JA, Arakawa Y, *et al*. Long term outcomes in patients with intracranial germinomas: a single institution experience of irradiation with or without chemotherapy. *J Neurooncol* 2008;**88**:161–7.
5. Shono T, Natori Y, Morioka T, *et al*. Results of a long-term follow-up after neuroendoscopic biopsy procedure and third ventriculostomy in patients with intracranial germinomas. *J Neurosurg* 2007;**107**(3 Suppl):193–8.

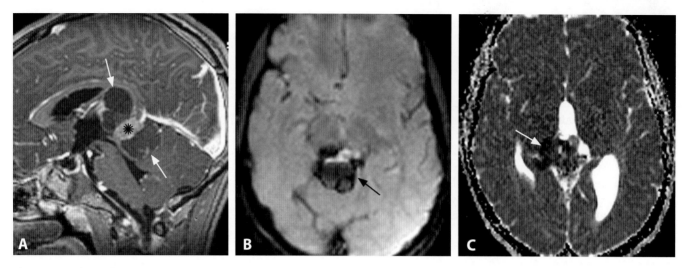

Figure 1. Midsagittal post-contrast T1W1 (A) shows a large mass centered at the pineal region with a solid enhancing component (*) and peripheral cystic-appearing portions (arrows). On axial T2*-weighted image (B) a cystic portion of the lesion contains fluid levels with dependent very low signal (arrow), consistent with hemorrhage. Axial ADC map (C) through the enhancing solid component reveals a predominantly very low signal, darker than the brain (arrow).

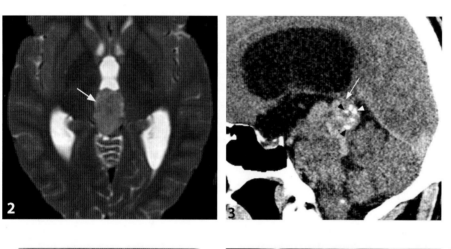

Figure 2. Axial fat-saturated T2WI image shows a pineal region mass (arrow) of signal intensity similar to the gray matter and hydrocephalus.

Figure 3. Non-enhanced CT image reconstructed in the sagittal plane shows a hyperdense mass (arrow) with characteristic scattered pineal gland calcifications (arrowheads). Ventriculomegaly is also present.

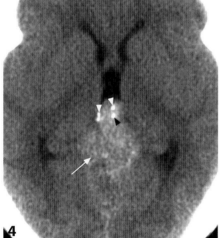

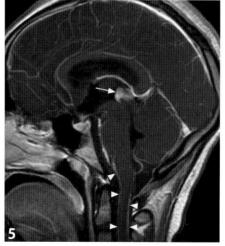

Figure 4. Axial non-enhanced CT image in another patient shows a hyperdense mass (arrow) in the pineal region with a more subtle appearance of "exploded" pineal gland calcifications (arrowheads).

Figure 5. Midsagittal post-contrast T1WI shows incompletely enhancing pineal gland lesion (arrow). Note seeding along ventral surfaces of the brainstem and surrounding the upper spinal cord (arrowheads).

Pineoblastoma

MAURICIO CASTILLO AND ZORAN RUMBOLDT

Specific Imaging Findings

The lesions arise from the pineal gland and are typically hyper-dense on non-contrast CT with variable enhancement. Tumors often contain calcifications, particularly in their periphery (so-called "exploded" calcifications), which is the most specific imaging finding. On MRI, the solid portions show very low ADC values and tend to be T2 iso to hypointense. Cysts and hemorrhage are not uncommon. After contrast administration, enhancement is the rule. Hydrocephalus is frequently present. Screening of the entire craniospinal axis before surgery is needed to rule out CSF tumor spread. MR spectroscopy shows marked elevation of choline, low-to-absent NAA, lactate, lipids and occasionally a specific peak at 3.4 ppm on short echo time studies, thought to represent taurine. On perfusion studies these masses show high relative cerebral blood volume.

Pertinent Clinical Information

Pineoblastomas are generally found in children and young adults. Some series report a slightly increased incidence in females. Because of their location, compression of the aqueduct of Sylvius leads to early onset of hydrocephalus and compression of the brainstem. Symptoms include elevated intracranial pressure, headaches, nausea/vomiting, ataxia and Parinaud syndrome. Nearly a half of the patients, regardless of their age presentation, will be found to have CSF tumor spread and thus many treatment protocols assume that all patients have it and treat the entire craniospinal axis. The main modes of treatment are initial tumor resection/debulking followed by chemotherapy and in older patients a combined chemo-radiation protocol. Despite aggressive treatment prognosis is poor, with survival rates around 50% at 5 years after the initial diagnosis.

Differential Diagnosis

Germ Cells Tumors (Germinoma) (67)
- engulfed or displaced instead of "exploded" pineal calcification
- generally found in (teenage) males
- similar to the brain on ADC maps

Papillary Tumor of the Pineal Region (PTPR)
- may be hyperintense on pre-contrast T1-weighted images
- centered on the posterior commissure

Astrocytoma (62)
- more commonly arises from tectum, very rare in pineal gland
- higher ADC, no taurine on MRS, lower perfusion

Pineocytoma
- tumor of older individuals
- absence of "exploded" pineal calcification
- higher ADC, no taurine on MRS, lower perfusion

Metastatic Neoplasm
- frequently heterogenous and necrotic
- additional lesions may be present
- usually in older individuals

Teratoma
- may contain fat
- younger patients, typically a neonatal tumor

Atypical Teratoid–Rhabdoid Tumor (ATRT)
- younger patients, typically a neonatal tumor
- may be indistinguishable from pineoblastoma

Background

Pineoblastomas are primitive neuroectodermal cell tumors (containing numerous small blue cells) and are highly malignant (WHO grade 4). Often these tumors contain necrosis and hemorrhage. They probably arise from the pineal precursor cells and comprise about 15–30% of all pineal gland tumors, particularly in younger patients. Overall, they represent less than 1% of all intracranial malignancies.

Papillary tumor of the pineal region (PTPR) has recently been added to the WHO classification of CNS tumors. This is an uncommon neoplasm for which origin from specialized ependymocytes of the subcommissural organ was postulated. It appears to be characteristically T1 hyperintense and with cystic areas on MR imaging. The clinical course of PTPR is characterized by frequent postoperative local recurrence.

REFERENCES

1. Smith AB, Rushing EJ, Smirniotopoulos JG. From the archives of the AFIP: lesions of the pineal region: radiologic–pathologic correlation. 2010;**30**:2001–20.

2. Dumrongpisutikul N, Intrapiromkul J, Yousem DM, Distinguishing between germinomas and pineal cell tumors on MR imaging. *AJNR* 2012;**33**:550–5.

3. Al-Hussaini M, Sultan I, Abuirmileh N, et al. Pineal gland tumors: experience from the SEER database. *J Neurooncol* 2009;**94**:351–8.

4. Yazici N, Varan A, Söylemezoğlu F, et al. Pineal region tumors in children: a single center experience. *Neuropediatrics* 2009;**40**:15–21.

5. Chang AH, Fuller GN, Debnam JM, et al. MR imaging of papillary tumor of the pineal region. *AJNR* 2008;**29**:187–9.

Brain Imaging with MRI and CT, ed. Zoran Rumboldt *et al.* Published by Cambridge University Press. © Cambridge University Press 2012.

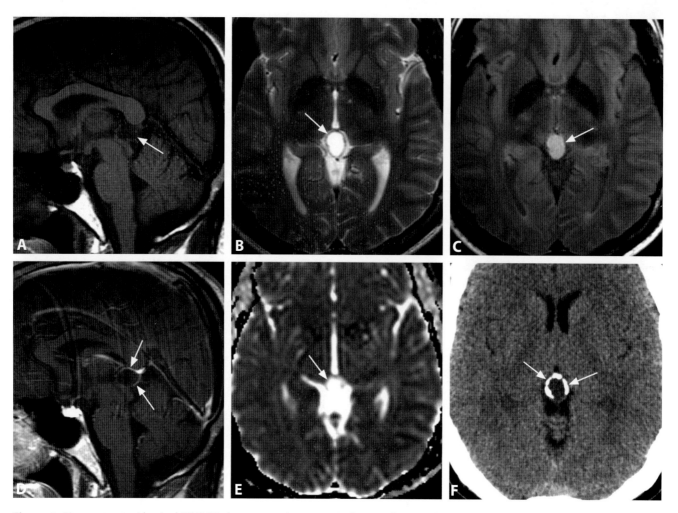

Figure 1. Non-contrast midsagittal T1WI (A) shows an oval structure in the pineal region (arrow) with a smooth capsule and no tectal compression. The central portion is similar to the CSF. Axial T2WI (B) also shows CSF-like signal of the contents (arrow), suggesting a cyst. Corresponding FLAIR image (C) shows high signal intensity (arrow). Post-contrast midsagittal T1WI (D) reveals no internal enhancement and enhancing displaced veins (arrows). ADC map shows high diffusion within the cyst (arrow), indistinguishable from the CSF. Axial CT image (F) shows peripheral calcifications (arrows) and slightly hyperdense contents.

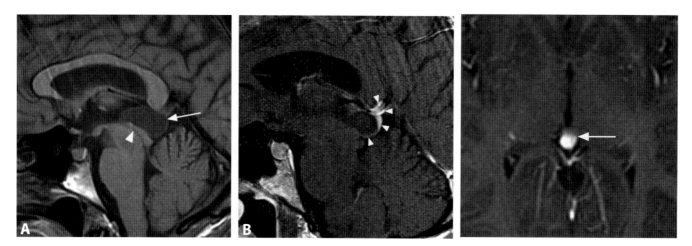

Figure 2. Non-contrast midsagittal T1WI (A) shows a larger cyst (arrow) of the pineal gland with minimal compression of the cephalad-most aqueduct (arrowhead) but no hydrocephalus. Note that the cyst is slightly brighter than the CSF. Post-contrast T1WI (B) shows enhancing veins (arrowheads) around the cyst, which does not enhance.

Figure 3. Axial post-contrast T1WI shows enhancement within a pineal cyst in this delayed image. A subtle fluid level (arrow) is appreciated with contrast being dependent.

140

Specific Imaging Findings

Pineal cysts are common and generally less than 15 mm in greatest dimension. When larger, they may compress the tectal plate and aqueduct resulting in hydrocephalus. Pineal cysts usually follow the signal intensity of CSF on T1- and T2-weighted images, occasionally having higher T1 signal. On FLAIR images they are usually brighter than the CSF. The contents are homogenous and follow the CSF on diffusion imaging. Their capsule is thin, less than 2 mm in thickness and devoid of nodularity. Cysts may contain internal septations which are also thin. The details of their capsule are more evident with high-resolution volumetric acquisitions and at 3.0 T than at 1.5 T. After contrast administration, the capsule may show linear but never nodular enhancement. The veins around it enhance and may be confused with their capsule. Because they do not have a blood–brain barrier, on delayed post-contrast images they may show fluid levels or enhance in a near-complete fashion, making them difficult to differentiate from solid lesions. When they bleed (pineal apoplexy) they show varying signal intensities corresponding to the age of the blood. Enlarging or decreasing size of the pineal cysts are rare. Pineal cysts are less well seen on CT and a higher percentage of them appear falsely as solid masses.

Pertinent Clinical Information

Pineal cysts are usually incidental findings on imaging studies. It is estimated that up to 40% of the population has them and they are identified by MRI in 7–15% of adults. Pineal cysts usually have no clinical implications and remain asymptomatic for years. Symptomatic cysts vary in size from 7 to 45 mm and they may produce symptoms of headache, vertigo, visual and oculomotor disturbances, obstructive hydrocephalus, and Parinaud syndrome due to compression of the dorsal midbrain. If they acutely bleed internally, they may suddenly enlarge and produce all of these symptoms, which is known as pineal apoplexy.

Differential Diagnosis

Epidermoid (143)
- very bright "light bulb" on DWI

Pineocytoma
- at least some nodular contrast enhancement is present

Pineoblastoma (68)
- predominantly solid contrast enhancement
- low ADC values
- "exploded" pineal calcification on CT

Germ Cell Tumor (Germinoma) (67)
- solid contrast enhancement
- ADC values similar to the brain

Metastatic Neoplasm
- solid or at least partial nodular enhancement is present

Background

Pineal cysts are non-neoplastic glial, fluid-filled structures. Their capsule is composed of an inner gliotic layer, an intermediate layer of pineal tissues and an outer one of connective tissue. It is not clear how they form. Some think that they represent an invagination of the pineal recess of the third ventricle into the gland. Other proposed etiologies include the presence of pre-existing lacunae which are invaded by differentiated glial cells (ependymal) or surface invaginations inviting CSF to accumulate within them. Normal pineal glands typically contain small cystic areas on histology. High-resolution heavily T2- and T1-weighted 3D sequences increase the detection rate of pineal cysts to the levels reported in autopsy series while decreasing the diagnostic uncertainty. Their management is controversial, as the outcome of surgery is variable with some patients improving when others remain equally symptomatic. Some cysts will change in size over time, but these changes are minimal and on average 2–3 mm. It has been suggested that incidentally identified pineal region cystic lesions, both typical and atypical, can be followed clinically and not with MRI.

REFERENCES

1. Pu Y, Mahankali S, Hou J, *et al.* High prevalence of pineal cysts in healthy adults demonstrated by high-resolution, noncontrast brain MR imaging. *AJNR* 2007;**28**:1706–9.
2. Fakhran S, Escott EJ. Pineocytoma mimicking a pineal cyst on imaging: true diagnostic dilemma or a case of incomplete imaging? *AJNR* 2008;**29**:159–63.
3. Fleege MA, Millder GM, Fletcher GP, *et al.* Benign pineal cysts of the pituitary gland: unusual imaging characteristics with histologic correlation. *AJNR* 1994;**15**:161–6.
4. Barboriak DP, Lee L, Provenzale JM. Serial MR imaging of pineal cysts: implications for natural history and follow-up. *AJR* 2001;**176**:737–43.
5. Cauley KA, Linnell GJ, Braff SP, Filippi CG. Serial follow-up MRI of indeterminate cystic lesions of the pineal region: experience at a rural tertiary care referral center. *AJR* 2009;**193**:533–7.

Brain Imaging with MRI and CT, ed. Zoran Rumboldt *et al.* Published by Cambridge University Press. © Cambridge University Press 2012.

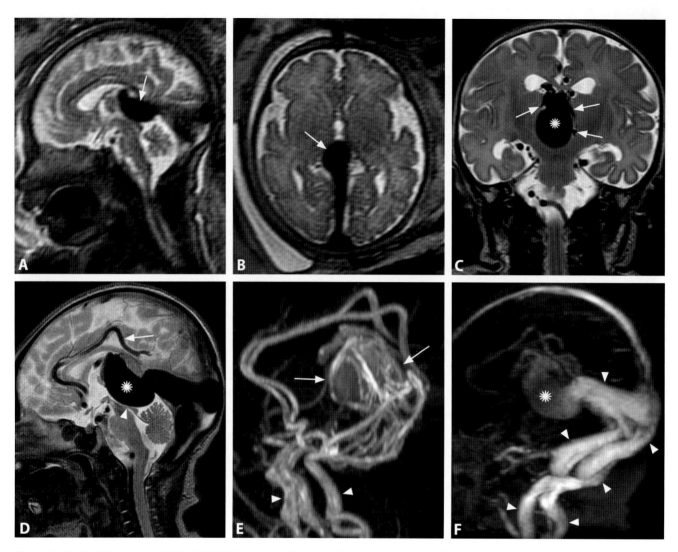

Figure 1. Sagittal (A) and axial (B) fetal MR T2WIs show a dilated vascular structure (arrows). The brain parenchyma is normal. Postnatal coronal T2WI (C) shows the midline dilated venous pouch (*) and adjacent choroidal feeders (arrows). Brain parenchyma is normal and lateral ventricles are minimally dilated. Sagittal T2WI (D) shows the large pouch (*) causing aqueductal compression (arrowhead). Note markedly dilated pericallosal arteries (arrow). MRA (E) reveals enlarged internal carotid and basilar arteries (arrowheads) and multiple feeders from the anterior choroidal, posterior cerebral, and pericallosal arteries converging towards the pouch (arrows). MRV (F) shows the pouch (*) and dilated venous drainage pathways (arrowheads).

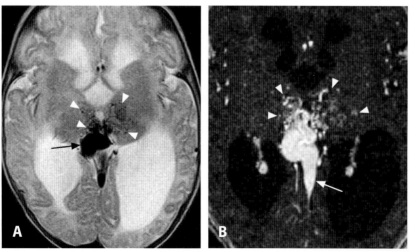

Figure 2. Axial T2WI (A) in an infant shows a large midline vascular structure (arrow) in the location of the vein of Galen. Numerous small flow-voids (arrowheads) converging to this venous pouch are arterial feeders. Note moderate hydrocephalus. Post-contrast MRA source image (B) again reveals multiple small arterial feeders (arrowheads) of the malformation, and its drainage into the falcine sinus (arrow).

Vein of Galen Aneurysmal Malformation (VGAM)

ANDREA ROSSI

Specific Imaging Findings

Prenatal ultrasound in vein of Galen aneurysmal malformation (VGAM) shows a midline cystic structure in the region of the quadrigeminal plate with intraluminal flow. Prenatal MRI shows the dilated pouch and draining sinus, hypointense on all imaging sequences due to flow phenomena. On postnatal MRI a dilated rounded to ovoid or tubular venous ampulla in the region of the quadrigeminal cistern and velum interpositum is again hypointense on all sequences, of variable, usually quite large dimensions. The arterial feeders are seen as multiple small flow-voids surrounding the ampulla; on MRA they appear to converge to the VGAM, whereas distal flow in the main cerebral arteries is not well seen. The draining vein is a persistent falcine sinus (instead of the nondeveloped straight sinus). Relative stenosis of the outflowing vein is often seen at the tentorial hiatus just below the callosal splenium. Patency of the draining vein and sinuses, especially at the sigmoid–jugular junction, must be assessed. The brain parenchyma should be carefully scrutinized for signs of injury including encephalomalacia, atrophy, subcortical calcifications, and ventriculomegaly. Herniation of cerebellar tonsils may be a consequence of venous hypertension. Catheter angiography elucidates the anatomy and pathophysiology of VGAM, but should be reserved for endovascular treatment.

Pertinent Clinical Information

Neonates with VGAM present with congestive cardiac failure – tachycardia, respiratory distress and cyanosis. During early infancy, macrocrania may appear as a consequence of maturational delay of the dural sinuses and granulations, or due to cerebral aqueduct compression by the dilated pouch, leading to hydrocephalus and intracranial hypertension. Older children usually present with chronic headache and hydrocephalus or seizures. Treatment is by transarterial embolization, and the optimal therapeutic window at 4–5 months of age has shown the best efficacy in controlling the malformation and allowing the brain to normally mature and develop. Earlier treatment carries a higher risk of failure and comorbidity; it may be contemplated in rapidly progressive cases with unresponsive heart failure. Severe diffuse brain injury is a contraindication for endovascular treatment. Spontaneous VGAM thrombosis has been described in rare cases.

Differential Diagnosis

Vein of Galen Aneurysmal Dilation
- arteriovenous malformation or dural fistula drain into the true vein of Galen

- the nidus is typically located in a paramedian pial location
- exceedingly uncommon in neonates

Aneurysm
- uncommon in children, especially neonates
- often arises within AVM nidus (venous aneurysm)
- may be partially thrombosed with layered appearance

Background

VGAM is the most common arteriovenous malformation of infancy, more prevalent in males (1.7 : 1 male to female ratio). The term VGAM is actually a misnomer, as the abnormality involves the median prosencephalic vein, the embryonic precursor of the vein of Galen. The abnormal flow through the connection blocks the normal involution of this vein and prevents the development of the vein of Galen. The arterial feeders are derived from the choroidal arteries that shunt into the venous pouch (commonly referred to as the "Galen ampulla") at the level of the choroidal fissure. The pouch is located in the midline in the region of the velum interpositum and receives bilateral and often symmetrical supply, although in the presence of a stronger unilateral feeder it will mildly shift to the opposite side. VGAM is categorized in two variants depending on angioarchitecture. The choroidal type is characterized by a large number of feeders from several choroidal arteries forming a network of vessels opening into the venous pouch, while the mural type is characterized by a smaller number of feeders (four or less). The venous drainage in both forms is towards the dilated median vein of the prosencephalon, which drains through a falcine sinus into the posterior third of the superior sagittal sinus as well as into occipital and marginal sinuses.

REFERENCES

1. Alvarez H, Garcia Monaco R, Rodesch G, et al. Vein of Galen aneurysmal malformations. *Neuroimaging Clin N Am* 2007;**17**:189–206.
2. Brunelle F. Arteriovenous malformation of the vein of Galen in children. *Pediatr Radiol* 1997;**27**:501–13.
3. Kalra V, Malhotra A. Fetal MR diagnosis of vein of Galen aneurysmal malformation. *Pediatr Radiol* 2010;**40** *(Suppl* 1):155.
4. Khullar D, Andeejani AM, Bulsara KR. Evolution of treatment options for vein of Galen malformations. *J Neurosurg Pediatr* 2010;**6**:444–51.

Brain Imaging with MRI and CT, ed. Zoran Rumboldt *et al.* Published by Cambridge University Press. © Cambridge University Press 2012.

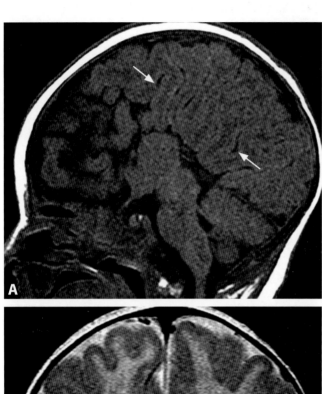

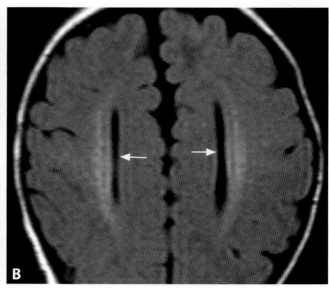

Figure 1. Sagittal T1WI (A) shows abnormal radial configuration of the parasagittal gyri (arrows) with completely absent corpus callosum. Axial FLAIR image (B) shows abnormal parallel configuration of the lateral ventricles (arrows). Coronal (C) T2WI shows the bundles of Probst (arrows) along the superior and medial aspect of the lateral ventricles and rounded hippocampi (arrowheads). Note the "trident" or "Viking helmet" appearance of the lateral ventricles and the interhemispheric fissure.

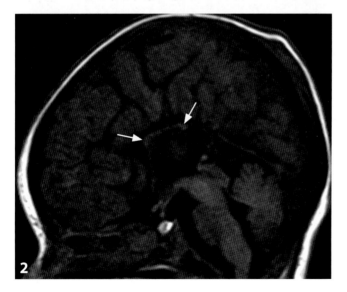

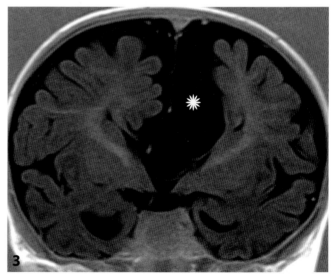

Figure 2. Midsagittal T1WI shows only a thin band of white matter (arrows) representing severe corpus callosum hypoplasia.

Figure 3. Coronal inversion recovery T1WI shows absent corpus callosum and an associated interhemispheric cyst (*).

Corpus Callosum Dysgenesis

MARIA GISELE MATHEUS

Specific Imaging Findings

Callosal dysgenesis (CD) is a spectrum of congenital defects of the corpus callosum (CC), which can be complete or partial. In complete CD, the CC, hippocampal commissure, and in half of the cases the anterior commissure are absent. In partial CD, the anterior commissure is always present as well as portions of CC. Multiplanar MR imaging is necessary to assess the CD abnormalities. With complete CC agenesis the morphology of the lateral ventricles is modified, as they become widely separated and lose the medially converging configuration, assuming an abnormal parallel appearance. The occipital horns are also enlarged. The interhemispheric fissure extends downwards to the roof of the third ventricle, which bulges upward. The midline cortical pattern is altered with the cingulate gyrus appearing absent and radially arrayed gyri converging to the roof of the third ventricle. The parietal and occipital sulci are shallow, and the hippocampi show round configuration. A parallel bundle of parasagittal white matter tracts is seen in the medial superior aspect of the lateral ventricles with relatively high T1 and low T2 signal intensity (bundle of Probst). On coronal images the constellation of findings leads to "trident" or "Viking helmet" appearance. Associated other abnormalities are frequently found with CD (in about three-quarters of cases), the most common ones being lipoma, interhemispheric cyst, and cortical dysplasia.

Pertinent Clinical Information

CD is often accompanied by other midline structural abnormalities, hypertelorism, neuronal migrational disorders, metabolic abnormalities, and a number of syndromes. These associated abnormalities lead to symptoms such as seizures, developmental delay, and pituitary/hypothalamic disfunctions. On the other hand, the majority of patients with isolated CC agenesis show only subtle cognitive, behavioral, and synchronous coordination deficits.

Differential Diagnosis

Acquired Defects of the CC
- focal defect or reduction in size, usually with associated signal abnormality
- adjacent gliosis and sometimes hemosiderin staining
- history of ischemia, trauma, ventricular shunting, or callosotomy

Severe Hydrocephalus (92–Figure 1)
- marked enlargement of the lateral ventricles

- significant loss of hemispheric brain parenchyma
- marked CC thinning, not absence, sometimes with additional acquired focal defect

Wallerian Degeneration (78)
- focal defect with abnormal signal
- related to distant (cortical hemispheric) neuronal damage

Background

CC development is a complex process that has not been completely elucidated. It starts developing from the lamina reunions when special glial cells with molecules capable to attract and repel axons form a bridge-like midline structure. These cells originate from the germinal matrix, migrate medially, and create a bridge across the medial interhemispheric meninx primitiva. The first callosal axons then grow following the surface of this bridge toward the contralateral hemisphere along the anterior comissure. Other fibers follow and accumulate by a process of fasciculation, which includes integration with early fibers using them as a support. The CC development starts at the genu, followed by body, isthmus, splenium and rostrum. By 12–13 weeks of embryological development, a well-defined callosal plate is obvious and CC is completely formed by week 20. Genetic/molecular events controlling commissuration and insults involving these structures result in CD.

REFERENCES

1. Kuker W, Mayrhofer H, Mader I, et al. Malformation of the midline commissures: MRI findings in different forms of callosal dysgenesis. *Eur Radiol* 2003;**13**:598–604.

2. Barkovich AJ, Kjos BO. Normal postnatal development of the corpus callosum as demonstrated by MR imaging. *AJNR* 1988;**9**:487–91.

3. Tang PH, Bartha AI, Norton ME, et al. Agenesis of the corpus callosum: an MR imaging analysis of associated abnormalities in the fetus. *AJNR* 2009;**30**:257–63.

4. Paul LK, Brown WS, Adolphs R, et al. Agenesis of the corpus callosum: genetic, developmental and functional aspects of connectivity. *Nat Rev Neurosci* 2007;**8**:287–99.

5. Wahl M, Strominger Z, Jeremy RJ, et al. Variability of homotopic and heterotopic callosal connectivity in partial agenesis of the corpus callosum: a 3T diffusion tensor imaging and Q-ball tractography study. *AJNR* 2009;**30**:282–9.

Brain Imaging with MRI and CT, ed. Zoran Rumboldt *et al.* Published by Cambridge University Press. © Cambridge University Press 2012.

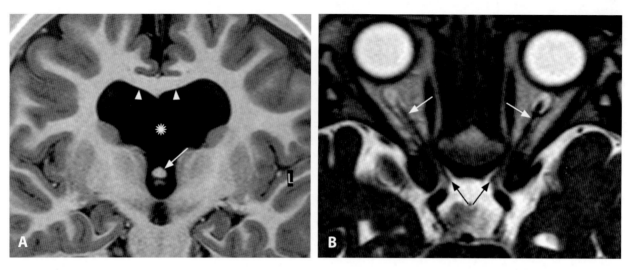

Figure 1. Coronal T1W IR (A) shows agenesis of the septum pellucidum (*) with flat roof of frontal horns (arrowheads) and fused fornices (arrow). Axial high resolution 3D T2WI (B) reveals thin optic nerves (arrows).

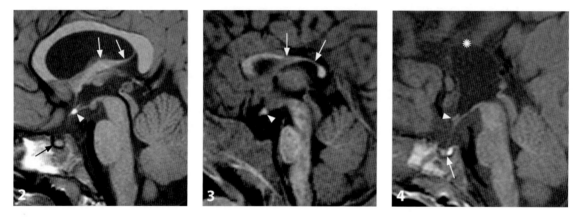

Figure 2. Midsagittal T1WI depicts low-lying fused fornices (white arrows) associated with a small pituitary gland (black arrow) and ectopic posterior pituitary lobe (white arrowhead).

Figure 3. Midsagittal T1WI shows a small corpus callosum with segmental dysgenesis (arrows), extreme anterior pituitary hypoplasia, ectopic posterior lobe (arrowhead), and pituitary stalk interruption.

Figure 4. Midsagittal T1WI reveals complete callosal agenesis (*) associated with a small pituitary gland (arrow) and a very thin optic chiasm (arrowhead).

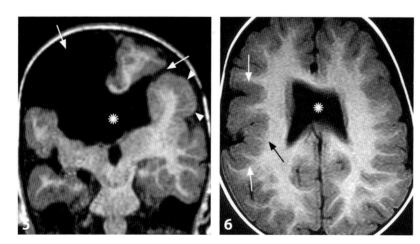

Figure 5. Coronal T1WI shows septal agenesis (*) and bilateral open lips schizencephaly (arrows). The adjacent cortex is polymicrogyric (arrowheads).

Figure 6. Axial T1WI in another patient reveals a focal fronto-parietal area of polymicrogyria (arrows) and absent septum pellucidum (*).

Septo-Optic Dysplasia

MARIASAVINA SEVERINO

Specific Imaging Findings

The wide spectrum of imaging findings in septo-optic dysplasia (SOD) includes variable combinations of defects involving the midline brain structures, pituitary gland, optic nerves and eyes, olfactory bulbs, as well as other brain structures. Midline brain defects classically consist of complete or partial absence of the septum pellucidum with fused midline fornices (60% of cases) and/or corpus callosum abnormalities, such as agenesis, dysplasia or hypoplasia. The presence of a normal septum pellucidum does not rule out SOD. Pituitary gland malformations include anterior pituitary hypoplasia and/or ectopic posterior lobe and/or thin or interrupted pituitary stalk. Another characteristic feature is the hypoplasia of the optic nerves and chiasm, more commonly bilateral than unilateral. Frequently associated ocular anomalies include coloboma, anophthalmia, and microphthalmia. The olfactory bulbs may be absent or hypoplastic. Other brain malformations commonly associated with SOD are schizencephaly (so-called SOD-plus), polymicrogyria, gray matter heterotopia, and hippocampal malformations.

Pertinent Clinical Information

The diagnosis of SOD is clinical and made when two or more features of the classical triad of optic nerve hypoplasia, pituitary hormone abnormalities and midline brain defects are present. Only a third of patients present with all cardinal features of SOD. Visual deficits (nystagmus, diminished visual acuity, color blindness) due to optic nerve hypoplasia and ocular malformations are usually the first presenting feature of the condition, while endocrine dysfunction may become apparent later on. The extent of pituitary–hypothalamic dysfunction (60–80% of cases) is highly variable, ranging from isolated pituitary hormone deficit (in particular growth hormone deficiency) to panhypopituitarism. Neurological deficits are common and range from global retardation to focal deficits such as epilepsy or hemiparesis. Associated features include anosmia, obesity, sleep disorders, sensorineural hearing loss, autistic spectrum disorder, limb abnormalities such as syndactyly, and cardiac anomalies.

Differential Diagnosis

Kallmann Syndrome
- aplasia/hypoplasia of the olfactory bulbs/tracts and/or the olfactory sulci

Lobar Holoprosencephaly (73)
- absent septum pellucidum, anterior midline falx and fissure with midline continuous frontal neocortex
- fully developed cerebral lobes with separation of deep gray nuclei

Isolated Pituitary Malformations
- absent midline brain anomalies and optic nerve hypoplasia

Background

SOD, also known as de Morsier syndrome, is a highly heterogeneous disorder affecting 1 in 10 000 live births. Most cases are sporadic and several environmental factors have been suggested to contribute to the pathogenesis, including young maternal age (with a preponderance of primigravida mothers) and drug or alcohol abuse during pregnancy. Currently, genetic abnormalities are identified in <1% of the patients with recessive or dominant mutations in early developmental genes (HESX1, SOX2, SOX3, OTX2). These factors are essential for normal early forebrain/pituitary development around 4–6 weeks of gestation. Hormonal replacement and neurodevelopmental support are the main forms of treatment.

REFERENCES

1. Raybaud C. The corpus callosum, the other great forebrain commissures, and the septum pellucidum: anatomy, development, and malformation. *Neuroradiology* 2010;**52**:447–77.
2. Webb EA, Dattani MT. Septo-optic dysplasia. *Eur J Human Genet* 2010;**18**:393–7.
3. Barkovich AJ, Fram EK, Norman D. Septo-optic dysplasia: MR imaging. *Radiology* 1989;**171**:189–92.
4. Miller SP, Shevell MI, Patenaude Y. Septo-optic dysplasia plus: a spectrum of malformations of cortical development. *Neurology* 2000;**54**:1701–3.
5. Riedl S, Vosahlo J, Battelino T, *et al*. Refining clinical phenotypes in septo-optic dysplasia based on MRI findings. *Eur J Pediatr* 2008;**167**:1269–76.

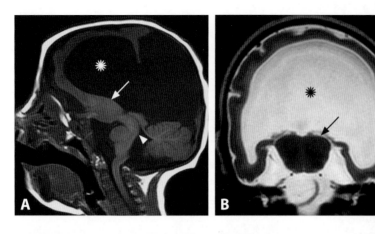

Figure 1. Midsagittal T1WI (A) shows a large single ventricle (*) that communicates posteriorly with a cyst. Posterior fossa is preserved, except for dorsal brainstem distortion (arrowhead). A pseudomass (arrow) is seen – coronal T2WI (B) reveals that this is due to a lack of separation between the thalami and hypothalamus (arrow). There is complete absence of midline structures (*) and brain is reduced to a rudimentary structure with shallow sulcation surrounding the holoventricle.

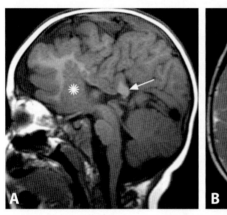
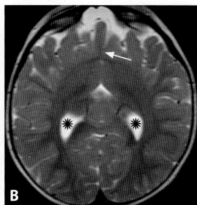

Figure 2. Midsagittal T1WI (A) shows a rudimentary callosal splenium (arrow). There is abnormal frontal gyration and midline heterotopic gray matter (*). The posterior fossa is normal. Axial T2WI (B) shows cleavage of the parieto-occipital lobes with an intervening interhemispheric fissure and falx. The more anterior regions are hypoplastic and uncleaved, with continuity of gray and white matter across the midline (arrow). There are rudimentary lateral trigones (*), while the frontal horns are not formed.

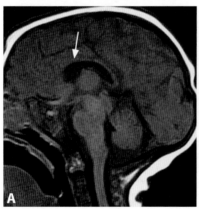
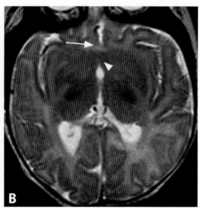

Figure 3. Midsagittal T1WI shows absent anterior portion (arrow) of the corpus callosum. Normal posterior fossa. Axial T2WI (B) demonstrates normal posterior cleavage of the brain. There is lack of separation of the striatum (arrowhead) and basal frontal white matter (arrow). The lateral trigones and third ventricle are relatively well formed. The frontal horns were present but not separated (not shown). Note a more normal head shape and sylvian fissures compared to 2B.

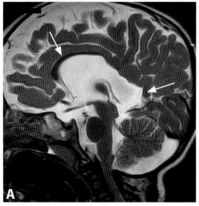
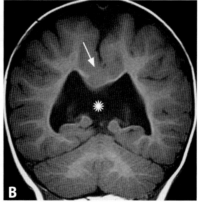

Figure 4. Midsagittal T2WI (A) shows that corpus callosum is separated in two portions (arrows) due to the absence of the body and anterior splenium, with intervening brain tissue representing segmental lack of separation. Coronal T1WI (B) reveals heterotopic gray matter bridging across the midline (arrow) in the region of uncleavage. Septum pellucidum is absent (*). Normal posterior fossa.

Holoprosencephaly

ANDREA ROSSI

Specific Imaging Findings

Holoprosencephaly (HPE) is characterized by lack of separation of the cerebral hemispheres and absence of midline structures. Several forms are identified based on the severity and extent of abnormalities.

- *Alobar HPE.* Complete absence of hemispheric separation and midline structures results in a so-called holosphere. A single monoventricle communicates posteriorly with a dorsal cyst. The hypothalamus is noncleaved to some degree, and the deep gray matter structures are nonseparated in almost all cases.
- *Semilobar HPE.* The occipital and, to some extent, parietal lobes are separated with posteriorly present interhemispheric fissure and falx, as well as the callosal splenium. The trigones and occipital horns of the lateral ventricles are formed, but the frontal horns and septum pellucidum are absent.
- *Lobar HPE.* Lack of separation involves basal frontal regions and, variably, basal ganglia and hypothalamus; thalami are completely separated. Corpus callosum extends more anteriorly, with presence of splenium and at least a part of the body. Rudimentary frontal horns are fused in the midline due to absent septum pellucidum.
- *Middle interhemispheric HPE (syntelencephaly).* Lack of separation involves the perirolandic region with complete separation both anteriorly and posteriorly. Consequently, an intermediate portion of the falx and interhemispheric fissure are absent and the corpus callosum is split into two portions, separated by brain tissue. Septum pellucidum is absent and lateral ventricles are dysmorphic.
- *Septo-preoptic HPE.* Lack of separation involves only a limited zone at the preoptic (subcallosal) and septal (suprachiasmatic–hypothalamic) regions. Partial posterior hypoplasia of the corpus callosum is common.

Pertinent Clinical Information

Affected patients have a variable clinical picture depending on the extent and severity of the malformation. In many cases, HPE is suspected because of associated craniofacial abnormalities, ranging from cyclopia and ethmocephaly to cleft lip/palate, hypotelorism, and single central incisor. Microcrania is common, and a trigonocephalic skull configuration may result from premature metopic suture fusion, due to lack of growth of the frontal lobes. Neurological abnormalities are variable, but often striking. Patients often present in the neonatal period with seizures, apnoic spells, and difficulty swallowing. Psychomotor delay is common. Less severe cases may have a noticeably minor involvement or even normal psychomotor functions.

Differential Diagnosis

Callosal Agenesis with Interhemispheric Cyst (71)
- large midline cyst may communicate with ventricles, simulating dorsal sac
- the falx, while frequently displaced, is present

Schizencephaly (84)
- bilateral clefts are often associated with septum pellucidum agenesis
- polymicrogyric cortex lines the clefts
- interhemispheric fissure and falx are present

Hydranencephaly (95)
- thalami are separated
- interhemispheric fissure and falx are present

Septo-Optic Dysplasia (72)
- complete cleavage of the cerebral hemispheres with presence of the falx
- hypoplastic optic nerves and chiasm

Background

HPE is the most common malformation of the human forebrain, with an incidence of 1 in 250 conceptions decreasing to 1 : 10000 births, owing to a high rate of spontaneous abortions. It occurs during the stage of ventral induction (4–5 gestational weeks), with lack of cleavage and formation of midline structures. Causes of HPE are manifold, including chromosomal abnormalities and syndromic forms, which are more common and associated with high perinatal mortality. Other causes include environmental factors (including maternal diabetes mellitus) and deletions/mutations in the genes known to be involved in HPE. At least 13 different HPE loci or chromosomal regions, nine of which include known HPE genes, have been identified. The most common HPE gene is *Sonic Hedgehog* (*SHH*, OMIM 600725) on 7q36. This, and another three (*ZIC2*, *SIX3*, and *TGIF*) genes, comprise approximately one-quarter of all HPE cases.

Different forms, including more recently described middle interhemispheric and septo-preoptic HPE, rather than representing separate variants, in fact constitute a continuous spectrum, with individual cases frequently showing overlapping features.

REFERENCES

1. Biancheri R, Rossi A, Tortori-Donati P, *et al*. Middle interhemispheric variant of holoprosencephaly: a very mild clinical case. *Neurology* 2004;**63**:2194–6.

2. Hahn JS, Barnes PD. Neuroimaging advances in holoprosencephaly: refining the spectrum of the midline malformation. *Am J Med Genet C Semin Med Genet* 2010;**154C**:120–32.

3. Hahn JS, Barnes PD, Clegg NJ, Stashinko EE. Septopreoptic holoprosencephaly: a mild subtype associated with midline craniofacial anomalies. *AJNR* 2010;**31**:1596–601.

4. Kauvar EF, Muenke M. Holoprosencephaly: recommendations for diagnosis and management. *Curr Opin Pediatr* 2010;**22**:687–695.

Brain Imaging with MRI and CT, ed. Zoran Rumboldt *et al.* Published by Cambridge University Press. © Cambridge University Press 2012.

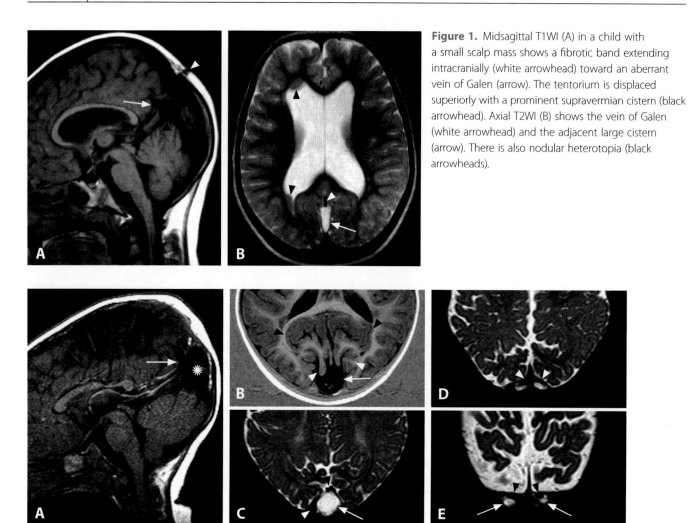

Figure 1. Midsagittal T1WI (A) in a child with a small scalp mass shows a fibrotic band extending intracranially (white arrowhead) toward an aberrant vein of Galen (arrow). The tentorium is displaced superiorly with a prominent supravermian cistern (black arrowhead). Axial T2WI (B) shows the vein of Galen (white arrowhead) and the adjacent large cistern (arrow). There is also nodular heterotopia (black arrowheads).

Figure 2. Midsagittal T1WI (A) shows embryonic vertical position of the straight sinus (arrow) and large supravermian cistern (*). Axial IR T1WI (B) shows the enlarged cistern (arrow) along with aberrant occipital gyration (arrowheads). T2WI (C) reveals duplicated falcine sinus (black arrowhead) extending toward the superior sagittal sinus (white arrowhead) along the supravermian cistern (arrow). More cephalad T2WIs (D, E) reveal the course of venous structures (arrowheads) inside the parietal foramina (arrows).

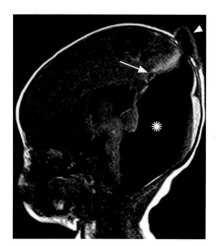

Figure 3. Sagittal T1WI shows the flow-void of persistent falcine sinus (arrow) extending toward a subtle defect in the calvarium and subcutaneous tissues (arrowhead).

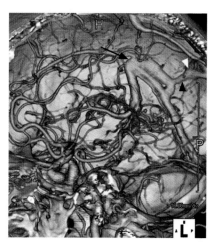

Figure 4. Lateral view of volume-rendered CTA shows incidental persistent falcine sinus (arrowheads), vertical vein of Galen and fenestrated straight sinus (arrow).

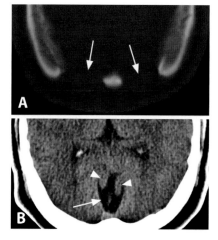

Figure 5. Bone window CT (A) reveals large parietal foramina (arrows). A more caudal CT (B) shows aberrant gyration (arrowheads) and a large supravermian cistern (arrow).

150

Atretic Parietal Encephalocele

MARIA GISELE MATHEUS

Specific Imaging Findings

Atretic parietal encephaloceles (APE) are located at the midline superior to the posterior fontanel. Non-enhanced CT images show a sharply marginated central calvarial defect (cranium bifidum) with associated extracranial soft tissue mass located under the scalp. Small cranium bifidum may only be seen with thin slices and 3D reconstructions. MRI shows an extracranial/subscalp mass just above the lambda with heterogeneous T1 signal intensity and hyperintense T2 signal. The APE may insinuate intracranially or show a fibrous band extending into the cranium bifidum. There is embryonic vertical positioning of the straight sinus, which is seen as a flow void connecting the vein of Galen with the superior sagittal sinus (SSS). There may be a "cigar-shaped" CSF tract within the interhemispheric fissure and fenestration of the SSS. The lower posterior aspect of the SSS shows a bifid configuration, best appreciated on axial or coronal T2WI. The tentorium is displaced upward with a large superior cerebellar cistern and prominent suprapineal recess of the third ventricle, giving a "spinning-top" configuration to the tentorial incisura. Variations of occipital cortical infolding may be present. The position of the dural venous sinuses with respect to the encephalocele is best seen on post contrast images. APE can be associated with other anomalies, such as callosal dysgenesis, heterotopia, Dandy–Walker syndrome, Walker–Walburg syndrome, and holoprosencephaly. Persistent falcine venous sinus (horizontally connecting the vein of Galen with the SSS) and parietal foramina (persistent bilateral symmetric calvarial defects) may be the only findings in individuals with incidentally found APE.

Pertinent Clinical Information

APE usually presents as a small (5–15 mm), hairless, midline scalp mass near the vertex, with or without associated angiomatous formation. Individuals with enlarged parietal foramina may warrant imaging of brain parenchyma and vasculature, as APE is frequently present. Patients with additional associated brain abnormalities manifest specific neurological symptoms, which are not directly related to the APE. However, APE may also be an incidental finding in developmentally normal children or adults.

Differential Diagnosis

Sinus Pericranii
- subscalp mass with internal venous flow
- communication between the intra and extracranial venous compartments
- avid contrast enhancement
- occur anteriorly and posteriorly, not limited to parietal region

Epidermoid (143)
- scalloping remodeling of the outer table of the skull
- characteristically hyperintense on DWI

Dermoid (75)
- may be indistinguishable/associated with APE

Hemangioma/Venous Malformation
- lobulated mass within the scalp with intact adjacent skull
- dense contrast enhancement
- prominent extracranial draining vein and feeding artery may be present

Background

The etiology of APE is not clear. The atretic masses are formed by dermal, meningeal and glial elements as well as fibrous tissue. The current hypothesis to explain APE includes: (a) involution of true meningoceles or encephaloceles formed early in fetal life; (b) persistence of a fetal nuchal bleb caused by early embryonic cerebral "blow-out"; and (c) persistence of neural crest remnants. It is thought that by one or more of these three mechanisms a midline strand connecting mesencephalic tectum to the overlying membranous cranium is formed. This interrupts the regular embryological movement of the straight sinus and marginal sinuses and is responsible for the characteristic appearance of the sinuses in APE. Atretic encephaloceles are also encountered in the occipital region. Pathologic examination reveals glial, meningeal (arachnoid), fibrous, and dermal elements. The prognosis does not depend on the existence of the APE itself, but rather on the associated brain anomalies.

REFERENCES

1. Patterson RJ, Egelhoff JC, Crone KR, Ball WS Jr. Atretic parietal cephaloceles revisited: an enlarging clinical and imaging spectrum? *AJNR* 1998;**19**:791–5.

2. Morioka T, Hashiguchi K, Samura K, *et al.* Detailed anatomy of intracranial venous anomalies associated with atretic parietal cephaloceles revealed by high-resolution 3D-CISS and high-field T2-weighted reversed MR images. *Childs Nerv Syst* 2009;**25**:309–15.

3. Yamazaki T, Enomoto T, Iguchi M, Nose T. Atretic cephalocele – report of two cases with special reference to embryology. *Childs Nerv Syst* 2001;**17**:674–8.

4. Reddy AT, Hedlund GL, Percy AK. Enlarged parietal foramina: association with cerebral venous and cortical anomalies. *Neurology* 2000;**54**:1175–8.

5. Martinez-Lage JF, Sola J, Casas C, *et al.* Atretic cephalocele: the tip of the iceberg. *J Neurosurg* 1992;**77**:230–5.

Brain Imaging with MRI and CT, ed. Zoran Rumboldt *et al.* Published by Cambridge University Press. © Cambridge University Press 2012.

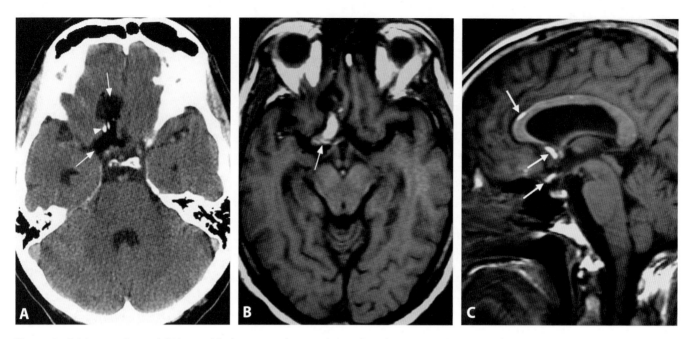

Figure 1. Axial non-enhanced CT image (A) shows a predominantly very low density mass (arrows) in the right suprasellar and basal frontal region with a few coarse, peripheral calcifications (arrowhead). Corresponding axial T1WI (B) demonstrates predominantly very high signal of the lesion (arrow). Midsagittal T1WI (C) reveals scattered droplets of lipid in the suprasellar region and along the superior surface of the corpus callosum (arrows), consistent with rupture of the mass and dissemination of its contents.

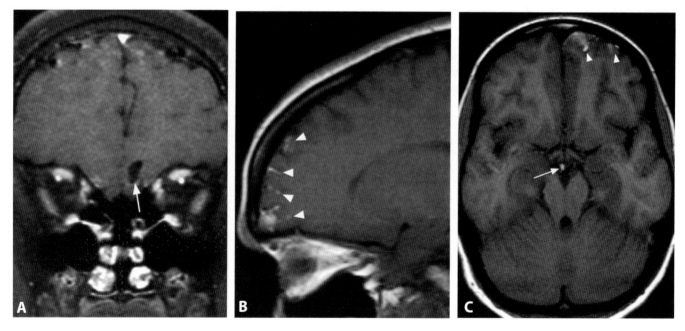

Figure 2. Post-contrast coronal T1WI with fat saturation (A) in a different patient shows a dark, non-enhancing lesion (arrow) in the anterior basal left frontal region, which was bright on the pre-contrast T1WI. Sagittal (B) non-enhanced T1WI reveals multiple small areas of hyperintensity along the frontal cortical sulci (arrowheads), representing subarachnoid spread of cyst contents. Axial non-contrast T1WI again shows the left frontal hyperintensities (arrowheads) as well as a suprasellar bright lesion (arrow).

Dermoid Cyst

BENJAMIN HUANG

Specific Imaging Findings

Intracranial dermoid cysts usually occur at or near the midline, most frequently in a parasellar, frontonasal, or posterior fossa location. Frontonasal and posterior fossa dermoids may be associated with a dermal sinus tract. The cysts usually follow imaging characteristics of fat, being typically hypodense on CT and T1 hyperintense. The capsule of the cyst frequently contains calcification. There is no contrast enhancement. Some dermoids may contain teeth (easily identified on CT) or hair which may appear as thin, curvilinear, low-signal intensity structures on T2-weighted images. If dermoid cysts rupture the fat droplets scatter throughout the subarachnoid spaces and in severe cases fat-fluid levels may be present within the ventricles. Post-contrast imaging may show extensive leptomeningeal enhancement when leakage of cyst contents leads to chemical meningitis. CT hyperdense dermoid cysts are very rare and occur exclusively in the posterior fossa.

Pertinent Clinical Information

Dermoids are uncommon, representing only about 0.5% of intracranial tumors. Clinical presentation is usually during the third decade of life with headaches, seizures, or symptoms related to compression of adjacent tissues (e.g. visual changes from optic chiasm compression); however, they are often asymptomatic. Cyst rupture may cause aseptic meningitis, seizure, ischemic symptoms and infarctions secondary to vasospasm, as well as acute hydrocephalus. Cyst rupture is actually more common than previously thought and it may also cause only minimal symptoms or be even completely asymptomatic. The goal of treatment is surgical removal of the cyst, although adherence of the cyst capsule to the nearby neurovascular structures may preclude complete resection. Nevertheless, dermoids are overall less likely to recur than epidermoid tumors.

Differential Diagnosis

Lipoma (76)
- homogeneous fat density/intensity
- may be indistinguishable

Epidermoid (143)
- usually off midline
- resembles CSF on CT, T1- and T2-weighted images, "dirty" appearance on FLAIR
- pathognomonic bright "light bulb" appearance on DWI

Teratoma
- usually contains enhancing soft tissue component
- more commonly in the pineal region

Craniopharyngioma (44)
- cystic with enhancing soft tissue components
- cyst contents do not demonstrate characteristics of fat

Background

Dermoid cysts are ectodermal inclusion cysts, which arise from the entrapment of ectodermally committed cells at the time of neural tube closure. The capsules of the cysts consist of stratified squamous epithelium that contains dermal appendages such as hair follicles and sebaceous glands. The cysts enlarge slowly due to desquamated epithelium and sebaceous secretions. The fat signal seen on MRI is due to the presence of liquid cholesterol derived from the breakdown of epithelial cells. High protein and calcium content with low lipids may be responsible for the high attenuation of rare CT hyperdense posterior fossa dermoids. Rupture of dermoid cysts is usually spontaneous. Although the mechanism of rupture is unknown, it has been hypothesized that glandular secretions, which may increase with age-dependent hormonal changes, lead to rapid cyst enlargement with subsequent capsule perforation. Malignant transformation (into squamous cell carcinoma) is very rare, but highly aggressive.

REFERENCES

1. Liu JK, Gottfried ON, Salzman KL, et al. Ruptured intracranial dermoid cysts: clinical, radiographic, and surgical features. *Neurosurgery* 2008;**62**:377–84.
2. Orakcioglu B, Halatsch ME, Fortunati M, et al. Intracranial dermoid cysts: variations of radiological and clinical features. *Acta Neurochir* 2008;**150**:1227–34.
3. Osborn AG, Preece MT. Intracranial cysts: radiologic–pathologic correlation and imaging approach. *Radiology* 2006;**239**:650–4.
4. Messori A, Polonara G, Serio A, et al. Expanding experience with spontaneous dermoid rupture in the MRI era: diagnosis and follow-up. *Eur J Radiol* 2002;**43**:19–27.
5. Hamlat A, Hua ZF, Saikali S, et al. Malignant transformation of intra-cranial epithelial cysts: systematic article review. *J Neurooncol* 2005;**74**:187–94.

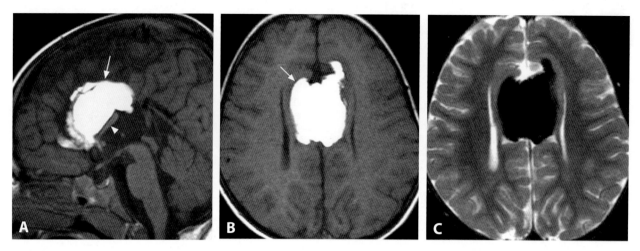

Figure 1. Midsagittal (A) and axial (B) T1WIs show a homogeneously hyperintense mass (arrow) with signal similar to the subcutaneous fat. There is associated callosal dysgenesis with only a thin remnant of the corpus callosum evident anteriorly (arrowhead). There is complete signal loss on fat-suppressed T2WI (C).

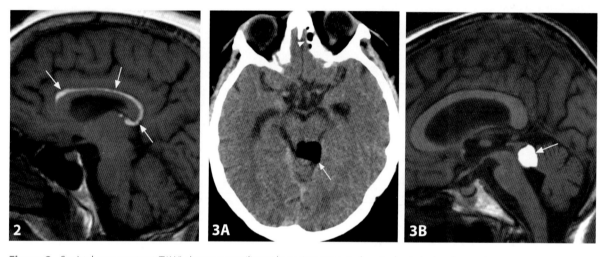

Figure 2. Sagittal non-contrast T1WI shows a curvilinear hyperintense interhemispheric lesion (arrows).

Figure 3. Axial CT (A) demonstrates a very low density mass (arrow) in the quadrigeminal plate cistern. The lesion can be difficult to discern from gas (air), as in the left ethmoid (arrowhead) on brain windows. In the setting of trauma this may be misinterpreted as pneumocephalus, if not viewed with bone window (or HU measured). On midsagittal non-contrast T1WI (B) the lesion (arrow) is homogeneously hyperintense.

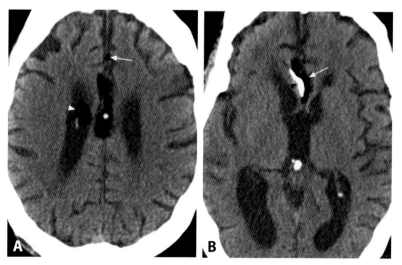

Figure 4. Axial non-enhanced CT image (A) shows a very dark pericallosal mass (*) with extension into the right lateral ventricle (arrowhead). There is also a similar tiny left parafalcine lesion (arrow), a common incidental finding. CT image at the level of the third ventricle (B) demonstrates curvilinear calcification (arrowhead) along the right lateral aspect of the hypodense mass (arrow).

Lipoma

BENJAMIN HUANG

Specific Imaging Findings

Most intracranial lipomas occur at or near the midline, are very small and completely incidental. Large lipomas are most frequently pericallosal in location and are typically subdivided into tubulonodular and curvilinear types. Tubulonodular ones are bulky, usually situated anteriorly and associated with callosal agenesis or severe hypogenesis. Curvilinear lipomas are a thin ribbon of fat along the dorsum of the corpus callosum with extension around the splenium or a small retrosplenial button of fat and may be associated with splenial hypoplasia. Extension into the lateral ventricles is not uncommon. Other typical locations are quadrigeminal plate/superior cerebellar cistern and suprasellar/intrapeduncular cistern. On CT, lipomas are sharply marginated with markedly low density, usually below –40 HU. Central or peripheral calcification may be present. Ossification may also occur, particularly in suprasellar and interpeduncular lipomas. Lipomas are uniformly T1 hyperintense and maintain signal isointense to fat on all pulse sequences. Chemical shift artifact is observed around the edges and fat suppression sequences lead to complete signal dropout. Flow-voids of encased vessels may sometimes be present. Chemical shift artifact also allows for distinction of small lipomas from aneurysms on TOF MRA images.

Pertinent Clinical Information

The vast majority of lipomas are asymptomatic. Headaches, seizures, psychomotor retardation, and cranial nerve deficits have all been reported in association with intracranial lipomas. Sylvian fissure lipomas appear to be associated with epilepsy and hydrocephalus has been reported with quadrigeminal plate lipomas. Symptoms are usually due to associated malformations which are seen in over half of large lipomas and, in addition to callosal dysgenesis, include absence of septum pellucidum, vermian hypoplasia, aqueductal stenosis, and cortical malformations.

Differential Diagnosis

Dermoid Cyst (75)

- may rupture and spill fat droplets into the subarachnoid space
- may be indistinguishable, except for possible growth on follow-up imaging

Teratoma

- usually located in pineal or suprasellar regions
- usually contains an enhancing soft tissue component

Subacute Hemorrhage

- hyperintense T1 signal but will not follow fat signal on other pulse sequences
- hyperdense on CT

Background

Intracranial lipomas are congenital malformations rather than neoplasms, believed to occur as a result of abnormal persistence and maldifferentiation of the meninx primitiva. The meninx is the mesenchymal precursor of the meninges and subarachnoid spaces. The characteristic locations of intracranial lipomas correspond to locations where the meninx persists the longest in fetal life. The last place to become clear of the primitive meninx is the lamina reunions, the thickened dorsal portion of the lamina terminalis which serves as a bed for ingrowing fibers of the corpus callosum. Persistence and lipomatous maldifferentiation of the meninx is hypothesized to cause incomplete formation of the corpus callosum. Large lipomas are readily detected on prenatal ultrasound. Surgical resection of lipomas is rarely indicated and is hazardous as blood vessels and nerves may be coursing through the lesions.

REFERENCES

1. Jabot G, Stoquart-Elsankari S, Saliou G, et al. Intracranial lipomas: clinical appearances on neuroimaging and clinical significance. J Neurol 2009;256:851–5.
2. Truwit CL, Barkovich AJ. Pathogenesis of intracranial lipoma: an MR study in 42 patients. AJR 1990;155:855–64.
3. Yildiz H, Hakyemez B, Koroglu M, et al. Intracranial lipomas: importance of localization. Neuroradiology 2006;48:1–7.
4. Ickowitz V, Eurin D, Rypens F, et al. Prenatal diagnosis and postnatal follow-up of pericallosal lipoma: report of seven new cases. AJNR 2001;22:767–72.
5. Kemmling A, Noelte I, Gerigk L, et al. A diagnostic pitfall for intracranial aneurysms in time-of-flight MR angiography: small intracranial lipomas. AJR 2008;190:W62–7.

SECTION 3

Parenchymal Defects or Abnormal Volume

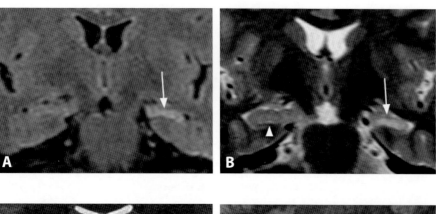

Figure 1. Coronal oblique FLAIR (A) and T2WI (B) in a patient with partial complex epilepsy show high signal and asymmetric volume loss of the left hippocampus (arrows). Compare to the normal right hippocampus (arrowhead).

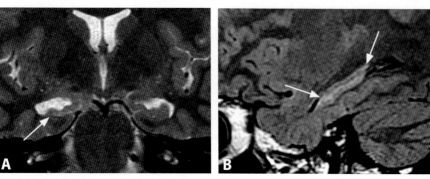

Figure 2. Coronal oblique T2WI (A) shows diminished volume of the right hippocampal head (arrow). Sagittal FLAIR image (B) shows abnormal high signal in the entire right hippocampus (arrow).

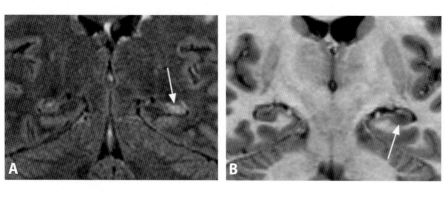

Figure 3. There is mild hyperintensity with subtle loss of internal architecture (arrow) in the left hippocampus on FLAIR image (A). IR T1WI (B) reveals low signal and lack of gray–white differentiation in its inferior portion (arrow), without volume loss.

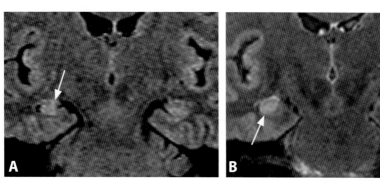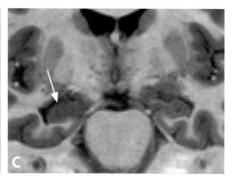

Figure 4. Coronal oblique FLAIR image acquired on a 1.5 T scanner (A) demonstrates possible subtle increased signal of the right hippocampus (arrow). The scan repeated on a 3 T scanner (B) reveals clear hyperintensity and loss of internal differentiation (arrow). IR T1WI at 3 T (C) shows loss of normal architecture in the right hippocampal head (arrow).

Hippocampal Sclerosis

ALESSANDRO CIANFONI

Specific Imaging Findings

Hippocampal sclerosis (HS) is defined by volume loss and T2 hyperintensity of the affected hippocampus. The atrophy may be of a variable degree and is frequently accompanied by more subtle signs: loss of internal architecture; atrophy of the ipsilateral parahippocampal gyrus, fornix, and mammillary body. Dedicated high-resolution FLAIR imaging in the oblique coronal plane perpendicular to the hippocampus is the single best technique to diagnose HS. Heavily T1-weighted inversion recovery images demonstrate the loss of volume and internal architecture. There is no contrast enhancement. Asymmetric bilateral hippocampal atrophy, and even symmetric bilateral involvement may be found in some cases. "Dual pathology", the coexistence of HS with another epileptogenic focus, is reported in 10–20% of surgical epilepsy patients, prompting search for possible additional foci.

Pertinent Clinical Information

HS, also known as mesial temporal sclerosis (MTS), is the most common abnormality in adults with refractory seizures. Patients have a history of intractable partial complex epilepsy and the treatment is partial temporal lobectomy, typically with open surgery. Resection leads to positive outcome when MRI and EEG findings are concordant, or if both volume loss and T2 hyperintensity are present without EEG correlation. Hyperperfusion in the ipsilateral mesial temporal lobe may be observed with ictal SPECT, while hypometabolism is found on inter-ictal FDG-PET; again, concordance with MRI correlates with better surgical outcomes. Lateralization of memory and language is ascertained before surgery, with a Wada test or f-MRI.

Differential Diagnosis

Choroidal Fissure Cyst
- enlarged choroidal fissure with CSF signal, may distort subjacent hippocampus
- no abnormal signal or hippocampal atrophy
- typically asymptomatic

Hippocampal Sulcus Remnant
- very small multiple cysts with CSF signal along the hippocampus
- asymptomatic

Mesial Temporal Lobe Neoplasms (166)
- mass effect rather than atrophy
- abnormality is not limited to the hippocampus

Post-Ictal Changes (104)
- swelling instead of volume loss
- other parts of the brain may be involved

Viral Encephalitis, including HSE (20)
- hippocampal swelling
- possible enhancement and hemorrhage
- short clinical history, acute to subacute onset of symptoms

Limbic Encephalitis (21)
- hippocampal swelling in the acute phase
- hippocampal atrophy without T2 hyperintensity in the chronic phase
- enhancement may be present
- usually known malignancy (paraneoplastic syndrome), subacute course
- may be indistinguishable

Alzheimer Dementia (89)
- usually bilateral
- no T2 hyperintensity

Chronic Anoxic Injury
- additional lesions in the deep gray matter and perirolandic cortex
- characteristically bilateral
- clinical history usually known

Background

Volume loss in HS corresponds to neuronal loss, and high T2 signal to gliosis, primarily in the dentate gyrus and Ammon's horn. History of complicated febrile seizures in early childhood is present in 9–50% of cases, but only 2–7% of children with febrile seizure develop epilepsy. The disease is most likely the end result of various processes: the cause of febrile convulsions or the seizures themselves might induce damage to the hippocampus, establishing a vicious cycle between the cause and the effect of seizures, as the post-ictal MRI findings may suggest. Also, a relatively frequent incidence of dual pathology suggests that HS in these patients is the result of chronic seizures originating from another focus. While the visual MRI assessment has a very high sensitivity and specificity for HS, additional techniques, such as hippocampal volumetry, T2-relaxometry, and MRS (showing decreased NAA levels) can increase accuracy, but are rarely used in clinical practice. The use of 3 T scanners may offer superior sensitivity for the subtle loss of hippocampal architecture, further improved with double inversion recovery sequence.

REFERENCES

1. Van Paesschen W. Qualitative and quantitative imaging of the hippocampus in mesial temporal lobe epilepsy with hippocampal sclerosis. *Neuroimaging Clin N Am* 2004;**14**:373–400.
2. Thom M, Mathern GW, Cross JH, Bertram EH. Mesial temporal lobe epilepsy: how do we improve surgical outcome? *Ann Neurol* 2010;**68**:424–34.
3. Hashiguchi K, Morioka T, Murakami N, *et al.* Utility of 3-T FLAIR and 3D short tau inversion recovery MR imaging in the preoperative diagnosis of hippocampal sclerosis: direct comparison with 1.5-T FLAIR MR imaging. *Epilepsia* 2010;**51**:1820–8.
4. Li Q, Zhang Q, Sun H, *et al.* Double inversion recovery magnetic resonance imaging at 3 T: diagnostic value in hippocampal sclerosis. *J Comput Assist Tomogr* 2011;**35**:290–3.

Brain Imaging with MRI and CT, ed. Zoran Rumboldt *et al.* Published by Cambridge University Press. © Cambridge University Press 2012.

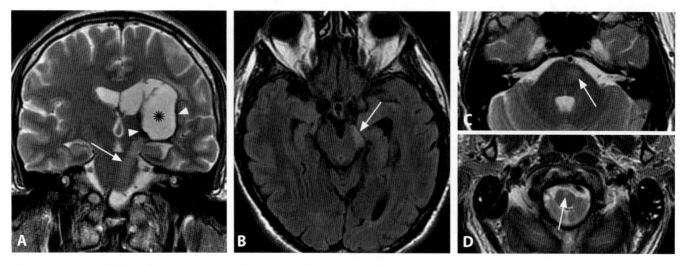

Figure 1. Coronal T2WI (A) shows a large area of encephalomalacia (*) in the left lenticulo-capsular region, with hemosiderin deposition (arrowheads) along its margins, representing chronic sequela of an old hemorrhage. There is also a linear hyperintensity along the left brainstem (arrow). Axial FLAIR image (B) shows the hyperintensity and volume loss of the left cerebral peduncle (arrow). The high signal and volume loss (arrows) corresponding to the left cortico-spinal tract extend throughout the brainstem, as seen on T2WIs at the pons (C) and at the pyramidal decussation in the medulla oblongata (D).

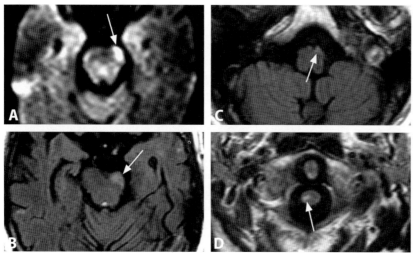

Figure 2. Axial DWI (A) 10 days after left middle cerebral artery territory infarction shows high signal in the left cerebral peduncle. Follow-up axial FLAIR images (B–D) reveal atrophy and hyperintensity of the cerebral peduncle (arrow in B), which extends inferiorly along the cortico-spinal tract into the medulla (arrow in C). Below the decussation within the spinal cord the hyperintensity is located on the right side (arrow in D).

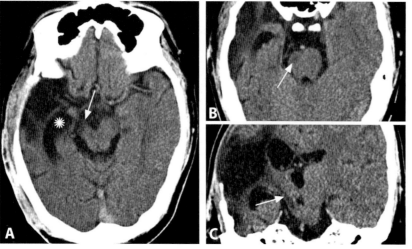

Figure 3. Non-enhanced axial CT (A) shows right temporal encephalomalacia with ex vacuo ventricular dilation (*), as well as decreased volume and attenuation of ipsilateral cerebral peduncle (arrow). Atrophy and hypodensity (arrow) are also seen in the pons on a more caudal image (B). CT reconstructed in the coronal plane (C) reveals linear hypodensity (arrow) extending along the right cortico-spinal tract from encephalomalacia to the brainstem.

Wallerian Degeneration

ALESSANDRO CIANFONI

Specific Imaging Findings

Abnormal MRI signal is found with Wallerian degeneration (WD) along the course of a major white matter tract (such as corticospinal tract, corticopontine tract, optic radiation, and corpus callosum), ipsilateral to a proximal cortical or subcortical lesion, most commonly ischemic, hemorrhagic, or traumatic. The abnormality is visible as a round to ovoid area of altered signal on multiple images that are perpendicular to the white matter tract, or as an oblongated or stripe-like lesion on images parallel to the tract. Around 4 weeks after the injury WD is seen as hypointense on PD/T2-weighted images, T1 hyperintense and possibly hypodense on CT, without contrast enhancement. This is followed over the following days to weeks with low T1 signal and the characteristic T2 hyperintensity and volume loss. Reduced diffusion is an early but transient finding, with in 1–2 weeks from the injury, in adults as well as neonates and it should not be confused with a new infarction. Most commonly WD is observed along the corticospinal tract (CST) in the posterior limb of the internal capsule, cerebral peduncle, ventro-lateral pons, and pyramidal decussation. Decreasing ADC values peak at 7 days. The cerebral peduncle and the hemipons are of decreased volume in the chronic stage.

Pertinent Clinical Information

WD indicates irreversible neuronal function loss and death, and its presence suggests poor recovery while the extent of CST WD correlates with the severity of the permanent motor deficit. Awareness of this pathological process should prevent misdiagnosis of new or distant lesions in the settings of infarcts, hemorrhages, demyelinating disease, or gliomas.

Differential Diagnosis

Ischemic Infarct (152)
- reduced diffusivity shortly after the onset of symptoms, not delayed for 1–2 weeks

Gliomas (162)
- mass effect instead of volume loss in the affected white matter tracts
- may be indistinguishable in the early phases

Demyelinating Lesions (112, 115)
- demyelinating lesions are typically focal, round or ovoid, and not elongated

Amyotrophic Lateral Sclerosis (15)
- bilateral symmetric CST T2 hyperintensity

Normal Corticospinal Tracts
- bilateral symmetric subtle and ill-defined T2 hyperintensity within the internal capsules and cerebral peduncles, more prominent with 3 T scanners
- absence of volume loss

Background

WD is caused by breakdown of axons and myelin, followed by irreversible gliosis and atrophy at a distance from the primary lesion. It is a result of severe proximal neuronal injury or axonal destruction along the corresponding white matter tract. CNS responds in a different way and has a lower chance of repair compared to the peripheral nervous system. Diffusion tensor imaging (DTI) reveals WD changes within days after the injury, with reduced fractional anisotropy (FA). DTI appears to differentiate primary ischemic (reduced FA and increased mean diffusivity MD) from secondary degenerative (reduced FA and normal MD) injury in the chronic stage. The FA and MD values in the degenerated CST stabilize within 3 months after stroke. The CST ADC values decrease in a time-dependent fashion in patients with poor motor outcome but not in those with good outcome. Recognition of this imaging marker may improve early outcome prediction and patient selection for rehabilitation and neuroprotection trials.

REFERENCES

1. Uchino A, Imada H, Ohno M. MR imaging of Wallerian degeneration in the human brain stem after ictus. *Neuroradiology* 1990;**32**:191–5.
2. DeVetten G, Coutts SB, Hill MD, *et al*; MONITOR and VISION study groups. Acute corticospinal tract Wallerian degeneration is associated with stroke outcome. *Stroke* 2010;**41**:751–6.
3. Uchino A, Takase Y, Nomiyama K, *et al*. Brainstem and cerebellar changes after cerebrovascular accidents: magnetic resonance imaging. *Eur Radiol* 2006;**16**:592–7.
4. Mazumdar A, Mukherjee P, Miller JH, *et al*. Diffusion-weighted imaging of acute corticospinal tract injury preceding Wallerian degeneration in the maturing human brain. *AJNR* 2003;**24**:1057–66.
5. Yu C, Zhu C, Zhang Y, *et al*. A longitudinal diffusion tensor imaging study on Wallerian degeneration of corticospinal tract after motor pathway stroke. *Neuroimage* 2009;**47**:451–8.

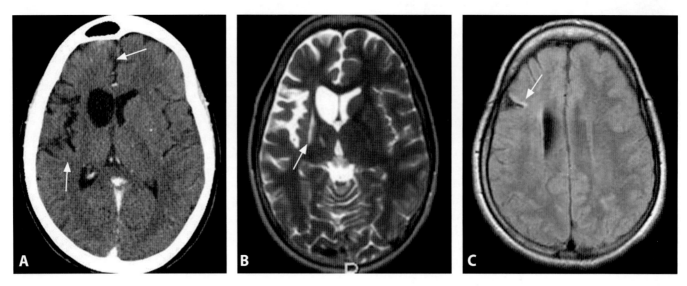

Figure 1. Enhanced axial CT scan (A) in a child with intractable seizures and left hemiplegia shows prominent volume loss of the anterior right hemisphere (arrows) with widening of the frontal horn, sylvian fissure and cortical sulci. There is no abnormal enhancement. Axial T2WI at a similar level (B) again demonstrates asymmetric atrophy. Chronic encephalomalacia with high signal is noted in the right putamen (arrow), while the right caudate head is missing. There is a lacunar lesion in the right thalamus. CT is equal to MRI in detecting atrophy, but MRI better shows deep gray matter abnormalities. Axial FLAIR image at a more cephalad level (C) shows hyperintensity (arrow) of the right frontal cortex in addition to atrophy.

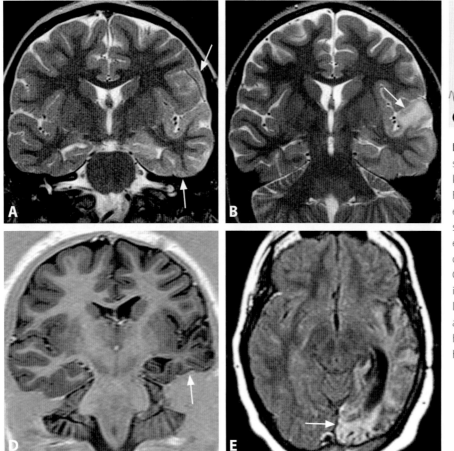

Figure 2. Coronal T2WI (A) in a child with seizures shows minimal hyperintensity of the left temporal and frontal cortex (arrows). Follow-up T2WI (B) after partial complex status epilepticus shows more prominent focal swelling and hyperintensity (arrow). Short echo time (TE 30 ms) MRS (C) reveals decreased NAA peak (arrow) and increased Glx level (arrowhead); choline and *myo*-inositol are mildly increased. IR T1WI two years later (D) shows prominent atrophy of the affected brain (arrow). Atrophy and T2 hyperintensity also involve the posterior left hemisphere (arrow) on axial FLAIR image (E).

Rasmussen Encephalitis

CHEN HOFFMAN AND ZORAN RUMBOLDT

Specific Imaging Findings

Rasmussen encephalitis is an inflammatory process affecting one cerebral hemisphere. The initial scans are normal or may in some cases show mild swelling and T2 hyperintensity of the involved cortical and subcortical areas, commonly in the frontal and temporal lobes. This is followed by progressive deterioration with gradual development of atrophy, predominantly in the affected hemisphere, but can also occur in the contralateral hemisphere. CT usually demonstrates asymmetrical atrophy, with or without brain infarcts. MRI can better demonstrate the atrophy and the abnormal tissue, before the formation of encephalomalacia on CT images. The cortical gray matter and subcortical white matter of the affected hemisphere are of abnormal high T2 signal. The basal ganglia may also be involved with progressive atrophy. There is typically no contrast enhancement and no hemorrhage. Diffusion tensor imaging shows increased ADC values and decreased fractional anisotropy (FA) in the affected hemisphere; there is also decreased perfusion as well as decreased metabolic activity on FDG-PET scans. MR spectroscopy typically shows a low NAA level, whereas elevated choline peak and lactate may also be found. Glutamine and glutamate (Glx peak) are usually increased, likely due to seizures. Atrophy and hypoperfusion of the contralateral cerebellar hemisphere (crossed cerebellar diaschisis) may also be present.

Pertinent Clinical Information

The age of onset is in childhood, usually between 1 and 14 years of age. An adult form has been recognized recently. The initial presentation is with seizures, which keep increasing in frequency and evolve into intractable epilepsia partialis continua, typically accompanied by progressive hemiparesis/hemiplegia and cognitive decline. Hemiparesis usually becomes fixed months to years after the onset of seizures. Patients may develop a variety of involuntary movements. The prognosis is poor, with cognitive and neurological deterioration, but relatively better in older individuals. In some patients, immunoglobulin or corticosteroids reduce seizure frequency in the short term. Biopsy is performed for definitive diagnosis. Seizures are refractory to antiepileptic medications and currently the only treatment is surgical. Functional hemispherectomy (or possibly cortical resection) may lead to seizure control and prevent further progression of neurological impairment and cognitive deterioration.

Differential Diagnosis

Mitochondrial Disorders (MELAS) (164)
- more acute onset
- frequently bilateral scattered lesions
- lesions may be reversible and new lesions are common

Perinatal Stroke
- radiological findings are stable and not progressive
- no cognitive and neurological deterioration

Sturge–Weber Syndrome (86)
- cortical calcifications
- pial venous enhancement
- enlarged choroid plexus may be present
- port-wine facial hemangioma

Unihemispheric Chronic Vasculitis
- contrast enhancement of the affected brain parenchyma

Background

Rasmussen encephalitis (Rasmussen encephalopathy, Rasmussen syndrome) is a rare disease of unknown etiology. It occurs following a viral disease in about half of the cases; therefore, viral etiology has been proposed. Another theory is autoimmune disease, with or without association with prior viral infection. Histopathologic examination reveals a characteristic triad of findings: perivascular lymphocytic cuffing of round cells, gliosis, and microglial nodules in the cortical layers and white matter.

A comparison of neuropathological findings and MRI revealed that the central areas of lesions contain only chronic and resolving abnormalities, while active inflammation is present at the margins and in areas of subtle MRI signal abnormality. This study suggests that the margin of the abnormality may be the ideal site for biopsy.

REFERENCES

1. Chiapparini L, Granata T, Farina L, et al. Diagnostic imaging in 13 cases of Rasmussen's encephalitis: can early MRI suggest the diagnosis? *Neuroradiology* 2003;**45**:171–83.
2. Geller E, Faerber EN, Legido A, et al. Rasmussen encephalitis: complementary role of multitechnique neuroimaging. *AJNR* 1998;**19**:445–9.
3. Fiorella DJ, Provenzale JM, Coleman RE, et al. (18) F-fluorodeoxyglucose positron emission tomography and MR imaging findings in Rasmussen encephalitis. *AJNR* 2001;**22**:1291–9.
4. Caraballo R, Bartuluchi M, Cersósimo R, et al. Hemispherectomy in pediatric patients with epilepsy: a study of 45 cases with special emphasis on epileptic syndromes. *Childs Nerv Syst* 2011;**27**:2131–6.
5. Kim SJ, Park YD, Hessler R, et al. Correlation between magnetic resonance imaging and histopathologic grades in Rasmussen syndrome. *Pediatr Neurol* 2010;**42**:172–6.

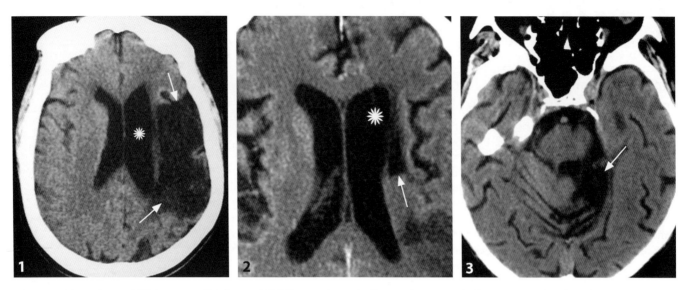

Figure 1. Non-enhanced CT shows a well-delineated CSF-like area (arrows) affecting the gray and white matter with volume loss and ex-vacuo enlargement of the lateral ventricle (*).

Figure 2. Non-enhanced CT image shows a CSF-like low attenuation in the left caudate nucleus (arrow) and associated dilation of the adjacent ventricle (*).

Figure 3. Axial non-enhanced CT image shows a prominent hypodensity in the superior left cerebellum (arrow) with attenuation values of the CSF, consistent with encephalomalacia.

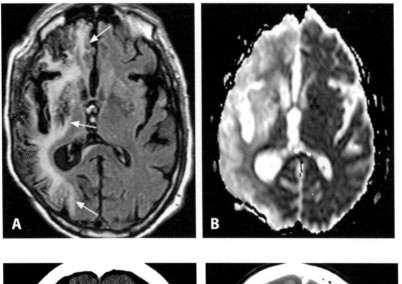

Figure 4. Axial FLAIR image (A) demonstrates a large area of volume loss involving the entire right anterior circulation (arrows) with white matter hyperintensity suggestive of gliosis. Corresponding ADC map (B) reveals very bright signal of the affected brain parenchyma, consistent with high diffusivity that is approaching the values of the CSF.

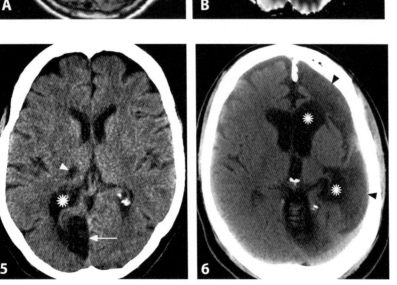

Figure 5. CT shows a CSF-like well-defined hypodensity affecting the right occipital gray and white matter (arrow) and dilated adjacent occipital horn (*). The additional smaller lesion is in the right thalamus (arrowhead).

Figure 6. CT shows atrophy and low attenuation of the left cerebral hemisphere (arrowheads) and enlarged lateral ventricle (*). The left half of the calvarium is also small indicating a remote injury early in life.

Chronic Infarct

ALESSANDRO CIANFONI

Specific Imaging Findings

Chronic infarcts are areas of variable size, shape, and location, usually with cortical and subcortical involvement, characterized by CSF-like density on CT and signal intensity on MRI. There is shrinking and/or amputation of the cerebral parenchyma, with passive (ex vacuo) dilation of adjacent CSF-containing spaces (such as ventricles and cortical sulci). Along the edges of the CSF-like area of encephalomalacia, there is an ill-defined rim of relatively higher CT attenuation, representing gliosis. FLAIR images show to better advantage the gliotic margins, which are bright between the CSF-like encephalomalacia and isointense normal white matter. Chronic infarct is also bright on ADC maps. CT and T2*WI may show chronic microhemorrhages and rarely distrophic calcifications, as bright and dark areas, respectively. There is no contrast enhancement and vascular paucity is usually present in the affected area. Curvilinear hyperintensity of the cerebral cortex corresponding to laminar necrosis may be seen on T1-weighted and FLAIR images, especially if the underlying white matter was not infarcted. Infarcts affecting large white matter tracts also show atrophy along the entire tract, remote from the primary injury (Wallerian degeneration). Atypical location and distribution of encephalomalacia and gliosis should raise possibility of a different etiology, such as prior traumatic contusion, surgery, venous infarct, vasculitis or metabolic disorders.

Pertinent Clinical Information

History of stroke with chronic stable neurological deficit is the most commonly encountered clinical scenario, but incidental finding of chronic infarcts also occurs in patients with minimal or absent symptoms and signs. This is explained by compensation (especially for in-utero or early postnatal lesions), and/or involvement of non-eloquent areas. Cardio-cerebro-vascular risk factors should be investigated in patients with cerebral infarcts, in order to reduce risk of new injuries or progressive deterioration. Location and shape of the lesion can suggest the causative mechanism: thromboembolic events of major arteries distal to the circle of Willis show a wedge or rectangular shape, within the corresponding vascular distribution; occlusions of perforating arteries cause subcortical (lacunar) infarcts, confined to the deep gray matter and/or white matter; embolic and hemodynamic infarcts, caused by occlusion of arteries proximal to the circle of Willis or emboli from these vessels or the heart, tend to involve the border zones between adjacent vascular territories ("watershed" areas).

Differential Diagnosis

Porencephalic cyst (83)
- may be indistinguishable, as majority of the cysts are chronic infarcts
- adjacent to/communicating with a ventricular cavity

Dilated Perivascular Spaces (168)
- absence of bright gliotic rim on FLAIR images
- large ones may show mass effect

Postoperative Encephalomalacia (82)
- signs of craniotomy, usually adjacent to the encephalomalacia/gliosis
- history

Post-traumatic Encephalomalacia (81)
- nonvascular distribution, typically antero-inferior frontal and temporal location
- frequently bilateral

Arachnoid Cyst (142)
- minimal or absent mass effect on the adjacent sulci with preserved cortical gray matter – absence of gliosis along the margins
- inner table of the adjacent bone may be scalloped due to cyst pulsatility

Epidermoid (143)
- presence of mass effect
- very bright on DWI, may be different from the CSF on FLAIR images
- preserved adjacent cortical gray matter, no gliosis

Background

Brain infarcts start involuting towards the chronic phase around the fourth week, by the sixth week the swelling and mass effect have disappeared, while encephalomalacia, cystic cavitation, and gliosis have ensued. The parenchymal volume loss causes asymmetric passive widening of the adjacent subarachnoid and ventricular CSF-containing spaces. Contrast enhancement, especially along the cortical gyri, can at times persist up to the eighth week and beyond.

REFERENCES

1. Cooper JA. Chronic cerebral infarction. In: *Diagnostic Imaging: Brain*. Osborn AG, *et al.*, eds. Amirsys, Salt Lake City, UT, 2004.

2. Giele JL, Witkamp TD, Mali WP; SMART Study Group. Silent brain infarcts in patients with manifest vascular disease. *Stroke* 2004;**35**:742–6.

3. Tsushima Y, Tamura T, Unno Y, *et al.* Multifocal low-signal brain lesions on T2*-weighted gradient-echo imaging. *Neuroradiology* 2000;**42**:499–504.

4. Kinoshita T, Ogawa T, Yoshida Y, *et al.* Curvilinear T1 hyperintense lesions representing cortical necrosis after cerebral infarction. *Neuroradiology* 2005;**47**:647–51.

5. Momjian-Mayor I, Baron JC. The pathophysiology of watershed infarction in internal carotid artery disease: review of cerebral perfusion studies. *Stroke* 2005;**36**:567–77.

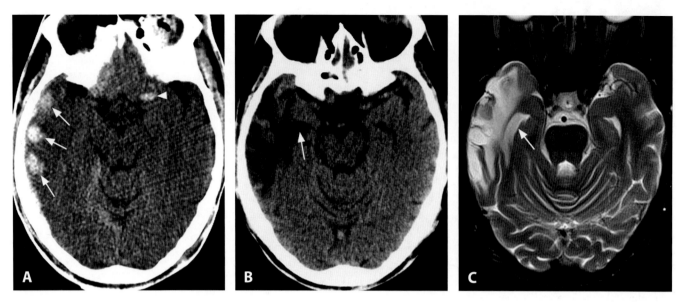

Figure 1. Axial non-enhanced CT (A) following acute head trauma shows several hemorrhagic areas in the right temporal lobe consistent with hemorrhagic contusions (arrows). At least one frontal contusion is also seen (arrowhead). Head CT obtained several years later (B) demonstrates development of encephalomalacia, indicated by the right temporal decreased density and parenchymal volume loss. Notice the ex-vacuo enlargement of the right temporal horn (arrow). Corresponding T2WI (C) also shows right temporal atrophy with enlarged temporal horn (arrow). Hyperintense areas correspond to low attenuation on CT and are consistent with encephalomalacia and gliosis.

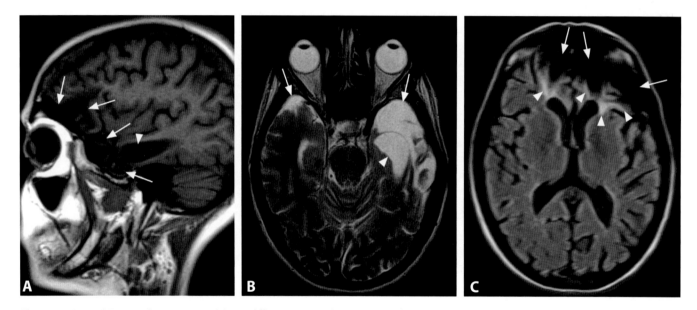

Figure 2. Sagittal T1WI without contrast (A) in a different patient shows anterior frontal and temporal hypointense areas (arrows) with loss of the cortical ribbon. The temporal horn is dilated (arrowhead). Axial T2WI at the level of the temporal lobes (B) reveals bilateral anterior hyperintensity (arrows), left greater than right, consistent with encephalomalacia and gliosis. There is a prominent ex-vacuo dilation of the left temporal horn (arrowhead). Axial FLAIR image at the level of the lateral ventricles (C) shows bifrontal hypointense CSF-like areas of encephalomalacia (arrows) and adjacent underlying hyperintense gliosis (arrowheads).

Post-Traumatic Atrophy

BENJAMIN HUANG

Specific Imaging Findings

Atrophy following traumatic brain injury can be divided into two types: focal atrophy and diffuse brain atrophy. Focal atrophy may manifest as either encephalomalacia or porencephaly. Characteristic locations for post-traumatic encephalomalacia parallel those of cortical contusions and include the orbitofrontal regions of the frontal lobes and the antero-inferior temporal lobes. Encephalomalacia can develop within weeks of the traumatic event, appearing as a relatively well-demarcated area of low density on CT with low T1 and high T2 signal on MRI, with associated parenchymal volume loss. Cystic replacement of brain parenchyma is occasionally seen on MRI. Areas of encephalomalacia are characteristically bordered by gliosis, which is also hypodense but usually of slightly higher attenuation on CT. Gliosis is best seen as a hyperintense rim adjacent to CSF-like hypointense encephalomalacia on FLAIR images.

Diffuse brain atrophy becomes evident months or years after brain trauma, even in relatively mild cases in which the initial imaging studies revealed no abnormalities. In these patients, delayed CT and MR imaging demonstrate first ventricular enlargement – particularly of the third ventricle and temporal horn, followed by diffuse widening of the cortical sulci and cerebellar fissures. Atrophy of corpus callosum is also a common finding. Diffuse post-traumatic volume loss in young children may develop at a very rapid rate, within days and weeks.

Pertinent Clinical Information

The long-term sequelae of traumatic brain injury are extremely varied and depend upon a number of factors including patient age, mechanism of trauma, injury severity, neurologic condition at presentation, and concomitant extracranial injuries. Most patients with mild brain injury may become asymptomatic after weeks to months, but as many as one-third have persistent symptoms such as headache, amnesia, visual or olfactory disturbances, dizziness, depression, and difficulty concentrating. Patients with moderate or severe head trauma (which is usually accompanied by abnormalities on initial brain imaging) can suffer from more severe and debilitating long-term deficits which include motor or sensory impairment, gait and balance disturbances, ataxia, or seizures. In general, the degree of atrophy appears to correlate with neurocognitive outcome following a traumatic brain injury.

Differential Diagnosis

Arachnoid Cyst (142)
- preserved adjacent cortex, the brain is displaced and not replaced
- absence of encephalomalacia and gliosis

Low-Grade Glioma (162)
- shows increased parenchymal volume rather than atrophy
- absence of CSF-like encephalomalacia

Remote Infarct (80)
- areas of encephalomalacia correspond to arterial territory, not the typical antero-inferior frontal and temporal frequently bilateral location

Post-Surgical Defect (82)
- evidence of overlying craniotomy

Background

Approximately 80% of nontraumatic brain injuries in the US are classified as "mild", but it has become increasingly clear that even these mild injuries can result in significant long-term sequelae. The fact that many develop persistent neurologic symptoms and early brain atrophy following relatively mild trauma suggests that microstructural damage, which is not detectable with conventional imaging techniques, has occurred in these patients. Autopsy studies of mild traumatic brain injury suggest that microscopic diffuse axonal injury occurs, which is supported by findings on newer structural and functional imaging techniques, such as DTI (decreased fractional anisotropy in normal-appearing white matter), proton MR spectroscopy (reduced levels of NAA), and magnetization transfer imaging (decreased white matter magnetization transfer ratios). These acute microstructural changes subsequently lead to a prolonged phase of neuronal degeneration above and beyond cell damage that occurs in the acute setting, but the exact mechanism of this delayed cell death remains to be fully elucidated.

REFERENCES

1. Zee CS, Hovanessian A, Go JL, *et al.* Imaging of sequelae of head trauma. *Neuroimag Clin N Am* 2002;**12**:325–38.

2. Belanger HG, Vanderploeg RD, Curtiss G, *et al.* Recent neuroimaging techniques in mild traumatic brain injury. *J Neuropsychiatry Clin Neurosci* 2007;**19**:5–20.

3. Cohen BA, Inglese M, Rusinek H, *et al.* Proton MR spectroscopy and MRI-volumetry in mild traumatic brain injury. *AJNR* 2007;**28**:907–13.

4. MacKenzie JD, Siddiqi F, Babb JS, *et al.* Brain atrophy in mild or moderate traumatic brain injury: a longitudinal quantitative analysis. *AJNR* 2002;**23**:1509–15.

5. Warner MA, Youn TS, Davis T, *et al.* Regionally selective atrophy after traumatic axonal injury. *Arch Neurol* 2010;**67**:1336–44.

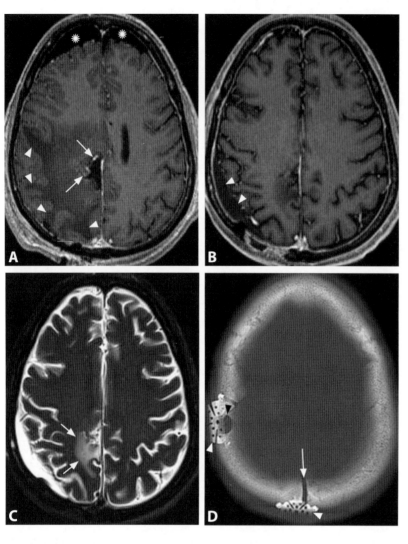

Figure 1. Post-contrast T1WI (A) obtained one day after a large metastatic tumor removal shows thin linear enhancement (arrows) along the margins of the resection site. Note vasogenic edema (arrowheads) and bifrontal pneumocephalus (*). Post-contrast T1WI 3 months later (B) demonstrates resolution of enhancement around a small parenchymal defect and an ipsilateral subdural collection (arrowheads), likely ex-vacuo. Corresponding T2WI (C) demonstrates hyperintense gliosis (arrows) in the surgical bed, as well as the subdural collection. CT image displayed with bone algorithm and window (D) shows the typical changes associated with craniotomy, with smoothly marginated lucency (arrow) through the calvarium that is fixed with titanium plates (white arrowheads). A burr hole is also present (black arrowhead).

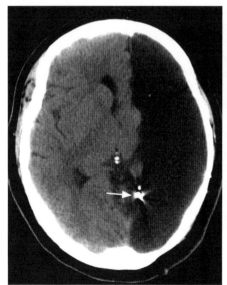

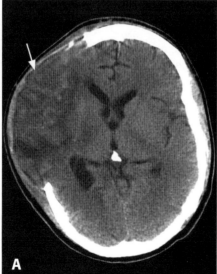

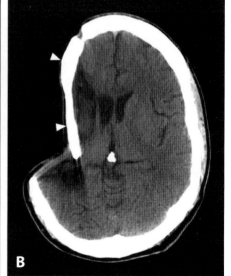

Figure 2. CT image obtained many years after a left hemispherectomy was performed. Note surgical clip (arrow) with associated artifact.

Figure 3. Non-enhanced axial CT image (A) shows status post-craniectomy for a large right middle cerebral artery infarction (arrow). A follow-up CT image (B) after delayed cranioplasty with bone flap replacement (arrowheads) reveals sunken appearance with underlying encephalomalacia.

Postoperative Defects

BENJAMIN HUANG

Specific Imaging Findings

Postoperative changes in the brain vary depending upon the amount of time elapsed between surgery and imaging. In all cases, calvarial changes consistent with a craniotomy or craniectomy indicate that the underlying parenchymal abnormalities are at least in part postoperative. In the acute postoperative setting, unenhanced CT demonstrates variable amounts of extra-axial fluid, blood and gas within the resection cavity. Edema and hemorrhage in the soft tissues overlying the craniotomy are also usually present. On MRI, gas appears as foci (frequently round) of low T1 and T2 signal and hemorrhage has a variable appearance depending on the age of blood products (usually iso- to hyperintense on T1WI). Rim of reduced diffusion along the periphery of the resection site may also represent blood products, in which case there is corresponding signal loss on T2* imaging; without T2* findings reduced diffusion is consistent with post-operative infarct. Intracranial air should resolve by 3 weeks, extra-axial fluid may be evident for up to a month. In high-grade gliomas biodegradable chemotherapeutic wafers may be left within the resection cavity. These wafers appear linear on imaging and are usually radiopaque on CT and hypointense on all MR sequences. With time, progressive local encephalomalacia and gliosis develop at the margins of a resection cavity, which may become filled with CSF.

Parenchymal contrast enhancement along the resection margins may begin to appear on MR by 24 h and is present in virtually all cases by day 7. Over subsequent days to weeks, this enhancement may become increasingly thick and nodular, but it usually resolves by 2–3 months. In rare instances, enhancement may persist for up to 8 months. Dural thickening and enhancement can persist for years and may be diffuse, not limited to the surgical bed.

Pertinent Clinical Information

In patients undergoing resection of brain tumors, it is recommended that the first postoperative MR be performed within the first 24 h of surgery, as the likelihood that benign enhancement will be seen increases from roughly 40% in the first postoperative day to 100% by day 7. Thin linear enhancement within the first 24 h after surgery may be normal in the majority of cases, but the presence of thick or nodular enhancement on an early postoperative scan generally indicates that residual enhancing tumor was left behind. The sensitivity and specificity of early postoperative MRI for predicting tumor regrowth have been reported to be 91% and 100%, respectively. Perioperative MR imaging is also commonly requested to rule out complications of surgery including infarcts, interval rehemorrhage, CSF leak, or infection.

Differential Diagnosis

Remote Infarct or Hemorrhage (80, 177)
- no evidence of prior craniotomy

Remote Trauma (81)
- no evidence of prior craniotomy
- characteristic locations of contusions include anterior and inferior frontal and temporal lobes

Arachnoid Cyst (142)
- no evidence of craniotomy
- normal adjacent brain parenchyma is displaced

Empyema or Operative Site Abscess (134, 156)
- persistent extra-axial fluid and/or gas
- peripheral contrast enhancement
- fluid may demonstrate reduced diffusivity on DWI/ADC

Background

Various mechanisms have been postulated for the development of postoperative parenchymal enhancement, including local disruption of the blood–brain barrier, neovascularity, luxury perfusion, and contrast extravasation along the surgical wound. Histologic studies have demonstrated development of granulation tissue containing large numbers of small blood vessels at resection margins at 1 week with subsequent development of vascular proliferation in the surrounding brain by 2–3 weeks. By 8–10 weeks, these parenchymal vascular elements become less prominent, paralleling the time course of resolving enhancement on imaging.

REFERENCES
1. Sinclair AG, Scoffings DJ. Imaging of the post-operative cranium. *Radiographics* 2010;**30**:461–82.
2. Elster AD, DiPersio DA. Cranial postoperative site: assessment with contrast-enhanced MR imaging. *Radiology* 1990;**174**:93–8.
3. Sato N, Bronen RA, Sze G, *et al.* Postoperative changes in the brain: MR imaging findings in patients without neoplasms. *Radiology* 1997;**204**:839–46.
4. Oser AB, Moran CJ, Kaufman BA, *et al.* Intracranial tumor in children: MR imaging findings within 24 hours of craniotomy. *Radiology* 1997;**205**:807–12.

Brain Imaging with MRI and CT, ed. Zoran Rumboldt *et al.* Published by Cambridge University Press. © Cambridge University Press 2012.

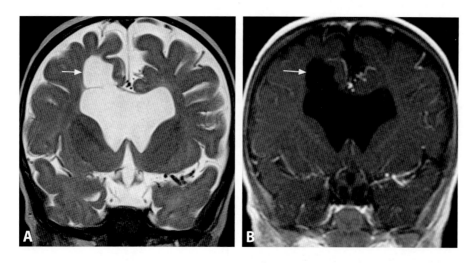

Figure 1. Coronal T2WI (A) and post-contrast T1WI (B) show a lesion (arrow) that follows the CSF signal intensity, abutting and probably communicating with the right lateral ventricle. The surrounding white matter is of normal signal. This cyst was a consequence of perinatal parenchymal hemorrhage. There is also absence of septum pellucidum and very thin corpus callosum.

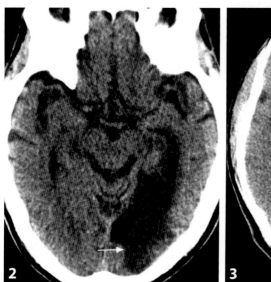
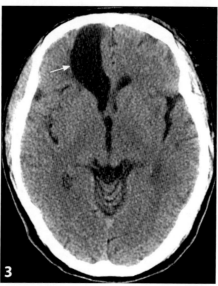

Figure 2. Axial non-enhanced CT image demonstrates a cyst (arrow) communicating with the occipital horn of the left lateral ventricle in a patient with a remote left posterior cerebral artery infarct.

Figure 3. Axial CT shows sharp margins of the right frontal cyst (arrow) and wide communication with the lateral ventricle. The cyst appears to extend to the surface of the brain.

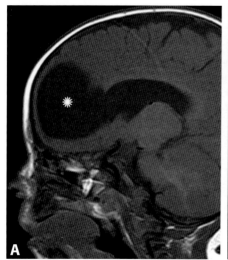
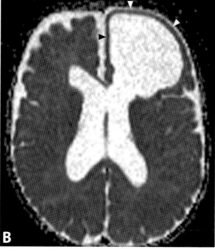

Figure 4. Sagittal T1WI without contrast (A) shows a frontal cyst (*) that communicates with the left lateral ventricle. There is no adjacent signal abnormality. Axial ADC map (B) reveals a thin cortical ribbon surrounding the cyst (arrowheads). The diffusion is identical within the cyst and inside the lateral ventricles.

Porencephalic Cyst

BENJAMIN HUANG

Specific Imaging Findings

Porencephalic cysts are smooth-walled CSF-filled cavities within the substance of the brain which abut with an enlarged lateral ventricle or the subarachnoid space. The cysts may be enclosed by a thin membrane or communicate directly with ventricles or/and other CSF-containing spaces. When large they may appear as a direct communication between the lateral ventricle and the subarachnoid space. Porencephalic cysts are lined by a thin layer of gliotic white matter, and the surrounding tissue often has normal signal characteristics. The contents of the cysts follow CSF on CT and on all MRI sequences and there is no enhancement after contrast administration.

Pertinent Clinical Information

Porencephalic cysts are primarily found in children, although they can occur in adults. As they are often the result of hemorrhage or ischemia, perinatally acquired cysts are associated with cerebral palsy, epilepsy, and psychomotor retardation. The presence and severity of symptoms depends on the location and extent of tissue destruction.

Differential Diagnosis

Schizencephaly (84)
- dysplastic gray matter lines the cleft

Arachnoid Cyst (142)
- tissue subjacent to the cyst is displaced and compressed but the cortical stripe is preserved
- no communication with lateral ventricles

Ependymal Cyst (146)
- entirely intraventricular
- may be difficult to distinguish when large but will not communicate with the subarachnoid space

Background

Porencephalic cysts may occur pre- or postnatally and both result from destruction of cerebral tissue from trauma, infarction, infection, or hemorrhage. Antenatally derived porencephalic cysts most commonly result from periventricular hemorrhage, followed by cerebral infarction and CNS infection during the late second or early third trimester. Associations with exposure to teratogens such as cocaine, vitamin A, and valproate have been reported, and a hereditary form has also been described. The area of destroyed tissue is eventually replaced with CSF, a process that may take up to 8 weeks. Depending on the cause the cysts differ in locations while those due to venous hemorrhagic infarctions communicate with an enlarged lateral ventricle and may spare the cortical mantle. Cysts caused by arterial infarctions always open to the subarachnoid space, due to occlusion of pial cerebral arteries and subsequent destruction of the subcortex, and may not extend to the lateral ventricle, usually located in the middle cerebral artery territory. Porencephalic cysts typically require no treatment, but in rare instances shunting or fenestration may relieve significant or progressive mass effect.

REFERENCES
1. Aprile I, Iaiza F, Lavaroni A, *et al.* Analysis of cystic intracranial lesions performed with fluid-attenuated inversion recovery MR imaging. *AJNR* 1999;**20**:1259–67.
2. Govaert P. Prenatal stroke. *Semin Fetal Neonatal Med* 2009; **14**:250–66.
3. Grant EG, Kerner M, Schellinger D, *et al.* Evolution of porencephalic cysts from intraparenchymal hemorrhage in neonates: sonographic evidence. *AJR* 1982;**138**:467–70.
4. Koch CA, Moore JL, Krähling KH, *et al.* Fenestration of porencephalic cysts to the lateral ventricle: experience with a new technique for treatment of seizures. *Surg Neurol* 1998; **49**:532–3.
5. Mancini GMS, de Coo IFM, Lequin MH, *et al.* Hereditary porencephaly: clinical and MRI findings in two Dutch families. *Eur J Paediatr Neurol* 2004;**8**:45–54.

Brain Imaging with MRI and CT, ed. Zoran Rumboldt *et al.* Published by Cambridge University Press. © Cambridge University Press 2012.

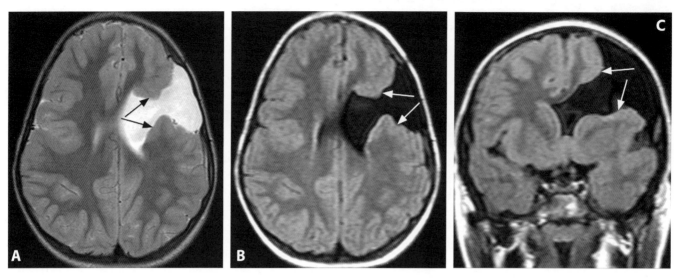

Figure 1. Axial T2WI (A), axial FLAIR (B), and coronal FLAIR (C) show a large full thickness left frontal hemisphere defect filled by CSF, lined by the gray matter (arrows) and extending from the surface to the lateral ventricle.

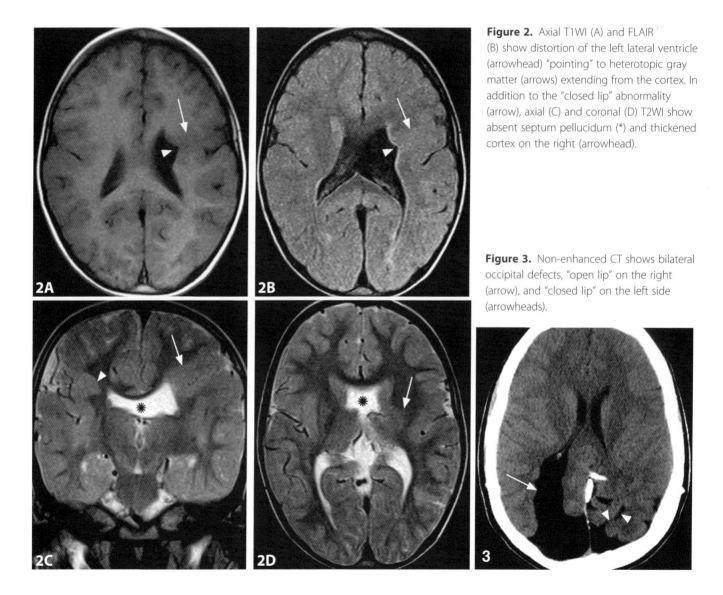

Figure 2. Axial T1WI (A) and FLAIR (B) show distortion of the left lateral ventricle (arrowhead) "pointing" to heterotopic gray matter (arrows) extending from the cortex. In addition to the "closed lip" abnormality (arrow), axial (C) and coronal (D) T2WI show absent septum pellucidum (*) and thickened cortex on the right (arrowhead).

Figure 3. Non-enhanced CT shows bilateral occipital defects, "open lip" on the right (arrow), and "closed lip" on the left side (arrowheads).

Schizencephaly

ALESSANDRO CIANFONI

Specific Imaging Findings

Schizencephaly is a hemispherical cerebral cleft that extends from the cortex to the ependymal surface of the lateral ventricles and is lined by the gray matter. The gray matter lining the cleft is morphologically abnormal, with pachygyric or micropolygyric appearance, and its continuity with the sulcal cortex gives the appearance of "diving gyri". The cleft can be large, filled by CSF (open lips or type II schizencephaly), or small, virtually invisible, with gray matter lining the cleft apposed on both sides of the defect (closed lips or type I schizencephaly). In type I schizencephaly, when a cleft is not clearly visible, a small focal deformity of the lateral ventricle, with the ependyma "pointing" to the schizencephaly, can offer a clue to the diagnosis. Another helpful finding is that of prominent venous vasculature overlying the cleft. In large clefts, remnants of the brain parenchyma or ependymal lining are visible in the form of so-called "roofing membranes", or "cords". Schizencephaly can be uni- or bilateral, most commonly found in the insula and/or the perirolandic gyri. Associated abnormalities, which are often visible on MRI, are hypoplasia of optic chiasm and pituitary gland, and dysgenesis septum pellucidum and corpus callosum (together forming septo-optic dysplasia); opercular syndromes with hypoplastic sylvian fissure and perisylvian polymicrogyria, and hippocampal abnormalities with temporal horns enlargement. Rarely gliosis and/or calcifications can be observed in the adjacent areas.

Pertinent Clinical Information

Clinical presentation of schizencephaly is highly variable: some individuals are asymptomatic, but more frequently it manifests with seizures (often intractable), developmental delay, mental retardation, and congenital motor deficits (spasticity, hemiparesis, or quadriparesis). The clinical picture tends to be more severe in patients with type II schizencephaly, with bilateral involvement, and with the cleft in the perirolandic region. The extent and severity of the associated brain abnormalities also influence the clinical presentation.

Differential Diagnosis

Nodular Heterotopia (117)
• abnormal gray matter is usually adjacent to a ventricle with normal surrounding white matter

• no ependymal deformity pointing to the cleft, no evidence of a CSF cleft

Focal Cortical Dysplasia (106)
• a thin straight line extends from the abnormal cortex toward ventricular surface
• no ependymal deformity, no cleft

Clastic Schizencephaly/Porencephalic Cyst (83)
• the cleft is not bordered by gray matter (it occurred after neuronal migration)
• adjacent gyri appear atrophic
• cleft might have gliotic changes along its margins (bright on FLAIR images)

Background

Genetic factors are held responsible for some cases of schizencephaly, such as familial series. Vascular, infectious, toxic, and autoimmune injuries during the particularly critical interval in the seventh week of gestational age as well as during the neuronal migration in the third trimester have been postulated as the likely etiology of schizencephaly in a majority of affected individuals. Fetal ultrasound is usually able to diagnose this condition *in utero*, especially the open lips type.

REFERENCES

1. Oh KY, Kennedy AM, Frias AE Jr, Byrne JL. Fetal schizencephaly: pre- and postnatal imaging with a review of the clinical manifestations. *Radiographics* 2005;**25**:647–57.

2. Barkovich AJ, Norman D. MR imaging of schizencephaly. *AJNR* 1988;**9**:297–302.

3. Barkovich AJ, Kjos BO. Schizencephaly: correlation of clinical findings with MR characteristics. *AJNR* 1992;**13**:85–94.

4. Hayashi N, Tsutsumi Y, Barkovich AJ. Morphological features and associated anomalies of schizencephaly in the clinical population: detailed analysis of MR images. *Neuroradiology* 2002; **44**:418–27.

5. Pilz D, Stoodley N, Golden JA. Neuronal migration, cerebral cortical development, and cerebral cortical anomalies. *J Neuropathol Exp Neurol* 2002;**61**:1–11.

Brain Imaging with MRI and CT, ed. Zoran Rumboldt *et al.* Published by Cambridge University Press. © Cambridge University Press 2012.

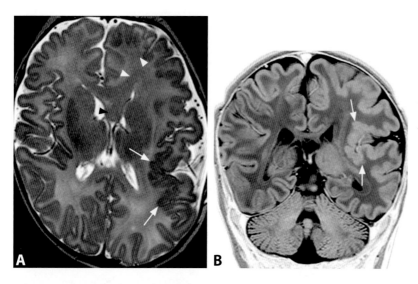

Figure 1. Axial T2WI (A) in a 1-month-old boy shows enlarged left cerebral hemisphere with perisylvian polymicrogyria (arrows). Subcortical frontal white matter and genu of the corpus callosum are hypointense (white arrowheads). Note thickening of the fornix (black arrowhead). Coronal IR T1WI (B) confirms enlarged left hemisphere and perisylvian polymicrogyria (arrows). The cerebellum is normal with symmetric hemispheres.

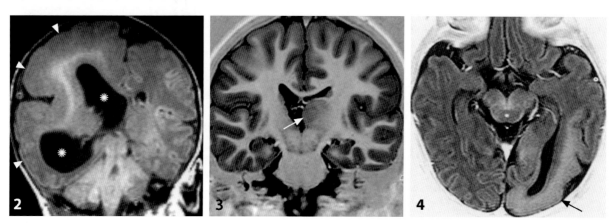

Figure 2. Coronal T1WI in a newborn with epilepsy shows enlarged right cerebral hemisphere including the lateral ventricle (*) with a diffusely lissencephalic appearance (arrowheads).

Figure 3. Coronal IR T1WI (B) in an 11-year-old girl with mild psychomotor delay shows enlarged left thalamus (arrow) within a minimally enlarged left cerebral hemisphere with normal cerebral cortex.

Figure 4. Axial IR T1WI in a different patient shows focal enlargement of the left occipital lobe with a lissencephalic appearance (arrow).

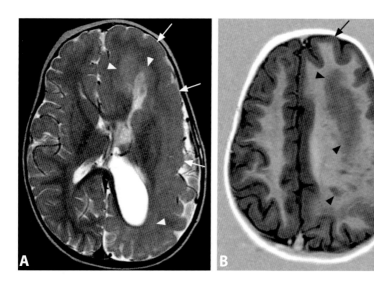

Figure 5. Axial T2WI (A) at the level of lateral ventricles in a 3-year-old boy with intractable seizures shows enlargement of the entire left cerebral hemisphere with dysplasia involving both the cortex (arrows) and white matter (arrowheads). IR T1WI at a higher level (B) also shows dysplastic gray (arrows) and white (arrowheads) matter. High T2 and low T1 signal of the white matter are due to demyelination and gliosis.

Hemimegalencephaly

ANDREA ROSSI

Specific Imaging Findings

Hemimegalencephaly (HME) is characterized by gross brain asymmetry with enlargement of all or part of one hemisphere and possible concomitant enlargement of the ipsilateral half of the brainstem and cerebellar hemisphere. Midline shift can be present, either total or limited to the occipital area. The cerebral cortex is thickened and shows a variable spectrum of abnormalities, ranging from lissencephaly to polymicrogyria. The most severe end of this spectrum has been termed hemilissencephaly. In milder cases, the cortical mantle may be grossly normal. The affected white matter shows abnormal signal intensity that varies with patient age: in neonates, T1 and T2 shortening (T1 bright, T2 dark) reflects abnormally advanced myelination for the age, whereas in older children the white matter becomes T2 hyperintense due to gliosis and lack of myelin. The lateral ventricle in the affected hemisphere shows variable abnormalities, including a straightened or collapsed frontal horn, colpocephalic dilation of the occipital horns, and global enlargement. In some cases, only a portion of the cerebral hemisphere, usually corresponding to a single lobe, is enlarged. Serial imaging studies may show progressive atrophy of the involved hemisphere, so that it eventually becomes smaller than the unaffected one.

Pertinent Clinical Information

Affected patients have a variable clinical picture depending on the extent and severity of the malformation. Most present during the first days or weeks of life with medically intractable seizures, severe psychomotor delay, and contralateral hemiparesis. Management of these children is difficult. Seizure control may not be achieved by pharmacologic treatment, and adverse side effects may be severe. Hemispherectomy has been advocated for patients with frequent, refractory, intractable seizures. Less severe cases may present with mild to moderate psychomotor delay.

Differential Diagnosis

Unilateral Polymicrogyria (103)
· affected hemisphere is smaller than the unaffected one

Rasmussen Encephalitis (79)
· patients with status epilepticus
· progressive hemiatrophy of involved cerebral hemisphere

Sotos Syndrome
· excessively rapid growth, acromegalic features, advanced bone age
· nonprogressive mental retardation
· large brain with normal gyration

Background

HME is a hamartomatous congenital malformation of the brain, involving dysplastic overgrowth limited to one cerebral hemisphere resulting from an imbalance between proliferation and apoptosis of neuronal and glial precursors in the germinal matrix. While it is suggested that HME represents a genetically programmed developmental disorder related to cellular lineage and establishment of symmetry, no chromosomal abnormalities have been found and the genetic background remains unknown. The severity of the malformation ranges from so-called total HME, in which there is concomitant ipsilateral enlargement of a cerebral hemisphere, half of the brainstem, and cerebellar hemisphere, to focal HME which involves a single cerebral lobe. Histologically, the cortex shows lack of alignment in the horizontal layers and an indistinct demarcation from the underlying white matter. Giant, dysplastic neurons and balloon cells identical to those seen in focal cortical dysplasia are scattered throughout the cortex and subcortical white matter. The cortical abnormality may range from a lissencephalic structure with little or absent gyration to a more frequent polymicrogyric arrangement that typically involves the perisylvian region but may extend to other areas. The white matter is also frequently abnormal; neonatal cases may show areas of abnormally increased myelination, whereas striking demyelination of all or part of the centrum semiovale is frequently seen in older patients. Less severe cases may be characterized by an enlarged but structurally normal cortical mantle, white matter, and deep gray matter nuclei. HME may be isolated or syndromic, associated with neurocutaneous disorders including tuberous sclerosis, neurofibromatosis type 1, Klippel–Trenaunay–Weber, the nevus sebaceous syndrome, hypomelanosis of Ito, and Proteus syndromes; some of these entities involve hypertrophy of a part or the entire ipsilateral half of the patient's body.

REFERENCES

1. Barkovich AJ, Chuang SH. Unilateral megalencephaly: correlation of MR imaging and pathologic characteristics. *AJNR* 1990;**11**:523–31.
2. Wolpert SM, Cohen A, Libenson MH. Hemimegalencephaly: a longitudinal MR study. *AJNR* 1994;**15**:1479–82.
3. Yagishita A, Arai N, Tamagawa K, Oda M. Hemimegalencephaly: signal changes suggesting abnormal myelination on MRI. *Neuroradiology* 1998;**40**:734–8.
4. Sato N, Yagishita A, Oba H, *et al*. Hemimegalencephaly: a study of abnormalities occurring outside the involved hemisphere. *AJNR* 2007;**28**:678–82.
5. Abdel Razek AA, Kandell AY, Elsorogy LG, *et al*. Disorders of cortical formation: MR imaging features. *AJNR* 2007;**30**:4–11.

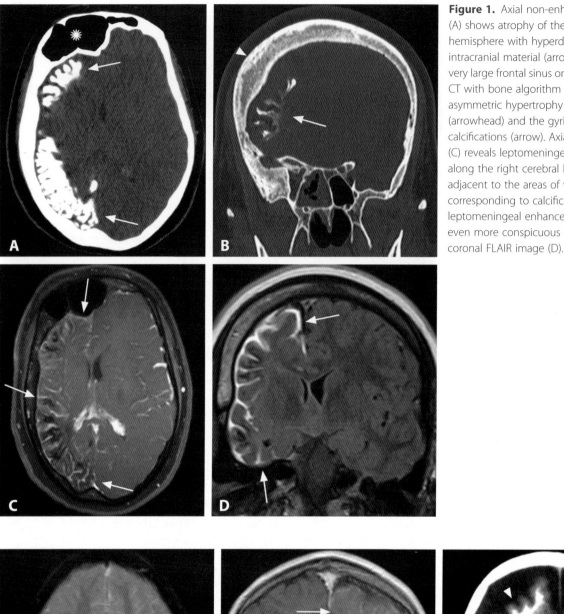

Figure 1. Axial non-enhanced CT image (A) shows atrophy of the right cerebral hemisphere with hyperdense bone-like intracranial material (arrows). There is also a very large frontal sinus on the right (*). Coronal CT with bone algorithm (B) shows the asymmetric hypertrophy of the right skull (arrowhead) and the gyriform intracranial calcifications (arrow). Axial post-contrast T1WI (C) reveals leptomeningeal enhancement along the right cerebral hemisphere (arrows), adjacent to the areas of very low signal corresponding to calcifications. The leptomeningeal enhancement (arrows) is even more conspicuous on post-contrast coronal FLAIR image (D).

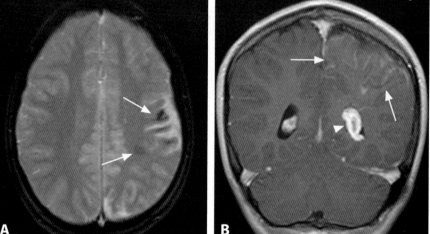

Figure 2. Axial T2*WI (A) shows mild volume loss of the left cerebral hemisphere with fronto-parietal cortical hypointense areas (arrows) consistent with calcification. Axial enhanced T1WI (B) shows left hemisphere leptomeningeal enhancement (arrows) and prominent left choroid plexus (arrowhead).

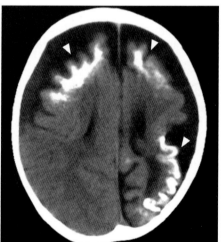

Figure 3. Axial non-enhanced CT shows atrophy of the left cerebral hemisphere and right frontal lobe with associated calcifications (arrowheads).

Sturge–Weber Syndrome

MARIA GISELE MATHEUS

Specific Imaging Findings

Sturge–Weber syndrome (SWS) shows a spectrum of findings related to leptomeningeal angiomatous changes, which consequently affect the brain parenchyma. There is atrophy of the affected brain, seen as widening of the cortical sulci and enlargement of the ventricles. Cortical gyriform calcifications are hyperdense on CT and hypointense on all MR sequences. There is an avid leptomeningeal contrast enhancement in the affected area, prominent medullary veins and enlargement of the ipsilateral choroid plexus, which can be seen on post-contrast CT or MRI. T2*-weighted MR sequences readily show calcifications, and susceptibility-weighted images (SWI) can show prominent medullary veins and sometimes the angiomatous changes without contrast administration. Intracranial SWS findings are usually unilateral, with a subtle predilection for the posterior portions of the brain, but may affect the whole cerebral hemisphere. However, SWS can also be bilateral or focal/isolated to one or a few lobes. Hypertrophy of the skull and paranasal sinuses (Dyke–Davidoff–Masson syndrome), and globe enlargement with abnormal enhancement, may also be present. Infratentorial pial angiomas are common but usually very subtle.

Pertinent Clinical Information

Patients with SWS generally develop normally until the onset of seizures, which over time become progressively refractory to medication. The overwhelming majority have a port-wine stain, usually along the V1 segment of the trigeminal nerve distribution, ipsilateral to the intracranial angiomatous changes. However, cases of SWS without port-wine stain have been described. Most patients are mentally retarded and 30% have hemiparesis. The ocular manifestations include choroidal and scleral or episcleral telangiectasia with glaucoma and enlarged globe. Progression in neurologic deficits occurs in some patients, but this is quite variable. Mild cases with subtle imaging findings that are discovered later in childhood and with minimal symptoms have also been described.

Differential Diagnosis

Meningioangiomatosis (189)
- cortical calcifications are typically restricted to a focal area
- leptomeningeal enhancement is variable and may extend into the brain via perivascular spaces
- absence of associated atrophy

Rasmussen Encephalitis (79)
- no abnormal contrast enhancement
- no calcifications
- progressive atrophy with T2 hyperintensity

Wyburn-Mason syndrome
- facial vascular nevus with associated intracranial or visual pathway arteriovenous malformations, may mimic leptomeningeal angiomatous changes
- absence of atrophy and leptomeningeal enhancement

Celiac Disease
- bilateral calcifications of the occipital lobes
- absence of facial or intracranial angiomatous abnormalities

Background

SWS is defined by the association of a facial capillary malformation (port-wine stain) with a vascular malformation of the eye causing congenital glaucoma and/or leptomeningeal angioma of the brain. Variants exist where only one of these three structures is involved with the vascular malformation. SWS is congenital and occurs sporadically, with the estimated incidence ranging around 1 in 20–50 000 live births. The cause remains obscure, and the primary lesion appears to be a capillary/post-capillary angiomatous abnormality with impaired venous drainage. The intracranial manifestations are primarily due to these abnormal vessels and secondary recruitment of collateral venous drainage. The medullary veins are recruited to drain the cortex in a reversed, centripetal direction, followed by progressive atrophy and superficial calcification of the affected cerebral hemisphere, most likely related to ischemia. Perfusion MRI, along with SPECT and PET studies, suggests that decreased brain blood flow combined with altered hemodynamics during prolonged seizures contributes to the neurologic decline in SWS patients. Several controversies exist in the management of seizures and other impairments in SWS, including the timing of surgery – early "prophylactic" operation versus later interventions. Complete excision of the angiomatous cortex is the primary surgical procedure in patients with focal lesions, while hemispherectomy is the treatment of choice in children with extensive hemispheric abnormalities.

REFERENCES

1. Smirniotopoulos JG. Neuroimaging of phakomatoses: Sturge–Weber syndrome, tuberous sclerosis, von Hippel–Lindau syndrome. *Neuroimaging Clin N Am* 2004;**14**:171–83.

2. Adams ME, Aylett SE, Squier W, Chong W. A Spectrum of unusual neuroimaging findings in patients with suspected Sturge–Weber syndrome. *AJNR* 2009;**30**:276–81.

3. Comi AM. Advances in Sturge–Weber syndrome. *Curr Opin Neurol* 2006;**19**:124–8.

4. Di Rocco C, Tamburrini G. Sturge–Weber syndrome. *Childs Nerv Syst* 2006;**22**:909–21.

5. Tong KA, Ashwal S, Obenaus A, *et al.* Susceptibility-weighted MR imaging: a review of clinical applications in children. *AJNR* 2008;**29**:9–17.

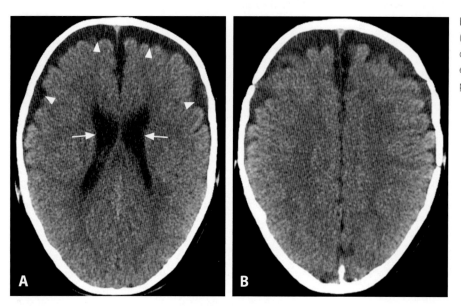

Figure 1. Non-enhanced axial CT images (A, B) of a 6-month-old child with macrocrania demonstrate bifrontal subarachnoid space enlargement (arrowheads) along with mild prominence of the lateral ventricles (arrows).

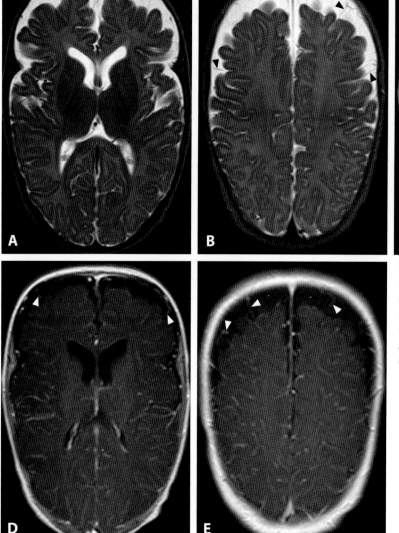

Figure 2. Axial T2WIs (A, B) demonstrate enlarged bifrontal subarachnoid spaces and mild increase in size of the lateral ventricles. Linear structures (arrowheads) likely represent transversing veins. FLAIR image (C) confirms CSF-like signal of the collections, without any signs of blood products. Post-contrast T1WIs (D, E) show enhancing transversing veins (arrowheads).

Benign External Hydrocephalus

MARIA VITTORIA SPAMPINATO

Specific Imaging Findings

Benign external hydrocephalus (BEH) is characterized by an increased amount of fluid in the subarachnoid spaces (SAS), with density and signal intensity following CSF, typically in the bilateral frontal regions and along the interhemispheric fissure. Enlarged SAS follow the contour of gyri and appear symmetric between the two hemispheres. Additional imaging features include widening of the suprasellar cistern and normal to slightly increased ventricular size. The distance between the frontal gyri and the skull and between the mesial frontal gyri and the anterior interhemispheric fissure measures more than 5 mm. MRI or Doppler ultrasound can confirm the presence of transversing leptomeningeal vessels within the extra-axial collections. MRI can rule out associated chronic subdural hematomas or hygromas.

Pertinent Clinical Information

Increased head circumference above the 95th percentile, full fontanelles, and frontal bossing are the most common clinical findings. Patients are usually referred for imaging when the head size has rapidly increased over the course of months. A family history of macrocephaly is often present. BEH is usually diagnosed between 3 and 8 months of age and is more common in male infants. Transient gross motor delay can be observed and is usually attributed to the added head weight in the macrocephalic infant. Otherwise BEH is usually not associated with developmental delay or neurological deficit. Once the diagnosis of BEH is established, clinical follow-up is required to confirm normal development and no treatment is necessary. In selected cases, follow-up imaging at 18–24 months of age can be considered and should show resolution of the abnormality.

Differential Diagnosis

Brain Atrophy
- diffuse sulcal enlargement without frontal predominance
- proportionally dilated ventricles

Subdural Hematoma (133)
- extra-axial collection with density/signal intensity of blood products
- no leptomeningeal vessels crossing the collections

Non-Accidental Trauma
- subdural hematomas of different age
- retinal hemorrhages and abnormal skeletal survey

Glutaric Aciduria Type 1 (16)
- enlarged sylvian fissures
- abnormal deep gray and/or white matter

Background

BEH is also known as benign enlargement of the SAS, extraventricular obstructive hydrocephalus, and benign extra-axial collections of infancy. The precise cause of the CSF accumulation in the SAS in infancy has not been established. Delayed functional maturity of arachnoid granulations is the most commonly cited explanation. Due to immaturity of arachnoid granulations, absorption of CSF may not keep pace with CSF production for a period of time in children under 2 years of age, resulting in CSF accumulation in the SAS, leaving the ventricles normal or only mildly prominent. Alternatively, BEH may be caused by amplification of the physiologic imbalance between skull and brain growth occurring in normal infants between 3 months and 1 year of age. Enlarged SAS represent a risk factor for the development of subdural hematomas following minimal or no trauma. This is thought to be caused by stretching of the bridging veins in the subdural space due to enlarged CSF spaces. BEH also results in increased incidence of chronic subdural effusions. Enlargement of SAS can occur in the setting of genetic conditions, such as mucopolysaccharidosis, achondroplasia, Sotos syndrome, and glutaric aciduria type I. In mucopolysaccharidosis the abnormal enlargement of the SAS persists beyond 18–24 months of age with progression to ventriculomegaly and communicating hydrocephalus. In glutaric aciduria type I, the sylvian fissure and the anterior SAS are preferentially enlarged. These genetic diseases should be considered in patients with enlargement of the SAS who do not fit the expected normal pattern of development, or in whom the finding does not resolve after 18–24 months of age.

REFERENCES

1. McNeely PD, Atkinson JD, Saigal G, *et al.* Subdural hematomas in infants with benign enlargement of the subarachnoid spaces are not pathognomonic for child abuse. *AJNR* 2006;**27**:1725–8.
2. Hellbusch LC. Benign extracerebral fluid collections in infancy: clinical presentation and long-term follow-up. *J Neurosurg* 2007;**107**(2 Suppl):119–25.
3. Paciorkowski AR, Greenstein RM. When is enlargement of the subarachnoid spaces not benign? A genetic perspective. *Pediatr Neurol* 2007;**37**:1–7.
4. Papasian NC, Frim DM. A theoretical model of benign external hydrocephalus that predicts a predisposition towards extra-axial hemorrhage after minor head trauma. *Pediatr Neurosurg* 2000;**33**:188–93.
5. Chen CY, Chou TY, Zimmerman RA, *et al.* Pericerebral fluid collection: differentiation of enlarged subarachnoid spaces from subdural collections with color Doppler US. *Radiology* 1996;**201**:389–92.

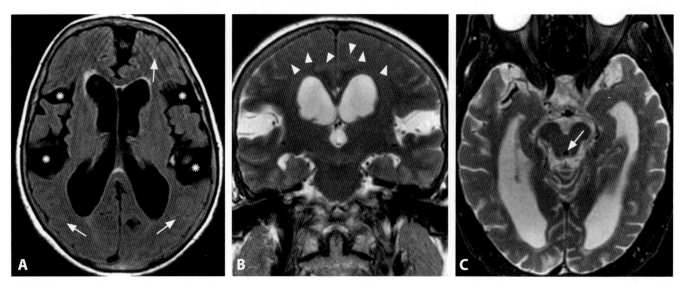

Figure 1. Axial FLAIR image (A) shows a striking disproportion between wide lateral ventricles and sylvian fissures (*) compared to effaced subarachnoid spaces along the convexities (arrows). Coronal T2WI (B) better shows this "gyral crowding" (arrowheads). Axial T2WI (C) reveals aqueductal flow void (arrow).

Figure 2. Axial FLAIR image (A) demonstrates dilated lateral ventricles and extensive confluent white matter hyperintensities (arrows), consistent with deep white matter ischemia, often associated with chronic communicating hydrocephalus. Midsagittal T2WI (C) shows prominent flow-void within the cerebral aqueduct (arrow), suggesting hyperdynamic CSF flow.

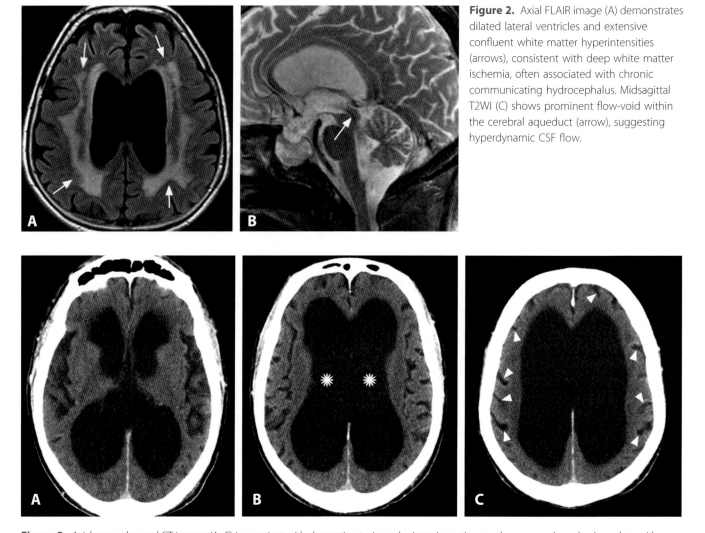

Figure 3. Axial non-enhanced CT images (A–C) in a patient with dementia, ataxia, and urinary incontinence show parenchymal volume loss with very wide supratentorial ventricles (*). The ventricles are clearly dilated more than the cortical sulci (arrowheads). Note absence of periventricular edema.

Normal Pressure Hydrocephalus

ALESSANDRO CIANFONI

Specific Imaging Findings

Dilated supratentorial ventricular system (triventricular hydrocephalus), with rounded frontal horns, enlarged temporal horns, bowing of the corpus callosum, and ballooning of the third ventricle are characteristic for normal pressure hydrocephalus (NPH), while the fourth ventricle is of normal size and cerebral aqueduct is patent. The Evans' index (ratio between the maximum widths of the frontal horns and the skull, measured along the inner table of the calvarium) is >0.3. There is disproportion between the ventricular size and the width of the sulci, especially in the mesial temporal regions and adjacent to the falx along the convexities, where the sulci may be effaced. This is known as "gyral crowding" and is best appreciated on coronal images. The sylvian fissures and the basal cisterns are, on the other hand, wide. Evidence of periventricular CSF resorption is frequently seen as periventricular areas that are hypodense on CT, of high T2 signal, and with increased ADC values. Flow-sensitive MR sequences characteristically reveal increased flow within the aqueduct. Parenchymal atrophy and leukoaraiosis can coexist or develop in the late phases. MRS may show lactate within the ventricles.

Pertinent Clinical Information

The original description of this entity included the triad of ataxia, dementia, and incontinence. It is estimated that 5–10% of cases of dementia are caused by idiopathic NPH (iNPH), and this is the only surgically treatable dementia (by CSF shunting). The diagnosis is made in the presence of gait disturbance accompanied by at least one of the other two elements of the triad in a patient over 40 years of age with gradual onset of symptoms, neuroimaging of triventricular hydrocephalus with patent sylvian aqueduct, and CSF opening pressure between 70 and 245 mm H_2O. Patients with a history of prior head trauma, intracranial hemorrhage or infection are classified as secondary NPH. Prognostic criteria for a positive response to shunting have not yet been validated; among the most reliable are the evidence of hyperdynamic flow in the aqueduct, large volume CSF tap test, and infusion tests, performed through ventricular catheters.

Differential Diagnosis

Brain Atrophy
- the width of the ventricles is proportional to the degree of sulcal widening
- parahippocampal and parafalcine sulcal enlargement
- absence of hyperdynamic flow within the aqueduct

Non-Communicating Hydrocephalus
- obstructing mass causing hydrocephalus

Aqueductal Stenosis (55)
- obstructing web or narrowing of the aqueduct

Background

Numerous theories try to explain the pathophysiology of iNPH. There is a very common association of iNPH, arterial hypertension and cerebrovascular disease, and multi-infarct dementia needs to be ruled out to diagnose iNPH. Individuals with "benign extra-axial collections of infancy" may be predisposed for iNPH, possibly indicating defective CSF resorption mechanisms. It has been proposed that in these subjects a part of the CSF drainage is through a periventricular interstitial pathway, which decompensates if deep white matter ischemia occurs later in life. Defective intracranial venous compliance has also been postulated as a causative mechanism, possibly leading to impaired CSF pulsation and resorption. Cognitive impairment in iNPH might be mediated by periventricular interstitial edema, leading to hypoperfusion and hypometabolism in the frontal pathways. PET and perfusion MR studies have shown global hypometabolism and regionally decreased cerebral blood flow. Gait disturbances might be explained by alterations in the basal ganglia and/or compression of the brainstem structures. Urinary symptoms of iNPH are caused by detrusor overactivity.

REFERENCES

1. Shprecher D, Schwalb J, Kurlan R. Normal pressure hydrocephalus: diagnosis and treatment. *Curr Neurol Neurosci Rep* 2008;**8**:371–6.
2. Sasaki M, Honda S, Yuasa T, et al. Narrow CSF space at high convexity and high midline areas in idiopathic normal pressure hydrocephalus detected by axial and coronal MRI. *Neuroradiology* 2008;**50**:117–22.
3. Scollato A, Tanenbaum R, Bahl G, et al. Changes in aqueductal CSF stroke volume and progression of symptoms in patients with unshunted idiopathic normal pressure hydrocephalus. *AJNR* 2008;**29**:192–7.
4. Bateman GA. The pathophysiology of idiopathic normal pressure hydrocephalus: cerebral ischemia or altered venous hemodynamics? *AJNR* 2008;**29**:198–203.
5. Bradley WG, Bahl G, Alksne JF, et al. Idiopathic normal pressure hydrocephalus may be a "two hit" disease: benign external hydrocephalus in infancy followed by deep white matter ischemia in late adulthood. *J Magn Reson Imaging* 2006;**24**:747–55.

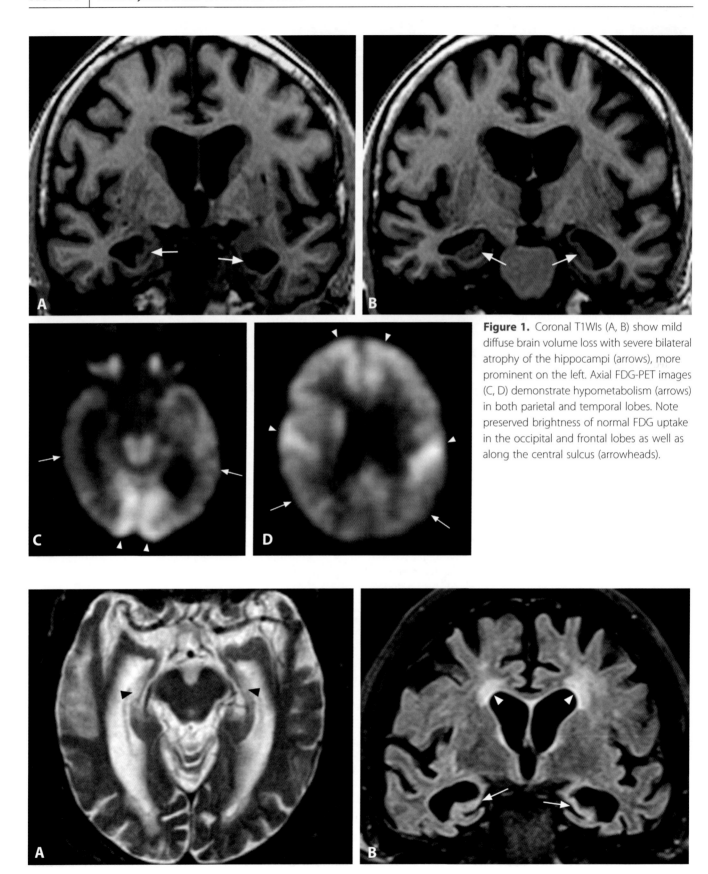

Figure 1. Coronal T1WIs (A, B) show mild diffuse brain volume loss with severe bilateral atrophy of the hippocampi (arrows), more prominent on the left. Axial FDG-PET images (C, D) demonstrate hypometabolism (arrows) in both parietal and temporal lobes. Note preserved brightness of normal FDG uptake in the occipital and frontal lobes as well as along the central sulcus (arrowheads).

Figure 2. Axial T2WI (A) in another patient shows diminutive hippocami (arrowheads) with otherwise relatively mild brain volume loss. Coronal FLAIR image (B) more clearly demonstrates prominent bilateral hippocampal atrophy (arrows). There is mild cerebral periventricular hyperintensity (arrowheads), which may be suggestive of microangiopathy.

Alzheimer Disease

MARIA VITTORIA SPAMPINATO

Specific Imaging Findings

The role of imaging in the evaluation of Alzheimer disease (AD) is to exclude other forms of dementia and identify early cases of AD which could benefit from treatment. Morphometric and metabolic measurements of the mesial temporal regions are the best imaging biomarkers for early diagnosis. In the appropriate clinical setting the diagnostic accuracy of MRI in the diagnosis of AD is approximately 87%. Typical MR findings consist of temporal and parietal cortical volume loss with prominent hippocampal atrophy. Angled coronal images perpendicular to the long axis of the hippocampus best show atrophy of the hippocampi and parahippocampal gyri with enlargement of the parahippocampal fissures.

Fluorodeoxyglucose (FDG) Positron Emission Tomography (PET) findings in the AD brain include decreased glucose uptake in the temporal and parietal lobes with sparing of the occipital and frontal lobes, while the posterior cingulate is typically affected first. FDG PET helps differentiate AD from other forms of dementia, such as vascular dementia and frontotemporal dementia, although advanced Parkinson's disease may present with a regional metabolic pattern not distinguishable from AD.

Pertinent Clinical Information

The diagnosis of AD is based on the criteria of the National Institute of Neurological and Communicative Disorders and Stroke – AD and Related Disorders Association. These standards require: insidious onset; gradual progression of memory impairment; deficits of recent memory in the early stages; impairment of orientation, judgment, problem-solving, community and home living, and personal care present later on. Clinical criteria have greater than 90% sensitivity for the diagnosis of dementia of any type, with specificity of less than 70% for the actual diagnosis of AD. Cognitive functions are measured by means of a battery of clinical and psychometric tests, including the mini mental status examination (MMSE) and clinical dementia rating (CDR). Other neurodegenerative processes leading to dementia also show a similar decline in cognitive functions and can mimic AD on the basis of clinical criteria alone. For this reason, increased emphasis has been placed on the role of neuroimaging techniques.

Differential Diagnosis

Frontotemporal Dementia (90)
- frontal and anterior temporal hypometabolism and brain volume loss

Corticobasal Degeneration
- basal ganglia and frontoparietal hypometabolism

Vascular Dementia
- chronic ischemic changes with multiple chronic infarcts
- absence of selective hippocampal atrophy

Creutzfeld–Jacob Disease (12)
- almost pathognomonic deep gray matter and cortical DWI hyperintensity
- absence of selective hippocampal atrophy

Parkinson Disease
- absence of selective hippocampal atrophy
- may be indistinguishable on PET

Background

AD is the most common type of dementia currently affecting more than four million people in the United States alone. The pathological hallmark of AD is the progressive deposition of neuritic plaques and neurofibrillary tangles in the brain which is believed to occur decades before the development of clinical symptoms. Neuropathological changes typical of AD, in particular neurofibrillary tangles, follow a predictable distribution at different stages of the disease. Initially, neurofibrillary tangles occur predominantly in the perirhinal region of the temporal lobe (Braak stages I–II, clinically silent), later on in the limbic system (Braak stages III–IV, incipient AD), and in the advanced stages of the disease they affect the neocortex (Braak stages V–VI, fully developed AD). Identification of individuals at risk before the clinical appearance of dementia has become a priority due to the potential benefits of early therapeutic intervention. Overlap with vascular dementia has been increasingly recognized.

REFERENCES

1. Karow DS, McEvoy LK, Fennema-Notestine C, *et al.* Alzheimer's Disease Neuroimaging Initiative. Relative capability of MR imaging and FDG PET to depict changes associated with prodromal and early Alzheimer disease. *Radiology* 2010;**256**:932–42.

2. Ramani A, Jensen JH, Helpern J. Quantitative MR imaging in Alzheimer disease. *Radiology* 2006;**241**:26–44.

3. Spampinato MV, Rumboldt Z, Hosker RJ, *et al.* Apolipoprotein E and gray matter volume loss in patients with mild cognitive impairment and Alzheimer disease. *Radiology* 2011;**258**:843–52.

4. Braak H, Braak E. Evolution of neuronal changes in the course of Alzheimer's disease. *J Neural Transm Suppl* 1998;**53**:127–40.

5. McKhann G, Drachman D, Folstein M, *et al.* Clinical diagnosis of Alzheimer's disease: report of the NINCDS-ADRDA Work Group* under the auspices of Department of Health and Human Services Task Force on Alzheimer's Disease. *Neurology* 1984;**34**:939–44.

Brain Imaging with MRI and CT, ed. Zoran Rumboldt *et al.* Published by Cambridge University Press. © Cambridge University Press 2012.

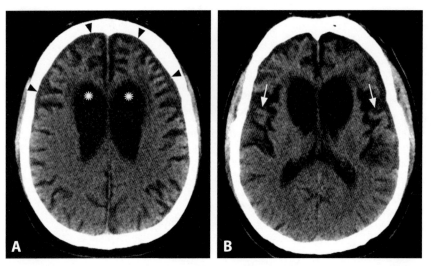

Figure 1. Axial non-enhanced CT image (A) in a 64-year-old patient with dementia shows prominent atrophy of the bilateral frontal lobes (arrowheads). The cortical sulci are very wide and there is also ex-vacuo dilation of the lateral ventricles (*). CT image at a lower level (B) reveals atrophy of the temporal lobes (arrows), in addition to the frontal parenchymal volume loss.

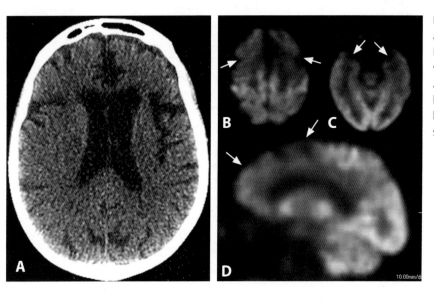

Figure 2. Axial non-enhanced CT image (A) in another patient with personality changes and impulsive behavior demonstrates mild brain volume loss without clear regional predominance. Axial (A, B) and sagittal (C) FDG-PET images reveal hypometabolism in both frontal and temporal lobes (arrows), which are not as bright as the other supra- and infratentorial parts of the brain.

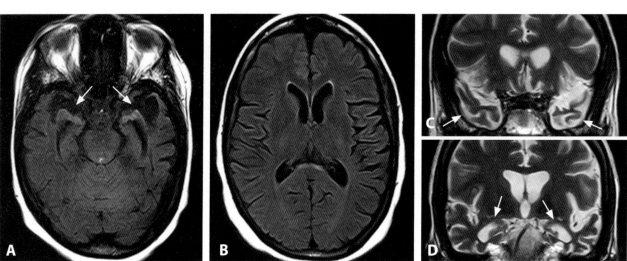

Figure 3. Axial FLAIR image (A) in a patient with progressive dysphasia shows prominent atrophy of the anterior temporal lobes (arrows). FLAIR image at a higher level (B) reveals absence of frontal lobe atrophy. Coronal T2WIs (C, D) show striking temporal lobe atrophy (arrows), left greater than right.

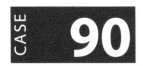

Frontotemporal Lobar Degeneration

MARIA VITTORIA SPAMPINATO

Specific Imaging Findings

The role of imaging in the evaluation of frontotemporal lobar degeneration (FTLD) is to exclude other forms of dementia such as Alzheimer disease and vascular dementia. FTLD typically shows selective atrophy of the anterior temporal and frontal lobes with relatively preserved occipital and parietal lobes. The involvement is often asymmetric, with the dominant hemisphere more severely affected. Diffuse brain atrophy may also be observed. FDG-PET in FTLD demonstrates decreased glucose uptake in the frontal and temporal cortices.

Pertinent Clinical Information

FTLD is the second most common type of dementia in individuals under 65 years of age with a prevalence of 15 per 100 000 in the 45–64 year age range. It is a primary neurodegenerative disease characterized by the development of progressive behavioral change, executive dysfunction and language deficits with relatively preserved memory in the early stages. FTLD comprises three clinical subtypes: (1) frontotemporal dementia (FTD, also known as Pick's disease) or the frontal variant, the most common form, characterized by early personality changes such as apathy and indifference, impulsive behaviors and disinhibition, and poor judgment; (2) semantic dementia (SD) characterized by early loss of word meaning but fluent speech; (3) progressive nonfluent aphasia (PNFA) characterized by loss of speech fluency with anomia (primary progressive aphasia). The differential diagnosis between AD and FTLD can be difficult in the early stages and the clinical overlap between these conditions highlights the importance of neuroimaging, along with neuropsychological testing.

Differential Diagnosis

Huntington Disease (91)
- atrophy of bilateral caudate nucleus and putamen, without significant cortical atrophy
- possible T2 hyperintensity of bilateral caudate and putamen

Alzheimer Disease (89)
- prominent hippocampal atrophy on MRI
- frontal and parietal hypometabolism (decreased FDG uptake on PET)
- absence of anterior frontal and temporal hypometabolism

Corticobasal Degeneration
- basal ganglia and frontoparietal hypometabolism

Vascular Dementia
- chronic ischemic changes with multiple chronic infarcts
- absence of prominent frontal and anterior temporal atrophy

Creutzfeld–Jacob Disease (12)
- almost pathognomonic deep gray matter and cortical DWI hyperintensity
- absence of prominent frontal and anterior temporal atrophy

Background

Typical pathologic features of FTLD include circumscribed lobar atrophy with abrupt transition between affected and unaffected brain and relative preservation of the hippocampus, when compared with AD. These syndromes encompass a large variety of neuropathologic appearances, including spongiform degeneration and gliosis, the classic tau-positive and ubiquitin-positive cytoplasmatic inclusions known as Pick's bodies, and ubiquitin-positive and tau-negative inclusions, the latter being found in most patients. In familial cases with mutation of the tau gene (chromosome 17), tau heavily accumulates in neurons and glial cells. Patients with FTLD show selective atrophy in anterior cingulate, frontal insula, subcallosal gyrus, and striatum suggesting degeneration of a paralimbic fronto-insular–striatal network. The subdivision into the three subtypes is primarily based on the characteristic clinical symptoms while MRI findings appear to be concordant: a predominant temporal atrophy discriminates SD from the other two subtypes. A more prominent right-sided frontal atrophy is suggestive of FTD whereas left-sided atrophy is more characteristic of PNFA. Management includes a trial of symptomatic medications and a multifaceted approach, including environmental modification and long-term care planning. Pathologically and clinically FTLD overlaps with progressive supranuclear palsy, corticobasal degeneration and amyotrophic lateral sclerosis. Average survival after the diagnosis is around 10 years.

REFERENCES

1. Rabinovici GD, Seeley WW, Kim EJ, et al. Distinct MRI atrophy patterns in autopsy-proven Alzheimer's disease and frontotemporal lobar degeneration. Am J Alzheimers Dis Other Demen 2007–2008;22:474–88.
2. Ibach B, Poljansky S, Marienhagen J, et al. Contrasting metabolic impairment in frontotemporal degeneration and early onset Alzheimer's disease. Neuroimage 2004;23:739–43.
3. Lindberg O, Ostberg P, Zandbelt BB, et al. Cortical morphometric subclassification of frontotemporal lobar degeneration. AJNR 2009;30:1233–9.
4. Cairns NJ, Bigio EH, Mackenzie IR, et al. Neuropathologic diagnostic and nosologic criteria for frontotemporal lobar degeneration: consensus of the Consortium for Frontotemporal Lobar Degeneration. Acta Neuropathol 2007;114:5–22.
5. Arvanitakis Z. Update on frontotemporal dementia. Neurologist 2010;16:16–22.

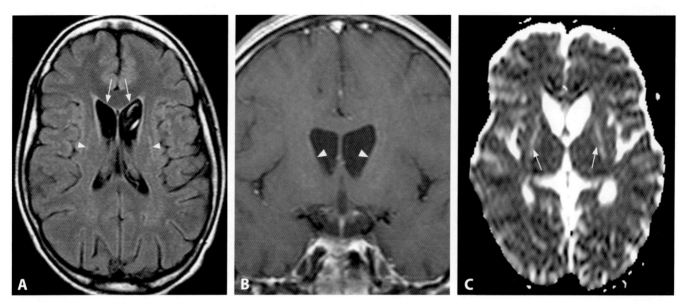

Figure 1. Axial FLAIR image (A) shows enlarged frontal horns (arrows) of the lateral ventricles with straight lateral contours and without perceptible adjacent caudate nucleus head. There are also very small putamina (arrowheads). Post-contrast coronal T1WI (B) reveals enlarged frontal horns with straight lateral contours (arrowheads) to a better advantage. There is no signal abnormality and no pathologic enhancement. Axial ADC map at a slightly lower level than the FLAIR image reveals increased diffusion in both putamina (arrows).

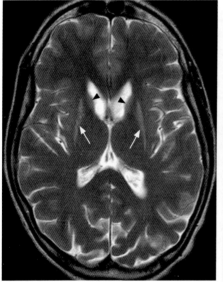

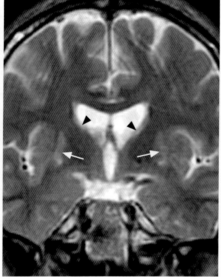

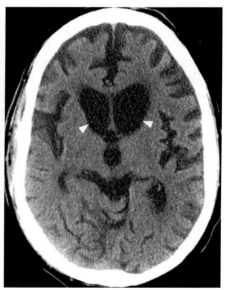

Figure 2. Axial T2WI in a 17-year-old patient shows a diminutive size of the bilateral caudate head (arrowheads) and putamen (arrows). There is associated hyperintensity, which is more prominent in the putamina.

Figure 3. Coronal T2WI in a teenager demonstrates dilated frontal horns with straightened and mildly convex contour (arrowheads) adjacent to the atrophic caudate heads. Also seen is bilaterally small and mildly hyperintense putamen (arrows).

Figure 4. CT shows advanced disease with prominent volume loss of the caudate heads and enlarged "boxed-out" appearance of the frontal horns (arrowheads). There is diffuse atrophy, but much more prominent in the deep gray matter.

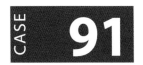

Huntington Disease

ZORAN RUMBOLDT AND BENJAMIN HUANG

Specific Imaging Findings

The characteristic imaging finding of Huntington disease (HD) is bilateral striatal (caudate nucleus and putamen) atrophy, particularly involving the heads of the caudate nuclei. This leads to symmetric enlargement of the adjacent frontal horns with flattening of their lateral contour. Signal abnormalities are not typically seen in adults. In the juvenile form of the disease, T2 hyperintensity may be observed in the caudate nucleus and putamen. Diffuse cerebral atrophy with white matter volume loss, generally more pronounced in the frontal lobes, is evident late in the course of the disease. Decreases in tissue volume are accompanied by increasing ADC values within the caudate nucleus, putamen, and periventricular white matter.

Pertinent Clinical Information

HD (also known as Huntington's chorea) is a neurodegenerative disorder characterized by the triad of fully penetrant dominant inheritance, progressive movement disorder, and dementia. Onset of symptoms is typically in the mid-30s to mid-40s, but it may occur as early as the first (juvenile form) and as late as the tenth decade of life. Chorea with brief, abrupt involuntary movements is prototypical for HD, with a much broader spectrum of possible motor signs. As the disease progresses, chorea is superseded by dystonia or akineto-rigid parkinsonian features. The disease is relentlessly progressive, resulting in death within 10–20 years after symptom onset, or less with the juvenile form. The diagnosis is made on the basis of characteristic motor signs and a positive family history, confirmed by genetic testing.

Differential Diagnosis

Normal Pressure Hydrocephalus (88)
- diffuse enlargement of supratentorial ventricles in older patients (usually > 60 years)
- lactate detected in lateral ventricles on MRS

Frontotemporal Dementia (Pick's Disease) (90)
- frontal and temporal lobe atrophy in older patients (mid-50s to mid-60s)

Alzheimer Dementia (89)
- characteristic PET findings in older patients
- parietal lobe, temporal lobe, and hippocampal atrophy with enlarged temporal horns

Background

The genetic abnormality causing Huntington disease is a trinucleotide (CAG) repeat expansion in the gene which encodes huntingtin protein with more than 38 repeats being fully penetrant and diagnostic. The normal huntingtin protein is widely expressed in the human brain, but its exact function is unknown, and the mechanism of HD is unclear. Neuronal loss in HD affects the striatum and layers III, IV, and V of the cortex. Histologically, the disease is characterized by the presence of intranuclear inclusion bodies made up of aggregates of the mutant huntingtin protein and other proteins. Decrease in volume as measured on volumetric MRI studies and increase in ADC of the caudate nuclei appear to correlate with disease severity. The magnetization transfer (MT) ratio is significantly decreased in presymptomatic HD carriers, reflecting gray matter degeneration. A longitudinal MRI study has shown that extrapolating backwards in time smaller caudate volumes were already evident 14 years before the onset of motor symptoms in HD carriers. To date, there is no effective treatment, and management revolves primarily upon relief of symptoms.

REFERENCES

1. Ho VB, Chuang HS, Rovira MJ, Koo B. Juvenile Huntington disease: CT and MR features. *AJNR* 1995;**16**:1405–12.

2. Simmons JT, Pastakia B, Chase TN, Shults CW. Magnetic resonance imaging in Huntington disease. *AJNR* 1986;**7**:25–8.

3. Cardoso F. Huntington disease and other choreas. *Neurol Clin* 2009;**27**:719–36.

4. Hobbs NZ, Barnes J, Frost C, *et al*. Onset and progression of pathologic atrophy in Huntington disease: a longitudinal MR imaging study. *AJNR* 2010;**31**:1036–41.

5. Ginestroni A, Battaglini M, Diciotti S, *et al*. Magnetization transfer MR imaging demonstrates degeneration of the subcortical and cortical gray matter in Huntington disease. *AJNR* 2010;**31**:1807–12.

Brain Imaging with MRI and CT, ed. Zoran Rumboldt *et al.* Published by Cambridge University Press. © Cambridge University Press 2012.

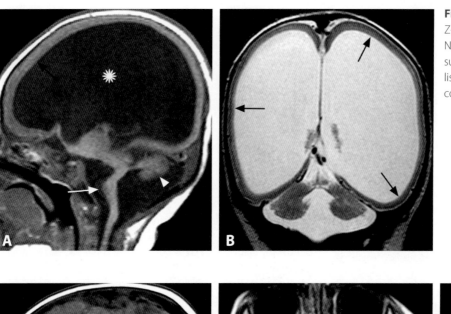

Figure 1. Sagittal T1WI (A) shows a typical Z-shaped hypoplastic brainstem (white arrow). Notice also cerebellar hypoplasia (arrowhead), supratentorial hydrocephalus (*), and diffuse lissencephaly (black arrows), as confirmed on coronal T2WI (B). Courtesy of Anna Nastro.

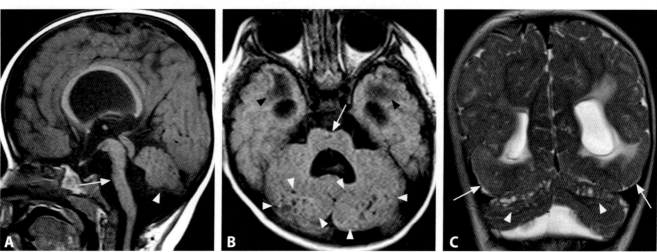

Figure 2. Sagittal T1WI (A) shows hypoplastic brainstem (arrow) with absent pontine protuberance and hypoplastic inferior vermis (arrowhead). Axial FLAIR image (B) shows multiple subcortical microcysts (white arrowheads) in both cerebellar hemispheres; the pons is hypoplastic with a midline cleft (arrow). White matter of the temporal poles is abnormally hypointense (black arrowheads) and the temporal horns are enlarged. Coronal T2WI (C) confirms subcortical bilateral cerebellar microcysts (arrowheads); the cerebellum is also hypoplastic. Note pachygyric appearance of bilateral basal temporo-occipital cortex (arrows) and extensive white matter signal abnormality.

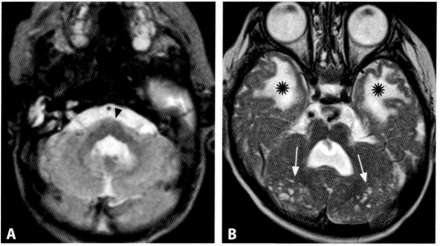

Figure 3. Progression of findings in a patient with muscle–eye–brain disease. Axial T2WI at neonatal age (A) shows hypoplastic pons (arrowhead) and essentially normal cerebellum. T2WI at 16 months of age (B) shows that multiple subcortical cerebellar microcysts (arrows) have formed. Also note hyperintense white matter (*) of the temporal poles.

Specific Imaging Findings

Hindbrain abnormalities in congenital muscular dystrophies (CMD) comprise a variable association of brainstem and cerebellar hypoplasia and dysplasia. In Walker–Warburg syndrome (WWS), the brainstem shows a typical posterior kink, resulting in a broad inverted S-shape on sagittal MR images; the cerebellum is profoundly hypoplastic, sometimes with a configuration that resembles a Dandy–Walker malformation, and the cerebellar cortex is dysplastic. In both Fukuyama CMD (FCMD) and muscle–eye–brain disease (MEB), the brainstem is hypoplastic, with a marked reduction in size of the pontine protuberance and presence of pontine clefts in MEB; the cerebellum is also hypoplastic, usually with a greater degree of involvement of the vermis than the hemispheres. Furthermore, CSF-isointense microcysts are found in both cerebellar hemispheres in a subcortical location. Supratentorially, the appearance of the cortex ranges from complete lissencephaly in WWS to a variable pachygyric or polymicrogyric irregularly bumpy and knobbed "cobblestone" appearance in FCMD and MEB, which is variably associated with white matter dysmyelination and ventricular enlargement. However, the supratentorial compartment may be completely normal.

Pertinent Clinical Information

Affected patients present with hypotonia, weakness, variably severe congenital joint contractures, and dystrophic changes on muscle biopsy. Serum creatine kinase is moderately elevated. Neurological involvement mainly comprises variably severe psychomotor delay and convulsions. Ocular findings include microphthalmia, cataracts, congenital glaucoma, persistent hyperplastic primitive vitreous, retinal detachment, and optic nerve atrophy.

Differential Diagnosis

Dandy–Walker Malformation (93)

- counter-clockwise rotation of hypoplastic vermis
- posterior fossa is variably expanded
- cerebellar hemispheres comparatively less hypoplastic than vermis
- normal brainstem

Pontocerebellar Hypoplasia

- hypoplastic cerebellar hemispheres abut the tentorium with a butterfly appearance on coronal images
- pontine protuberance is variably reduced, without longitudinal clefts
- subcortical cavitations may be present in the most severe cases

Cerebellar Atrophy

- cerebellar bulk loss results in a skeleton appearance
- progressive volume loss

- cerebellar cortex may be T2 hyperintense due to gliosis
- intact brainstem

Background

CMDs are a heterogeneous group of disorders characterized by hypotonia of prenatal onset and frequent congenital contractures associated with histological findings of muscular dystrophy. A common group of CMDs is associated with aberrant glycosylation of α-dystroglycan (αDG); these are therefore called dystroglycanopathies. They are classified into Walker–Warburg syndrome (WWS), Fukuyama congenital muscular dystrophy (FCMD), muscle–eye–brain disease (MEB), isolated, and limb-girdle CMD. Mutations in six different genes: protein-O-mannosyl transferase 1 (POMT1), protein-O-mannosyl transferase 2 (POMT2), protein-O-mannose 1,2-N-acetylglucosaminyltransferase 1 (POMGnT1), fukutin, fukutin-related protein, and LARGE, have been detected in patients affected with dystroglycanopathies. These gene products are involved in the glycosylation of αDG, a cellular receptor expressed in neurons and oligodendrocytes that is implicated in normal basement membrane formation and neuronal migration. The term "cobblestone lissencephaly" is used to describe the cortical malformation typical of dystroglycanopathies, where the irregularly bumpy and knobbed cortical surface results from the overmigration of neurons beyond cortical layer 1 and into the leptomeninges through gaps in the glial limiting membrane. This cortex has a disorganized unlayered appearance on histology. Posterior fossa abnormalities are a hallmark of dystroglycanopathies, and comprise a variable association of brainstem deformation, hypoplasia, and cerebellar hypodysplasia. Cerebellar subcortical microcysts represent subarachnoid spaces engulfed by the fusion of disorganized folia at the boundary between normal and polymicrogyric cortices. These cysts may progressively increase in size.

REFERENCES

1. Aida N, Tamagawa K, Takada K, et al. Brain MR in Fukuyama congenital muscular dystrophy. AJNR 1996;**17**:605–13.
2. Barkovich AJ, Millen KJ, Dobyns WB. A developmental classification of malformations of the brainstem. Ann Neurol 2007;**62**:625–39.
3. Clement E, Mercuri E, Godfrey C, et al. Brain involvement in muscular dystrophies with defective dystroglycan glycosylation. Ann Neurol 2008;**64**:573–82.
4. van der Knaap MS, Smit LM, Barth PG, et al. Magnetic resonance imaging in classification of congenital muscular dystrophies with brain abnormalities. Ann Neurol 1997;**42**:50–9.

Brain Imaging with MRI and CT, ed. Zoran Rumboldt *et al.* Published by Cambridge University Press. © Cambridge University Press 2012.

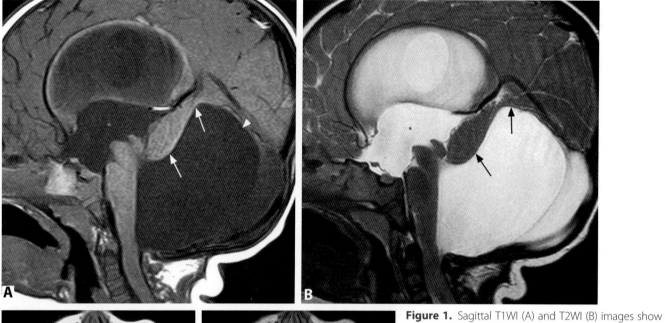

Figure 1. Sagittal T1WI (A) and T2WI (B) images show hypoplastic vermis with verticalization and elevated tentorial insertion (arrows). The fourth ventricle is markedly enlarged and extends posteriorly, forming a retrocerebellar cyst (arrowhead). Axial T1WI (C) and T2WI (D) images show hypoplastic cerebellar hemispheres (arrows) that are winged outwards against the petrous ridges with a markedly enlarged fourth ventricle. The cerebellar falx (arrowhead) is normal. There is associated hydrocephalus (*).

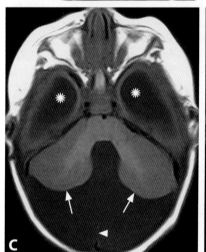 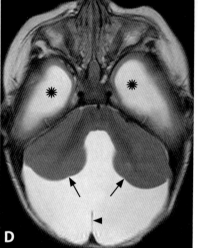

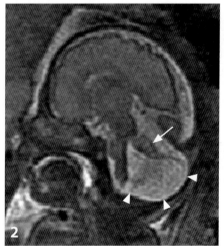 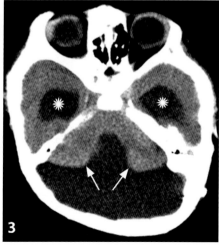

Figure 2. Fetal MRI at 32 weeks gestational age. Sagittal T2WI (A) shows enlarged posterior fossa with hypoplastic, elevated vermis (arrow) and enlarged fourth ventricle (arrowheads).

Figure 3. CT image in another patient shows a markedly enlarged fourth ventricle with hypoplastic cerebellar hemispheres (arrows) and hydrocephalus (*), resembling Figure 1 C and D.

Specific Imaging Findings

The hallmark of Dandy–Walker malformation (DWM) is vermian hypoplasia with verticalization (counter-clockwise rotation) of the vermis; as a consequence, the vermis lies behind the quadrigeminal plate. The foliation of the vermis is rudimentary and sometimes dysplastic. The cerebellar hemispheres are displaced bilaterally but are not significantly hypoplastic. The brainstem is generally not affected. The fourth ventricle is markedly enlarged and bulges posteriorly, forming a large pseudocyst; in some cases, it extends upward through a congenital dehiscence of the tentorium, thereby occupying a space between the occipital lobes. Inferiorly, the cyst may bulge into the foramen magnum, whereas laterally, the extension of the fourth ventricle is limited by the reflection of the pia mater over the posterior surface of the cerebellar hemispheres. The entire posterior fossa is enlarged. Supratentorial hydrocephalus is frequently associated but does not technically form a constituting element of the malformation.

Pertinent Clinical Information

Patients with DWM often present with macrocephaly in the neonatal period. Infants may elicit medical attention because of hydrocephalus, developmental delay, or ataxia. Apnea and seizures are seen frequently, whereas developmental delay and mental retardation are highly variable. Mortality is significant in patients with severe obstructive hydrocephalus or multiple associated congenital anomalies. Incidental DWM in asymptomatic adults has been reported.

Differential Diagnosis

Vermis Hypoplasia
- normal position of the cerebellar vermis relative to the brainstem or minimal upward rotation
- no elevation of the tentorium cerebelli, posterior fossa not enlarged

Mega Cisterna Magna
- infracerebellar CSF collection that communicates with subarachnoid spaces
- normal cerebellar vermis, normal posterior fossa size
- no hydrocephalus
- incidental finding

Persistent Blake's Pouch (Blake's Pouch Cyst)
- infra-retrocerebellar cyst that communicates with the fourth ventricle but not with the subarachnoid spaces
- tetraventricular hydrocephalus with related clinical symptoms
- normal vermis

Arachnoid Cyst (142)
- excluded from CSF circulation, may behave as a mass
- compression of normally developed cerebellum, fourth ventricle

Joubert Syndrome (57)
- molar tooth sign (thickened elongated superior cerebellar peduncles)
- posterior fossa is not enlarged

Background

The initial description by Dandy and Blackfan was in 1914, although the term DWM was only introduced 40 years later. The characteristic triad of DWM consists of complete or partial agenesis of the vermis with upward ("counter-clockwise") rotation, dilatation of the fourth ventricle which extends posteriorly as a retrocerebellar cyst, and enlarged posterior fossa with upward displacement of transverse sinuses, tentorium, and torcular. Hydrocephalus is a common complication but not a true component of the malformation. The question as to how large a posterior fossa should be to meet the DWM definition is still debated, and the terminology "Dandy–Walker variant", once widely used to describe cases with partial agenesis or hypoplasia and vermis rotation with no substantial enlargement of the posterior fossa, has been subsequently discarded because of its variable definitions, lack of specificity, and confusion with classic DWM. DWM is believed to occur from a failure of development of the rhombencephalic roof during the second embryonal month, with persistence of its superior portion (called the anterior membranous area) between the caudal edge of the developing vermis and the cranial edge of the developing choroid plexus. This results in a midline defect with partial agenesis or hypoplasia of the vermis, which is then displaced superiorly by the outpouching of the underlying fourth ventricle. Recent genetic evidence suggests that DWM, along with a range of posterior fossa anomalies including vermis hypoplasia and mega cisterna magna, may be caused by mesenchymal–neuroepithelial signalling defects, including *FOXC1* (a gene expressed only in the posterior fossa mesenchyme overlying the cerebellum) and *ZIC1*–*ZIC4*, which are expressed in the dorsal developing CNS, including cerebellum and spinal cord.

REFERENCES

1. Barkovich AJ, Millen KJ, Dobyns WB. A developmental and genetic classification for midbrain–hindbrain malformations. *Brain* 2009;**132**:3199–230.
2. Parisi MA, Dobyns WB. Human malformations of the midbrain and hindbrain: review and proposed classification scheme. *Mol Genet Metab* 2003;**80**:36–53.
3. Garel C, Fallet-Bianco C, Guibaud L. The fetal cerebellum: development and common malformations. *J Child Neurol* 2011;**26**:1483–92.
4. Maria BL, Bozorgmanesh A, Kimmel KN, *et al.* Quantitative assessment of brainstem development in Joubert syndrome and Dandy–Walker syndrome. *J Child Neurol* 2001;**16**:751–8.

Brain Imaging with MRI and CT, ed. Zoran Rumboldt *et al.* Published by Cambridge University Press. © Cambridge University Press 2012.

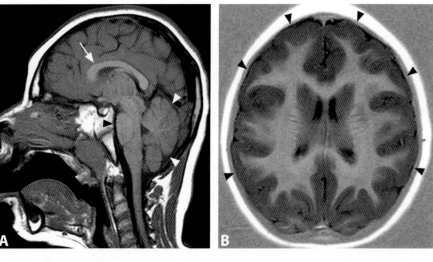

Figure 1. Midsagittal T1WI shows reduced craniofacial proportions and slightly small corpus callosum (arrow), but relatively normal hindbrain (arrowheads). Axial IR T1WI (B) shows simplified gyral pattern (arrowheads) with normal cortical thickness.

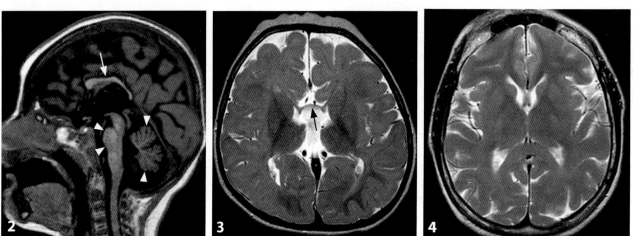

Figure 2. Sagittal T1WI in another patient reveals marked reduction of brain volume associated with small dysmorphic corpus callosum (arrow) and pontocerebellar hypoplasia (arrowheads).

Figure 3. Axial T2WI reveals mildly simplified gyral pattern associated with extreme partial corpus callosum agenesis (arrow).

Figure 4. T2WI shows diffuse abnormal high signal of the white matter consistent with reduced myelination.

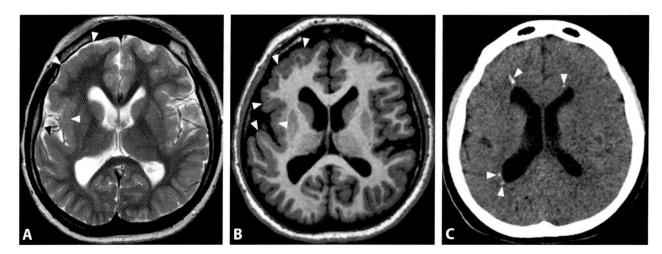

Figure 5. A patient with congenital TORCH infection. Axial T2WI (A) and T1WI (B) reveal right frontal, insular and anterior temporal polymicrogyria (arrowheads). CT image (C) at a slightly more cephalad level demonstrates multiple periventricular calcifications (arrowheads).

Microcephaly

MARIASAVINA SEVERINO

Specific Imaging Findings

Microcephaly is characterized by a reduced (at least <30%) cranio-facial ratio compared with age-matched normocephalic children. Primary congenital microcephaly refers to a small head size with relatively preserved brain architecture. Microcephaly with simplified gyral pattern shows a reduced number of gyri and shallow sulci (one-quarter to one-half of normal depth) without thickening of the cerebral cortex (cortical thickness <4 mm). There is a correlation between the degree of microcephaly, the volume of white matter and the presence of simplified gyral pattern. Reduced white matter bulk and enlarged extra-axial spaces are frequent accompanying features. Other developmental brain anomalies are often associated, including callosal agenesis, dysgenesis or hypoplasia, periventricular nodular heterotopias, pontocerebellar hypoplasia, and abnormal myelination. Cortical malformation such as lissencephaly and polymicrogyria may also be present. Secondary microcephaly may present white matter T2 hyperintensities (consistent with gliosis, cavitations, demyelination), cortical malformations, and calcifications.

Pertinent Clinical Information

Microcephaly is a clinical observation defined as a head circumference over 2 standard deviations below the mean for age and gender; severe microcephaly is characterized by a head circumference over 3 standard deviations below the mean. Microcephaly may be present at birth, or it may become evident in the first few years of life when the head fails to grow while the face continues to develop at a normal rate, producing a child with a small head, a relatively large face, and slanted forehead. Patients may present with mental retardation (50%), epilepsy (40%), cerebral palsy (20%), and ophthalmologic disorders (20–50%). Children with severe microcephaly are more likely to have imaging abnormalities and more severe developmental impairments than those with milder microcephaly. Finally, microcephalic patients may present extracerebral malformations suggestive of a chromosomal abnormality or syndromes.

Differential Diagnosis

Lissencephaly (19)
- the affected cortex is agyric
- cortical thickness usually at least 1 cm
- brain circumference may be normal or reduced

Pachygyria
- few sulci are present and the gyri are broad
- cortical thickness usually 6–9 mm

Background

Microcephaly is due to inadequate brain growth resulting in a small head size. Many different genetic causes or noxious agents affecting the brain during prenatal, perinatal or early postnatal period can lead to microcephaly. It can be divided into two major categories: primary (genetic) and secondary (acquired). Acquired microcephalies are usually the result of ischemia, congenital infections (such as TORCH), trauma, and metabolic or toxic insults (such as fetal alcohol syndrome). Genetic etiologies have been reported in 15–53% of microcephalic children with a remarkable genetic heterogeneity. Seven loci associated with autosomal recessive microcephaly have been described (*MCPH1*, *WDR62*, *CDK5RAP2*, *CEP152*, *ASPM*, *CENPJ* and *STIL*). Moreover, microcephaly is present in many genetic syndromes, such as Down (21 trisomy), Edward (18 trisomy), Cri-du-chat (5p-), and Cornelia de Lange syndromes. No clear genotype–phenotype correlation has yet emerged. Many of the mutated proteins localize to the centrosome, which is a final integration point for many regulatory pathways affecting prenatal neurogenesis. Microcephaly is a disorder of cell proliferation, implying that either the number of cycles of cell proliferation is reduced or the programmed cell death is increased. The gyral simplification seems to reflect reduced tension on the cortex due to a decreased number of axons and is considered at least partly a consequence of microcephaly and not a separate, unrelated feature. There is no specific treatment for microcephaly.

REFERENCES

1. Adachi Y, Poduri A, Kawaguch A, *et al*. Congenital microcephaly with a simplified gyral pattern: associated findings and their significance. *AJNR* 2011;**32**:1123–9.

2. Vermeulen RJ, Wilke M, Horber V, Krägeloh-Mann I. Microcephaly with simplified gyral pattern: MRI classification. *Neurology* 2010; **74**;386–91.

3. Ashwal S, Michelson D, Plawner L, *et al*. Practice parameter: evaluation of the child with microcephaly (an evidence-based review): report of the Quality Standards Subcommittee of the American Academy of Neurology and the Practice Committee of the Child Neurology Society. *Neurology* 2009;**73**:887–97.

4. Basel-Vanagaite L, Dobyns WB. Clinical and brain imaging heterogeneity of severe microcephaly. *Pediatr Neurol* 2010; **43**:7–16.

5. Mochida GH. Genetics and biology of microcephaly and lissencephaly. *Semin Pediatr Neurol* 2009;**16**:120–6.

Brain Imaging with MRI and CT, ed. Zoran Rumboldt *et al*. Published by Cambridge University Press. © Cambridge University Press 2012.

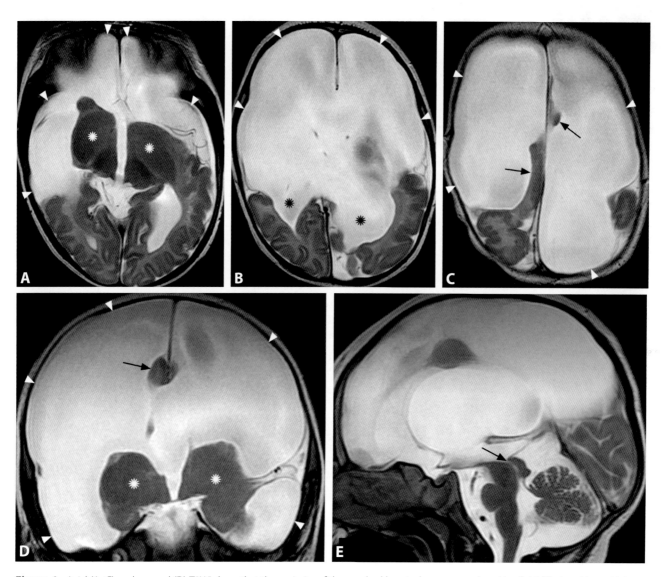

Figure 1. Axial (A–C) and coronal (D) T2WI show that the majority of the cerebral hemispheres are replaced by fluid-filled cavities, which appear to widely communicate with remnants of the lateral ventricles (black *) posteriorly. There are remnants of the cerebral hemispheres in the basal temporal and parieto-occipital regions and along the falx (arrows). Note that, although most of the residual cerebral cortex is dysplastic, the fluid-filled cavities are not lined by cortex (arrowheads). The basal ganglia are absent, while the thalami are preserved (white *). Sagittal T2WI (E) shows essentially normal infratentorial structures although the brainstem is mildly thinned due to Wallerian degeneration. The cerebral aqueduct is patent (arrow).

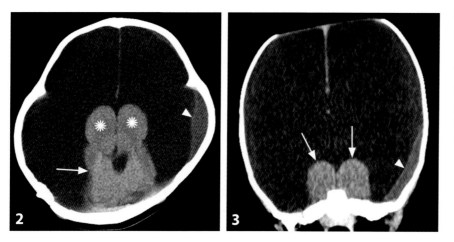

Figure 2. Axial CT shows bilateral thalami (*) and infratentorial brain structures (arrow), without any evidence of cerebral hemispheres. A small extra-axial collection (arrowhead).

Figure 3. Reconstructed coronal CT in another patient shows preserved thalami (arrows) without other brain parenchyma, and an extra-axial collection (arrowhead).

Hydranencephaly

ANDREA ROSSI

Specific Imaging Findings

Hydranencephaly presents as a replacement of the cerebral hemispheres by large, fluid-filled cystic cavities that are widely communicating with rudiments of the lateral ventricles posteriorly. Remnants of the basal portions of the temporal lobes and of the posterior parts of the occipital and parietal lobes are usually present, and the cortex may be normal or dysplastic. The cerebral falx is intact and appears to float within the cystic cavities; typically, one or more parafalcine cerebral rudiments are found. The basal ganglia are absent, whereas the thalami are notably present and abut the overlying cavitations. The brainstem is normally developed, but is usually thinned as a result of Wallerian degeneration; the cerebellum is also normal. MR angiography can show abrupt cut-off or hypoplasia of the vessels distal to the supraclinoid internal carotid arteries, but can also display an entirely patent, albeit stretched, craniocervical arterial tree. The skull may be enlarged as a consequence of CSF pulsation.

Pertinent Clinical Information

During pregnancy there is usually no obvious maternal illness or distress. The diagnosis is postnatal in a majority of cases, and may be delayed due to a surprisingly silent clinical course despite the severe pathological findings. Patients may elicit medical attention because of progressive increase of head circumference during the first weeks or months of life. Seizures may also appear. The prognosis is usually dismal with death in infancy in most cases. However, prolonged survival has also been reported and very rare cases of hemi-hydranencephaly, where only one cerebral hemisphere is affected, have been incidentally discovered in adults.

Differential Diagnosis

Severe Hydrocephalus (92)
- a rim of cortex is present around the dilated ventricles

Bilateral Open-Lip Schizencephaly (84)
- the cleft is bordered by polymicrogyric cortex
- middle cerebral artery distribution

Alobar Holoprosencephaly (73)
- absent falx cerebri
- rudimentary uncleaved brain anterior to the cyst cavity
- partial or complete fusion of thalami

Background

Hydranencephaly refers to massive necrosis of one or, more frequently, both cerebral hemispheres occurring during the fetal period or, rarely, after birth. The hemispheres are replaced by large, fluid-filled cavities that appear to widely communicate with remnants of the ventricular system. These cavities are bordered by a thin membrane that lies against the dura mater. This membrane may contain islands of preserved cortex and is continuous with the molecular layer of adjacent preserved portions of the cerebral hemispheres, which are typically located in the territory of the posterior cerebral arteries. The pathogenesis of hydranencephaly is related to an obstruction of the internal carotid arteries, typically at the supraclinoid segments, resulting in liquefaction and resorption of cerebral tissue. Putative causal factors include infection, anoxia, twin–twin transfusion, or thrombophilia. The arteries may then become recanalized so that no evident arterial abnormalities may be detected on postnatal imaging or autopsy. Preservation of the vertebrobasilar circulation explains sparing of the posterior vascular territories. Hydranencephaly may rarely be isolated to only one cerebral hemisphere and exceptional cases of infratentorial involvement have been reported. Hydranencephaly occurs as an isolated defect without other associated malformations. Nearly all cases are sporadic, affecting approximately 1 in 5000 pregnancies.

REFERENCES

1. Govaert P. Prenatal stroke. *Semin Fetal Neonatal Med* 2009;**14**:250–66.
2. Quek YW, Su PH, Tsao TF, et al. Hydranencephaly associated with interruption of bilateral internal carotid arteries. *Pediatr Neonatol* 2008;**49**:43–7.
3. Taori KB, Sargar KM, Disawal A, et al. Hydranencephaly associated with cerebellar involvement and bilateral microphthalmia and colobomas. *Pediatr Radiol* 2011;**41**:270–3.
4. Kelly TG, Sharif UM, Southern JF, et al. An unusual case of hydranencephaly presenting with an anterior midline cyst, a posterior calcified mass, cerebellar hypoplasia and occlusion of the posterior cerebral arteries. *Pediatr Radiol* 2011;**41**:274–7.
5. Ulmer S, Moeller F, Brockmann MA, et al. Living a normal life with the nondominant hemisphere: magnetic resonance imaging findings and clinical outcome for a patient with left-hemispheric hydranencephaly. *Pediatrics* 2005;**116**:242–5.

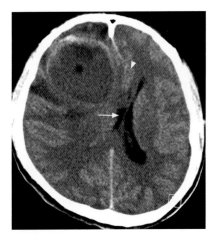

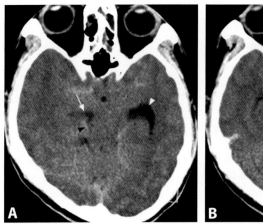

Figure 1. Axial CT in a patient with abscess (*) shows leftward shift with compressed right lateral ventricle (arrow) and paramedian frontal cortex displaced across the midline (arrowhead) beyond the free margin of the falx.

Figure 2. Axial CT (A) in a traumatized patient reveals diffuse SAH and effaced suprasellar cisterns (*). There is medial displacement of the right temporal horn (arrow) past the tentorial edge (black arrowhead). The left temporal horn is dilated (white arrowhead) indicating trapped left lateral ventricle. A more caudal CT image (B) shows inferior herniation of the mesial right temporal lobe along with the tip of the temporal horn (arrow).

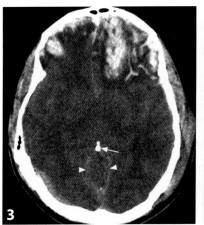

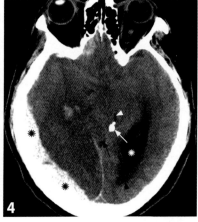

Figure 3. Axial CT reveals inferior displacement of the pineal gland (arrow) to the level of tentorial incisura (arrowheads). Also bilateral frontal contusions, diffuse edema and right-sided subdural hematoma.

Figure 4. CT shows medial displacement of the right temporal lobe (black arrow) past tentorial edge, and inferior pineal gland dislocation (white arrow), adjacent to the cerebral aqueduct (white arrowhead). Dilated left lateral ventricle (white *) with adjacent edema (black arrowhead), subdural hematoma (black *), and contusions.

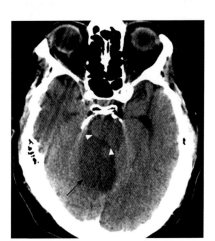

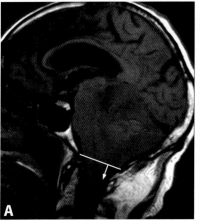

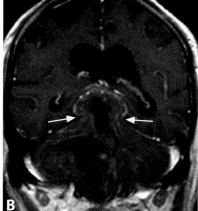

Figure 5. Axial CT in a patient with a large cerebellar infarction shows upward herniation of the infarcted tissue (black arrow) with brainstem compression (arrowheads).

Figure 6. Midsagittal T1WI (A) in a patient with cerebellar hemorrhage shows effacement of the superior cerebellar cistern, along with compressed fourth ventricle and brainstem. Cerebellar tonsils are pushed inferiorly (arrow) through the foramen magnum (white line). Coronal post-contrast T1WI (B) reveals upward vermian herniation through the tentorial incisura (arrows).

Acquired Intracranial Herniations

BENJAMIN HUANG

Specific Imaging Findings

Subfalcine herniation is the most common type of acquired cerebral herniation with cingulate gyrus being displaced beneath the inferior free margin of the falx cerebri on imaging. The degree of midline shift can be quantified by measuring displacement of the septum pellucidum. Transtentorial herniation can be either descending or ascending, of which the former can be subdivided into lateral and central types. In lateral descending transtentorial herniation, the mesial temporal lobe is displaced inferomedially through the tentorial incisura, with the early imaging findings of effaced ipsilateral suprasellar cistern and widened ipsilateral ambient cistern. Central transtentorial herniation is caused by a central or bilateral mass leading to downward displacement of the brain, best seen as the inferiorly pushed pineal gland calcification, located much lower than the choroid plexus calcifications (for two or more 5-mm slices). In ascending transtentorial herniation the cerebellum is displaced upward through the tentorial hiatus. Imaging findings include effacement of the superior cerebellar cistern, protrusion of the vermis through the incisura, and brainstem compression. Inferior displacement of the cerebellar tonsils through the foramen magnum is referred to as tonsillar herniation and is best depicted on sagittal images with the tonsils more than 5 mm below the foramen magnum. Hydrocephalus can occur with herniations as a result of obstructed CSF flow.

Pertinent Clinical Information

Cerebral herniations are frequently responsible for the presenting neurologic symptoms of the underlying pathologic processes. Subfalcine herniation can result in infarction of the anterior cerebral artery territory due to compression against the falx. With lateral transtentorial herniation, a lateralized, fixed and dilated ipsilateral or contralateral pupil due to cranial nerve III compression and occipital lobe infarcts due to posterior cerebral artery compression can occur. Central descending transtentorial herniation results in a fairly typical sequence of clinical signs as a result of brainstem compression occuring in an orderly rostral to caudal fashion. Ascending transtentorial herniation can compress the posterior cerebral or superior cerebellar arteries, resulting in infarctions or can cause hydrocephalus due to compression of the aqueduct. Tonsillar herniation can lead to loss of consciousness due to compression of the medulla by the displaced tonsils, hydrocephalus from obstruction of the outlet foramina of the fourth ventricle, or infarcts due to compression of the posterior inferior cerebellar artery.

Differential Diagnosis

Chiari 1 Malformation
- absence of space-occupying lesions
- isolated herniation of cerebellar tonsils through the foramen magnum

Intracranial Hypotension (37)
- diffuse dural thickening and enhancement
- sagging brain appearance
- absence of focal lesions

Background

Any space-occupying intracranial process can potentially cause brain herniation. As the cranial vault is essentially a fixed-volume compartment and the brain is essentially an incompressible structure, any increase in intracranial mass or pressure can only be compensated for by reductions in CSF or intravascular volume. These compensatory mechanisms are very limited in capacity and, when exceeded, readily give way to cerebral herniation. A number of variables also influence the degree of herniation and its neurologic sequelae, including the focality and location of the mass, size of the mass, intracranial pressure, degree of underlying brain atrophy, and certainly the rate at which changes in pressure occur. It is important to keep in mind that frequently multiple types of herniation occur simultaneously. Acquired tonsillar herniation may occur over time in patients with craniosynostosis syndromes due to disproportionately slow growth of the skull, impaired venous drainage, and hydrocephalus, which all lead to elevated intracranial pressure.

REFERENCES

1. Johnson PL, Eckard DA, Chason DP, *et al*. Imaging of acquired cerebral herniations. *Neuroimag Clin N Am* 2002;**12**:217–28.
2. Laine FJ, Shedden AI, Dunn MM, Ghatak NR. Acquired intracranial herniations: MR imaging findings. *AJR* 1995;**165**:967–73.
3. Server A, Dullerud R, Haakonsen M, *et al*. Post-traumatic cerebral infarction. Neuroimaging findings, etiology and outcome. *Acta Radiol* 2001;**42**:254–60.
4. Gentry LR. Imaging of closed head trauma. *Radiology* 1994;**191**:1–17.
5. Ranger A, Al-Hayek A, Matic D. Chiari type 1 malformation in an infant with type 2 Pfeiffer syndrome: further evidence of acquired pathogenesis. *J Craniofac Surg* 2010;**21**:427–31.

SECTION 4

Abnormalities Without Significant Mass Effect

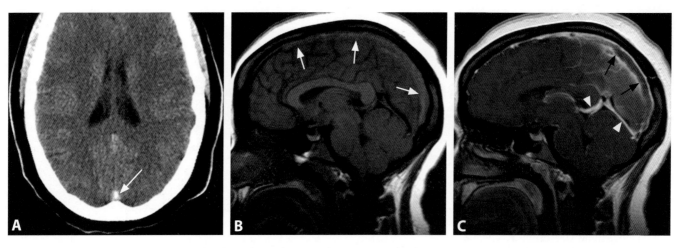

Figure 1. Non-enhanced axial CT image (A) shows hyperdensity in the superior sagittal sinus (arrow). Sagittal T1WI (B) reveals increased signal within the sinus (arrows). Corresponding (slightly tilted anteriorly) post-contrast T1WI (C) shows lack of normal enhancement (arrows) within the sinus. Compare to normal enhancing vein of Galen and straight sinus (arrowheads).

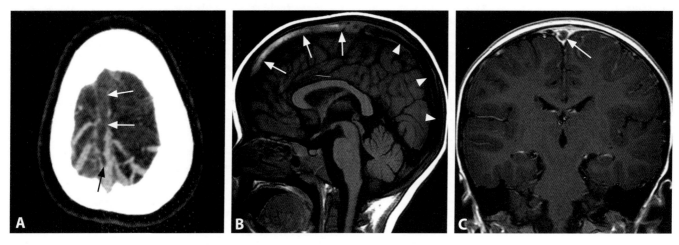

Figure 2. Enhanced axial CT image (A) shows a filling defect (arrows) in the superior sagittal sinus. Sagittal T1WI (B) shows increased intensity of the anterior superior sagittal sinus (arrows). Compare to normal posterior aspect of the sinus (arrowheads). Peripheral enhancement around the sinus filling defect (arrow) is seen on coronal post-contrast T1WI (C).

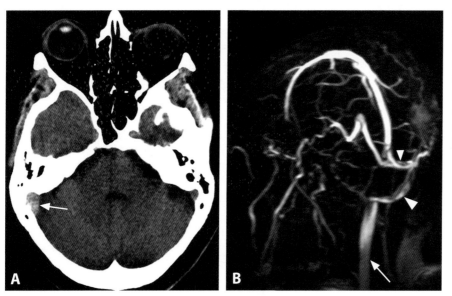

Figure 3. Non-enhanced axial CT image (A) shows hyperdensity of the right sigmoid sinus (arrow). Posterior right oblique MIP from post-contrast MRV (B) demonstrates absence of the right transverse and sigmoid sinuses as well as the internal jugular vein. Note normal left transverse sinus (small arrowhead), sigmoid sinus (large arrowhead), and internal jugular vein (arrow).

Dural Venous Sinus Thrombosis

GIULIO ZUCCOLI

Specific Imaging Findings

Increased density in the occluded sinus leading to a "cord sign" is the classic imaging finding of dural venous sinus thrombosis (DVST) on unenhanced CT images. However, a high variability in the degree of thrombus density is responsible for a low sensitivity of this sign. Thus, evaluation with CT angiogram, MR and MRV may be required to confirm the diagnosis. The "empty delta" sign consisting of a triangular area of enhancement with a relatively low-density center is seen in 25–30% of cases on contrast-enhanced CT scans. On MRI, acute thrombus is T1 isointense, T2 and T2* hypointense. Of note, this T2 hypointensity may mimic normal flow-void. Peripheral enhancement is seen around the acute hypointense clot corresponding to the empty delta CT sign. Subacute thrombus becomes T1 and T2 hyperintense. Chronic thrombus is most commonly T1 isointense and T2 hyperintense. DWI/ADC signal of the thrombus is variable, as is the degree of enhancement in organized thrombus. Visible serpiginous intrathrombus flow-voids on T2WI, corresponding areas of flow signal on TOF-MRV, and brightly enhancing channels on post-contrast MRV are present in most cases of chronic partial recanalization. Thrombosis shows no flow-related signal on phase contrast MRV, and absent to diminished enhancement on post contrast MRV and CTV. Engorged collateral veins may be present, primarily in the chronic phase. TOF-MRV of a subacute T1 bright clot may potentially misrepresent sinus patency.

Pertinent Clinical Information

DVST has a large spectrum of clinical manifestations as it may present with headache, seizure, papilledema, altered mental status, and focal neurological deficit including cranial nerve palsies. Unilateral headache is more common than diffuse headache. However, pain location is not associated with the site of thrombosis. Affected patients may initially show subarachnoid hemorrhage sparing the basal cisterns.

Differential Diagnosis

Normal Dural Venous Sinuses
- blood in venous sinuses is usually slightly hyperdense; especially in newborns, physiologic polycythemia in combination with unmyelinated brain makes the dural sinuses appear hyperdense

Acute Subdural Hematoma (133)
- blood along the entire tentorium of the cerebellum, not limited to the periphery

Congenital Hypoplasia/Atresia
- unilateral transverse sinus, variant anatomy of the torcular herophili
- focal areas of narrowing may be indistinguishable

Prominent Arachnoid Granulations (Pacchioni's Granulations) (130)
- typically round or ovoid filling defect of CSF density/intensity
- transverse and superior sagittal sinus locations are typical

Background

DVST is a rare cause of stroke affecting all age groups and accounting for 1–2% of strokes in adults. While age distribution is uniform in men, a peak incidence is reported in women aged 20–35 years which may be related to pregnancy and use of contraceptives. DVST should always be considered in the differential diagnosis in patients with severe headache, focal neurological deficits, idiopathic intracranial hypertension and intracranial hemorrhage. Many causative conditions have been described in DVST including infections, trauma, hypercoagulable states, hyperhomocysteinemia, hematologic disorders, collagenopathies, inflammatory bowel diseases, use of medications, and intracranial hypotension. Thrombosis most frequently affects the superior sagittal sinus. However, multiple locations, particularly in the contiguous transverse and sigmoid sinuses, are found in as many as 90% of patients. Focal brain abnormalities have been found in as many as 57% of patients. Bleeding represents a non-negligible complication of thrombolytic therapy, potentially affecting patients' outcome.

REFERENCES

1. Leach JL, Fortuna RB, Jones BV, Gaskill-Shipley MF. Imaging of cerebral venous thrombosis: current techniques, spectrum of findings, and diagnostic pitfalls. *Radiographics* 2006;**26**(*Suppl* **1**):S19–41.

2. Meckel S, Reisinger C, Bremerich J, *et al*. Cerebral venous thrombosis: diagnostic accuracy of combined, dynamic and static, contrast-enhanced 4D MR venography. *AJNR* 2010;**31**:527–35.

3. Leach JL, Wolujewicz M, Strub WM. Partially recanalized chronic dural sinus thrombosis: findings on MR imaging, time-of-flight MR venography, and contrast-enhanced MR venography. *AJNR* 2007;**28**:782–9.

4. Oppenheim C, Domingo V, Gauvrit JY, *et al*. Subarachnoid hemorrhage as the initial presentation of dural sinus thrombosis. *AJNR* 2005;**26**:614–7.

5. Dentali F, Squizzato A, Gianni M, *et al*. Safety of thrombolysis in cerebral venous thrombosis. A systematic review of the literature. *Thromb Haemost* 2010;**104**:1055–62.

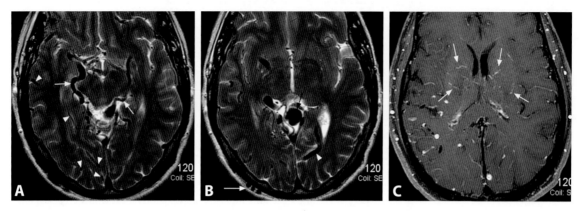

Figure 1. Axial T2WI (A) shows large tortuous basal veins of Rosenthal (arrows) and vessels within the right temporo-occipital sulci (arrowheads). Slightly more cephalad (B) a large vein of Galen (black arrow), tortuous sulcal signal voids (arrowhead) and large subgaleal veins (white arrow) are seen. Post-contrast T1WI (C) shows enhancement of leptomeningeal vessels on the right and bilateral medullary veins (arrows).

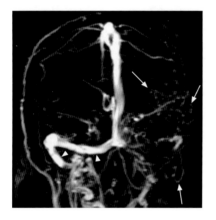

Figure 2. Contrast-enhanced MRV reveals multiple small curvilinear structures (arrows) on the left. Left transverse and sigmoid sinuses show areas of narrowing and occlusion. Normal right transverse and sigmoid sinuses (arrowheads).

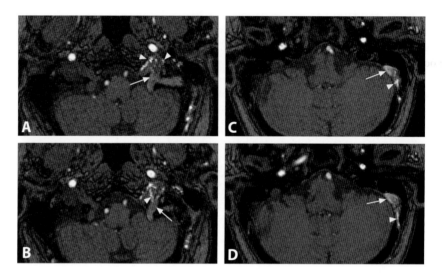

Figure 3. 3D TOF MRA source images (A, B) show multiple high-intensity structures (arrowheads) adjacent to left jugular bulb (arrows) with extension into the bulb. At a more cephalad level (C, D) bright linear structures (arrowheads) are adjacent and extending into the left sigmoid sinus (arrow). Note mild hyperintensity of left sigmoid sinus and jugular bulb.

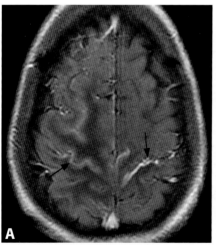
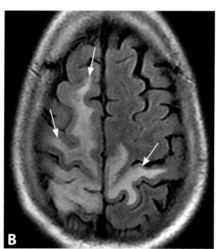

Figure 4. Axial post-contrast T1WI (A) shows enhancing prominent venous structures (arrows) and adjacent hypointense edema in the subcortical white matter. Corresponding FLAIR image (B) more clearly shows the hyperintensity of edema (arrows) caused by venous hypertension.

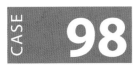

Dural Arteriovenous Fistula

MATTHEW OMOJOLA AND ZORAN RUMBOLDT

Specific Imaging Findings

Dural arteriovenous fistula (DAVF) may not be visualized on routine CT or MRI images. MRI findings of larger or high-flow DAVFs include: multiple extra axial linear or tortuous flow-voids on T2WI, either at the base of the brain, around the tentorial incisura, in the basal cisterns, or in the sulci along the convexity, which are even better visualized with susceptibility-weighted imaging (SWI). Major deep and superficial draining veins may be enlarged. Large tortuous signal voids may be present in the scalp of the affected side. Post-contrast images may show prominent tortuous vessels within the sulci indicating retrograde cortical venous drainage. Large deep medullary (white matter) veins and white matter T2 hyperintensity are indicative of venous hypertension. Perfusion studies show increased relative cerebral blood volume (rCBV) in all of these patients. CT demonstrates complications, primarily subarachnoid, subdural, parenchymal, or occasionally intraventricular hemorrhages. MRA or CTA in the high-flow DAVF often show enlarged tortuous arterial and venous structures. Findings of high intensity structures adjacent to the sinus wall on 3D TOF MRA appear to be diagnostic of DAVF. MRV confirms enlarged venous structures and may show evidence of venous sinus thrombosis or occlusion. DSA demonstrates the exact fistula site, is very useful for treatment planning and offers endovascular treatment options.

Pertinent Clinical Information

DAVFS occur in adults, more commonly females. They may be clinically silent and incidentally found at imaging. Pulsatile tinnitus, audible bruit, headache, cognitive impairment, seizures, cranial nerve palsies and focal neurologic deficit may all occur in patients with DAVF. Lesions located in the cavernous sinus region present with ophthalmoplegia, eye pain, orbital congestion or features of carotid cavernous fistula. Development of venous hypertension frequently leads to progressive dementia. Acute symptoms may be due to intracranial hemorrhages, which occur in DAVFs with retrograde cortical flow. Therefore, the presence of retrograde cortical flow represents a clear indication for treatment of these lesions.

Differential Diagnosis

Arteriovenous Malformation (AVM) (182)

- usually parenchymal in location with a focal nidus ("bag of worms") best seen on T2-weighted images

Venous Thrombosis (97)

- presence of intraluminal clot
- may lead to DAVF

Background

DAVF is thought to represent acquired pachymeningeal connection between arteries and veins without an intervening nidus. The true incidence is not known, but has been reported to represent about 10–15% of all intracranial vascular malformations. Common locations are tentorial, parasellar, along the transverse sinuses and falx. Dural sinus thrombosis and trauma are considered responsible for development of these lesions. DAVF may occur and occlude spontaneously. There are various classification methods of DAVF based upon the venous outflow pattern and associated outflow restrictions, which might influence the clinical presentation and treatment outcomes. Retrograde flow into cortical veins results in deep venous engorgement, leading to venous hypertension, which in turn leads to ischemia and hemorrhage.

Recent developments in rapid 4D contrast-enhanced MR angiography technique are very promising and it may eventually obviate the need for diagnostic catheter angiography.

REFERENCES

1. Kwon BJ, Han MH, Kang HS, Chang KH. MR imaging findings of intracranial dural arteriovenous fistulas: relations with venous drainage patterns. *AJNR* 2005;**26**:2500–7.

2. Noguchi K, Melhem ER, Kanazawa T, *et al.* Intracranial dural arteriovenous fistulas: evaluation with combined 3D time-of-flight MR angiography and MR digital subtraction angiography. *AJR* 2004;**182**:183–90.

3. Meckel S, Maier M, San Millan Ruiz D, *et al.* MR angiography of dural arteriovenous fistulas: diagnosis and follow-up after treatment using a time-resolved 3D contrast-enhanced technique. *AJNR* 2007;**28**:877–84.

4. Nishimura S, Hirai T, Sasao A, *et al.* Evaluation of dural arteriovenous fistulas with 4D contrast-enhanced MR angiography at 3T. *AJNR* 2010;**31**:80–5.

5. Noguchi K, Kuwayama N, Kubo M, *et al.* Intracranial dural arteriovenous fistula with retrograde cortical venous drainage: use of susceptibility-weighted imaging in combination with dynamic susceptibility contrast imaging. *AJNR* 2010;**31**:1903–10.

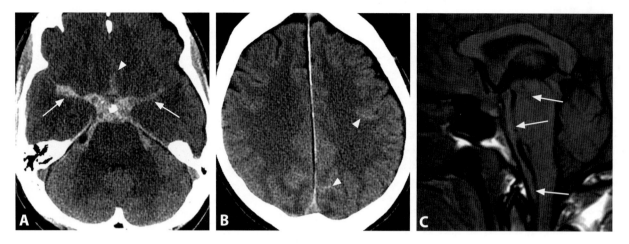

Figure 1. Non-enhanced CT (A) shows hyperdensity throughout basal cisterns extending into sylvian (arrows) and interhemispheric (arrowhead) fissures. A more cephalad CT (B) shows subtle sulcal iso- to hyperdensity (arrowheads). Midsagittal T1WI (C) reveals isodense material within the cisterns (arrows).

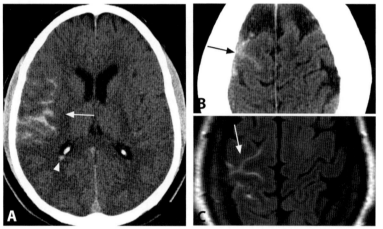

Figure 2. Non-enhanced CT (A) shows hyperintensity within the right sylvian fissure (arrow) and layering in the lateral ventricle (arrowhead). CT along the convexity (B) shows subtle sulcal hyperintensities (arrow), better seen (arrow) on corresponding FLAIR image (C).

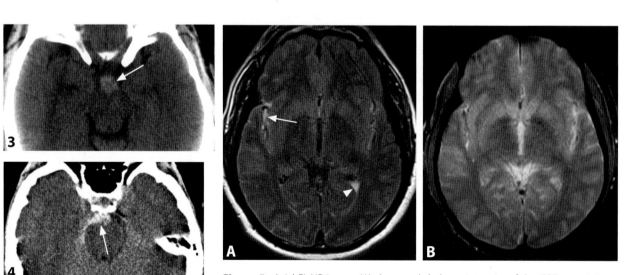

Figures 3 and 4. Non-enhanced CT images in two patients show perimesencephalic hemorrhage (arrows), limited to basal cisterns.

Figure 5. Axial FLAIR image (A) shows subtle hyperintensity of the CSF-containing spaces along the brain surface (arrow) and within ventricles (arrowhead). Corresponding hypointensity is not well appreciated on T2*WI (B).

Subarachnoid Hemorrhage

MATTHEW OMOJOLA

Specific Imaging Findings

On CT, subarachnoid hemorrhage (SAH) characteristically presents as hyperdense material filling the basal cisterns and/or fissures and cortical sulci. The density and extent depend on the volume of blood. If sufficiently diluted by the CSF, a small SAH may not be seen on CT. Dilution and redistribution may lead to intraventricular extension and the hyperdensity gradually fades away. Diluted SAH can appear as effacement of the cortical sulci. Traumatic SAH may be associated with other injuries such as parenchymal and extra-axial hematomas. The most common cause of nontraumatic SAH is aneurysmal rupture, usually presenting with diffuse SAH, while a filling defect within the hyperdense clot may indicate the aneurysm location. An associated parenchymal hematoma may also be present. Nonaneurysmal SAH (NASAH) is most commonly perimesencephalic, located almost exclusively in the basal cisterns with possible minimal extension into the interhemispheric and sylvian fissures. Other types of NASAH tend to be located along the convexity – apart from trauma, vasculitis, cortical vein thrombosis, Moyamoya, and cerebral amyloid angiopathy may present this way. On MRI, SAH is best seen with FLAIR sequence, which is more sensitive than CT. T2*WI tend to show hypointensity, but this is variable. Hyperacute SAH (within the first few hours), similar to hyperacute hematoma, is extremely T2 hyperintense, brighter than the CSF; it becomes hypointense in the acute phase. T1 signal varies but is always hyperintense compared to the CSF. Leptomeningeal enhancement may be present. In patients with nontraumatic SAH and either the perimesencephalic pattern or no blood on CT, negative CTA is reliable in ruling out aneurysms. DSA is indicated for diffuse SAH with negative CTA.

Pertinent Clinical Information

Acute nontraumatic SAH typically presents with a sudden onset "thunderclap" headache described as "the worst headache ever". Prodromal or sentinel headache is reported by many patients. Nausea and vomiting are common, photophobia and neck stiffness may be present. Hydrocephalus and vasospasm are the main complications of SAH. The presence of three or more separate areas of SAH in traumatized patients is a poor prognostic indicator.

Differential Diagnosis

Diffuse Brain Edema
- diffuse hypodensity of the brain with loss of differentiation between gray and white matter
- cerebellum usually spared, appears relatively hyperdense
- fading SAH may resemble cerebral edema due to effacement of cortical sulci

Meningitis (120)
- high protein content of CSF may be indistinguishable from SAH on FLAIR
- not CT hyperdense, no signal loss on T2* images

Collateral Leptomeningeal Vessels in Arterial Occlusions (Moyamoya) (122)
- vascular structures can usually be identified
- uncommon in basal cisterns

Cortical Vein Thrombosis (181)
- localized sulcal CT hyperdensity and T2* hypointensity corresponding to cortical vein
- adjacent parenchymal infarct and/or hemorrhage may be present

Background

The most common cause of nontraumatic SAH is by far rupture of intracranial aneurysm (about 85% of cases). Mortality of aneurysmal SAH is very high at about 30–40% with permanent neurological deficit in another third of patients. Recent advances in diagnosis and treatment appear to have somewhat mitigated the morbidity and mortality of SAH. CT is diagnostic in about 100% of patients within the first 12 h of a major SAH. About 10% of SAH may not be detectable after 24 h. A negative CT scan in the appropriate clinical setting should be followed by a lumbar puncture. CTA has become the main technique for detection of aneurysms. DSA offers both diagnostic confirmation and endovascular embolization treatment. Around 8–10% of patients have NASAH, most commonly perimesencephalic, which has excellent prognosis.

REFERENCES

1. Agid R, Andersson T, Almqvist H, *et al*. Negative CT angiography findings in patients with spontaneous subarachnoid hemorrhage: when is digital subtraction angiography still needed? *AJNR* 2010;**31**:696–705.

2. Brinjikji W, Kallmes DF, White JB, *et al*. Inter and intra observer agreement in CT characterization of non aneurysmal perimesencephalic subarachnoid hemorrhage. *AJNR* 2010;**31**:1103–5.

3. van Asch CJJ, van der Schaaf IC, Rinkel GJE. Acute hydrocephalus and cerebral perfusion after aneurysmal subarachnoid hemorrhage. *AJNR* 2010;**31**:67–70.

4. Cuvinciuc V, Viguier A, Calviere L, *et al*. Isolated acute nontraumatic cortical subarachnoid hemorrhage. *AJNR* 2010;**31**:1355–62.

5. Boesiger BM, Shiber JR. Subarachnoid hemorrhage diagnosis by computed tomography and lumbar puncture: are fifth generation CT scanners better at identifying subarachnoid hemorrhage? *J Emerg Med* 2005;**29**:23–7.

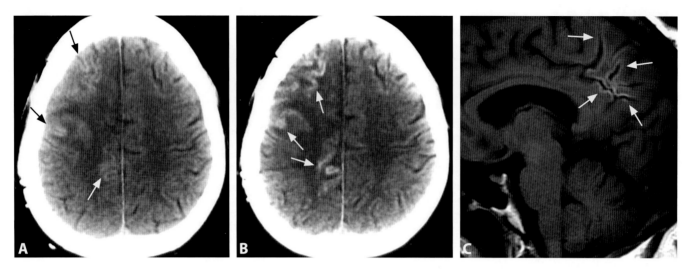

Figure 1. Axial non-enhanced CT image (A) a few days following gunshot injury in a young man shows subtle gyral high-density areas (arrows). Further follow-up CT (B) demonstrates extensive gyral hyperdensity (arrows) in the right hemisphere. Sagittal non-contrast T1WI (C) reveals gyral hyperintense signal along the parafalcine right parietal cortex (arrows).

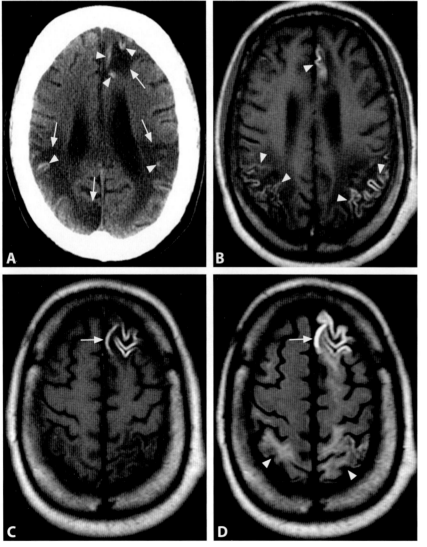

Figure 2. Non-enhanced axial CT image (A) in a patient with sequelae of a remote severe untreated posterior reversible encephalopathy syndrome (PRES) shows bilateral predominantly posterior hypodense areas of encephalomalacia (arrows) with focal gyral cortical hyperdensities (arrowheads). Bright cortical lesions (arrowheads) are more conspicuous on a non-contrast T1WI at a similar level (B). A more superior T1WI (C) reveals a prominent left frontal cortical hyperintensity (arrow), which is further accentuated on the corresponding FLAIR image (D). Note bilateral areas of gliosis (arrowheads), with low T1 signal and hyperintensity on FLAIR image.

Laminar Necrosis

MATTHEW OMOJOLA

Specific Imaging Findings

Acute to subacute laminar necrosis (LN) on CT cannot be differentiated from brain swelling/edema and often occurs in the setting of hypoxic–ischemic changes and other lesions that lead to cerebral edema/swelling. Follow-up CT shows resolution of edema with possible local volume loss. Chronic LN demonstrates cortical hyperdensity in the affected gyri. MRI of LN in the acute to subacute setting shows reduced diffusion of the involved cortical regions, frequently with T2 hyperintensity and effacement of the sulci. Subcortical U fibers are usually affected by the edema. There is no evidence of blood products on T2*-weighted images. Associated deep gray matter changes may be present depending on the cause of the LN. Gyral enhancement on post-contrast T1WI may occur, usually in the subacute stage. Chronic LN is classically visualized as T1 hyperintense gyri with surrounding volume loss. The hyperintensity may be even more prominent on FLAIR images while diffusion imaging is unremarkable. Cortical hypointensity is present on T2* images in some cases. Findings of LN start fading away on long follow-up studies. Encephalomalacia and gliosis of the adjacent or other areas of the brain may be present, depending on the underlying etiology.

Specific Clinical Information

LN tends to occur in the setting of hypoxic–ischemic encephalopathy from any cause, infarction, and hypoglycemia. It is seen with seizures, posterior reversible encephalopathy syndrome (PRES), mitochondrial disorders, osmotic myelinolysis, CNS lupus, and brain injury. Extensive changes have a poor prognosis and tend to be associated with death or vegetative state.

Differential Diagnosis

Cortical Hemorrhage (178, 179, 181)
- usually focal and mass-like
- signal loss on T2* MRI

Hemorrhagic Conversion of Infarct
- usually associated with larger acute infarction
- not limited to the gray matter
- signal loss on T2* MRI

Cortical Calcifications/Mineralization (188, 189, 191)
- may be permanent on follow-up
- may be indistinguishable on CT and T2*-weighted MRI (calcification and mineralization have been demonstrated in LN)

Background

The cortical and deep gray matter is hypermetabolic and as such is more susceptible to ischemia or anoxia than the white matter, with the cortical layer 3 being the most vulnerable. LN is a manifestation of selective vulnerability of the gray matter and may therefore occur in the absence of white matter changes. However, severe hypoxic–ischemic changes tend to also affect the white matter and result in associated encephalomalacia. Histologically, LN has been described as pan necrosis with fat-laden macrophages. Presence of mineralization such as calcification with traces of iron has also been demonstrated. Acute LN changes could be missed at imaging: brain swelling may mask the changes on CT while improper windowing on MR may produce a 'superscan' that may initially be mistaken for a normal study. Recently described findings on susceptibility-weighted imaging (SWI) are absence of blood products in a large proportion of pediatric patients, while dotted or laminar hemorrhages are found in a minority of cases. LN in a setting of hypoxic–ischemic encephalopathy, especially in adults, shows linear gyral and basal ganglia hypointensities.

REFERENCES

1. Niwa T, Aida N, Shishikura A, et al. Susceptibility weighted imaging findings of cortical laminar necrosis in pediatric patients. AJNR 2008;29:1795–8.

2. Kesavadas C, Santhosh K, Thomas B, et al. Signal changes in cortical laminar necrosis – evidence from susceptibility-weighted magnetic resonance imaging. Neuroradiology 2009;51:293–8.

3. Siskas N, Lefkopoulos A, Ioannidis I, et al. Cortical laminar necrosis in brain infarcts: serial MRI. Neuroradiology 2003;45:283–8.

4. McKinney AM, Teksam M, Felice R, et al. Diffusion-weighted imaging in the setting of diffuse cortical laminar necrosis and hypoxic–ischemic encephalopathy. AJNR 2004;25:1659–65.

5. Takahashi S, Higano S, Ishii K, et al. Hypoxic brain damage: cortical laminar necrosis and delayed changes in white matter at sequential MR imaging. Radiology 1993;189:449–56.

Brain Imaging with MRI and CT, ed. Zoran Rumboldt *et al.* Published by Cambridge University Press. © Cambridge University Press 2012.

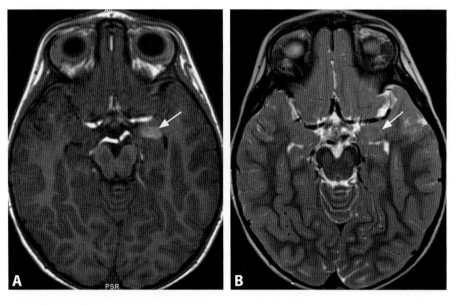

Figure 1. Axial T1WI (A) in a child with seizures shows hyperintense abnormality (arrow) in the left amygdala, without significant mass effect or perifocal edema. T2WI (B) at a similar level fails to reveal any abnormal signal in the left amygdala (arrow).

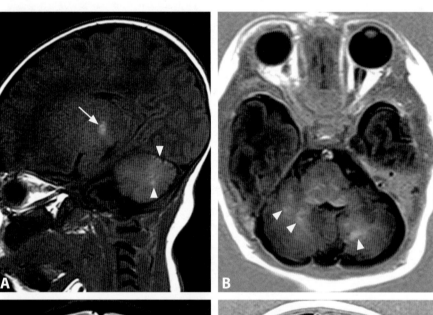

Figure 2. Sagittal T1WI (A) in a neonate shows hyperintense areas in the cerebellum (arrowheads) and supratentorial brain (arrow). Axial IR T1WI (B) also shows the cerebellar lesions (arrowheads), without mass effect. T2WI (C) shows a subtle left thalamic hypointensity (arrow). IR T1WI (D) reveals corresponding hyperintensity (arrow). Follow-up IR T1WI at a similar level a year later (E) shows interval white matter myelination with decreased conspicuity of the left thalamic lesion (arrow).

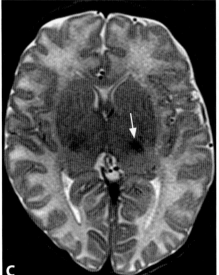
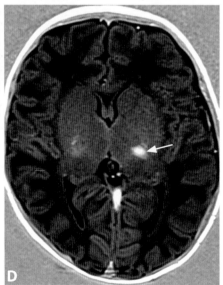
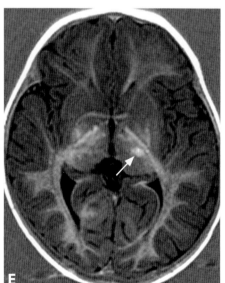

Neurocutaneous Melanosis

MAJDA THURNHER

Specific Imaging Findings

Neurocutaneous melanosis (NCM) appears to involve the brain in specific locations; most commonly, melanocytic lesions are detected in the anterior temporal lobe (amygdala) and cerebellum, followed by the pons and medulla oblongata. Round or oval shaped lesions are best seen on T1-weighted images as areas of high signal intensity (due to melanin). The lesions are T2 iso- or hypointense and do not enhance with contrast. The T1 hyperintensity is more conspicuous within the first months of life, before the myelination appears complete on T1-weighted images. In patients with leptomeningeal involvement FLAIR images show sulcal/leptomeningeal hyperintensity and enhancement of the thickened leptomeninges is seen on post-contrast images, especially prominent along the basal cistern, tentorium, brainstem, inferior vermis and folia of the cerebellar hemispheres. NCM lesions are slightly hyperdense on CT; very high density may suggest associated hemorrhage. Echogenic foci may be seen on neonatal head ultrasound exam.

Pertinent Clinical Information

NCM typically presents early in childhood. Neurological manifestations of NCM are most commonly related to increased intracranial pressure, communicating hydrocephalus (due to the leptomeningeal melanocytic tumors) and epilepsy. Cranial nerve palsies are frequently associated. The risk for NCM is high in children with large congenital melanocytic nevi, in particular those over the trunk and neck with multiple satellite lesions. The criteria for diagnosing NCM are: (a) large or numerous pigmented nevi in association with leptomeningeal melanosis, (b) no evidence of malignant transformation of the cutaneous lesions, and (c) no malignant melanoma in other organs.

Differential Diagnosis

Metastatic Melanoma (180)
- intracerebral metastases show perifocal edema and/or necrosis
- leptomeningeal enhancement is usually nodular

Meningeal Carcinomatosis (119)
- typically focal linear and/or nodular leptomeningeal contrast enhancement
- additional parenchymal enhancing lesions are frequently present

Infectious and Inflammatory Meningeal Processes (118, 120, 160)
- enhancing meningeal and intraparenchymal enhancing lesions are T1 hypo- to isointense
- associated hydrocephalus, abscess, and/or empyema may be present

Subarachnoid Hemorrhage (99)
- sulcal hyperintensity on FLAIR images is usually more focal and not diffuse
- typically sudden onset of symptoms

Moyamoya (122)
- prominent flow-voids within the subarachnoid spaces
- parenchymal T1 hyperintensities only if associated with infarct and/or hemorrhage

Background

Primary melanocytic lesions of the CNS arise from melanocytes located within the leptomeninges, and this group includes diffuse melanocytosis and meningeal melanomatosis, melanocytoma, and malignant melanoma. NCM or Touraine syndrome is a rare, noninherited congenital phakomatosis characterized by the presence of congenital melanocytic nevi and a benign or malignant pigmented cell tumor of the leptomeninges. Giant cutaneous melanocytic nevi (GCMN) and leptomeningeal melanocytosis (LM) are caused by proliferation of melanin-producing cells. Intra-axial benign or malignant melanotic brain lesions are found in approximately 50% of individuals with NCM. The overall risk for malignant transformation of nevi is 12%. Symptomatic patients generally have very poor prognosis. NCM may be associated with other neurocutaneous syndromes such as Sturge–Weber or von Recklinghausen disease. Features of Dandy–Walker complex are also present in some cases. NCM is considered to follow from neurulation disorders, which could account for the associated developmental malformations. Although NCM is seen almost exclusively in children with congenital nevi, rare cases with or without dermatologic lesions have been described in young adults, in the third and fourth decades of life.

REFERENCES

1. Hayashi M, Maeda M, Maji T, et al. Diffuse leptomeningeal hyperintensity on fluid-attenuated inversion recovery MR images in neurocutaneous melanosis. AJNR 2004;25:138–41.

2. Barkovich AJ, Frieden IJ, Williams ML. MR of neurocutaneous melanosis. AJNR 1994;15:859–67.

3. Smith AB, Rushing EJ, Smirniotopoulos JG. Pigmented lesions of the central nervous system: radiologic–pathologic correlation. Radiographics 2009;29:1503–24.

4. Sutton BJ, Tatter SB, Stanton CA, Mott RT. Leptomeningeal melanocytosis in an adult male without large congenital nevi: a rare and atypical case of neurocutaneous melanosis. Clin Neuropathol 2011;30:178–82.

5. Marnet D, Vinchon M, Mostofi K, et al. Neurocutaneous melanosis and the Dandy–Walker complex: an uncommon but not so insignificant association. Childs Nerv Syst 2009;25:1533–9.

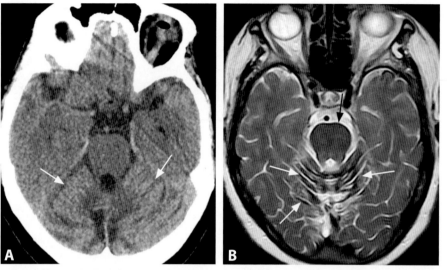

Figure 1. Axial non-enhanced CT image (A) in a patient with progressive sensorineural hearing loss shows only atrophy of the cerebellum (arrows). Axial T2WI at a similar level (B) reveals very dark regions (arrows) that are lining the surface of the superior vermis and adjacent cerebellar hemispheres (white arrows) as well as the pons (black arrow).

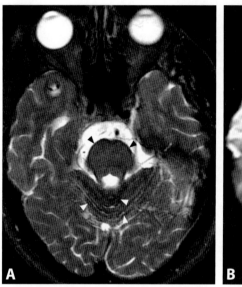
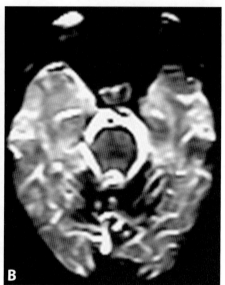

Figure 2. Axial FSE T2WI with fat suppression (A) in another patient shows linear areas of very low signal in the superior vermis (white arrowheads) and along the pons (black arrowheads). Corresponding GRE T2*WI (B) demonstrates a marked loss of signal intensity along the superior cerebellum and the brainstem.

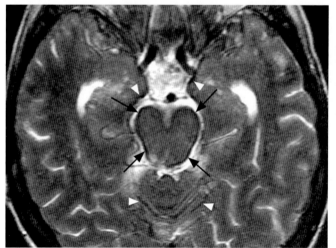

Figure 3. Axial T2WI reveals dark lining (arrows) along the midbrain surface. A more subtle dark lining is present along the mesial temporal lobes and vermis (arrowheads).

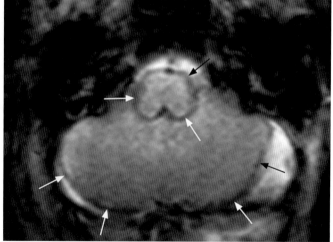

Figure 4. Axial T2*WI in a young child with history of germinal matrix hemorrhage shows hypointensity along the surface of the brainstem and cerebellum (arrows).

Superficial Siderosis

MAURICIO CASTILLO

Specific Imaging Findings

MRI using T2-weighted sequences is the imaging method of choice, particularly with gradient-recalled echo T2* techniques. Susceptibility effects induced by superficial siderosis (SS) are more obvious at 3.0 T than at 1.5 T. A black line follows the contour of the cerebellum, medulla, pons, and midbrain and to a lesser extent the supratentorial regions such as the temporal lobes (particularly the sylvian and interhemispheric fissures). The cisternal portions of the cranial nerves may also appear dark. The surface of the spinal cord can also show SS. The cerebellum commonly shows atrophy particularly in its vermis and the anterior aspects of the hemispheres. The cerebral hemispheres may also be atrophic. Occasionally, dystrophic calcifications develop in areas of chronic SS, which is better seen on CT. Contrast enhancement may rarely occur. The most important role of imaging is to look for the underlying cause of SS. If the brain study does not reveal obvious causes the next step is spinal MRI. If all MRI studies are non-conclusive a myelogram and post-myelogram CT may be done to identify causes of CSF leak in spinal axis. Occasionally cerebral and spinal angiography may be used as the last resort in attempting to find out the reason for SS.

Pertinent Clinical Information

Classically, SS presents in adults with progressive gait ataxia and other cerebellar abnormalities as well as sensorineural hearing loss and other cranial nerve deficits. Pyramidal signs and loss of bladder control are observed in a small number of patients and at the end of the disease, dementia will develop in about 25% of patients. SS should be excluded in all patients with signs of cerebellar degeneration. CSF analysis may reveal xanthochromia, high iron concentrations, red blood cells and increased proteins. The peripheral nervous system is not affected but involvement of spinal nerve roots may give rise to conflicting clinical symptoms.

Differential Diagnosis

Leptomeningeal Seeding with Inflammatory, Infectious and Neoplastic Processes (118, 119, 120, 135)
- prominent contrast enhancement
- T2 hypointensity is rare
- possible nodularity

Background

SS refers to deposition of chronic blood products, particularly hemosiderin, in the pia and subpial regions of the brain and spinal cord. Repeat bouts of hemorrhage are needed for SS to occur. Chronic exposure of brain cells (particularly microglia and oligodendrocytes) to hemosiderin leads to their production of ferritin, which worsens the process. The cells that are more prone to produce ferritin are found in the cerebellum (Bergman glia), explaining why SS occurs there with a higher frequency and severity. The causes of SS are multiple and may include repeated hemorrhages from amyloidosis, cavernomas, tumors (ependymoma, meningioma, oligodendroglioma, pineocytoma), dural AV fistulae, aneurysms, AVMs, repeated trauma (boxing, use of jackhammer), dural tears, post-operative (post-hemispherectomy, chronic suboccipital subdural hematoma), encephalocele, intracranial hypotension, anticoagulation, and nerve root avulsions. The end result is neuronal loss, gliosis and demyelination. Schwann cells are particularly prone to damage, which explains frequent sensorineural hearing loss in these patients. There is no specific treatment of SS and the use of chelating drugs is unclear with reports of deferiprone, a lipid-soluble iron chelator, leading to improvement of symptoms. Treatment should be guided towards the underlying disease (if identified) that resulted in SS. Because the cochlea is spared, implantation may improve hearing loss in some individuals.

REFERENCES

1. Kumar N. Neuroimaging in superficial siderosis: an in-depth look. *AJNR* 2010;**31**:5–14.
2. Linn J, Herms J, Dichgans M, *et al.* Subarachnoid hemosiderosis and superficial cortical hemosiderosis in cerebral amyloid angiopathy. *AJNR* 2008;**29**:184–6.
3. Hsu WC, Loevner LA, Forman MS, Thaler ER. Superficial siderosis of the CNS associated with multiple cavernous malformations. *AJNR* 1999;**20**:1245–8.
4. Kakeda S, Korogi Y, Ohnari N, *et al.* Superficial siderosis associated with a chronic subdural hematoma: T2-weighted MR imaging at 3T. *Acad Radiol* 2010;**17**:871–6.
5. Levy M, Llinas RH. Pilot safety trial of deferiprone in 10 subjects with superficial siderosis. *Stroke* 2012;**43**:120–4.

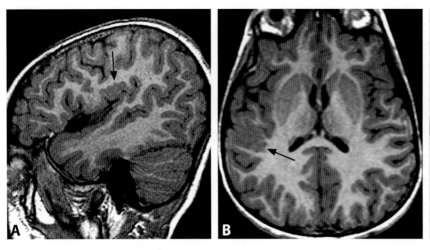

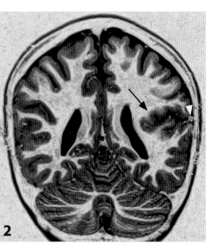

Figure 1. Sagittal (A) and reconstructed axial (B) T1WIs from a 3D acquisition in a 3-year-old patient with intractable seizures show a focal area of irregular cortical thickening along the right posterior perisylvian region (arrows).

Figure 2. Coronal IR T1WI shows irregular thickened cortex (arrow) along a deep left sylvian fissure. There is an adjacent anomalous enlarged vein (arrowhead).

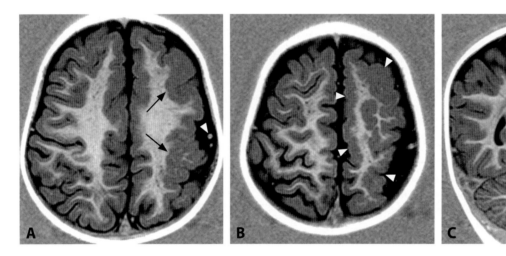

Figure 3. Axial IR T1WI (A) demonstrates thickened and irregular cortex of the left frontal and parietal lobes with absent or rudimentary cortical sulci (arrows). Note adjacent large venous structure (arrowhead). A more cephalad image (B) shows corrugated appearance of the affected cortex (arrowheads) and reduced sulci. Coronal IR T1WI (C) demonstrates indentation of the brain (arrowhead) in the region of abnormal cortex.

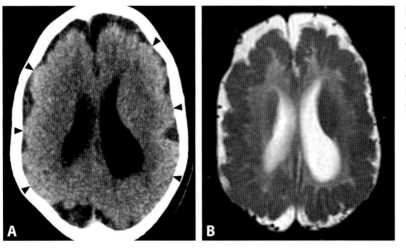

Figure 4. Non-enhanced axial CT image (A) in a 4-month-old child with infantile spasms reveals diffuse abnormal thickening of the cortical ribbon (arrowheads), reduced sulcation, and indistinct gray-white matter junction. Corresponding T2WI (B) shows diffuse bilateral thickening of the cortex with the appearance of cortical palisades.

Polymicrogyria

MARIA VITTORIA SPAMPINATO

Specific Imaging Findings

Polymicrogyria is characterized by an irregular cortical surface, apparent thickening of the cortex, "stippled" gray–white matter junction, and a greater than expected number of abnormally small gyri, usually without T2 signal abnormality in the myelinated brain. High-resolution images reveal that the cortical ribbon itself is thin, and the apparent thickening results from juxtaposition of the small folds. The perisylvian cortex is the site most commonly affected by polymicrogyria; however, any region of the cortical mantle can be involved. Cortical involvement can be restricted to a single focus or it can affect extended areas, as seen in cases of uni- or bilateral, symmetrical or asymmetrical, diffuse polymicrogyria. The imaging appearances of polymicrogyric cortex can be heterogeneous, ranging from multiple abnormal small gyri to a relatively smooth cortical surface and an overall coarse appearance. Diffuse coarse polymicrogyria can have the appearance of cortical palisades. The sulcation pattern is aberrant, without a recognizable pattern. Sulci may be shallow or deeply indent the parenchyma. Polymicrogyria may be associated with schizencephaly, corpus callosum dysgenesis, cerebellar hypoplasia, periventricular and subcortical heterotopias. An imaging protocol including volumetric T1-weighted images with thin sections (< 1.5 mm) and reconstruction in the three orthogonal planes is optimal for evaluation of these abnormalities.

Pertinent Clinical Information

Clinical manifestations and the age of presentation vary depending on the location of the malformation, the extent of cortical involvement (focal, multifocal, diffuse, unilateral, or bilateral), and the presence or absence of associated anomalies. Patients affected by unilateral or bilateral diffuse polymicrogyria present with moderate or severe intellectual impairment, mixed seizure types, and motor dysfunction. Individual clinical features include hemiparesis or tetraparesis, speech disturbance, dyslexia, and developmental delay. Neurological and development abnormalities can precede the onset of seizures. Coexistent anomalies include dysmorphic facial features, hand, foot, skin, palate, and cardiac abnormalities.

Differential Diagnosis

Classic Lissencephaly (19)
- abnormally thickened cortex (10–15 mm)
- smooth brain surface with areas of agyria and pachygyria
- shallow sylvian fissures

Cobblestone Complex (92)
- mixed cortical malformation with areas of polymicrogyria, agyria and pachygyria
- hydrocephalus, hypoplastic brain stem and cerebellum, dysplastic corpus callosum
- with congenital muscular dystrophies

Focal Cortical Dysplasia (FCD) (106)
- focal small lesion, frequently at the bottom of a sulcus
- high T2 signal of the cortex and/or underlying white matter is commonly present
- blurring of the gray–white matter junction in Type I
- tapered linear extension of T2 hyperintensity towards the ventricle (transmantle sign) may be present in Type II

Dysembryoplastic Neuroepithelial Tumor (DNET) (108)
- multicystic "bubbly" lesion
- typically sharply demarcated and wedge-shaped extending toward the ventricle

Low-Grade Glioma (Oligodendroglioma) (161)
- gray and white matter involvement
- presence of mass effect
- T2 hyperintensity

Background

Polymicrogyria is one of the most common malformations of cortical development. It is caused by disturbance of the late neuronal migration or early cortical organization. The deep neuronal layers do not develop normally, leading to overfolding and abnormal lamination of the cortex. As a result, the polymicrogyric cortex is either four-layered or unlayered. The development of these irregular undulations occurs as early as 18 gestational weeks, before the first primary sulci form at midgestation. Because it is a primary cortical disorder, both connectivity and gyration/sulcation of these regions are very abnormal. In addition, the overlying meninges are thickened and may demonstrate vascular proliferation of unclear etiology. Causes of polymicrogyria include congenital infection (especially cytomegalovirus infection), mutations of one or multiple genes, and in-utero ischemia. It can also occur with several chromosomal deletion and duplication syndromes (Aicardi, DiGeorge, and Delleman syndromes, among others).

REFERENCES

1. Barkovich AJ. Current concepts of polymicrogyria. *Neuroradiology* 2010;**52**:479–87.

2. Leventer RJ, Jansen A, Pilz DT, *et al*. Clinical and imaging heterogeneity of polymicrogyria: a study of 328 patients. *Brain* 2010;**133**:1415–27.

3. Chang B, Walsh CA, Apse K, Bodell A. Polymicrogyria overview. In: Pagon RA, Bird TD, Dolan CR, Stephens K, eds. *GeneReviews* [Internet]. Seattle (WA): University of Washington, Seattle; 1993–2005 Apr 18 [updated 2007 Aug 06].

4. Raybaud C, Widjaja E. Development and dysgenesis of the cerebral cortex: malformations of cortical development. *Neuroimaging Clin N Am* 2011;**21**:483–543.

5. Hehr U, Schuierer G. Genetic assessment of cortical malformations. *Neuropediatrics* 2011;**42**:43–50.

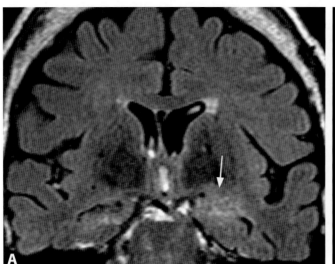
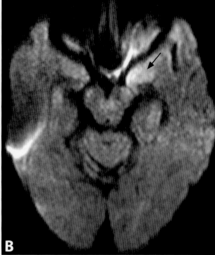

Figure 1. Coronal FLAIR image (A) shows swollen and bright left amygdala (arrow). Axial DWI (B) shows corresponding high signal intensity (arrow).

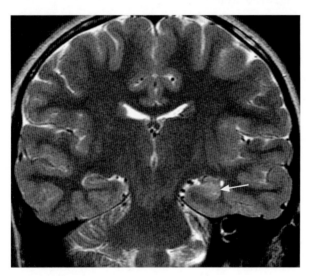

Figure 2. Coronal T2WI (A) in another patient after seizures shows a bright and somewhat expanded left hippocampus (arrow).

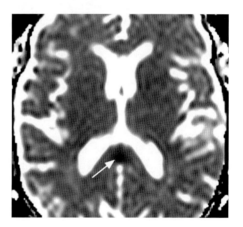

Figure 3. ADC map shows a focal low signal (arrow) in the splenium of corpus callosum.

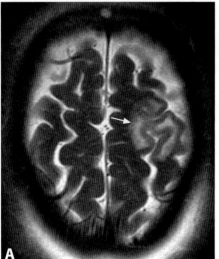
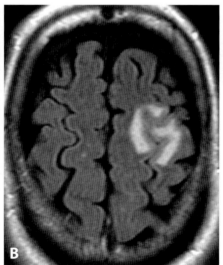
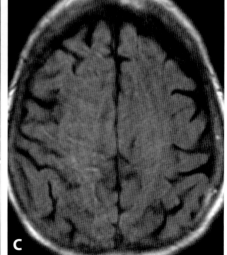

Figure 4. Axial T2WI (A) at the convexities shows high signal in the left posterior frontal lobe (arrow) involving gray and white matter, which corresponded to the epileptogenic focus on EEG. Matching FLAIR image (B) confirms findings and shows that the cortex is slightly swollen. Follow-up FLAIR image 2 months later (C) shows complete resolution of abnormalities.

Seizure-Related Changes (Peri-Ictal MRI Abnormalities)

MAURICIO CASTILLO

Specific Imaging Findings

The cortex involved is expanded and bright on T2 and FLAIR sequences. DWI shows high signal and on ADC maps values may be normal to slightly low. Mesial temporal lobes are typically affected but other parts of the brain may also be involved. Contrast enhancement is rare but has been described. Findings generally disappear from 2 weeks to 2 months after the ictus and the affected regions return to normal or become atrophic. MR spectroscopy may show normal choline, low n-acetyl aspartate (NAA) and lactate. Lactate tends to disappear within the first few days after the ictus. PET studies show increased fluoro-deoxyglucose uptake in corresponding sites. The abnormality may be localized in the splenium of the corpus callosum, also showing reduced diffusion. Occasionally the white matter can be diffusely affected, with T2 hyperintensity and reduced diffusion in a pattern similar to diffuse anoxia. In these patients, MR spectroscopy may show high glutamine and glutamate and low NAA. Patients with persistent low NAA after the first week have worse prognosis. This syndrome is called acute encephalopathy with biphasic seizures and late reduced diffusion (AESD).

Pertinent Clinical Information

Most patients have prolonged seizures which may be partial or generalized. The imaging findings are seen in the first 3 days that follow the seizure episode and thereafter tend to slowly normalize. Patients tend to be children, but these MRI findings may be seen at any age. These imaging abnormalities tend to correspond with sites of electroencephalographic ictal activity and increased radionuclide uptake on PET studies. Patients with AESD have a typical clinical course: a prolonged (> 30 min duration) usually febrile seizure followed by secondary seizures (generally clusters of partial complex ones) a few days later and encephalopathy. Infection and associated pathologic changes are considered responsible for AESD.

Differential Diagnosis

Herpes Encephalitis (20)
- no previous seizures, acute onset
- fever or viral-like illness, positive CSF

Gliomas (165, 166)
- may enhance and contain calcifications

- may be indistinguishable with follow-up needed, tumors that produce seizures may also induce cortical edema
- MR spectroscopy shows high choline levels

Focal Cortical Dysplasia (106)
- MR spectroscopy and ADC values are normal
- does not change over time

Global Anoxia (13)
- clinical history is typically suggestive of anoxic injury

Background

Seizure-induced abnormalities, also known as (transient) peri-ictal MRI abnormalities, tend to affect the cortex acutely, particularly the hippocampi. The hippocampi may be affected by the seizures directly or as a result of seizure activity elsewhere or high fever. The abnormalities are due to vasogenic, cytotoxic, or excitotoxic edema or a combination of any of these three processes. These underlying mechanisms probably include increased blood flow due to increased activity. This increased blood flow is unable to compensate the high regional metabolism and the end result is hypoxia, hypercarbia, lactic acidosis and vasodilation. Increased permeability may also play a role. Similar findings have been produced in experimental models of kainic acid-induced partial status epilepticus. As the condition progresses, the sodium–potassium pump fails and there is secondary intracellular accumulation of calcium which may induce cell death.

REFERENCES

1. Kim J-A, Chung JI, Yoon PH, *et al*. Transient MR signal changes in patients with generalized tonicoclonic seizure or status epilepticus: periictal diffusion-weighted imaging. *AJNR* 2001;**22**:1149–60.
2. Cox JE, Mathews VP, Santos CC, Elster AD. Seizure-induced transient hippocampal abnormalities on MR: correlation with positron emission tomography and electroencephalography. *AJNR* 1995;**16**:1736–8.
3. Castillo M, Smith JK, Kwock L. Proton MR spectroscopy in patients with acute temporal lobe seizures. *AJNR* 2001;**22**:152–7.
4. Takanashi J, Tada H, Terada H, Barkovich AJ. Excitotoxicity in acute encephalopathy with biphasic seizures and late reduced diffusion. *AJNR* 2009;**30**:132–5.
5. Gürtler S, Ebner A, Tuxhorn I, *et al*. Transient lesion in the splenium of the corpus callosum and antiepileptic drug withdrawal. *Neurology* 2005;**65**:1032–6.

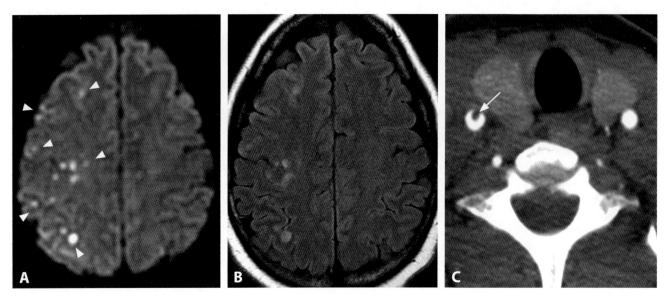

Figure 1. Axial DWI (A) and FLAIR image (B) through the level of the centrum semiovale show multiple small foci of cortical and subcortical hyperintensity (arrowheads) in the frontal and parietal lobes. Axial image from a neck CTA (C) demonstrates a filling defect (arrow) in the right common carotid artery consistent with a nonocclusive thrombus.

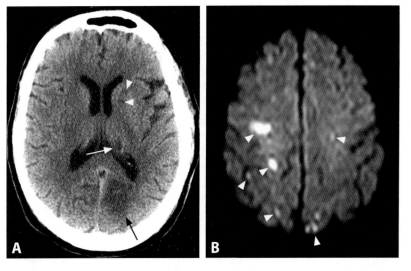

Figure 2. Axial CT image (A) in a patient with atrial fibrillation shows hypodense infarcts in the left occipital lobe (black arrow), thalamus (white arrow), and anterior limb of the internal capsule (arrowheads). DWI (B) at a higher level reveals many additional lesions (arrowheads) in bilateral cerebral hemispheres. Note involvement of multiple vascular territories and varying size of the lesions.

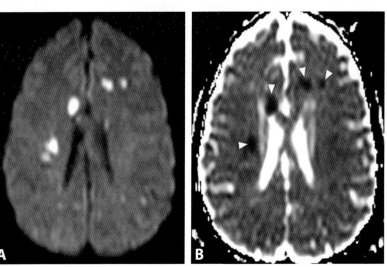

Figure 3. Axial DWIs (A) in another patient shows multiple bilateral small bright areas. Corresponding ADC map (B) demonstrates low signal (arrowheads) of the lesions, consistent with reduced diffusion and representing acute infarcts. Again note involvement of multiple vascular territories and varying size of the lesions.

Embolic Infarcts

BENJAMIN HUANG

Specific Imaging Findings

Embolic infarcts may be isolated or multiple and vary in size depending on the size of the dislodged thrombus. Small acute embolic infarcts are extremely difficult to detect prospectively on CT or conventional MR sequences, particularly in patients with pre-existing chronic ischemic lesions. The infarcts are hypodense on CT and T2 hyperintense, with little or no mass effect when small. Diffusion MRI is the most sensitive technique for early detection of infarcts, which are bright on trace DWI and dark on ADC maps, consistent with reduced diffusion. The infarcts are typically located peripherally in the cortex or subcortical white matter of the cerebral hemispheres, but involvement of deep structures such as the basal ganglia and centrum semiovale is not uncommon, as well as location along "watershed" areas between vascular territories. Most embolic infarcts occur in the middle cerebral artery territory due to preferential blood flow through the MCA. The presence of multiple infarctions involving more than one major arterial territory is highly suggestive of embolic etiology. Bilaterality and/or involvement of anterior and posterior circulations suggests a cardiac or aortic source, while multiple infarcts of differing ages suggest ongoing embolization. Like with other infarcts, enhancement may occur in the subacute period.

Pertinent Clinical Information

Signs and symptoms of embolic infarcts vary depending upon the size, number, and location, and can also be asymptomatic. Patients may present with a history of repeated transient ischemic attacks (TIAs) and 21–67% of patients presenting with TIA have focal signal abnormalities on DWI imaging in the acute setting; additional ischemic events occur in around 15% of these cases. Further evaluation of the heart and extracranial vessels is mandatory, as an underlying cardiac or vascular abnormality will be detected in roughly 78% of these patients. Approximately one-quarter of patients presenting with classical "lacunar stroke" syndromes (dysarthria–clumsy hand syndrome, pure motor stroke, pure sensory stroke, etc.) and normal CT scan show embolic stroke patterns with multiple lesions on DWI, indicating that the diagnosis of lacunar infarcts with clinical and CT findings is inaccurate.

Differential Diagnosis

Hemodynamic (Hypoperfusion) Infarctions
- infarcts are located in the watershed regions between vascular territories
- may be indistinguishable from embolic infarcts

CNS Vasculitis (123)
- can involve gray matter, subcortical white matter or deep white matter

- MRA frequently shows multifocal stenoses in large and medium vessel vasculitis
- scattered areas of pial enhancement may be found
- may present with subarachnoid hemorrhage

Small Vessel (Lacunar) Infarct
- a single lesion usually located in deep gray matter, internal capsule, pons, or corona radiata
- may be indistinguishable from an isolated embolic infaction

Septic Emboli
- often subcortical in location
- (rim) enhancement is commonly present early on (acute phase)

Fat Emboli
- usually history of a long bone fracture; petechial rash and respiratory distress present
- "starfield pattern" of innumerable punctate lesions predominantly in the "watershed" distribution

Background

Most ischemic cerebral infarcts are due to local thrombosis or thromboembolism, while a small minority has hemodynamic etiology. Thrombotic infarction occurs when thrombosis of an atherosclerotic or otherwise diseased vessel causes luminal occlusion, while embolic infarcts are caused by thrombus dislodgement and distal migration from an upstream location, the most common being carotid bifurcation and the heart. In patients with TIAs, early diffusion MRI abnormalities may be reversible and only evident during the first two days. This is presumably due to autolysis of clot and vessel recanalization. Diffusion MRI has also been used for the detection of frequently clinically silent embolic events associated with vascular and cardiac surgery as well as with diagnostic and interventional endovascular procedures.

REFERENCES

1. Kunst MM, Schaefer PW. Ischemic stroke. *Radiol Clin North Am* 2011;**49**:1–26.
2. Wessels T, Rottger C, Jauss M, *et al*. Identification of embolic stroke patterns by diffusion-weighted MRI in clinically defined lacunar stroke syndromes. *Stroke* 2005;**36**:757–61.
3. Moustafa RR, Izquierdo-Garcia D, Jones PS, *et al*. Watershed infarcts in transient ischemic attack/minor stroke with > or = 50% carotid stenosis: hemodynamic or embolic? *Stroke* 2010;**41**:1410–6.
4. Purroy F, Montaner J, Rovira A, *et al*. Higher risk of further vascular events among transient ischemic attack patients with diffusion-weighted imaging acute ischemic lesions. *Stroke* 2004;**35**:2313–9.
5. Ryu CW, Lee DH, Kim TK, *et al*. Cerebral fat embolism: diffusion-weighted magnetic resonance imaging findings. *Acta Radiol* 2005;**46**:528–33.

Brain Imaging with MRI and CT, ed. Zoran Rumboldt *et al*. Published by Cambridge University Press. © Cambridge University Press 2012.

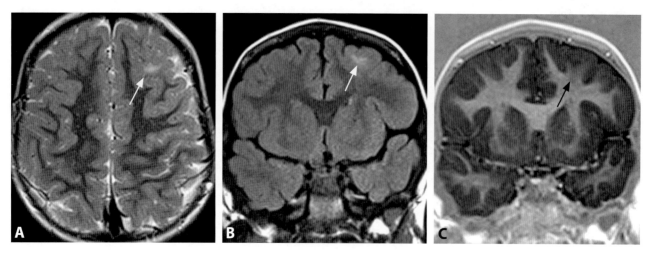

Figure 1. Axial T2WI (A) in a 4-year-old patient with intractable seizures shows a subtle left frontal subcortical hyperintensity (arrow). Coronal FLAIR image (B) also shows the subcortical hyperintensity (arrow). Coronal IR T1WI (C) reveals a slightly larger area of the subcortical decreased signal with blurring of the gray matter–white matter junction (arrow).

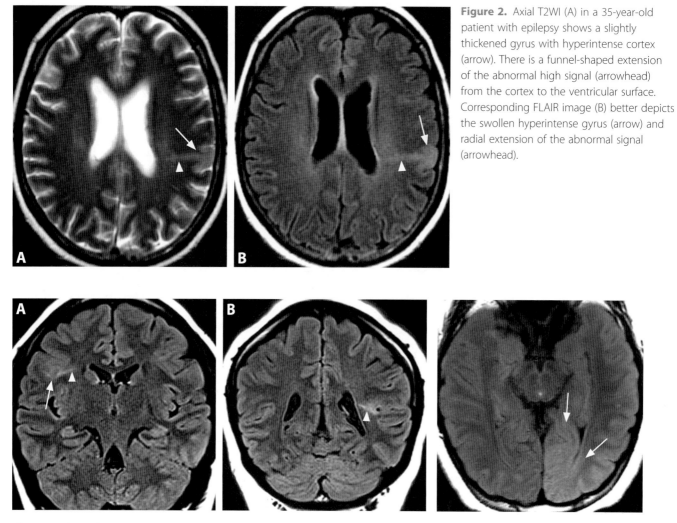

Figure 2. Axial T2WI (A) in a 35-year-old patient with epilepsy shows a slightly thickened gyrus with hyperintense cortex (arrow). There is a funnel-shaped extension of the abnormal high signal (arrowhead) from the cortex to the ventricular surface. Corresponding FLAIR image (B) better depicts the swollen hyperintense gyrus (arrow) and radial extension of the abnormal signal (arrowhead).

Figure 3. Coronal FLAIR image (A) reveals a subtle hyperintense cortical thickening (arrow) as well as extension of the abnormal signal (arrowhead) toward the ventricle. A more posterior FLAIR image (B) shows an additional similar lesion (arrowhead).

Figure 4. Axial FLAIR shows abnormal left hemisphere with prominent occipital hyperintensity (arrows).

218

Focal Cortical Dysplasia

ZORAN RUMBOLDT AND MARIA GISELE MATHEUS

Specific Imaging Findings

Focal cortical dysplasia (FCD) Type I shows only localized blurring of the gray–white matter junction and sometimes decreased volume of the subcortical white matter and cortex that may be detected with dedicated high spatial resolution heavily T1-weighted inversion recovery spin echo and 3D gradient echo images. The lesions are preferentially located at the bottom of an abnormally deep sulcus. The subcortical white matter may show hyperintense T2 signal, best depicted on high-resolution FLAIR images. These findings can be very subtle, typically not seen on CT and routine MRI scans, and in a significant number of cases not even on dedicated MR imaging. Functional studies (PET, SPECT and MEG) may be able to localize the seizure focus and tailored MRI of the suspicious area with a surface coil may then depict the lesion. Co-registration of PET and MR images substantially increases sensitivity. FCD Type II shows localized cortical thickening and T2 hyperintensity, which can characteristically extend in a tapered linear fashion towards the ventricle, known as the transmantle sign. Gray–white matter junction blurring and subtle white matter T1 hyointensity may be present. The gyral pattern may be abnormal with broad gyri and irregular sulci. A lesion detected on imaging is not necessarily the seizure focus, and FCD may occur in a multifocal and multilobar distribution.

Pertinent Clinical Information

FCD is the most common cause of epilepsy in children, and one of the more common etiologies of seizure disorders in adults. Seizures may start very early in infancy, and usually present within the first decade of life. Treatment aims at seizure control, and because the epilepsy is frequently refractory to medications, detection of the seizure focus is followed by surgical resection. Surgery is curative in a majority of patients, provided that the responsible cortical lesion is entirely removed.

Differential Diagnosis

Low Grade Glioma (161, 162)
- presence of mass effect
- absence of linear extension to the ventricular surface
- more common in temporal lobes

Dysembryoplastic Neuroepithelial Tumor (DNET) (108)
- multicystic "bubbly" lesion
- typically sharply demarcated and wedge-shaped

Ganglioglioma (166)
- mass is typically at least partly cystic
- contrast enhancement is usually present

- frequently contains calcifications
- rarely poorly delineated, solid and non-enhancing, but still with mass effect
- predilection for temporal lobe

Tuberous Sclerosis Complex (TSC) (107)
- cortical tubers are usually multiple
- presence of subependymal nodules, which calcify and may enhance with contrast
- solitary tuber is indistinguishable from FCD type II (on both histology and imaging)
- associated additional clinical and extracranial imaging findings

Background

With the improvement and increased utilization of modern imaging techniques, FCD has been increasingly recognized as a major cause of epilepsy. A recent consensus classification system by the International League against Epilepsy, based on the correlation of imaging data, electroclinical features and post-surgical seizure control with neuropathological findings, includes three subtypes: FCD Type I characterized by aberrant radial (Ia) or tangential (Ib) lamination of the neocortex affecting one or multiple lobes; FCD Type II characterized by cortical dyslamination and dysmorphic neurons without (IIa) or with balloon cells (IIb); FCD Type III occurs in combination with hippocampal sclerosis (IIIa), with neoplasms (IIIb), adjacent to vascular malformations (IIIc), and with other lesions (trauma, ischemia or encephalitis) obtained in early life (IIId). Histopathological features of FCD Type III are otherwise very similar to those in Type I. Small FCD not detected with MRI is often located in the depth of the frontal sulci.

REFERENCES

1. Colombo N, Salamon N, Raybaud C, et al. Imaging of malformations of cortical development. *Epileptic Disord* 2009;**11**:194–205.
2. Hofman PA, Fitt GJ, Harvey AS, et al. Bottom-of-sulcus dysplasia: imaging features. *AJR* 2011;**196**:881–5.
3. Abdel Razek AA, Kandell AY, Elsorogy LG, et al. Disorders of cortical formation: MR imaging features. *AJNR* 2009;**30**:4–11.
4. Blümcke I, Mühlebner A. Neuropathological work-up of focal cortical dysplasias using the new ILAE consensus classification system – practical guideline article invited by the Euro-CNS Research Committee. *Clin Neuropathol* 2011;**30**:164–77.
5. Wagner J, Urbach H, Niehusmann P, et al. Focal cortical dysplasia type IIb: completeness of cortical, not subcortical, resection is necessary for seizure freedom. *Epilepsia* 2011;**52**:1418–24.

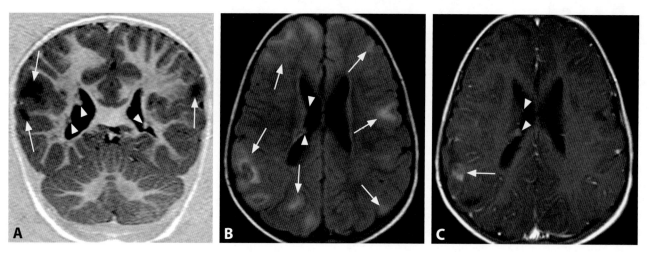

Figure 1. Coronal IR T1WI (A) shows bilateral cortico-subcortical areas of very low signal (arrows) and brighter nodules (arrowheads) protruding into the ventricles. Axial FLAIR image (B) shows multiple patchy cortico-subcortical hyperintensities (arrows). Subependymal nodules (arrowheads) are not well seen. The nodules (arrowheads) are enhancing on the matching post-contrast T1WI (C). Only one of the cortico-subcortical lesions enhances (arrow).

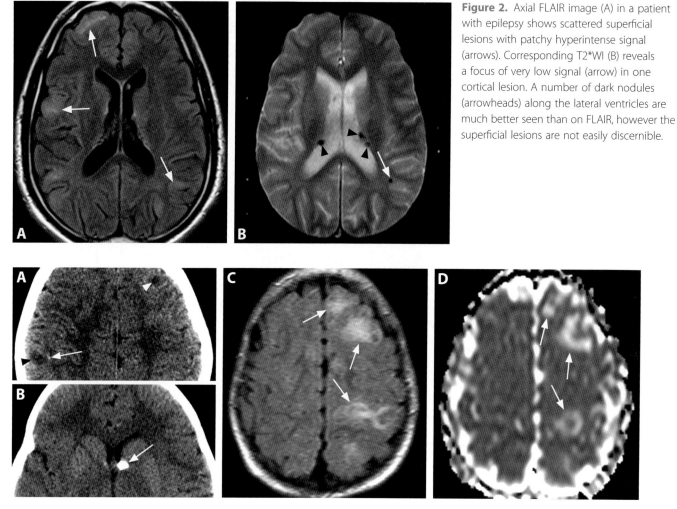

Figure 2. Axial FLAIR image (A) in a patient with epilepsy shows scattered superficial lesions with patchy hyperintense signal (arrows). Corresponding T2*WI (B) reveals a focus of very low signal (arrow) in one cortical lesion. A number of dark nodules (arrowheads) along the lateral ventricles are much better seen than on FLAIR, however the superficial lesions are not easily discernible.

Figure 3. Non-enhanced axial CT image (A) shows subtle cortico-subcortical hypodensities (arrowheads), one of which contains a peripheral calcification (arrow). Calcified subependymal nodules (arrow) are seen at a lower level (B). FLAIR (C) and ADC map (D) show patchy hyperintensity of the cortical tubers (arrows).

Tuberous Sclerosis Complex

MARIA GISELE MATHEUS

Specific Imaging Findings

Tuberous sclerosis complex (TSC) abnormalities of the CNS are cortical tubers, subependymal nodules, and subependymal giant cell astrocytomas (SEGA or SGCA). Cortical tubers are typically randomly scattered focal cortical and subcortical lesions of high T2 signal that are iso- to hypointense on T1-weighted images and primarily affecting supratentorial parenchyma, but may also be found in the cerebellum. They are best depicted on FLAIR images. The tubers generally show bright signal of increased diffusivity on ADC maps and decreased cerebral blood volume on perfusion studies. Calcifications may be present and some enhance with contrast. The white matter may show radial bands of hyperintense T2 signal and cystic degeneration (usually in the deep white matter). Subependymal nodules are multiple bilateral small (< 12 mm) sharply demarcated masses indenting the contours of the lateral ventricles. They show very low T2 signal, are frequently T1 hyperintense and enhance with gadolinium. A vast majority of subependymal nodules calcify and are hence well seen on CT and T2* MR images, as very bright and very dark nodules, respectively. SEGA are typically located at the subependymal surface of the caudate nucleus near the foramen of Monro. They are slow-growing > 12 mm minimally invasive masses with well-defined margins and avid homogeneous enhancement. Internal calcification and cysts are often present. The adjacent parenchyma is typically preserved unless anaplastic degeneration occurs. Hemimegalencephaly is also found more frequently in patients with TSC.

Pertinent Clinical Information

Epilepsy is the most prevalent clinical symptom, usually with increasing severity and frequency of seizures and poor response to medical therapy. Surgical excision of the established epileptogenic tubers is the treatment of choice. SEGA-related hydrocephalus is another important clinical concern. Patient is classified as "Definite TSC" when two major features or one major feature plus two minor features are present. "Probable TSC" and "Possible TSC" are also part of the diagnostic classification. Cortical tuber, subependymal nodule and SGCA are three distinct major features.

Differential Diagnosis

Focal Cortical Dysplasia Type IIb (Taylor's, Balloon Cell Type) (106)
- a single focus of cortical dysplasia with associated radial white matter abnormality
- no subependymal nodules
- FCD and TS are indistinguishable histologically

Subependymal Nodular Heterotopia (117)
- isointense signal to gray matter
- absence of calcifications
- no contrast enhancement

Congenital CMV Infection (184)
- periventricular calcification with multiple other brain abnormalities (polymicrogyria, white matter lesions)

Background

TSC is the second most common neurocutaneous syndrome, autosomal dominant with a de-novo mutation rate of up to 70%, characterized by the formation of hamartomatous lesions in multiple organs. The genes responsible for the disorder are tumor suppressor genes *TSC1* (9q34), which encodes the protein *hamarti*, and *TSC2* (16p13), which encodes the protein tuberin. These proteins have a role in regulation of cell growth and differentiation. The disease has complete penetrance but with a high phenotypic variability: some patients have obvious signs at birth, while others remain undiagnosed for many years. SGCA are primary brain tumors formed by astrocytes and giant cells that occur in TSC with a prevalence of 1.7–26%. Only a single cortical tuber may be present in some patients, which is indistinguishable from Type IIb focal cortical dysplasia (FCD), so TSC should be considered when FCD is associated with seizure onset in infancy, family history of seizures, and peridysplastic calcification. Around 20% of TSC patients do not have either *TSC1* or *TSC2* mutations. Diffusion tensor imaging unveils the microstructural abnormalities of the normal-appearing white matter, while FDG-PET is very helpful in determining the seizure foci.

REFERENCES

1. Griffiths PD, Hoggard N. Distribution and conspicuity of intracranial abnormalities on MR imaging in adults with tuberous sclerosis complex: a comparison of sequences including ultrafast T2-weighted images. *Epilepsia* 2009;**50**:2605–10.

2. Hirfanoglu T, Gupta A. Tuberous sclerosis complex with a single brain lesion on MRI mimicking focal cortical dysplasia. *Pediatr Neurol* 2010;**42**:343–7.

3. Garaci FG, Floris R, Bozzao A, *et al.* Increased brain apparent diffusion coefficient in tuberous sclerosis. *Radiology* 2004;**232**:461–5.

4. Widjaja E, Wilkinson ID, Griffiths PD. Magnetic resonance perfusion imaging in malformations of cortical development. *Acta Radiol* 2007;**48**:907–17.

5. Baskin HJ. The pathogenesis and imaging of tuberous sclerosis complex. *Pediatr Radiol* 2008;**38**:936–52.

Brain Imaging with MRI and CT, ed. Zoran Rumboldt *et al.* Published by Cambridge University Press. © Cambridge University Press 2012.

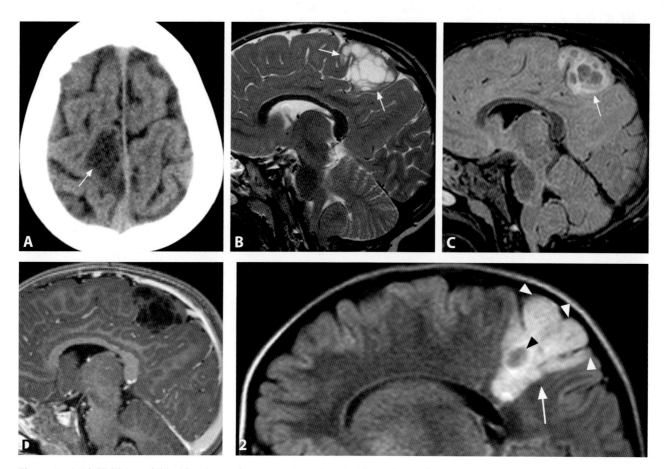

Figure 1. Axial CT (A) in a child with seizures shows a cortico-subcortical hypodensity (arrow) without mass effect and with subtle internal heterogeneity. Sagittal T2WI through the lesion (B) shows its bright cyst-like appearance with internal septations (arrow). Corresponding FLAIR image (C) reveals bright internal septa and lesion periphery producing a multicystic "bubbly" appearance. The cyst-like structures are hypointense and there is no enhancement on post-contrast T1WI (D).

Figure 2. A right parietal wedge-shaped hyperintensity (arrow) is detected on sagittal FLAIR image. The lesion shows enlarged but preserved gyrus-like configuration of the cortex (white arrowheads) with a subcortical pseudocyst (black arrowhead).

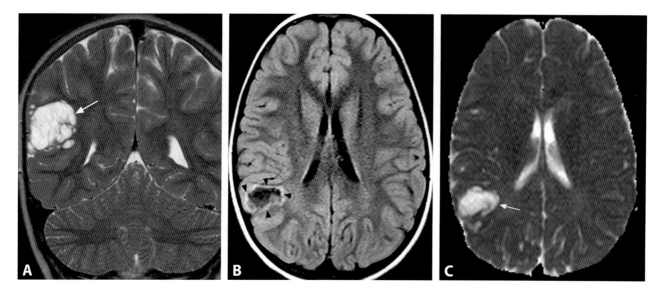

Figure 3. Coronal T2WI (A) in a 9-year-old girl shows a mass (arrow) in the right supramarginal gyrus with a multilobular, multicystic structure. There is no perifocal edema. On axial FLAIR image (B), the typical peripheral hyperintense rim (arrowheads) surrounding a hypointense core is present. Corresponding ADC map (C) shows the lesion to be very bright (arrow), reflecting a high degree of diffusivity.

Dysembryoplastic Neuroepithelial Tumor (DNT, DNET)

GIOVANNI MORANA

Specific Imaging Findings

On CT, dysembryoplastic neuroepithelial tumor (DNT or DNET) appears as a low density cortico-subcortical supratentorial area. Calcifications are rare. Remodeling of the adjacent calvarium is frequent with superficially located tumors. On MRI, the classic appearance is of a well-demarcated pseudocystic lesion, strongly T2 hyperintense and T1 hypointense with variable signal on FLAIR images. Mass effect is minimal to absent, there is no surrounding vasogenic edema. DNTs may have a triangular-shaped pattern with the base along the cortical surface with preserved gyral pattern. Thin hyperintense signal on FLAIR images is visible both along the surface (bright rim) and as stripes along thin internal septa, resulting in a very characteristic multicystic, "bubbly" appearance. Additional small cysts, separated from the main mass, are often located in the neighboring cortex or subcortical white matter. Some lesions may show a more heterogeneous signal consistent with solid, cystic, or semiliquid structures. Solid components may either be solitary or form a multinodular pattern interspersed within a cystic frame. Contrast enhancement is rare, variable, and more often ring-like. Bleeding is also rare. Tumors show increased diffusivity with high ADC values and low rCBV on perfusion imaging. The MRS pattern is nonspecific with increase in mI/Cr and Cho/NAA ratios. Lactate and lipid peaks are usually absent.

Pertinent Clinical Information

DNTs are usually diagnosed in patients under the age of 20 with a history of seizures that do not respond well to medication. The natural history of the lesion is characterized by very slow increase in size over time. The prognosis after complete surgical excision is favorable, and seizure control dramatically improves; neverthe-less, recurrence after surgical removal and/or malignant trans-formation have been reported.

Differential Diagnosis

Ganglioglioma (166)
- more mass effect and enhancement, edema may be present
- usually a single or a few "cysts", "bubbly" appearance rare
- calcifications are common

Angiocentric Glioma
- cortical rim of hyperintensity on T1-weighted images
- stalk-like extension to the adjacent ventricle on T2-weighted images

Focal Cortical Dysplasia (106)
- focal cortical thickening with loss of gray–white matter demarcation

- funnel-shaped high T2 signal in the subcortical white matter
- no contrast enhancement
- isolated tuber (calcifications extremely common)

Giant Perivascular Spaces; Neuroepithelial Cyst (168, 169)
- non-enhancing CSF-like cyst with minimal to no surrounding signal abnormality

Background

DNTs are classified as neuronal and mixed neuronal–glial tumors. The adjacent cortex usually shows a disordered architecture, with the tumor originating on a background of cortical dysplasia. They are preferentially located, in decreasing order, in the temporal, frontal, parietal, and occipital lobes; less common locations are extracortical areas such as the caudate nucleus, lateral ventricle, septum pellucidum, and fornix. Two main histological forms have been described – simple and complex variants. The simple form is characterized by a unique specific glioneuronal element, corresponding to pseudocysts on MRI. This glioneuronal unit is composed by oligodendrocyte-like tumor cells and floating neurons within a myxoid tumor matrix. The complex form is characterized by a more heterogeneous architecture composed of multiple glial nodules resembling astrocytomas, oligodendroglio-mas, or oligoastrocytomas, in addition to the distinctive glio-neuronal element. Neuropathological distinction of simple and complex DNT variants is not fully reflected on MRI, but calcifi-cations, hemorrhage, and contrast enhancement occur only in complex variants.

REFERENCES

1. Ostertun B, Wolf HK, Campos MG, et al. Dysembryoplastic neuroepithelial tumors: MR and CT evaluation. AJNR 1996;17:419–30.
2. Campos AR, Clusmann H, von Lehe M, et al. Simple and complex dysembryoplastic neuroepithelial tumor (DNT) variants: clinical profile, MRI, and histopathology. Neuroradiology 2009;51:433–43.
3. Daumas-Duport C. Dysembryoplastic neuroepithelial tumors. Brain Pathol 1993;3:255–68.
4. Bulakbasi N, Kocaoglu M, Sanal TH, Tayfun C. Dysembryoplastic neuroepithelial tumors: proton MR spectroscopy, diffusion and perfusion characteristics. Neuroradiology 2007;49:805–12.
5. Ray WZ, Blackburn SL, Casavilca-Zambrano S, et al. Clinicopathologic features of recurrent dysembryoplastic neuroepithelial tumor and rare malignant transformation: a report of 5 cases and review of the literature. J Neurooncol 2009;94:283–92.

Brain Imaging with MRI and CT, ed. Zoran Rumboldt *et al.* Published by Cambridge University Press. © Cambridge University Press 2012.

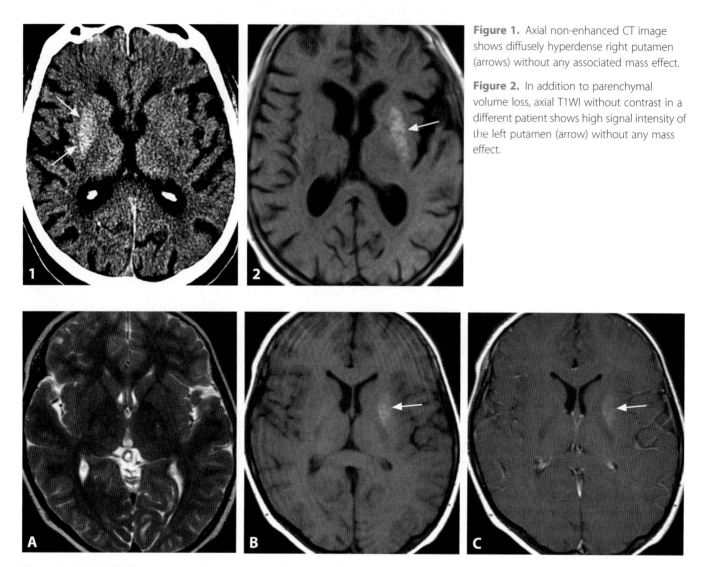

Figure 1. Axial non-enhanced CT image shows diffusely hyperdense right putamen (arrows) without any associated mass effect.

Figure 2. In addition to parenchymal volume loss, axial T1WI without contrast in a different patient shows high signal intensity of the left putamen (arrow) without any mass effect.

Figure 3. Axial T2WI (A) in a 63-year-old woman with diabetes mellitus and right-sided involuntary movements is unremarkable. T1WI (B) reveals hyperintense left putamen (arrow). There is no enhancement of the lesion (arrow) on post-contrast T1WI (C).

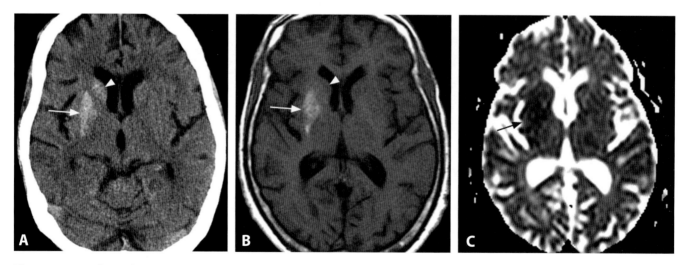

Figure 4. Non-enhanced CT image (A) in a 71-year-old patient with diabetes and left-sided chorea shows hyperdense putamen (arrow) and caudate nucleus head (arrowhead). T1WI without contrast (B) shows putaminal hyperintensity (arrow) and normal caudate head (arrowhead). Mildly decreased diffusivity of the putamen (arrow) is present on corresponding ADC map (C).

Nonketotic Hyperglycemia With Hemichorea–Hemiballismus

ZORAN RUMBOLDT

Specific Imaging Findings

T1 hyperintensity in the contralateral striatum, especially putamen, without edema or mass effect is the characteristic imaging finding of nonketotic hyperglycemia with hemichorea–hemiballismus (NK hyperglycemia with HCHB). CT commonly shows corresponding hyperdensity, while some lesions may remain isodense and therefore undetectable. Mild to moderate decrease in diffusion (low ADC signal) is commonly found, while increased susceptibility change (hypointensity) may also be present, suggesting paramagnetic mineral deposition. There is no contrast enhancement of the lesions, which demonstrate variable and frequently normal T2 signal. In addition to the putamen and caudate, globus pallidus and midbrain (subthalamic nucleus) may also be involved; bilateral lesions also occur (with bilateral clinical presentation) but are much less common. There is also decreased perfusion within the lesions and reduced FDG uptake on PET scans. MR spectroscopy shows decreased NAA, increased choline, and elevated lactate peak. The lesions may disappear with appropriate treatment or persist for years.

Pertinent Clinical Information

HCHB is usually a continuous, nonpatterned, involuntary movement disorder caused by basal ganglia dysfunction, described in nonketotic hyperglycemic patients. It occurs in elderly individuals with primary diabetes mellitus, more commonly in women and Asian populations. In most patients hemichorea improves along with the disappearance of the lesions. Correction of underlying hyperglycemia and supportive care results in resolution within days to weeks.

Differential Diagnosis

Hypertensive Hematoma (177)
- associated mass effect and edema
- clinical presentation without hemichorea–hemiballismus

Ischemic Infarction (152)
- presence of mass effect
- homogenously CT hyperdense/T1 hyperintense lesions selectively involving striatum would be highly unusual
- clinical presentation without hemichorea–hemiballismus

Leigh Disease (10)
- occurs in children and young adults
- hemichorea–hemiballismus is an unusual presentation

Methanol Intoxication (5)
- lesions are characteristically bilateral
- typical imaging findings of hemorrhage, when present
- clinical presentation without hemichorea–hemiballismus

Hypoxic Ischemic Encephalopathy (7)
- occurs in neonates
- bilateral involvement
- T1 hyperintensity around the posterior limb of the internal capsule including thalamus

Background

Despite characteristic imaging findings and clinical manifestations, the underlying mechanism is still unclear. The markedly reduced rates of cerebral glucose metabolism in the corresponding lesions on T1-weighted magnetic resonance images provide evidence of regional metabolic failure. Usually, both the clinical syndrome and neuroimaging abnormalities are reversible. A transient, reversible metabolic impairment within the basal ganglia has been considered a possible cause of this disorder. The imaging abnormalities may be a consequence of an ischemic episode caused by prolonged, uncontrolled hyperglycemia, and inflammation within the CNS may participate in the pathogenesis. The imaging findings are thought to be due to gemistocytic astrocyte accumulation. T1 hyperintensity may be from the protein hydration layer inside the cytoplasm of swollen gemistocytes appearing after an acute cerebral injury. These astrocytes also express metallothionein with zinc, which is thought to be the cause of asymmetric hypointensity of the posterior putamen that may be observed on susceptibility-weighted images (SWI).

REFERENCES

1. Cherian A, Thomas B, Baheti NN, et al. Concepts and controversies in nonketotic hyperglycemia-induced hemichorea: further evidence from susceptibility-weighted MR imaging. J Magn Reson Imaging 2009;29:699–703.

2. Lee EJ, Choi JY, Lee SH, et al. Hemichorea– hemiballism in primary diabetic patients: MR correlation. J Comput Assist Tomogr 2002;26:905–11.

3. Oh SH, Lee KY, Im JH, Lee MS. Chorea associated with non-ketotic hyperglycemia and hyperintensity basal ganglia lesion on T1-weighted brain MRI study: a meta-analysis of 53 cases including four present cases. J Neurol Sci 2002;200:57–62.

4. Lai PH, Chen PC, Chang MH, et al. In vivo proton MR spectroscopy of chorea–ballismus in diabetes mellitus. Neuroradiology 2001;43:525–31.

5. Wang JH, Wu T, Deng BQ, et al. Hemichorea–hemiballismus associated with nonketotic hyperglycemia: a possible role of inflammation. J Neurol Sci 2009;284:198–202.

Brain Imaging with MRI and CT, ed. Zoran Rumboldt et al. Published by Cambridge University Press. © Cambridge University Press 2012.

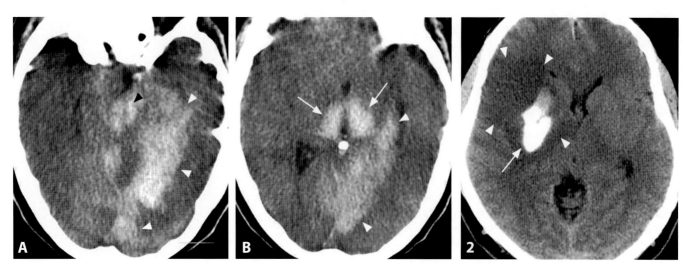

Figure 1. Non-enhanced CT images (A and B) obtained a few hours after attempted intra-arterial thrombolysis of a basilar artery thrombosis show high-density material in the brainstem (black arrowhead), left occipital and medial temporal lobes (white arrowheads), and bilateral thalami (arrows), which measures 70–90 HU.

Figure 2. Non-enhanced CT image immediately following endovascular recanalization of the right MCA occlusion. Very bright (HU over 200) material is present in the right basal ganglia (arrow). Note hypodensity and mass effect of the acute infarction (arrowheads).

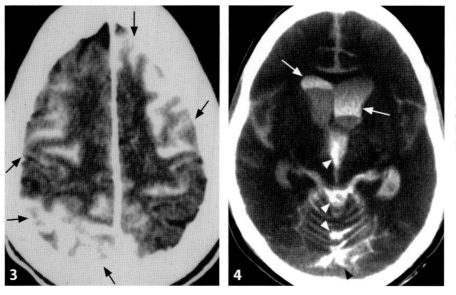

Figure 3. Non-enhanced CT obtained a few hours after coronary artery stenting shows marked hyperdensity of the subarachnoid spaces (arrows), measuring 80–160 HU.

Figure 4. CT image following SAH and subsequent embolization of three cerebral aneurysms shows fluid layering in the frontal horns, with the brighter fluid (arrows) on top. Note additional bright material (arrowheads).

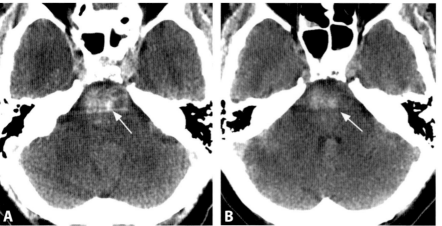

Figure 5. Non-enhanced CT image obtained a few hours after basilar artery endovascular recanalization (A) shows a very hyperdense material (arrow) within the pons, ill-defined and without notable mass effect. Follow-up CT image (B) acquired 12 h later reveals substantial interval decrease in the attenuation (arrow).

Hyperdensity Following Endovascular Intervention

ZORAN RUMBOLDT AND BENJAMIN HUANG

Specific Imaging Findings

Head CT scans obtained immediately following procedures involving intra-arterial injection of large volumes of iodinated contrast media may show parenchymal or subarachnoid space enhancement mimicking intracranial hemorrhage. The findings include diffuse parenchymal hyperintensity and increased subarachnoid space attenuation usually corresponding to the arterial territory injected, without associated gyral swelling. Occasionally, ventricular CSF may also demonstrate increased density. The presence of contrast does not exclude hemorrhage, as the two can coexist. Measuring the attenuation of the involved regions may be helpful, as contrast enhancement will usually demonstrate higher values (as high as 160 HU) than blood. Follow-up CT is also useful, as the contrast enhancement typically resolves completely within 24 h. In patients undergoing attempted endovascular revascularization for acute infarct, a hyperdense lesion with maximum HU > 90 that persists after 24 h is considered contrast extravasation and is highly associated with hematoma formation. On the other hand, the common finding of parenchymal, subarachnoid, and intraventricular hyperattenuation due to contrast accumulation following uneventful embolization of cerebral aneurysms is almost always clinically insignificant. In unclear cases parenchymal contrast stain may also be differentiated from hemorrhage by performing brain MRI. Dual-energy CT with 80 and 140 KV seems to reliably distinguish intracranial hemorrhage from iodinated contrast. In acute ischemic patients treated with intra-arterial thrombolysis, sulcal hyperintensity may be found on FLAIR images, which is likely caused by iodinated contrast medium. In rare patients with contrast-induced encephalopathy, early imaging demonstrates edema in addition to the cortical contrast enhancement, which usually resolves within a few days.

Pertinent Clinical Information

Rare cases of contrast-induced neurotoxicity have been reported following endovascular interventions which require large volumes of iodinated contrast (e.g. peripheral, visceral, coronary, or cerebral angiography), with both ionic and non-ionic low-osmolar contrast agents. The neurotoxicity typically manifests within a few hours of contrast injection. Patients may become acutely encephalopathic or experience focal neurologic symptoms such as weakness, numbness, aphasia, cortical blindness, or seizure. Symptoms typically begin to resolve within hours to days, and most patients experience a complete recovery. Asymptomatic contrast staining following endovascular intracranial interventions is much more common.

Differential Diagnosis

Acute Hemorrhage (177, 178, 179)
- no history of preceding endovascular procedure
- density lower than contrast (typically 40–60 HU)

- attenuation remains about the same or increases over the first 3 days (as the clot retracts)

Background

A small amount of contrast leakage into the CSF always occurs, but this is insufficient to produce radiographically detectable enhancement. The amount of injected contrast material has been associated with asymptomatic transient hyperdensity of the brain parenchyma and subarachnoid spaces that occurs after endovascular treatment of intracranial aneurysms. Large contrast leaks following intraarterial injections are believed to be due to disruption of the blood–brain barrier (BBB) caused by the osmotic effect of the contrast media on the vascular endothelium. As the solution draws water out of the endothelial cells, cell shrinkage causes the intervening tight junctions to separate, allowing spread of the contrast agent into the extracellular space. With contrast injections into recently infarcted tissue, as occurs during attempted revascularization for acute strokes, the BBB disruption may already have occurred. Sulcal hyperintensity on FLAIR images following intra-arterial thrombolysis has been associated with subsequent hemorrhagic transformation. The mechanism behind the occasional contrast encephalopathy remains unclear – it has been suggested that when contrast permeates the brain parenchyma it causes neuronal excitotoxicity and reversible cortical dysfunction. Contrast neurotoxicity may in rare cases result in irreversible injury.

REFERENCES

1. Brisman JL, Jilani M, McKinney JS. Contrast enhancement hyperdensity after endovascular coiling of intracranial aneurysms. *AJNR* 2008;29:588–93.
2. Yoon W, Seo JJ, Kim JK, et al. Contrast enhancement and contrast extravasation on computed tomography after intra-arterial thrombolysis in patients with acute ischemic stroke. *Stroke* 2004;35:876–81.
3. Phan CM, Yoo AJ, Hirsch JA, et al. Differentiation of hemorrhage from iodinated contrast in different intracranial compartments using dual-energy head CT. *AJNR* 2012; Mar 1. [Epub ahead of print].
4. Kim EY, Kim SS, Na DG, et al. Sulcal hyperintensity on fluid-attenuated inversion recovery imaging in acute ischemic stroke patients treated with intra-arterial thrombolysis: iodinated contrast media as its possible cause and the association with hemorrhagic transformation. *J Comput Assist Tomogr* 2005;29:264–9.
5. Guimaraens L, Vivas E, Fonnegra A, et al. Transient encephalopathy from angiographic contrast: a rare complication in neurointerventional procedures. *Cardiovasc Intervent Radiol* 2010;33:383–8.

Brain Imaging with MRI and CT, ed. Zoran Rumboldt et al. Published by Cambridge University Press. © Cambridge University Press 2012.

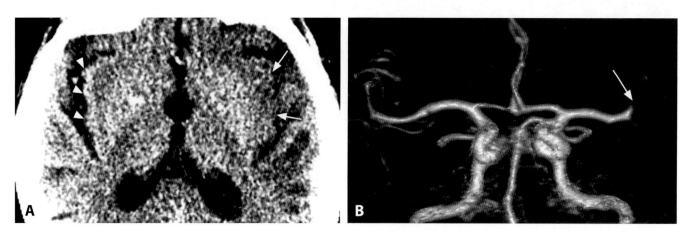

Figure 1. Non-enhanced axial CT image (A) viewed with stroke windows (W 30, L 30) shows loss of the normal gray matter density of the left insular ribbon (arrows). Compare to the normal cortical insular ribbon on the right (arrowheads). CTA (B) demonstrates occlusion of the left M2 branches (arrow).

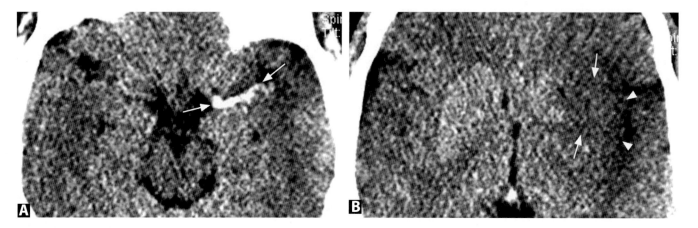

Figure 2. Non-enhanced axial CT (A) viewed on stroke windows shows a hyperdense left middle cerebral artery (arrows), indicative of acute thrombus. Image at the level of the basal ganglia (B) demonstrates loss of normal gray matter density in the left lateral lentiform nuclei (arrows) and in the left insula (arrowheads).

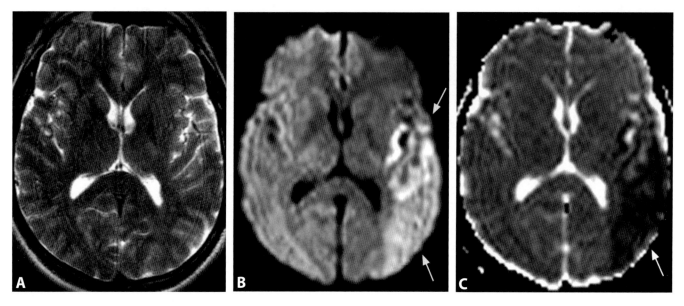

Figure 3. Axial T2WI (A) obtained within 3 h of ictus is normal. Corresponding DWI image (B) and ADC map (C) demonstrate reduced diffusion in the posterior left MCA territory (arrows).

Early (Hyperacute) Infarct

BENJAMIN HUANG

Specific Imaging Findings

In the hyperacute stage (< 6 h), non-contrast CT is negative in anywhere from 20 to 70% of cases, the earlier obtained after ictus the more likely it is to appear normal. Early changes of cerebral infarction on CT include loss of the gray–white matter (GM–WM) differentiation (loss of the insular ribbon, deep gray matter definition, and focal cortico-subcortical differentiation), effacement of the cortical sulci, and a hyperdense vessel (usually middle cerebral artery) suggestive of acute thrombus. Viewing with stroke windows (such as W 30, L 30) often improves the conspicuity of the findings, especially the loss of the GM–WM differentiation.

Diffusion MRI is by far the most sensitive technique for detection of hyperacute infarcts and becomes positive within 30 min after vessel occlusion. Infarcted tissue shows hyperintensity on DWI and low signal on ADC maps, consistent with reduced diffusion. Abnormalities on T2WI and FLAIR images usually become evident 3–6 h after onset, as increased signal intensity and mild swelling of the infarcted tissue. A hyperintense vessel may be seen on FLAIR, corresponding to CT hyperdensity. Contrast-enhanced T1WI may demonstrate arterial enhancement secondary to slow flow, collateral flow, or hyperperfusion following early recanalization. Parenchymal, frequently "gyriform" enhancement may occasionally appear early, suggesting higher hemorrhage risk. CTA and MRA demonstrate arterial occlusions and critical stenoses as well as the status of collateral vessels.

Pertinent Clinical Information

The most common presenting symptoms are sudden onset of unilateral weakness or numbness, dysphasia, and visual disturbances; dizziness, impairment of consciousness, and severe headache may be present. Although it is often clear when a patient is having a stroke, the clinical diagnosis can be incorrect in up to 20–30% of cases. Furthermore, decisions on whether to attempt intravenous or intra-arterial recanalization in part depend upon the imaging findings. The goals of imaging in the hyperacute period are therefore (1) detection of alternative explanation for symptoms (hematoma, neoplasm); (2) identification of contra-indications for attempted recanalization (hemorrhage or hypodensity in over one-third of the MCA territory); and (3) detection of large vessel occlusions. The window for intravenous thrombolysis according to the ECASS-III trial is up to 4.5 h after onset. Intra-arterial recanalization can generally be performed up to 6–12 h. CT and MR perfusion in hyperacute stroke patients may potentially allow differentiation of the infarct core from the salvageable ischemic penumbra (indicated by the area of perfusion mismatch), possibly guiding treatment decisions. The volume of DWI abnormality >70–100 ml indicates a high risk and poor outcome with recanalization.

Differential Diagnosis

Neoplasm (153, 161, 162)
- mass effect and vasogenic edema frequently present
- abnormality does not correspond to an arterial territory
- commonly enhance with contrast

Cerebritis
- abnormality does not correspond to an arterial territory
- may enhance

Venous Infarct (181)
- lesion in a nonarterial territorial distribution
- evidence of cortical vein or venous sinus thrombosis

Background

DWI changes in hyperacute ischemic stroke reflect cytotoxic edema caused by failure of cell membrane ATP-dependent Na^+/K^+ pump, which in turn results in an alteration of water homeostasis. Cell swelling (cytotoxic edema) occurs as water migrates from the extracellular into the intracellular space, resulting in a reduction of extracellular volume and restriction of overall water motion. These changes begin within minutes of ischemia onset, and because the overall water content remains constant, there is no change in volume in the very acute setting. ADC values continue to decrease with its nadir at 1–4 days. Tissue swelling and development of T2 hyperintensity represent the subsequent development of vasogenic edema caused by extravasation of water from vessels into the extracellular space; however, without the typical finger-like appearance on imaging studies. Some diffusion changes are reversible in the very early stages of ischemia, particularly following recanalization, but this may be only temporary as true DWI reversibility is overall very rare.

REFERENCES

1. Fiebach J, Jansen O, Schellinger P, *et al.* Comparison of CT with diffusion-weighted MRI in patients with hyperacute stroke. *Neuroradiology* 2001;**43**:628–32.
2. Gonzalez RG. Imaging-guided acute ischemic stroke therapy: from "time is brain" to "physiology is brain". *AJNR* 2006;**27**:728–35.
3. Kloska SP, Wintermark M, Englehorn T, *et al.* Acute stroke magnetic resonance imaging: current status and future perspective. *Neuroradiology* 2010;**52**:189–201.
4. Schaefer PW, Copen WA, Lev MH, *et al.* Diffusion-weighted imaging in acute stroke. *Neuroimag Clin N Am* 2005;**15**:503–30.
5. Mlynash M, Lansberg MG, De Silva DA, *et al.* Refining the definition of the malignant profile: insights from the DEFUSE-EPITHET pooled data set. *Stroke* 2011;**42**:1270–5.

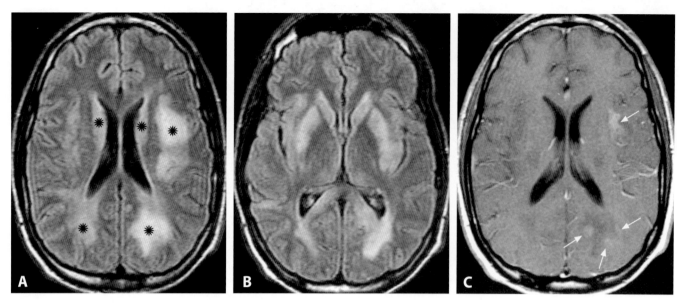

Figure 1. Axial FLAIR images (A and B) in a patient following a smallpox vaccination demonstrate bilateral areas of increased signal (*), predominantly affecting the white matter and the basal ganglia. Note the asymmetry in the distribution and size of white matter lesions. Axial post-contrast T1WI (C) at a similar level as A shows patchy areas of enhancement (arrows) within some of the lesions in the left cerebral hemisphere.

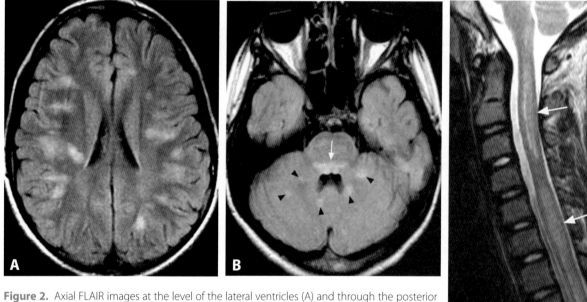
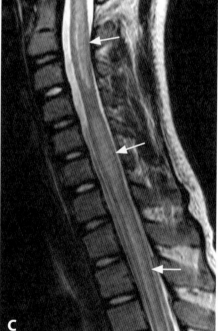

Figure 2. Axial FLAIR images at the level of the lateral ventricles (A) and through the posterior fossa (B) in a child demonstrate patchy bilateral, asymmetric areas of increased signal in the cerebral white matter, as well as in the dorsal pons (arrow) and cerebellar white matter (arrowheads). Sagittal T2WI through the cervical and upper thoracic spine (C) demonstrates long segments of intramedullary hyperintense signal (arrows) with associated spinal cord enlargement.

Acute Disseminated Encephalomyelitis (ADEM)

BENJAMIN HUANG

Specific Imaging Findings

CT is usually normal unless lesions are large, when they appear as subtle hypodensities. On MRI, lesions of acute disseminated encephalomyelitis (ADEM) are typically multiple and asymmetrically distributed, usually involving cerebral white matter and deep gray matter nuclei. Cortical gray matter and infratentorial involvement is also common. The lesions are T2 hyperintense and iso- to faintly hypointense on T1-weighted images, usually with little mass effect. Periventricular MS-like lesions and "black holes" on T1-weighted images are unusual. Contrast enhancement is uncommon and can have variable appearances. Diffusion findings vary, in part depending upon the stage of disease, with reduced diffusion more commonly observed in the acute stage. PWI shows reduced or normal rCBV within lesions. MRS will show lactate and normal or reduced levels of NAA in the acute stage, and reduced NAA and increased choline in the subacute stage. Approximately 30% of patients with ADEM will also have spinal cord involvement on MRI, usually extending over multiple levels with frequent enlargement of the brainstem and spinal cord.

Pertinent Clinical Information

ADEM is a monophasic disorder which typically begins within days to weeks after a prior infectious episode or vaccination. Although the syndrome can occur at any age, it is more common in children. Patients present with rapid onset encephalopathy which may be preceded by a prodromal phase of fever, malaise, headache, nausea, and vomiting. Neurologic symptoms of ADEM include unilateral or bilateral pyramidal signs, acute hemiplegia, ataxia, cranial nerve palsies, visual loss due to optic neuritis, seizures, impaired speech, paresthesias, signs of spinal cord involvement, and alterations in mental status, ranging from lethargy to coma.

Differential Diagnosis

Multiple Sclerosis (115, 125)

- absence of a diffuse bilateral lesion pattern
- two or more periventricular lesions (Dawson's fingers)
- presence of black holes
- deep gray matter involvement not typically seen

Encephalitis

- predominant gray matter involvement
- symmetric lesions are common

Background

ADEM is an immune-mediated inflammatory disorder with an autoimmune reaction to myelin. The exact pathogenesis is unclear, but two leading theories are recognized. The first proposes that structural similarity between a recently introduced pathogen and the host's own myelin proteins results in a cross-reactive anti-myelin immune response through molecular mimicry. The second theory suggests that CNS tissue damage from an infection causes segregated myelin antigens to leak into the systemic circulation through a damaged blood–brain barrier, eliciting a T-cell response which, in turn, further damages the CNS. Histologically, ADEM has a similar appearance to multiple sclerosis. On the basis of a single clinical episode, ADEM and MS may be impossible to distinguish from one another, while the accuracy of distinction using different MRI criteria may at best approach 90%. Recurrent and multiphasic forms of the disorder have been described. Up to 28% of patients initially diagnosed with ADEM go on to develop multiple sclerosis. With appropriate treatment (steroids, IVIg, and/or plasmapheresis), symptoms may rapidly resolve or may require weeks to months to improve. Most patients with ADEM make a complete recovery, but permanent neurologic sequelae occur in one-third of cases. Low ADC values and brainstem location of lesions may portray a worse prognosis.

REFERENCES

1. Balasubramanya KS, Kovoor JME, Jayakumar PN, et al. Diffusion-weighted imaging and proton MR spectroscopy in the characterization of acute disseminated encephalomyelitis. *Neuroradiology* 2007;**49**:177–83.
2. Bernarding J, Braun J, Koennecke HC. Diffusion- and perfusion-weighted MR imaging in a patient with acute demyelinating encephalomyelitis (ADEM). *J Magn Reson Imaging* 2002;**15**:96–100.
3. Rossi A. Imaging of acute disseminated encephalomyelitis. *Neuroimag Clin N Am* 2008;**18**:149–61.
4. Callen DJ, Shroff MM, Branson HM, et al. Role of MRI in the differentiation of ADEM from MS in children. *Neurology* 2009;**72**:968–73.
5. Donmez FY, Aslan H, Coskun M. Evaluation of possible prognostic factors of fulminant acute disseminated encephalomyelitis (ADEM) on magnetic resonance imaging with fluid-attenuated inversion recovery (FLAIR) and diffusion-weighted imaging. *Acta Radiol* 2009;**50**:334–9.

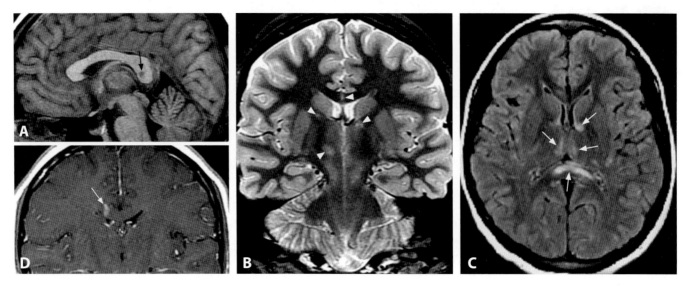

Figure 1. Midsagittal T1WI (A) shows a rounded hypointense lesion (arrow) in the substance of the splenium of the corpus callosum. Coronal fat saturated T2-weighted image (B) shows multiple moderately bright lesions (arrowheads) in the central white and gray matter. Axial FLAIR image (C) reveals multiple lesions including the deep gray matter nuclei and the callosal splenium (arrows). After contrast administration, there is enhancement of the right-sided periventricular lesion on a coronal T1WI (D).

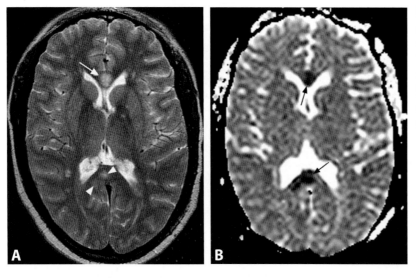

Figure 2. Axial T2WI (A) in a 29-year-old woman shows a hyperintense rounded lesion located centrally within the genu of the corpus callosum (arrow). There is another similar lesion within the splenium (arrowheads). A few additional punctuate areas of high T2 signal are present in the periventricular white matter and left internal capsule. ADC map (B) reveals dark signal of the corpus callosum lesions (arrows).

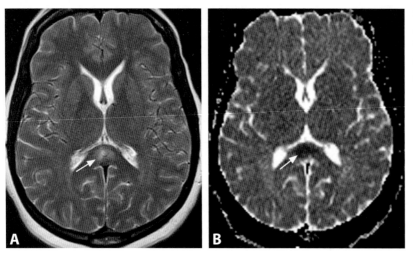

Figure 3. Axial T2WI (A) in a different patient demonstrates a hyperintense central lesion (arrow) within the splenium of the corpus callosum. Corresponding ADC map (B) shows very low signal consistent with associated reduced diffusivity (arrow).

Susac Syndrome

MAURICIO CASTILLO

Specific Imaging Findings

MR is the imaging method of choice and shows multiple small foci of high T2 signal intensity throughout the white and gray matter, supra- and infra-tentorially. Corpus callosum is always involved. Involvement of gray matter is more apparent within the basal ganglia and thalami but also occurs in the cortex. Many lesions enhance after contrast administration during the acute and subacute periods of the disease. Leptomeningeal contrast enhancement may also be seen and as the CSF has increased proteins its signal intensity on FLAIR images may be increased. During the acute period lesions tend to show reduced ADC. A pathognomonic finding for Susac syndrome is that of rounded lesions centrally within the corpus callosum (and not at the calloso-septal interface as in multiple sclerosis). Another typical finding is "string of pearls" – the studding of the internal capsules with microinfarcts on MRI. In the chronic stage the white matter lesions may become confluent and the brain suffers generalized atrophy.

Pertinent Clinical Information

The classic clinical triad includes: subacute encephalopathy, retinal artery branch occlusions and sensorineural hearing loss. Most patients are women between 20 and 40 years of age. Findings on brain MRI, audiogram, and funduscopy help reach the correct diagnosis. Unfortunately, the complete clinical triad is present in less than 5% of patients at the onset of the disease. Headache routinely accompanies the encephalopathy and may be constant, migrainous, or both. Bilateral long-tract signs commonly accompany the encephalopathy, which is laden with psychiatric features, confusion, memory loss, and other cognitive changes. It has been proposed that the diagnosis of Susac syndrome can be made when only the encephalopathy and pathognomonic MRI lesions are present.

Differential Diagnosis

Multiple Sclerosis (115, 125)
- look for involvement of the optic nerves and spinal cord
- less involvement of gray matter
- lesions tend to be larger and reduced diffusion is less common
- no leptomeningeal enhancement

Vasculitis (123)
- absence of rounded corpus callosum lesions
- leptomeningeal enhancement is typical, while parenchymal is rare

Background

The classic clinical triad of Susac syndrome (subacute encephalopathy, retinal artery branch occlusions and sensorineural hearing loss) was initially described in 1979. This rare syndrome may also be called RED-M, which stands for retinopathy, encephalopathy, deafness, and microangopathy. Another acronym is SICRET (small infarcts of cochlear, retinal, and encephalic tissues). From the clinical standpoint the differential diagnosis includes demyelinating disease, connective tissue disease, infection, procoagulant states, and ischemia. The etiology of the disease and the explanation for the types of tissues affected are not clear. Histology shows small brain infarcts and accompanying local inflammatory changes but no evidence of vasculitis. Because many lesions resolve they must be caused by other etiologies than infarction. The disease is usually monophasic, it may last up to several years, and leaves behind residual disabilities. Treatment varies from corticosteroids to other more potent immunosuppressive medications. The efficacy of any of these treatments has not been conclusively proven, but patients who are treated early seem to have a better prognosis.

REFERENCES

1. Susac JO, Murtagh FR, Egan RA, et al. MRI findings in Susac's syndrome. *Neurology* 2003;**61**:1783–7.

2. Do TH, Fisch C, Evoy F. Susac syndrome: report of four cases and review of the literature. *AJNR* 2004;**25**:382–8.

3. Xu MS, Tan CB, Umapathi T, Lim CC. Susac syndrome: serial diffusion-weighted MR imaging. *Magn Reson Imaging* 2004;**22**:1295–8.

4. White ML, Zhang Y, Smoker WRK. Evolution of lesions in Susac syndrome at serial MR imaging with diffusion-weighted imaging and apparent diffusion coefficient values. *AJNR* 2004;**25**:706–13.

5. Rennebohm R, Susac JO, Egan RA, Daroff RB. Susac's syndrome – update. *J Neurol Sci* 2010;**299**:86–91.

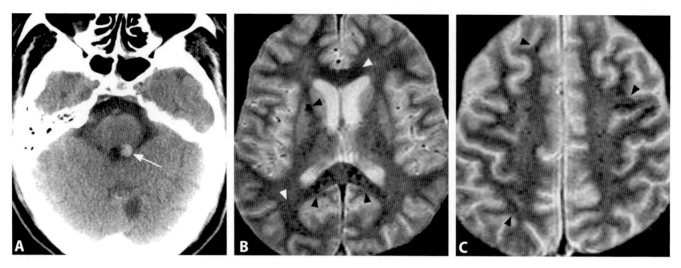

Figure 1. Non-enhanced CT (A) in a traumatized patient shows a hyperdense lesion in the left superior cerebellar peduncle (arrow). Follow-up T2*WI (B, C) reveals inumerable bilateral punctate dark lesions (arrowheads) primarily in the corpus callosum and at the gray–white matter junction.

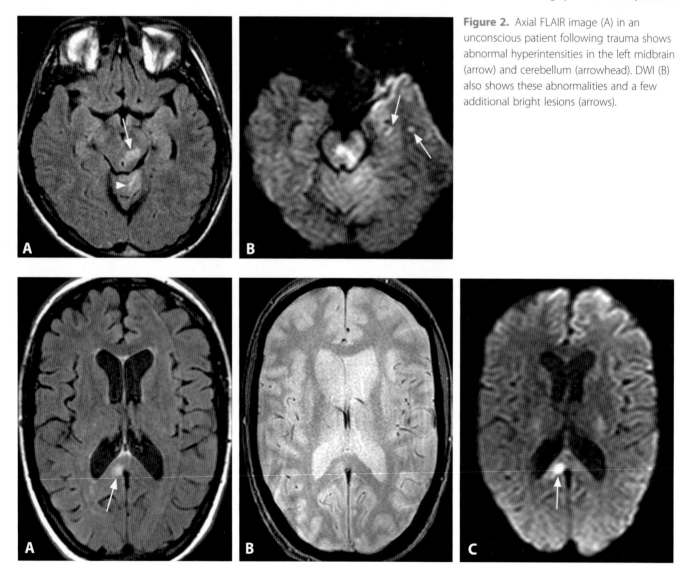

Figure 2. Axial FLAIR image (A) in an unconscious patient following trauma shows abnormal hyperintensities in the left midbrain (arrow) and cerebellum (arrowhead). DWI (B) also shows these abnormalities and a few additional bright lesions (arrows).

Figure 3. Axial FLAIR image (A) shows a hyperintense lesion (arrow) in the splenium of the corpus callosum, which is less conspicuous on T2*WI (B) but very prominent on DWI (C).

Diffuse Axonal Injury

MAJDA THURNHER

Specific Imaging Findings

Diffuse axonal injury (DAI, shear injury) on CT presents as small hypodense (nonhemorrhagic) or hyperdense (hemorrhagic) foci; however, the majority of DAI lesions are not detected on CT. Gray–white matter junction (especially paramedial), dorso-lateral midbrain, and corpus callosum (especially the splenium) are the most typical DAI locations. Multiple oval lesions 1–15 mm in diameter are detected on T2WI and FLAIR images. T2 signal intensity depends on the presence of hemorrhage: hemorrhagic lesions show low signal, while the nonhemorrhagic ones are T2 hyperintense. On T1WI the lesions are usually hypointense and not well seen, hyperintensity is present in sub-acute hemorrhagic lesions. T2* sequences detect susceptibility effects of hemoglobin degradation products as areas of signal loss in hemorrhagic lesions. The detection of acute or chronic hem-orrhagic DAI is improved by heavily T2*WI, such as with higher field strength and a longer echo time (TE), and even further with susceptibility-weighted imaging (SWI). Diffusion MR imaging is the most sensitive modality for DAI detection with bright signal on DWI in the acute phase. Some lesions may only be detected with DWI, some with T2* and a few with FLAIR. Presence of hemorrhage in the interpeduncular cistern on initial CT is a marker for possible brainstem DAI.

Pertinent Clinical Information

The main and classic DAI symptom is lack of consciousness; however, this is not always present. A conscious patient may show other signs of brain damage, depending on lesion location. Most patients (> 90%) with severe DAI remain in a persistent vegeta-tive state. Milder forms of DAI in the chronic phase may cause residual neuropsychiatric problems and cognitive deficits, focal neurologic lesions, memory loss, concentration difficulties, intel-lectual decline, psychiatric disturbances, headaches, and seizures.

Differential Diagnosis

Cerebral Amyloid Angiopathy (CAA) (178)
• preferential peripheral cortico-subcortical location of micro-bleeds, not seen on CT
• elderly patients, not in a setting of trauma

Chronic Systemic Hypertension (177)
• microbleeds typically in the deep gray and white matter, not seen on CT
• corpus callosum is usually spared

Embolic Infarcts (105)
• may enhance with contrast
• rarely hemorrhagic

Cerebral Cavernous Malformations (CCM, cavernomas) (183)
• characteristic T2WI appearance with central hyperintensity and dark rim of larger lesions

Vasculitis (123)
• areas of leptomeningeal enhancement may be present
• chronic/acute infarcts are common

Hemorrhagic Metastases (180)
• usually some nodular contrast enhancement

Background

DAI constitutes around 50% of all primary brain injuries. It results from the abnormal rotation or deceleration of the head affecting adjacent tissues that differ in density and rigidity. Gray and white matter move at different velocities and shearing forces develop at their interfaces, which causes stretching, twisting, or compression of axons. DAI occurs at the time of the accident and it can be hemorrhagic or nonhemorrhagic. Delayed (secondary) changes will evolve over a few minutes or hours after impact and additionally contribute to the axonal damage. The term DAI is actually a misnomer, as the injuries predominate in certain regions. DAI is subdivided according to the severity of pathology, clinical presentation, and likelihood of survival into three stages (Adams and Gennarelli): (1) gray–white matter junction; (2) lobar white matter and corpus callosum; (3) brainstem. Number and volume of lesions on DWI is also a predictor of patient outcome. Diffusion tensor imaging (DTI) shows promising results for the detection of abnormalities and evaluation of cog-nitive disorders in DAI patients.

REFERENCES

1. Hammoud DA, Wasserman BA. Diffuse axonal injuries: pathophysiology and imaging. *Neuroimaging Clin N Am* 2002;**12**:205–16.
2. Schaefer PW, Huisman TA, Sorensen AG, et al. Diffusion-weighted MR imaging in closed head injury: high correlation with initial Glasgow coma scale score and score on modified Rankin scale at discharge. *Radiology* 2004;**233**:58–66.
3. Parizel PM, Özsarlak Ö, Van Goethem JW, et al. Imaging findings in diffuse axonal injury after closed head trauma. *Eur Radiol* 1998;**8**:960–5.
4. Skadsen T, Kvistad KA, Solheim O, et al. Prevalence and impact of diffuse axonal injury in patients with moderate and severe head injury: a cohort study of early magnetic resonance imaging findings and 1-year outcome. *J Neurosurg* 2010;**113**:556–63.
5. Beretta L, Anzalone N, Dell'Acqua A, et al. Post-traumatic interpeduncular cistern hemorrhage as a marker for brainstem lesions. *J Neurotrauma* 2010;**27**:509–14.

Brain Imaging with MRI and CT, ed. Zoran Rumboldt *et al.* Published by Cambridge University Press. © Cambridge University Press 2012.

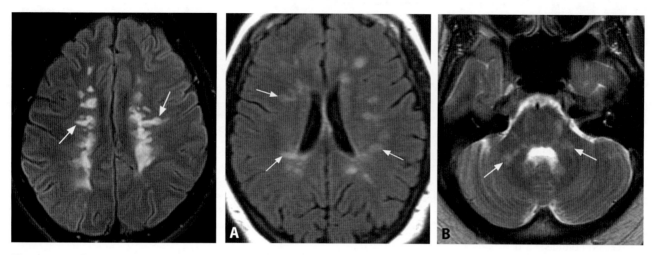

Figure 1. Axial FLAIR image shows multiple bilateral partly confluent hyperintense lesions in the centrum semiovale with orientation perpendicular to the location of the lateral ventricles (arrows).

Figure 2. FLAIR image (A) shows multiple WM hyperintensities – some finger-like radiating away from the ventricles (arrow). T2WI (B) reveals lesions in the brainstem and middle cerebellar peduncles (arrows).

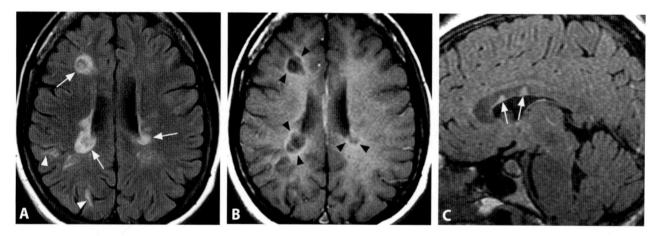

Figure 3. Axial FLAIR image (A) shows bilateral periventricular (arrows) and juxtacortical (arrowheads) lesions. Corresponding T1WI with magnetization transfer (B) reveals central low signal of the periventricular lesions with a hyperintense ring (arrowheads). Sagittal FLAIR image (C) shows two hyperintense lesions (arrows) extending superiorly from the calloso-septal interface.

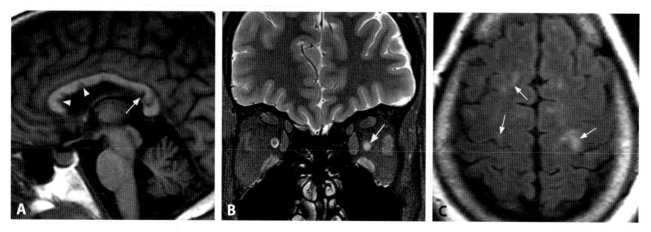

Figure 4. Midsagittal T1WI (A) reveals multiple hypointense corpus callosum lesions (arrowheads). A much darker lesion (arrow) represents a "black hole". Coronal T2WI with fat saturation (B) shows high signal of the enlarged left optic nerve (arrow). Some hyperintensities on FLAIR image (C) are juxtacortical (arrows).

Multiple Sclerosis

MATTHEW OMOJOLA AND ZORAN RUMBOLDT

Specific Imaging Findings

Multiple sclerosis (MS) lesions are T2 hyperintense and primarily located in the white matter. MS plaques are of varying shapes and sizes with the classical ovoid lesions radiating perpendicular from the ventricular wall ("Dawson's fingers"). This classic appearance needs to be present on axial images. Corpus callosum lesions at the calloso-septal interface are highly suggestive of MS, as are the ones within the brainstem and middle cerebellar peduncles. Juxtacortical white matter involvement is typical, while optic radiations and optic nerves are commonly affected. Multiple discreet lesions may coalesce and become smudgy. Active MS plaques may show reduced diffusion and, more reliably, enhancement with contrast. "Black holes", corresponding to chronic MS lesions, are very dark on T1WI, frequently with a thin peripheral bright rim, better seen with magnetization transfer. Larger demyelinating plaques show low attenuation on CT. The revised McDonald criteria require presence of at least two T2 hyperintense lesions in at least two of the four locations – juxtacortical, periventricular, infratentorial, and spinal cord, in the appropriate clinical setting. If brain MRI is not conclusive, spinal MRI may be helpful, as around 25% of patients present with isolated spinal cord lesions.

Pertinent Clinical Information

Patients are more commonly young females presenting with various symptoms and signs, such as tingling, numbness, weakness, fatigue, coordination and balance problems. Optic neuritis, a frequent presenting sign, is present in up to 50% of cases. CSF examination typically shows increased protein and oligoclonal bands. Symptoms can spontaneously resolve and come back or present in another part of the body. In Asian patients, the optic–spinal type is more frequent, older age group is affected, fewer cases are positive for oligoclonal bands, and total CSF protein is higher. MR imaging has an important role, excluding alternative diagnoses, and characterizing dissemination in space and time; however, it is currently not reliable for predicting the clinical disease evolution.

Differential Diagnosis

Incidental White Matter T2 Hyperintensities
- incidence 5–10% in 20–40 years age group, >30% over 50 years of age, most individuals over 80 years
- under 3 mm in size in a subcortical location is considered normal

Migraine; Connective Tissue Diseases
- white matter lesions without characteristic periventricular distribution
- lesions more common in frontal location

Chronic Hypertensive Encephalopathy (177)
- microhemorrhages on T2* images
- mostly cerebral periventricular and pontine lesions; involvement of corpus callosum, cerebellar peduncles, optic nerves or spinal cord is unusual

CADASIL (22)
- characteristic involvement of the temporal lobes and external capsule
- microhemorrhages on T2* MRI are common (around 40%)

ADEM (112)
- diffuse bilateral lesion pattern
- periventricular (Dawson's fingers) lesions are unusual
- deep gray matter involvement
- absence of black holes

Susac Syndrome (113)
- typical rounded central corpus callosum lesions
- reduced diffusion of lesions is common on ADC maps
- leptomeningeal enhancement may be present

CNS Vasculitis (123)
- usually prominent gray matter involvement
- leptomeningeal enhancement frequently present
- may be indistinguishable

Background

MS is an inflammatory demyelinating CNS disorder. Histology shows perivenular infiltrates of T cells and macrophages with associated perivenular demyelination. Four subtypes of MS are recognized: relapsing remitting, secondary progressive, primary progressive and progressive relapsing. The McDonald criteria, which incorporated MRI findings into the diagnostic criteria, have recently been revised. The lesions need to be disseminated in space, and in time (new lesion on follow up) in patients with clinical syndrome suggesting MS. Normal-appearing white matter and gray matter involvement has been increasingly reported and may correlate better with clinical findings. "Dawson's fingers" are named after James Walker Dawson, a Scottish pathologist who wrote about disseminated sclerosis in 1916. Susceptibility-weighted MRI (SWI) may reveal the location of MS plaques around cerebral veins, corresponding to Dawson's fingers.

REFERENCES

1. Rovira A, León A. MR in the diagnosis and monitoring of multiple sclerosis: an overview. *Eur J Radiol* 2008;**67**:409–14.

2. Polman CH, Reingold SC, Banwell B, *et al.* Diagnostic criteria for multiple sclerosis: 2010 revisions to the McDonald criteria. *Ann Neurol* 2011;**69**:292–302.

3. Lovblad KO, Anzalone N, Dorfler A, *et al.* MR imaging in multiple sclerosis: review and recommendations for current practice. *AJNR* 2010;**31**:983–9.

4. Moraal B, Wattjes MP, Geurts JJ, *et al.* Improved detection of active multiple sclerosis lesions: 3D subtraction imaging. *Radiology* 2010;**255**:154–63.

Brain Imaging with MRI and CT, ed. Zoran Rumboldt *et al.* Published by Cambridge University Press. © Cambridge University Press 2012.

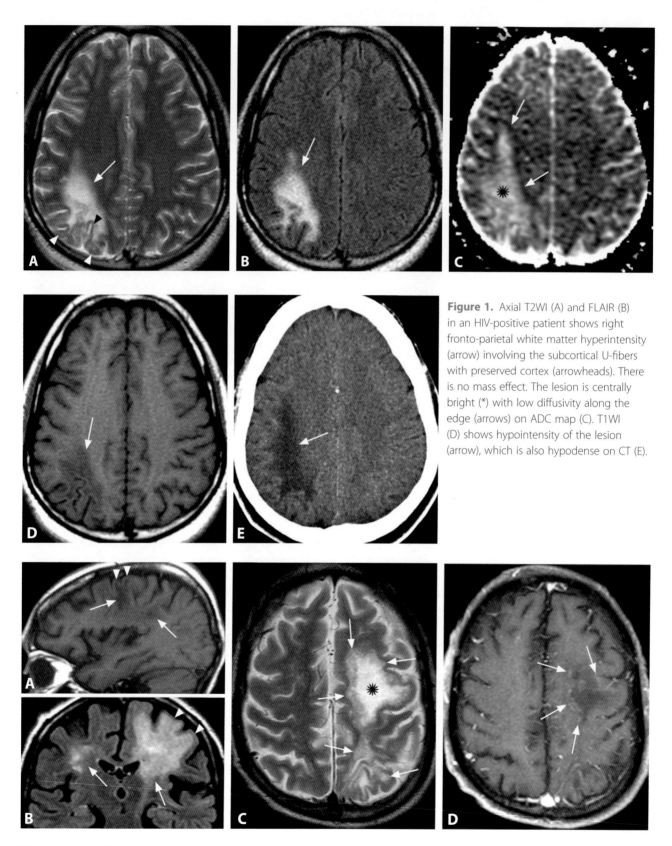

Figure 1. Axial T2WI (A) and FLAIR (B) in an HIV-positive patient shows right fronto-parietal white matter hyperintensity (arrow) involving the subcortical U-fibers with preserved cortex (arrowheads). There is no mass effect. The lesion is centrally bright (*) with low diffusivity along the edge (arrows) on ADC map (C). T1WI (D) shows hypointensity of the lesion (arrow), which is also hypodense on CT (E).

Figure 2. Sagittal T1WI (A) in a patient with Crohn's disease undergoing monoclonal antibody treatment and presenting with new neurologic deficits shows patchy subcortical hypointensity (arrow) with preserved overlying cortex (arrowheads). Coronal FLAIR (B) reveals bilateral hyperintense white matter lesions (arrows) with subcortical extension and sparing of the cortex (arrowheads). Axial T2WI (C) shows very high signal (*) in the center of the left hemisphere abnormality with peripheral mild hyperintensity (arrows). Corresponding post-contrast T1WI (D) shows subtle enhancement primarily along the lesion's edges (arrows).

Progressive Multifocal Leukoencephalopathy (PML)

ZORAN RUMBOLDT

Specific Imaging Findings

On CT, progressive multifocal leukoencephalopathy (PML) presents as patchy areas of low attenuation limited to the white matter, resembling vasogenic edema. MRI is the technique of choice showing high T2 signal of the lesions which are usually multifocal, commonly found in the parieto-occipital region, corpus callosum, and cerebellum, but they can be solitary and occur in any location. The lesions are characteristically of very low T1 signal, asymmetrical, and involving the subcortical U-fibers. In classic PML (cPML) enhancement is absent and hemorrhage is very unusual. At the center of active lesions, microcysts of very high T2 signal are sometimes seen. DWI shows a central low signal intensity core, surrounded by a rim of higher signal, with corresponding higher and lower ADC values, respectively. The advancing edge of reduced diffusivity represents active disease and may also contain incomplete T1 hyperintense rim. Perfusion studies show low rCBV of PML lesions. A severe reduction in NAA and increase in choline levels, along with lactate peak, is found on MRS. Inflammatory PML (iPML) lesions, which usually occur in the setting of immune reconstitution inflammatory syndrome (IRIS), show peripheral enhancement and/or mass effect. Advanced chronic stage of the disease demonstrates prominent atrophy of the involved white matter.

Pertinent Clinical Information

PML is an opportunistic infection caused by JC (after the patient John Cunningham) polyomavirus (JCV), which may affect any immunocompromised patient. The incidence has greatly increased with the AIDS epidemic and it also occurs as a side effect of monoclonal antibody medications. The clinical presentation includes gradually worsening hemiparesis, speech disturbances, limb incoordination, and visual impairment, without prominent dementia. The diagnosis suggested on imaging is confirmed by CSF polymerase chain reaction (PCR) for JC virus DNA. Therapy consists of cessation of immunosuppressive agents and restoration of the immune system.

Differential Diagnosis

HIV Encephalopathy (25)
- diffuse white matter T2 hyperintensity with preserved normal T1 signal
- only mild NAA decrease and choline increase, without prominent lactate on MRS

PRES (32)
- typically bilateral symmetric to almost symmetric
- usually posterior

IRIS (128)
- may coexist

Masses with Vasogenic Edema (Metastases, Abscesses) (155, 156)
- post-contrast enhancement of the lesion within vasogenic edema

Background

JCV is ubiquitous and infects at least 50% of the human population by adulthood. Despite this, PML remains exceptionally rare and essentially limited to patients with impaired T-cell function. JCV has a predilection for oligodendrocytes and the histopathological hallmark of PML is demyelination with enlarged oligodendroglial nuclei and bizzare astrocytes. Without treatment prognosis is very poor with overall survival of 6–12 months. Both clinical and radiological improvement occurs in approximately half of the AIDS patients who undergo highly active antiretroviral therapy (HAART). Progressive decrease of the abnormal signal on FLAIR and T1WI indicates good response with leukomalacia of burnt-out lesions. Increased ratio of *myo*-inositol to creatine on MRS also signifies favorable prognosis. Disease progression with contrast enhancement in iPML is usually secondary to IRIS. PML following treatment with monoclonal antibodies (primarily natalizumab) in patients with multiple sclerosis, Crohn's disease, and other autoimmune disease processes is usually iPML that occurs together with IRIS. Periodic brain MRI scans may allow detection of presymptomatic lesions in these patients. Post-transplantation PML has a higher case fatality and may have a higher incidence than reported in HIV patients on HAART or patients treated with natalizumab. PML can occur in patients with minimal or occult immunosuppression, including in the setting of sarcoidosis. JCV infection can also lead to neurotropic disease processes, different from PML.

REFERENCES

1. Bag AK, Curé JK, Chapman PR, *et al*. JC virus infection of the brain. *AJNR* 2010;**31**:1564–76.
2. Shah R, Bag AK, Chapman PR, Curé JK. Imaging manifestations of progressive multifocal leukoencephalopathy. *Clin Radiol* 2010;**65**:431–9.
3. Cosottini M, Tavarelli C, Del Bono L, *et al*. Diffusion-weighted imaging in patients with progressive multifocal leukoencephalopathy. *Eur Radiol* 2008;**18**:1024–30.
4. Thurnher MM, Post MJ, Rieger A, *et al*. Initial and follow-up MR imaging findings in AIDS-related progressive multifocal leukoencephalopathy treated with highly active antiretroviral therapy. *AJNR* 2001;**22**:977–84.
5. Berger. JR. The basis for modeling progressive multifocal leukoencephalopathy pathogenesis. *Curr Opin Neurol* 2011;**24**:262- 7.

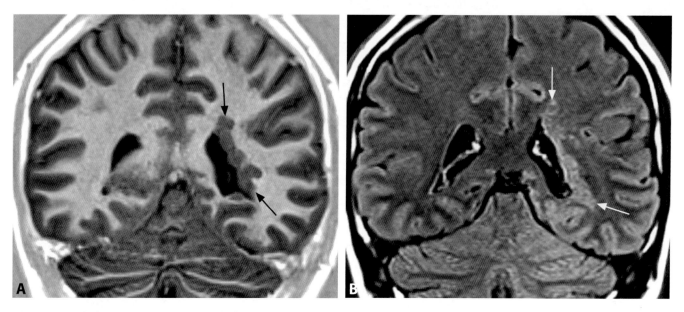

Figure 1. Coronal IR T1WI (A) shows a string of nodules (arrows) in the wall of the left lateral ventricle with the same signal intensity as the cortical gray matter. The curvilinear abnormality (arrows) has the same signal as the cortex on a coronal FLAIR image (B).

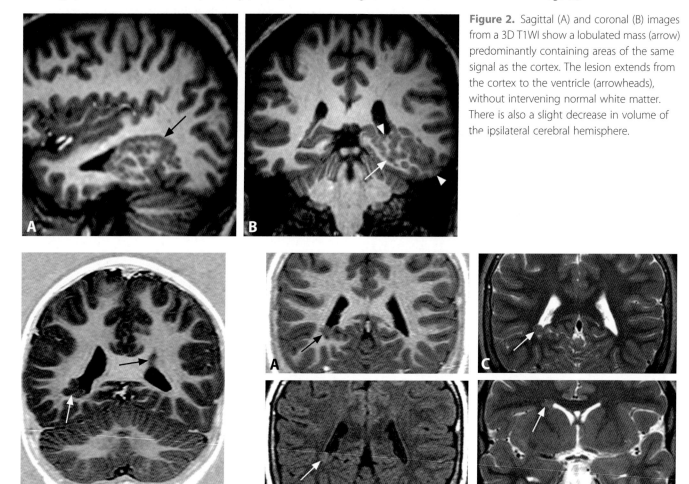

Figure 2. Sagittal (A) and coronal (B) images from a 3D T1WI show a lobulated mass (arrow) predominantly containing areas of the same signal as the cortex. The lesion extends from the cortex to the ventricle (arrowheads), without intervening normal white matter. There is also a slight decrease in volume of the ipsilateral cerebral hemisphere.

Figure 3. Coronal IR T1WI shows bilateral subependymal nodules (arrows) with signal intensity of the cortex.

Figure 4. Coronal IR T1WI (A), FLAIR (B), and T2WI (C) in a 10-year-old patient with pharmacoresistant epilepsy show a subependymal gray matter nodule (arrow). An additional lesion (arrow) is also present on a more anterior T2WI (D).

Nodular Heterotopia

MARIA GISELE MATHEUS

Specific Imaging Findings

Nodular heterotopia (NH) may be located in subependymal or subcortical locations. The subependymal type (periventricular nodular heterotopia, PNH) is the more common one. The lesions show signal intensity that follows the gray matter on all MRI sequences, best seen on T1-weighted inversion recovery and FLAIR images. The nodules do not calcify or enhance with contrast and there is no associated edema. PNH lesions are typically located along the walls of the lateral ventricles causing indentation of the lateral ventricular contours. PNH is most commonly found in the peritrigonal region, it may be unilateral or bilateral, and the number and distribution of lesions varies, from a single one to a few scattered heterotopias to almost continuous nodules. The surrounding white matter and the overall appearance of the cerebral hemisphere is otherwise normal. Subcortical NH (SNH), on the other hand, shows irregular lobulated masses in the subcortical white matter, usually continuous with the overlying cortex and underlying ventricular surface without intervening normal white matter. The overlying cortex is usually thin with shallow sulci. The size of SNH heterotopias varies from a focal small lesion to a conglomerate of abnormal gray matter that involves a large part of the hemisphere. The ipsilateral hemisphere and basal ganglia may be of decreased volume.

Pertinent Clinical Information

Bilateral NH is an X-linked dominant disorder with predominance in females due to a near total male mortality during embryogenesis. Clinical related symptoms are epilepsy, intelligence ranging from normal to borderline mental retardation, and coagulopathy. Sporadic heterotopias are associated with seizures and developmental delay, which varies with the severity of brain involvement. Heterotopias may be seen in conjunction with other brain malformations and syndromes, especially the subcortical type.

Differential Diagnosis

Congenital Cytomegalovirus Infection (184)
- heterotopic gray matter may be indistinguishable
- polymicrogyria, periventricular calcification, ventricular enlargement, cerebellar hyploplasia, and lissencephaly are frequently associated
- severity depends on timing of infection during gestation

Tuberous Sclerosis Complex (107)
- subependymal nodules usually exhibit prominent protrusion into the ventricle
- subependymal nodules are often calcified

- subependymal nodules may enhance with gadolinium
- additional lesions are present, primarily cortical hamartomas (tubers)

Background

Development of the cerebral cortex can be divided into three stages: (1) neuronal and glial proliferation in the ventricular and subventricular zones, (2) migration of immature but postmitotic neurons to the developing cerebral cortex, and (3) cortical organization. Migration is basically regulated by specialized radial glial cells and a complex molecular mechanism including cytoskeleton, anchor receptors, and signaling (initiation and stop biochemical signs). Heterotopia is a neuronal migration disorder characterized by clusters of disorganized neurons in abnormal locations and it is divided into three main groups: PNH, SNH, and marginal glioneural heterotopia. Breakdown in neuronal migration apparatus with consequent arrest of neurons along their path from the germinal matrix to the cortex and their ectopic accumulation appears to be the primary mechanism responsible for heterotopia. Presence of abnormal heterotopic germinal matrix and tangential path of the neurons have also been proposed as possible contributors in pathogenesis, especially for the subcortical type. The neuropathological analysis may distinguish two different groups of nodular heterotopias: group 1 nodular heterotopia is identified on MRI and shows projecting and local circuit neurons intermingled with glial cells; group 2 nodules are formed by projecting neurons without glial cells, located in the temporal lobe, small and undetected by MRI, and associated with hippocampal sclerosis or gangliogliomas. Cortical dysplasia is associated with both types.

REFERENCES

1. Barkovich AJ. Morphologic characteristics of subcortical heterotopia: MRI imaging study. *AJNR* 2000;**21**:290–5.
2. Abdel Razek AA, Kandell AY, Elsorogy LG, et al. Disorders of cortical formation: MR imaging features. *AJNR* 2009;**30**:4–11.
3. Verrotti A, Spalice A, Ursitti F, et al. New trends in neuronal migrational disorders. *Eur J Paediatr Neurol* 2010;**14**:1–12.
4. Battaglia G, Chiapparini L, Franceschetti S, et al. Periventricular nodular heterotopia: classification, epileptic history, and genesis of epileptic discharges. *Epilepsia* 2006;**47**:86–97.
5. Meroni A, Galli C, Bramerio M, et al. Nodular heterotopia: a neuropathological study of 24 patients undergoing surgery for drug-resistant epilepsy. *Epilepsia* 2009;**50**:116–24.

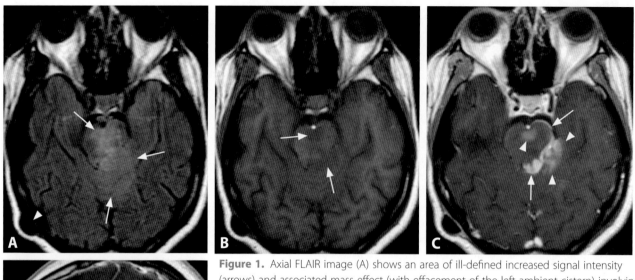

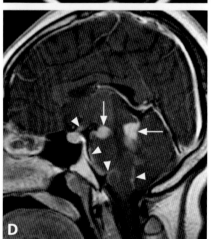

Figure 1. Axial FLAIR image (A) shows an area of ill-defined increased signal intensity (arrows) and associated mass effect (with effacement of the left ambient cistern) involving the brainstem and pons. Note the reservoir of a ventriculo-peritoneal shunt (arrowhead). Corresponding T1WI (B) shows mild hypointensity (arrows) of the involved areas. Post-contrast T1WI (C) reveals enhancement along the surface of the brain (arrows) of variable thickness and some nodularity. Enhancement also extends into the brain parenchyma (arrowheads). Sagittal post-contrast T1WI (D) demonstrates multiple areas of enhancement along the brainstem, cerebellum, and suprasellar cisterns. There are various patterns of enhancement along the brain surface – thicker and more nodular (arrows), as well as linear and isolated to the leptomeninges (arrowheads).

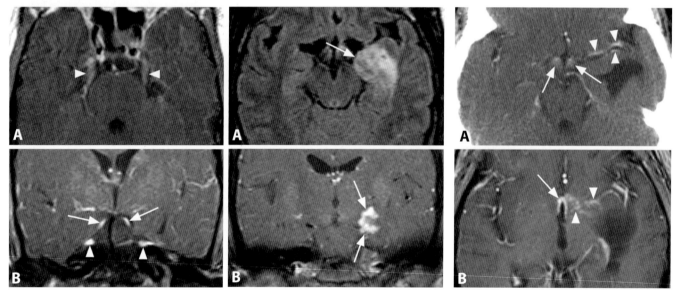

Figure 2. Axial post-contrast T1WI (A) shows bilateral trigeminal nerve enhancement (arrowheads). Coronal post-contrast T1WI with fat-saturation (B) reveals enhancement of the oculomotor nerves (arrows), in addition to the trigeminal nerves (arrowheads).

Figure 3. Axial FLAIR image (A) shows mild left mesial temporal swelling and hyperintensity (arrow). Coronal post-contrast T1WI with fat-sat (B) reveals enhancement (arrows) along the surface of the left mesial temporal lobe.

Figure 4. Post-contrast CT image (A) shows subtle enhancement along the suprasellar cisterns (arrows) and left sylvian fissure (arrowheads). Post-contrast T1WI with fat saturation (B) reveals patchy enhancement in similar areas (arrow and arrowheads).

Neurosarcoidosis

ZORAN RUMBOLDT

Specific Imaging Findings

MRI is the imaging modality of choice for neurosarcoidosis with the typical imaging feature of thickened and enhancing leptomeninges, primarily along the base of the brain with suprasellar and cranial nerve involvement. The leptomeningeal lesions are typically patchy, thick, and somewhat nodular, while smooth and diffuse enhancement is relatively rare. Infiltrating extension of the leptomeningeal enhancement along the surface of the brain (and/or spinal cord) into the parenchyma (along the perivascular spaces) is a relatively characteristic feature. Intra-axial, dural, and intraosseus granulomas may also be present, sometimes without associated leptomeningeal involvement. Granulomas are homogenous and without necrotic portions, enhance with contrast and are of characteristically low T2 signal. As with other inflammatory and infectious processes, perfusion studies show low cerebral blood volume of these lesions. FDG-PET may reveal other locations of the disease, primarily in the mediastinum, even with negative chest CT scans.

Pertinent Clinical Information

Neurosarcoidosis is a diagnostic challenge, especially in the absence of systemic involvement. Symptoms, when present, may be subtle and resemble those of other diseases. On the other hand, sarcoid-related imaging abnormalities are frequently not associated with correlating symptoms. The most common manifestations are cranial neuropathies, primarily affecting optic and facial nerves. Encephalopathy, seizures, diabetes insipidus and other endocrine manifestations may be encountered. The diagnosis is commonly established through a combination of chest imaging (CT), nuclear medicine scans (Gallium and FDG-PET), and laboratory findings: CSF analysis and serum angiotensin-converting enzyme (ACE) level. Imaging follow-up is recommended due to a high rate of progression and recurrence following treatment.

Differential Diagnosis

Tuberculosis (160)
- infarctions (from involvement of the arteries) are common
- involved meninges may be T1 hyperintense, which is accentuated with magnetization transfer
- MRS shows elevated lipids and lactate
- leptomeningeal and parenchymal lesions may be indistinguishable

Fungal Granulomas
- parenchymal granulomas may be indistinguishable
- abscesses, when present, may show low ADC signal of reduced diffusion

Secondary Lymphoma (135)
- leptomeningeal enhancement is typically smooth and more diffuse, not nodular and patchy
- rCBV may be increased on perfusion imaging

Leptomeningeal Carcinomatosis (119)
- high rCBV on perfusion imaging
- additional parenchymal metastases may be present
- may be indistinguishable

Meningitis (120)
- leptomeningeal enhancement is typically thin and smooth
- corresponding high signal of the sulcal subarachnoid spaces on FLAIR images

CNS Vasculitis (123)
- areas of leptomeningeal enhancement, when present, are smooth, thin and scattered
- focal parenchymal lesions are T2 hyperintense, without nodules of low T2 signal

Subacute Infarction (124)
- may be indistinguishable (sarcoidosis may lead to infarct)
- enhancement is usually smooth and thin, limited to the area of infarcted brain

Background

Sarcoidosis affects the CNS more frequently than previously appreciated with subclinical neurosarcoidosis being fairly common. It is estimated that 5–25% of patients with systemic sarcoidosis have CNS involvement. The diagnosis is often delayed, potentially leading to serious and disabling complications. CNS biopsy that shows sterile, noncaseating granuloma is the only definitive proof of disease. Adverse effects of high-dose systemic corticosteroids, the standard therapy, tend to discourage treatment in the absence of significant neurologic disease. However, other immunosuppressive medications and newer immunomodulators, such as anti-TNF-α agents, have emerged as an effective and well-tolerated alternative. During follow-up, MRI changes show excellent correlation with clinical improvement or worsening on immunosuppressive therapy. Patients with enhancing dural and parenchymal T2-hypointense lesions, which likely represent a reparative tissue response, frequently do not have correlating neurologic symptoms and are less likely to respond to treatment.

REFERENCES

1. Shah R, Roberson GH, Curé JK. Correlation of MR imaging findings and clinical manifestations in neurosarcoidosis. *AJNR* 2009;**30**:953–61.
2. Lury KM, Smith JK, Matheus MG, Castillo M. Neurosarcoidosis – review of imaging findings. *Semin Roentgenol* 2004;**39**:495–504.
3. Pickuth D, Spielmann RP, Heywang-Köbrunner SH. Role of radiology in the diagnosis of neurosarcoidosis. *Eur Radiol* 2000;**10**:941–4.
4. Spencer TS, Campellone JV, Maldonado I, *et al*. Clinical and magnetic resonance imaging manifestations of neurosarcoidosis. *Semin Arthritis Rheum* 2005;**34**:649–61.
5. Terushkin V, Stern BJ, Judson MA, *et al*. Neurosarcoidosis: presentations and management. *Neurologist* 2010;**16**:2–15.

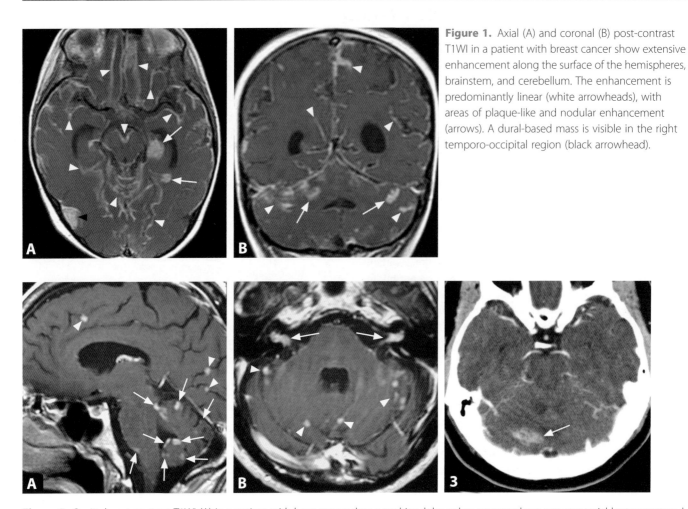

Figure 1. Axial (A) and coronal (B) post-contrast T1WI in a patient with breast cancer show extensive enhancement along the surface of the hemispheres, brainstem, and cerebellum. The enhancement is predominantly linear (white arrowheads), with areas of plaque-like and nodular enhancement (arrows). A dural-based mass is visible in the right temporo-occipital region (black arrowhead).

Figure 2. Sagittal post-contrast T1WI (A) in a patient with lung cancer shows multinodular enhancement along supratentorial leptomeningeal surfaces (arrowheads). The nodules are more concentrated along the cerebellar vermis and brainstem (arrows). Axial post-contrast T1WI (B) reveals enhancement within bilateral internal auditory canals (arrows), in addition to cerebellar lesions (arrowheads).

Figure 3. Axial contrast-enhanced CT image in another patient shows subtle enhancement along the superior cerebellar surface, with a focal more prominent lesion (arrow).

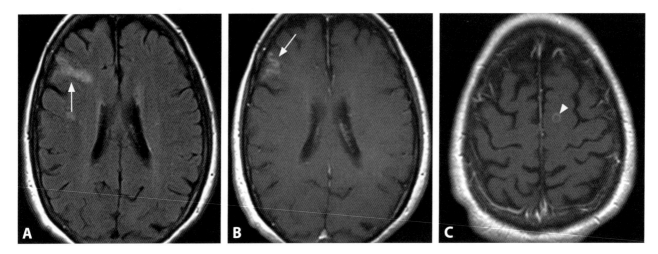

Figure 4. FLAIR image (A) shows a cortico-subcortical hyperintense area (arrow), suggestive of edema. Corresponding post-contrast T1WI reveals gyriform leptomeningeal enhancement (arrow) in this area. T1WI at a higher level (C) shows a subcortical rim-enhancing nodule, consistent with intra-axial metastasis.

Meningeal Carcinomatosis

ALESSANDRO CIANFONI

Specific Imaging Findings

Meningeal carcinomatosis on MR imaging presents as a focal or multifocal, frequently diffuse linear and/or nodular contrast enhancement along the leptomeninges – covering the surface of the brain: within the cortical sulci and the cerebellar folia, along the brainstem and cranial nerves. FLAIR images can show increased signal of the subarachnoid spaces, within the sulci, as well as hyperintense signal of edema in the adjacent brain. T2WI and unenhanced T1WI are usually unremarkable, unless vasogenic edema is present in the adjacent brain, either from advanced infiltrative disease, or from concurrent intra-axial lesions. Unenhanced CT is usually normal, while contrast-enhanced CT is positive usually only with advanced disease. The posterior fossa is a preferred site of involvement and spinal imaging often reveals spread of the disease along the entire neuraxis. Association with dural and intra-axial brain metastasis is commonly encountered. Perfusion imaging shows increased cerebral blood volume in larger lesions.

Pertinent Clinical Information

Leptomeningeal carcinomatosis most often presents late in the course of neoplastic disease, and carries a particularly dismal prognosis, especially if associated with solid tumors. The hallmark of clinical presentation is a cancer patient who complains of a focal neurologic dysfunction and is found to have multifocal signs on neurologic examination, commonly including a single or multiple cranial nerve dysfunction. The clinical course is relentlessly progressive; treatment is limited and cures are the subject of case reports. Treatment is palliative, and therapeutic options include radiation, systemic chemotherapy, intrathecal chemotherapy, and more recently immunotoxins and gene therapy.

Differential Diagnosis

Nonspecific Infectious Meningitis (120)
- less frequently nodular, may be indistinguishable from carcinomatosis with a linear enhancement pattern

Tuberculosis (160)
- basal cisterns are typically involved
- infarctions in the territories of the encased vessels are frequently present
- cerebral blood volume is not increased on perfusion imaging

Neurosarcoidosis (118)
- often associated with dural disease and infiltrative brain involvement
- cerebral blood volume is low to normal on perfusion imaging

Secondary Lymphoma (135)
- usually smooth and linear, less frequently nodular, may be indistinguishable

Primary CNS Tumor Dissemination (67, 68, 174)
- the primary tumor is almost always either present on images or/and the patient has a known history of a CNS neoplasm, most commonly medulloblastoma

Post-Ictal Leptomeningeal Enhancement
- absence of nodularity

Acute Infarct (152)
- leptomeningeal enhancement is smooth without nodularity

Subacute Infarct (124)
- gyriform enhancement without associated edema
- adjacent encephalomalacia
- absence of nodularity

Sturge–Weber Syndrome (86)
- typically unilateral cerebral involvement
- smooth and linear enhancement
- additional features: hemiatrophy, superficial calcifications, enlarged choroid plexus

Background

Leptomeningeal carcinomatosis has also been called neoplastic meningitis and carcinomatous meningitis, and a more correct and all-encompassing term is leptomeningeal metastasis, as it is not always associated with carcinomas nor inflammation. Leptomeningeal carcinomatosis per se is a form of metastatic spread in solid tumors (most frequently breast and lung cancer), while leptomeningeal metastasis also occurs with lymphoma and leukemia, or as a local dissemination of primary CNS tumors (drop metastasis). It represents spread of tumor cells through the CSF, or hematogenously to the pia mater and/or arachnoid. Contrast-enhanced MRI has the highest sensitivity (close to 100%), while CSF cytology (sensitivity of 85%) has the highest specificity. The main therapeutic problems are the diffuse nature of metastatic spread through the neuraxis, and the inability of most chemotherapeutic agents to penetrate the blood–brain barrier.

REFERENCES

1. Collie DA, Brush JP, Lammie GA, *et al.* Imaging features of leptomeningeal metastases. *Clin Radiol* 1999;**54**:765–71.

2. Smirniotopoulos JG, Murphy FM, Rushing EJ, *et al.* Patterns of contrast enhancement in the brain and meninges. *Radiographics* 2007;**27**:525–51.

3. Kesari S, Batchelor TT. Leptomeningeal metastases. *Neurol Clin* 2003;**21**:25–66.

4. Groves MD. New strategies in the management of leptomeningeal metastases. *Arch Neurol* 2010;**67**:305–12.

5. Clarke JL, Perez HR, Jacks LM, *et al.* Leptomeningeal metastases in the MRI era. *Neurology* 2010;**74**:1449–54.

Brain Imaging with MRI and CT, ed. Zoran Rumboldt *et al.* Published by Cambridge University Press. © Cambridge University Press 2012.

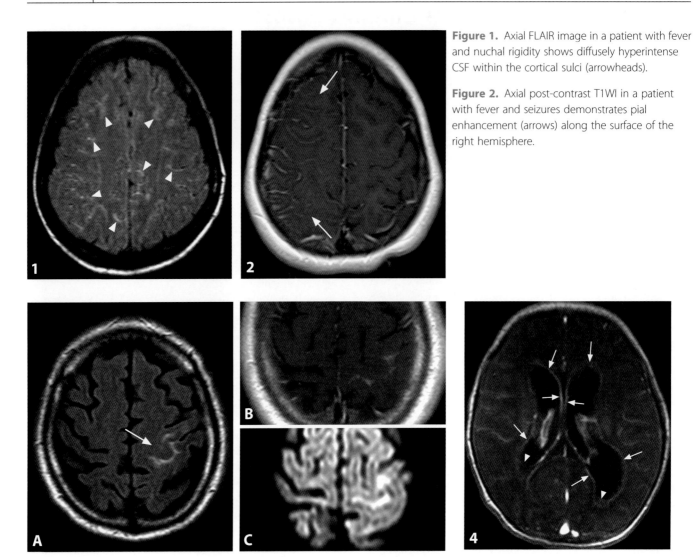

Figure 1. Axial FLAIR image in a patient with fever and nuchal rigidity shows diffusely hyperintense CSF within the cortical sulci (arrowheads).

Figure 2. Axial post-contrast T1WI in a patient with fever and seizures demonstrates pial enhancement (arrows) along the surface of the right hemisphere.

Figure 3. Axial FLAIR image (A) shows hyperintensity (arrow) within a few sulci along the left hemisphere. There is corresponding enhancement on post-contrast T1WI (B) and bright signal on DWI (C).

Figure 4. Post-contrast T1WI shows hydrocephalus and ventriculitis with ependymal enhancement (arrows) and debris (arrowheads).

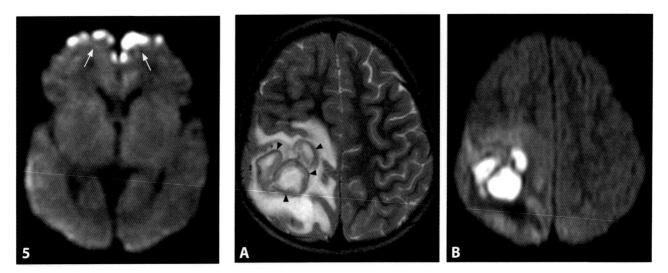

Figure 5. Axial DWI shows hyperintensity (arrows) in the frontal extra-axial spaces due to subdural empyemas.

Figure 6. T2WI (A) shows high signal in the central portions and in the surrounding edema, while the abscess rim is of low signal (arrowheads). Corresponding DWI (B) shows very high signal from the pus in the central portions.

Meningitis (Infectious)

MAURICIO CASTILLO

Specific Imaging Findings

The diagnosis of uncomplicated infectious meningitis is a clinical one and imaging is not indicated. If done, the most specific findings are high CSF signal intensity on FLAIR images and leptomeningeal/subarachnoid space contrast enhancement. Contrast enhancement may also be seen on CT, but not to the extent that it is shown by MRI. Patients suspected of having complications need to be imaged with MRI including DWI, post-contrast images, T2*-weighted images (to look for thrombosed cortical veins), MRV and MRA. Diffusion imaging is very helpful in demonstrating reduced diffusion in any local collection of pus (abscess, empyema, ventriculitis) and also in detecting acute infarctions. Ventricular debris with an irregular level is the most frequent sign of ventriculitis, while hydrocephalus and ependymal enhancement are less commonly encountered. Large subdural sterile fluid collections are typical in children with *Haemophilus influenza* meningitis. Tubercular meningitis has a predilection for involvement of basal cisterns, especially the interpeduncular fossa, typically with thick enhancing exudates, frequently leading to infarcts in the territories of the middle cerebral artery perforating vessels.

Pertinent Clinical Information

Infectious meningitis is more common in children and it can grossly be divided into bacterial (pyogenic), viral (lymphocytic) and tubercular. The last two may occasionally assume a chronic form. The diagnosis of meningitis is a clinical one (not an imaging one) and is based on abnormal CSF that shows: high numbers of white blood cells, high protein, and low glucose. The most important clinical symptoms are: fever, headaches, signs of increased intracranial pressure, nuchal rigidity, irritability, lethargy and altered mental status and seizures. Hyperreflexia may also be present. Complications of meningitis occur in up to 50% of patients, the most common ones being ventriculomegaly, subdural collection, and infarct.

Differential Diagnosis

Leptomeningeal Carcinomatosis (119)
- typically more focal
- thicker nodular enhancement is common (not with lymphoma)
- increased cerebral blood volume on perfusion studies
- history of primary cancer elsewhere

Sarcoidosis (118)
- less diffuse and more concentrated in basilar cisterns
- nodular areas of enhancement are common
- meningeal masses that may simulate meningiomas
- more common in black individuals, positive chest radiograph, different laboratory findings, involvement of eyes

Other Pathologic Causes of High CSF Signal on FLAIR Images (97,120, 122)
- hemorrhage, "ivy" sign in Moyamoya disease (collateral circulation), infarction, superior sagittal sinus thrombosis, adjacent tumors, status epilepticus, gadolinium accumulation in patients with renal impairment

Other Non-pathologic Causes of High CSF Signal on FLAIR Images
- supplementary oxygen, anesthesia, gadolinium from prior MRI study within 24–48 h in individuals with normal renal function, artifacts

Background

Meningitis usually reaches the brain via hematogeneous dissemination and affects the leptomeninges and subarachnoid spaces. It can also enter the brain directly or via continuity from infected sinonasal and temporal bone cavities. Although it may occur at any age, it is more common in children and its incidence appears to be increasing worldwide. Complications of meningitis include: hydrocephalus, subdural sterile and infected (empyemas) collections, brain abscesses, ventriculitis, venous and arterial thromboses, arteritis and infarctions. The infection may also extend into the inner ear and cause acute or chronic deafness secondary to fibrosing and eventually ossifying labyrinthitis, for which the earliest imaging signs may be observed as early as 4 weeks after the onset of meningitis. Worldwide, mortality is high, reaching 25% of affected individuals. Uncomplicated meningitis is medically treated while many of its complications require surgery. Steroid administration may help control symptoms particularly in chronic meningitis.

REFERENCES

1. Jaremko JL, Moon AS, Kumbla S. Patterns of complications of neonatal and infant meningitis on MRI by organism: a 10 year review. *Eur J Radiol* 2011;**80**:821–7.

2. Fukui MB, Williams RL, Mudigonda S. CT and MR imaging features of pyogenic ventriculitis. *AJNR* 2001;**22**:1510–6.

3. Tha KK, Terae S, Kudo K, Miyasaka K. Differential diagnosis of hyperintense cerebrospinal fluid on fluid-attenuated inversion recovery images of the brain. Part I: pathological conditions. *Br J Radiol* 2009;**82**:426–34.

4. Durisin M, Bartling S, Arnoldner C, *et al.* Cochlear osteoneogenesis after meningitis in cochlear implant patients: a retrospective analysis. *Otol Neurotol* 2010;**31**:1072–8.

5. Morris JM, Miller GM. Increased signal in the subarachnoid space on fluid-attenuated inversion recovery imaging associated with the clearance dynamics of gadolinium chelate: a potential diagnostic pitfall. *AJNR* 2007;**28**:1964–7.

Brain Imaging with MRI and CT, ed. Zoran Rumboldt *et al.* Published by Cambridge University Press. © Cambridge University Press 2012.

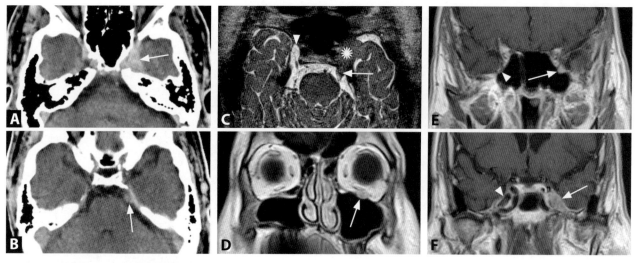

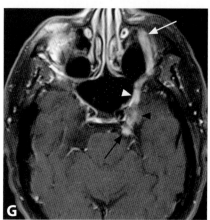

Figure 1. Enhanced axial CT (A) in a patient with new numbness and previously treated left cheek melanoma shows thickened left cavernous sinus (arrow). A more cephalad image (B) reveals a small extra-axial mass (arrow) along the course of the left trigeminal nerve. Axial T2WI from a 3D acquisition (C) shows isointense tissue filling the left Meckel's cave (*) and extending along the cisternal trigeminal nerve (arrow). Note normal left Meckel's cave (arrowhead). Coronal post-contrast T1WI (D) shows a thick enhancing left infraorbital nerve (arrow). A more posterior image (E) reveals enhancing enlarged maxillary nerve (arrow) at foramen rotundum. Compare to normal contralateral nerve (arrowhead). Further back (F), there is enhancing tissue in the left Meckel's cave (arrow). Note normal right counterpart (arrowhead). Axial post-contrast T1WI with fat saturation (G) demonstrates the abnormal enhancement (arrowheads) extending from the infraorbital foramen (white arrow) to the cisternal trigeminal nerve (black arrow) through foramen rotundum (white arrowhead) and Meckel's cave (black arrowhead).

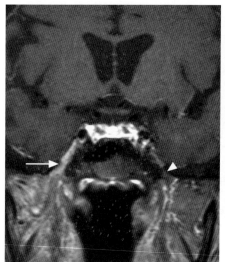

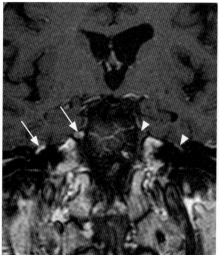

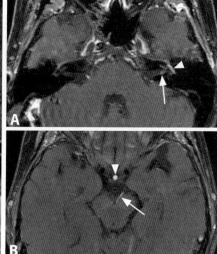

Figure 2. Coronal post-contrast T1WI with fat saturation shows a thickened enhancing right mandibular nerve (arrow) extending toward the cavernous sinus. Note normal left mandibular nerve at the foramen ovale (arrowhead).

Figure 3. Coronal post-contrast T1WI shows thickened enhancing right-sided facial and trigeminal nerves (arrows, right to left) around the skull base. Compare to normal contralateral counterparts (arrowheads).

Figure 4. Axial post-contrast fat saturated T1WI (A) shows enhancement in the left IAC (arrow) and tympanic facial nerve (arrowhead). Left oculomotor nerve (arrow) enhances at a more cephalad level (B). Normal enhancing pituitary stalk (arrowhead).

Perineural Tumor Spread

ZORAN RUMBOLDT

Specific Imaging Findings

Perineural tumor spread (PNS) typically occurs with head and neck cancers and may be seen on CT; however, MRI is far more sensitive, especially with dedicated high-resolution images. Maxillary (V2) and mandibular (V3) divisions of the trigeminal nerve, along with the facial nerve, are most commonly involved. Typical findings are obliteration of the fat planes at skull base foramina, contrast enhancement and/or enlargement of a nerve. Replacement of the normal fluid in the Meckel's cave and cavernous sinus enlargement are frequent additional findings. Muscle denervation atrophy is an indirect sign of (V3) PNS with T2 hyperintensity and enhancement in the early, and volume loss and T1 hyperintensity in the late phase. CT may show obliteration of the fat planes, primarily the pterygopalatine fossa, and expansion of the skull base foramina. Detection of a suspicious cavernous sinus mass should prompt a search for PNS and a head and neck malignancy. False positive enhancement occurs with other conditions that disrupt the blood–nerve barrier, primarily inflammation and edema, which are commonly present following surgery and radiotherapy. In addition to inflammatory and infectious processes, such as sarcoidosis, PNS rarely occurs with intracranial neoplasms, such as meningioma.

Pertinent Clinical Information

PNS is a common and a potentially devastating complication of head and neck malignancies; it may be the only evidence of the disease. As it is initially clinically silent in about a half of patients, imaging plays a crucial role in its detection and delineation. Undiagnosed, the cancer slowly progresses and eventually results in symptoms, usually facial weakness or numbness, sometimes 10 or more years after the initial cancer treatment. Facial pain and/ or paresthesias may also occur. Imaging evidence of PNS worsens prognosis; however, surgery followed by radiation results in a high cure rate (approximately 80%). In symptomatic patients aggressive treatment results in a cure rate of less than 50%.

Differential Diagnosis

Inflammatory and Infectious Processes (118)
- typically cannot be tracked along the nerve to the extracranial origin
- leptomeningeal involvement not limited to the cranial nerves
- may be indistinguishable

Nerve Sheath Tumors (Schwannoma, Neurofibroma) (141)
- focal and/or nodular lesions instead of smooth diffuse thickening of the nerve
- extracranial extension along the nerve is rare (except in NF1)

Cavernous Sinus Meningioma (47)
- extracranial extension is exceptional
- dural-based mass, presence of dural tail

Cavernous Sinus Hemangioma (48)
- very bright on T2WI
- very avid and early contrast enhancement, similar to vascular structures, progressive filling on dynamic studies

Tolosa–Hunt Syndrome (49)
- limited to the cavernous sinus, orbital apex and the dura, does not extend along trigeminal nerve branches
- pain is the prominent symptom, responds rapidly to corticosteroids

Background

PNS is the extension of tumor cells along the endoneurium or perineurium with overall incidence from 2.5% to 5%. The most common head and neck malignancies to spread perineurally are squamous cell carcinoma (SCC) of the skin and adenoid cystic carcinoma, but mucosal SCC, melanoma (especially desmoplastic), lymphoma, sarcomas, and virtually any malignant neoplasm may exhibit this behavior. Proliferating neoplastic cells initially lead to mild increase in nerve diameter, followed by destruction of the blood–nerve barrier that allows for accumulation of the contrast material on imaging. Correctly performed and interpreted MRI is essentially 100% sensitive for PNS, while the sensitivity of CT is under 90%. MRI may underestimate the full extent of the disease in a minority of cases.

REFERENCES

1. Maroldi R, Farina D, Borghesi A, *et al*. Perineural tumor spread. *Neuroimaging Clin N Am* 2008;**18**:413–29.
2. Ginsberg LE. MR imaging of perineural tumor spread. *Magn Reson Imaging Clin N Am* 2002;**10**:511–25.
3. Chang PC, Fischbein NJ, McCalmont TH, *et al*. Perineural spread of malignant melanoma of the head and neck: clinical and imaging features. *AJNR* 2004;**25**:5–11.
4. Hanna E, Vural E, Prokopakis E, *et al*. The sensitivity and specificity of high-resolution imaging in evaluating perineural spread of adenoid cystic carcinoma to the skull base. *Arch Otolaryngol Head Neck Surg* 2007;**133**:541–5.
5. Gandhi MR, Panizza B, Kennedy D. Detecting and defining the anatomic extent of large nerve perineural spread of malignancy: comparing "targeted" MRI with the histologic findings following surgery. *Head Neck* 2011;**33**:469–75.

Brain Imaging with MRI and CT, ed. Zoran Rumboldt *et al.* Published by Cambridge University Press. © Cambridge University Press 2012.

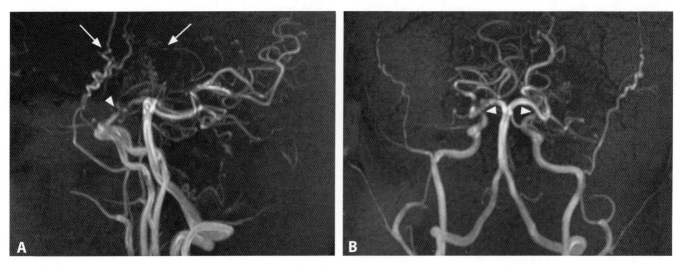

Figure 1. Lateral (A) and frontal (B) MIP reconstructions of a brain MR angiogram demonstrate bilateral supraclinoid internal carotid artery (ICA) narrowing (arrowheads), moyamoya collateral vessels (arrows), and preserved arteries of the posterior circulation.

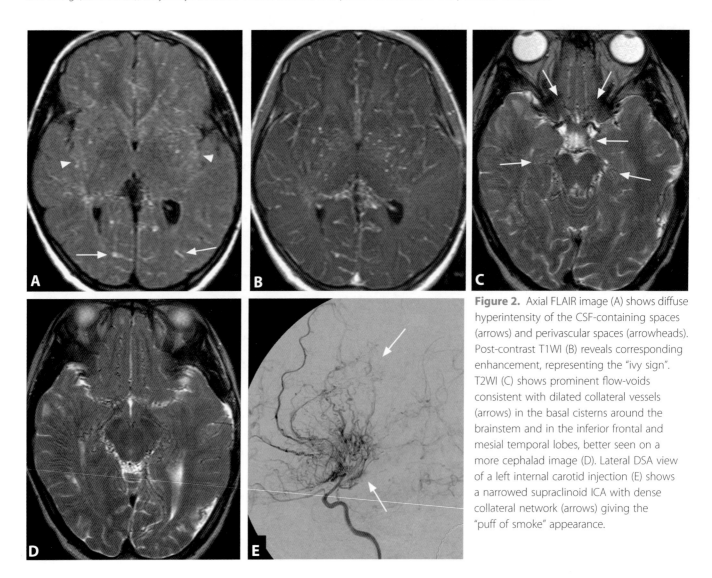

Figure 2. Axial FLAIR image (A) shows diffuse hyperintensity of the CSF-containing spaces (arrows) and perivascular spaces (arrowheads). Post-contrast T1WI (B) reveals corresponding enhancement, representing the "ivy sign". T2WI (C) shows prominent flow-voids consistent with dilated collateral vessels (arrows) in the basal cisterns around the brainstem and in the inferior frontal and mesial temporal lobes, better seen on a more cephalad image (D). Lateral DSA view of a left internal carotid injection (E) shows a narrowed supraclinoid ICA with dense collateral network (arrows) giving the "puff of smoke" appearance.

Subacute Infarct

BENJAMIN HUANG AND ZORAN RUMBOLDT

Specific Imaging Findings

The subacute period of ischemic infarcts lasts from 24 h to approximately 2 weeks. Infarcts become better defined as well-demarcated wedge-shaped areas of low density involving both gray and white matter. Mass effect with gyral swelling, compression of the adjacent ventricles, and possible herniations may initially increase but subsequently begin diminishing after approximately 1 week and usually resolve by 3 weeks. Hemorrhage is evident in up to 20% of ischemic infarcts. Between the second and third weeks, the infarct may become isodense, a phenomenon known as "fogging".

On MRI, ADC values continue to decrease during the hyperacute and acute periods reaching the nadir at around 4 days, and then begin to rise, returning to baseline at 1–2 weeks. Thereafter, the diffusion becomes elevated. The T2 signal intensity increases over the first 4 days and remains relatively stable, while T1 signal decreases and becomes similar to the CSF in the chronic period due to encephalomalacia. Some infarcts develop gyriform cortical T1 hyperintensity in the late subacute period (approximately 2 weeks), which peaks at 1–2 months and may resolve several months later. Patchy gyriform contrast enhancement is common, appearing at 2–6 days and persisting for up to 5 months. Sometimes cortical enhancement may be the only finding in subacute infarcts.

Pertinent Clinical Information

The dreaded complications of ischemic infarction in the subacute period are malignant edema, which occurs in up to 10% of supratentorial infarcts and if untreated carries a mortality rate of up to 80%, and hemorrhage. Patients with malignant supratentorial infarctions (typically involving > 2/3 of the MCA territory) show progressive deterioration of consciousness within 24–48 h as a result of increasing edema, commonly causing subfalcine and uncal herniation. The predisposing factors include abnormalities of the ipsilateral circle of Willis and insufficient leptomeningeal collateral vessels. Conservative treatment includes pharmacologic strategies and hypothermia. Patients who fail to respond to conservative management may require decompressive hemicraniectomies. Hemorrhagic transformation is seen in 6% of ischemic strokes within 3 days, in 17–26% within 5–7 days, and in 43% by 4 weeks, but in most cases it remains asymptomatic. Symptomatic hemorrhagic transformation occurs in up to 6.8% of untreated patients and in up to 11% of cases following intra-arterial thombolytic treatment.

Differential Diagnosis

Neoplasm (153, 155)
- vasogenic edema usually present

- contrast enhancement is mass-like, not gyriform
- at least some portions of the cortex appear spared

Encephalitis
- vasogenic edema may be present
- non-arterial distribution, typically bilateral
- clinical presentation usually differs

Venous Infarction (181)
- non-arterial distribution
- evidence of venous thrombosis usually present

Background

During the early subacute period, the release of inflammatory mediators from ischemic brain leads to increasing edema due to water extravasation into the interstitial space, resulting in increases in tissue volume and T2 signal. Because extracellular water molecules are relatively unrestricted, ADC begins to rise and becomes normal at 1–2 weeks. This process is referred to as pseudonormalization, referring to the fact that tissue is necrotic despite the normal ADC values. Hemorrhagic transformation of ischemic infarcts is believed to be due to disruption of the blood–brain barrier (BBB) and subsequent revascularization of the infarcted tissue. Extravasation then causes further parenchymal injury through compression, ischemia, and direct toxicity of blood components. The appearance of cortical necrosis was initially thought to represent cortical hemorrhage, but the absence of susceptibility on T2*-weighted sequences argues against this. Although the mechanism causing T1 shortening remains unclear, it is now felt to reflect neuronal damage and reactive tissue change, with gliosis and deposition of fat-laden macrophages. Enhancement in the subacute period is due to BBB breakdown.

REFERENCES

1. Lansberg MG, Thijs VN, O'Brien MW, et al. Evolution of apparent diffusion coefficient, diffusion-weighted, and T2-weighted signal intensity of acute stroke. *AJNR* 2001;**22**:637–44.

2. Shaefer PW, Copen WA, Lev MH, et al. Diffusion-weighted imaging in acute stroke. *Neuroimag Clin N Am* 2005;**15**:503–30.

3. Siskas N, Lefkopoulos A, Ioannidis I, et al. Cortical laminar necrosis in brain infarcts: serial MRI. *Neuroradiology* 2003;**45**:283–8.

4. Huttner HB, Schwab S. Malignant cerebral artery infarction: clinical characteristics, treatment strategies, and future perspectives. *Lancet Neurol* 2009; **8**:949–58.

5. Khatri P, Wechsler LR, Broderic JP. Intracranial hemorrhage associated with revascularization therapies. *Stroke* 2007;**38**:431–40.

Brain Imaging with MRI and CT, ed. Zoran Rumboldt *et al.* Published by Cambridge University Press. © Cambridge University Press 2012.

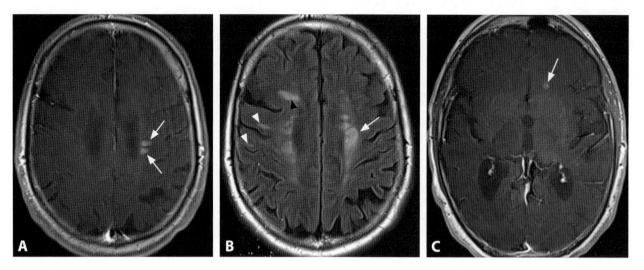

Figure 1. Axial post-contrast T1WI (A) shows two periventricular uniformly enhancing lesions (arrows), perpendicular to the ventricular surface. Corresponding FLAIR image (B) reveals confluent hyperintensity (arrow) at and around the enhancing areas. Finger-like (black arrowhead) and juxtacortical (white arrowhead) lesions are also present. Post-contrast T1WI at a lower level reveals a ring-enhancing lesion (arrow).

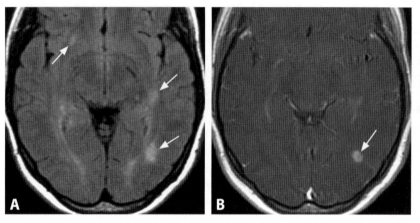

Figure 2. FLAIR image (A) shows multiple patchy hyperintensities (arrows). Corresponding post-contrast T1WI (B) reveals enhancement of the left optic radiation lesion (arrow).

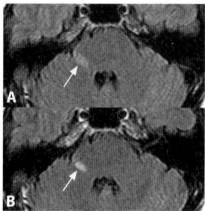

Figure 3. Axial FLAIR image through the pons (A) shows a subtle hyperintensity (arrow). Enhancement of the lesion (arrow) is present on post-contrast FLAIR image (B).

Figure 4. Axial post-contrast T1WI at the level of lateral ventricles (A) demonstrates a subtle punctuate periventricular area of enhancement (arrow). Corresponding DWI (B) reveals a prominent hyperintensity of the lesion (arrow). This was caused by a combination of increased T2 signal and reduced diffusion of the active plaque.

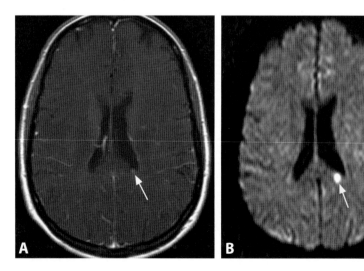

Active Multiple Sclerosis

MARIASAVINA SEVERINO

Specific Imaging Findings

Active multiple sclerosis (MS) plaques cause breakdown of the blood–brain barrier (BBB) and therefore enhancement on post-contrast MR images. Two enhancement patterns exist: uniform, reflecting the onset of a new lesion, and ringlike, indicating reactivation of an older lesion. Uniform enhancement may be faint, irregular, and with ill-defined margins. Peripheral ring-like enhancement is usually incomplete ("open"); however, it may form a full circle. There is no associated mass effect and no edema surrounding the enhancing area (except for tumefactive MS, which is discussed separately). Hyperacute plaques (first 24 h) may show restricted diffusion due to acute inflammation. On DWI acute lesions frequently show a ring pattern with hyperintense rim, while the center of the lesion has high ADC values. The diffusion findings and contrast enhancement, however, frequently do not coexist. Although MS plaques can be found throughout the brain, they have a predilection for periventricular white matter, corpus callosum, juxtacortical regions, optic radiations, as well as infra-tentorial locations. The enhancing lesions also follow this distribution. Ovoid appearance with orientation perpendicular to the ventricular surface is highly characteristic, but only on axial images. Microbleeds may be seen within MS plaques on T2* MR imaging, primarily with SWI. The detection rate of enhancing lesions is increased by delayed imaging, triple dose of contrast and use of magnetization transfer. The higher contrast dose may have a role in cases of diagnostic doubt following the standard dose.

Pertinent Clinical Information

The most common presentations of MS include: optic neuritis, ataxia, cranial nerve palsy, weakness, numbness, and fatigue. Suggestive clinical findings are symptom exacerbation upon exposure to a higher temperature (Uhthoff's phenomenon) and an electrical sensation running down the spine when bending the neck (Lhermitte's sign). CSF analysis shows increased protein and frequently oligoclonal bands. Approximately 80–85% of patients present with a relapsing–remitting course (RRMS), symptoms and signs evolve over days and improve over weeks. Around 5–10% have progressive MS from the onset (primary progressive MS: PPMS). Rarely patients show initially progressive course with subsequent relapses (progressive relapsing MS, PRMS). In some patients who do well for a long time (20 years) a "benign form" is retrospectively recognized.

Differential Diagnosis

Metastatic Neoplasms (155)
- perifocal edema with high T2 signal is almost always present, unless the lesions are punctate

Vasculitis (123)
- cortico-leptomeningeal contrast enhancement, especially in a multiple scattered pattern is highly characteristic; however, this is not always present
- cortical involvement is common
- calloseptal interface is spared

ADEM (112)
- very common involvement of gray matter, especially thalamus
- frequently larger patchy lesions

Background

MS is considered an inflammatory autoimmune neurologic disease characterized by disseminated CNS lesions. The peak onset is between 20 and 40 years of age, it may develop in children, and females are more commonly affected. Recent data suggest a complex multifactorial disorder that results from the interaction of genetic and environmental factors. Double inversion recovery (DIR) MR sequences improve detection of lesions, especially cortical ones. MR image subtraction reveals more active MS lesions with greater interobserver agreement, which is further improved with use of 3D sequences. Therapeutic approaches are based on altering the functions of the immune system, either by using broad immunosuppressive drugs or by modulating them more discreetly as with beta interferon. Early initiation of treatment offers benefits in most patients, and these benefits appear to persist for the long term. Monoclonal antibodies such as natalizumab are very specific and potent medications, and their use led to introduction of disease remission for the first time. Treatment with natalizumab, however, carries the risk of progressive multifocal leukoencephalopathy (PML).

REFERENCES

1. Lovblad KO, Anzalone N, Dorfler A, et al. MR imaging in multiple sclerosis: review and recommendations for current practice. AJNR 2010;**31**:983–9.

2. Uysal E, Erturk SM, Yildirim H, et al. Sensitivity of immediate and delayed gadolinium-enhanced MRI after injection of 0.5 M and 1.0 M gadolinium chelates for detecting multiple sclerosis lesions. AJR 2007;**188**:697–702.

3. Stecco A, Migazzo E, Saponaro A, et al. Gadolinium dose optimisation in patients with multiple sclerosis: intra- and inter-individual comparisons. Eur J Radiol 2006;**57**:37–42.

4. Moraal B, Wattjes MP, Geurts JJ, et al. Improved detection of active multiple sclerosis lesions: 3D subtraction imaging. Radiology 2010;**255**:154–63.

Brain Imaging with MRI and CT, ed. Zoran Rumboldt et al. Published by Cambridge University Press. © Cambridge University Press 2012.

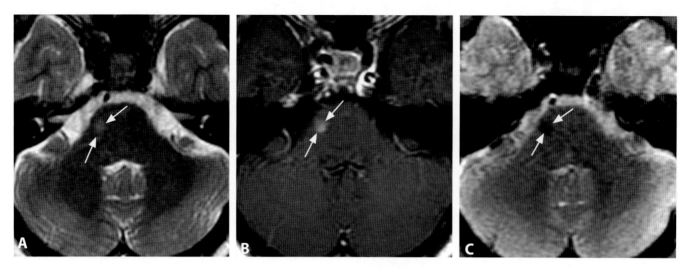

Figure 1. Axial MR images show a small area of abnormal signal (arrows) with ill-defined borders and no mass effect in the right pons, mildly hyperintense on T2WI (A), with "brush-like" enhancement on post-contrast T1WI (B), and mildly hypointense, with no blooming artifact on T2*WI (C).

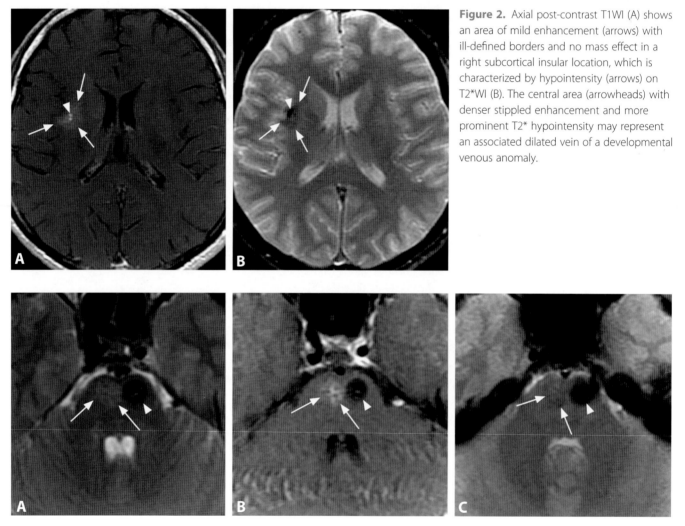

Figure 2. Axial post-contrast T1WI (A) shows an area of mild enhancement (arrows) with ill-defined borders and no mass effect in a right subcortical insular location, which is characterized by hypointensity (arrows) on T2*WI (B). The central area (arrowheads) with denser stippled enhancement and more prominent T2* hypointensity may represent an associated dilated vein of a developmental venous anomaly.

Figure 3. Axial T2WI (A), post-contrast T1WI (B), and T2*WI (C) reveal two adjacent round signal abnormalities in the pons, with different signal patterns. The right-sided abnormality (arrows) shows faint T2 hyperintensity, mild lacy enhancement, and mild T2* hypointensity. The left-sided abnormality is a cavernoma (arrowheads), with central mixed signal, peripheral dark hemosderin ring, and "blooming" artifact on T2*WI (C).

Capillary Telangiectasia

ALESSANDRO CIANFONI

Specific Imaging Findings

The characteristic MR imaging appearance of capillary telangiectasia is a small area with ill-defined margins of faint "brush-like", stippled, or "lacy" contrast enhancement, and without any mass effect, perifocal edema, or gliosis. In over half of the cases it is invisible on T2WI and FLAIR images, and in the remaining cases it shows mild T2 hyperintensity. The typical additional diagnostic clue, which is not always present, is a mild hypointensity on T2*-weighted images (GRE, SWI, EPI, PWI, BOLD), without clear "blooming" artifact. CT is almost always negative, while in rare cases it shows small calcifications. Angiography usually fails to reveal any abnormality. The most common location is in the pons, but it can be found anywhere in the brain and more rarely in the spinal cord. Capillary telangiectasia varies in size between a few millimeters and 2 cm; it may be associated with an adjacent developmental venous anomaly (DVA) and/or cavernoma (cavernous malformation).

Pertinent Clinical Information

Capillary telangiectasia is almost invariably an incidental, asymptomatic finding with very slow or absent growth. There are rare reports of symptomatic telangiectasias, which are usually larger than 1 cm in size. Clinical response and relapse on steroid treatment have been described. Hemorrhage is exceptional, and is thought to arise from commonly associated cavernous malformations. Capillary telangiectasia may also possibly be a radiation-induced vascular malformation. Due to its benign course, treatment and follow-up are not warranted. Misdiagnosis with metastatic neoplasms is common and should be avoided.

Differential Diagnosis

Metastasis and Other Enhancing Neoplasms (153, 155, 158)

- typically better defined with distinct margins
- mass effect and vasogenic edema are present except in some very small lesions
- intense contrast enhancement
- mild hypointensity on T2* images is uncommon

Subacute Lacunar Infarct

- T2 hyperintense

- high signal on ADC map consistent with increased diffusion
- enhancement is peripheral, if present

Developmental Venous Anomaly and Cavernoma (127, 183)

- often associated
- DVA has dilated enhancing veins, with "caput medusa"
- cavernoma has "popcorn appearance" – central mixed high and low T2 signal and lobulated appearance, peripheral hemosiderin ring

Background

Capillary telangiectasia is a slow-flow CNS vascular malformation, which was also classified as occult vascular malformation, before the advent of MR imaging. Typical microscopic features are clusters of thin-walled "capillary-type" ectatic blood vessels interspersed in a background of normal brain tissue. Typical mild T2* signal hypointensity is most likely related to high levels of paramagnetic deoxyhemoglobin due to slow flow and deoxygenation of blood. Hemorrhage, on the other hand, would be marked by presence of hemosiderin, and "blooming" artifacts. Its frequent association with other slow flow capillary–venous vascular malformations suggests common etiology, with hereditary and acquired factors, probably with a venous outflow restriction as a common denominator.

REFERENCES

1. Sayama CM, Osborn AG, Chin SS, Couldwell WT. Capillary telangiectasias: clinical, radiographic, and histopathological features. Clinical article. *J Neurosurg* 2010;**113**:709–14.
2. Castillo M, Morrison T, Shaw JA, Bouldin TW. MR imaging and histologic features of capillary telangiectasia of the basal ganglia. *AJNR* 2001;**22**:1553–5.
3. Yoshida Y, Terae S, Kudo K, *et al*. Capillary telangiectasia of the brain stem diagnosed by susceptibility-weighted imaging. *J Comput Assist Tomogr* 2006;**30**:980–2.
4. Scaglione C, Salvi F, Riguzzi P, *et al*. Symptomatic unruptured capillary telangiectasia of the brain stem: report of three cases and review of the literature. *J Neurol Neurosurg Psychiatry* 2001;**71**:390–3.
5. Pozzati E, Marliani AF, Zucchelli M, *et al*. The neurovascular triad: mixed cavernous, capillary, and venous malformations of the brainstem. *J Neurosurg* 2007;**107**:1113–9.

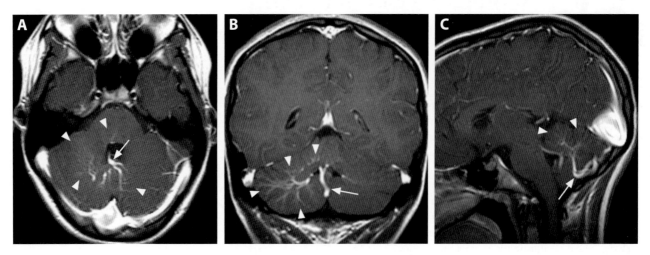

Figure 1. Post-contrast T1WIs in axial (A), coronal (B), and sagittal (C) planes show infratentorial linear enhancing structures (arrowheads) converging to a larger one (arrows), giving a "caput medusae" appearance.

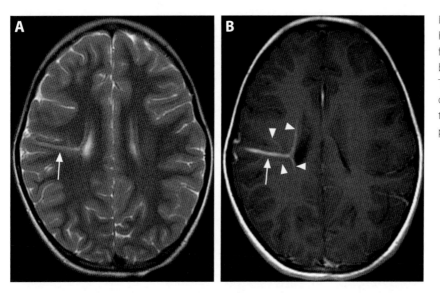

Figure 2. T2WI (A) in a different patient shows a hyperintense linear structure (arrow) that extends from the wall of the right lateral ventricle to the brain surface, corresponding to a draining vein. The vein is densely enhancing (arrow) on corresponding post-contrast T1WI (B). Some of the tributaries (arrowheads) are well seen on the post-contrast image.

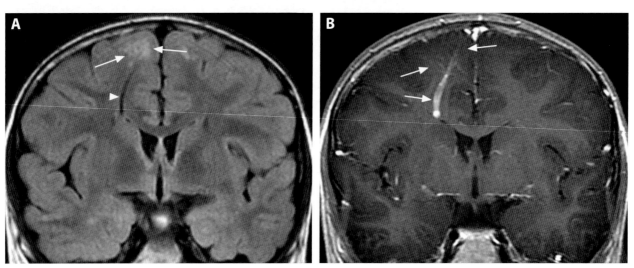

Figure 3. Hypointense flow-void (arrowhead) and hyperintense tributaries (arrows) are noted on coronal FLAIR image (A) in another patient. All these structures avidly enhance (arrows) on post-contrast T1WI (B).

Developmental Venous Anomaly

GIULIO ZUCCOLI

Specific Imaging Findings

Developmental venous anomalies (DVAs, venous angiomas, venous malformations) consist of dilated medullary veins draining centripetally and radially into a transcerebral collector that ultimately converges into the deep or superficial venous system in an area in which there is an absence of normal draining veins. The *caput medusae* (head of the Medusa) represents the typical morphological appearance of DVAs: contrast enhancement of the network of feeding veins converging into the single draining vein is caused by the slow flow on both CT and MR imaging. Size of DVAs is quite variable, and large DVAs draining an entire hemisphere may be occasionally observed. The draining vein of large DVAs can demonstrate flow-void (high-velocity signal loss best seen on T2WI), whereas medullary veins and smaller collecting veins are frequently seen as T2 hyperintensities, or they may remain imperceptible on non-contrasted MR images. If the vessel is obliquely oriented, a "yin–yang" symbol appearance may occur because of the characteristic spatial misregistration artifacts associated with venous flow. DWI/ADC findings are usually unremarkable. Brain parenchyma adjacent to DVAs is most commonly normal on standard images however, a minority of DVAs are associated with T2 hyperintensity in the drainage territory, usually in a periventricular location. DVAs are usually not visible on unenhanced CT.

Pertinent Clinical Information

DVAs are most commonly incidentally found on MR imaging and are estimated to occur in around 3% of individuals. There is an association with sporadic cavernous malformations but not with familial cavernomas. De-novo cavernomas have been described to occur adjacent to pre-existing DVAs. DVA is generally considered a benign finding. Notwithstanding, a variety of symptoms including headache, non-communicating hydrocephalus, tinnitus, and cranial nerve dysfunction have been described in association with DVAs. As with other venous structures, thrombosis may occur in DVAs. Hemorrhage in association with DVAs has been described, especially in the cerebellum.

Differential Diagnosis

Arteriovenous Malformation (AVM) (182)
- nidus of abnormal vascular structures – "bag of worms" best seen on T2WI
- absence of caput medusa appearance

Venous Thrombosis (97)
- stagnant flow within enlarged deep medullary, subependymal and cortical veins
- associated venous infarct may be present in the involved territory

Sturge–Weber Syndrome (86)
- atrophy of the involved cerebral hemisphere
- cortical gyriform calcifications
- enlargement of the ispilateral choroid plexus
- facial angiomas and enhancing pial angiomas coexist

Background

Once felt to be rare, DVAs are now considered to be the most common vascular malformation in the brain parenchyma, constituting approximately 60% of all vascular malformations at autopsy. The etiology of DVAs is unknown and it is currently accepted that early failure, abnormal development, or intrauterine occlusion of small veins may trigger the development of a compensatory system of the venous drainage. DVAs are commonly solitary, although it is not rare to find multiple DVAs in the same patient. Frontal, parietal, and brachium pontis-dentate nucleus represent the most common locations. DVAs serve as normal drainage routes of the brain because of the absence of the standard territorial venous drainage.

REFERENCES

1. Santucci GM, Leach JL, Ying J, et al. Brain parenchymal signal abnormalities associated with developmental venous anomalies: detailed MR imaging assessment. *AJNR* 2008;**29**:1317–23.
2. Pereira VM, Geibprasert S, Krings T, et al. Pathomechanisms of symptomatic developmental venous anomalies. *Stroke* 2008;**39**:3201–15.
3. Truwit CL. Venous angioma of the brain: history, significance, and imaging findings. *AJR* 1992;**159**:1299–307.
4. San Millán Ruíz D, Delavelle J, Yilmaz H, et al. Parenchymal abnormalities associated with developmental venous anomalies. *Neuroradiology* 2007;**49**:987–95.
5. Lee C, Pennington MA, Kenney CM 3rd. MR evaluation of developmental venous anomalies: medullary venous anatomy of venous angiomas. *AJNR* 1996;**17**:61–70.
6. Petersen TA, Morrison LA, Schrader RM, Hart BL. Familial versus sporadic cavernous malformations: differences in developmental venous anomaly association and lesion phenotype. *AJNR* 2010;**31**:377–82.

Brain Imaging with MRI and CT, ed. Zoran Rumboldt et al. Published by Cambridge University Press. © Cambridge University Press 2012.

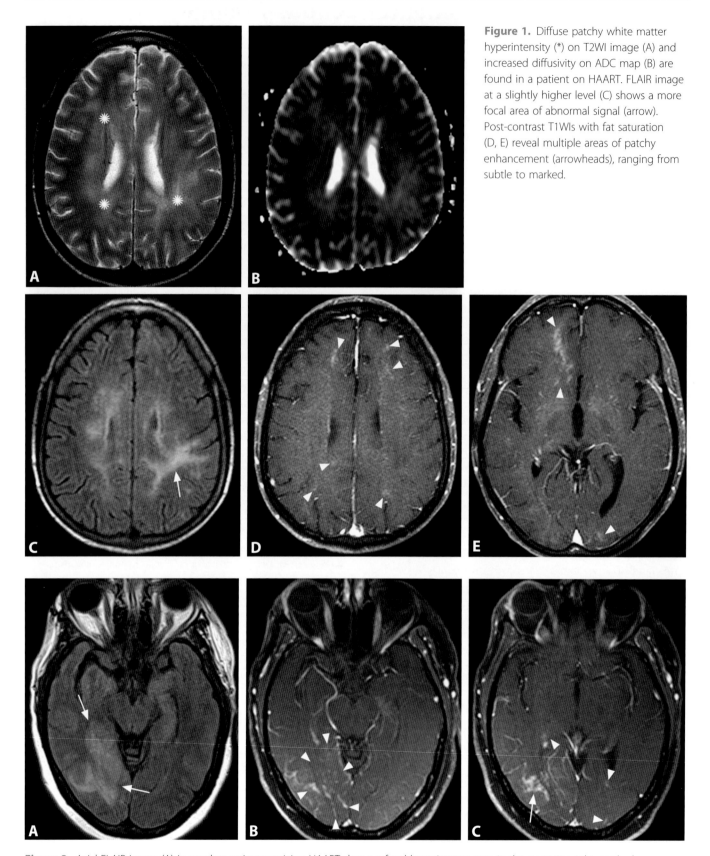

Figure 1. Diffuse patchy white matter hyperintensity (*) on T2WI image (A) and increased diffusivity on ADC map (B) are found in a patient on HAART. FLAIR image at a slightly higher level (C) shows a more focal area of abnormal signal (arrow). Post-contrast T1WIs with fat saturation (D, E) reveal multiple areas of patchy enhancement (arrowheads), ranging from subtle to marked.

Figure 2. Axial FLAIR image (A) in another patient receiving HAART shows a focal hyperintense area in the posterior right cerebral hemisphere (arrows), without mass effect. Corresponding post-contrast T1WI with fat saturation (B) reveals "lacy" patchy and punctuate areas of enhancement (arrowheads). A slightly more cephalad post-contrast image (C) shows a more densely enhancing area (arrow), along with additional bilateral subtle enhancing lesions (arrowheads).

Immune Reconstitution Inflammatory Syndrome (IRIS)

ZORAN RUMBOLDT

Specific Imaging Findings

Patchy and ill-defined, usually large areas of "lacy" enhancement within the white matter are characteristic of immune reconstitution inflammatory response (IRIS) on post-contrast MR imaging. These enhancing lesions may be focal or scattered throughout different areas of the brain and leptomeningeal enhancement may also be observed. There is usually associated white matter T2 hyperintensity, low T1 signal, increased diffusivity and minimal to mild mass effect. The new imaging findings frequently occur within or adjacent to the isolated pre-existing lesions, and may be associated with progressive multifocal leukoencephalopathy (PML).

Areas of abnormal signal and contrast enhancement do not necessarily correspond to each other and enhancement may be absent. Overall, the imaging findings in IRIS are diverse and frequently atypical so that this entity should be considered whenever an unusual MRI appearance is encountered in patients treated with HAART.

Pertinent Clinical Information

IRIS presents as clinical deterioration and imaging disease progression during immunologic recovery while the HIV infection is effectively treated with HAART. Criteria for diagnosis include prior response to antimicrobial therapy, return of original symptoms or new inflammatory syndromes after initiation of HAART, and negative CSF cultures. The patients at greatest risk have a low CD4$^+$ T-cell count prior to the initiation of HAART and show a rapid decrease in plasma HIV RNA during the first 3 months of therapy. IRIS may also occur following discontinuation of natalizumab in patients with multiple sclerosis.

Differential Diagnosis

HIV Encephalitis (25)
- T2 hyperintensity is diffuse and without corresponding T1 hypointensity
- absence of contrast enhancement

PML (116)
- contrast enhancement is rare and more subtle
- may be indistinguishable/the two entities may be present at the same time

Cryptococcal Meningitis (8)
- bilateral involvement of the deep gray matter is characteristic

CMV Encephalitis
- T2 hyperintensity and contrast enhancement limited to a thin subependymal area

Lymphoma (158)
- focal mass lesions with dense enhancement and mass effect
- low signal on T2WI and ADC maps

- increased FDG uptake on PET; cerebral blood volume may be increased on perfusion studies

Toxoplasmosis (157)
- focal enhancing lesions typically in the deep gray matter with prominent edema and mass effect
- eccentric target sign may be present on post-contrast images

Progression of Multiple Sclerosis (125)
- the lesions tend to show characteristic appearance and occur in typical locations
- new signal abnormality and/or enhancement is focal, even when extending from a pre-existing lesion

Background

IRIS represents a spectrum of clinicopathologic entities encountered in HIV-infected patients occurring weeks to months after initiation of HAART resulting in rapid CD4$^+$ cell count recovery and suppression of viral load, frequently in the context of opportunistic infections, primarily PML. It may be more common and more severe in patients with natalizumab-associated PML than it is in patients with HIV-associated PML. IRIS may also occur without any opportunistic infection as a T cell-mediated encephalitis. Brain biopsy helps to identify IRIS and diseases that mimic it. Histology demonstrates diffuse microglial hyperplasia and massive and diffuse perivascular and intraparenchymal infiltration, predominantly by CD8+/CD4− lymphocytes. In cases with a more favorable course, inflammation is mild with marked macrophage activation and presence of CD4+ lymphocytes. Severe inflammation in the lethal cases is mostly composed of CD8+ cytotoxic lymphocytes. Current recommendations for IRIS treatment include systemic corticosteroids along with continuation of HAART.

REFERENCES

1. Smith AB, Smirniotopoulos JG, Rushing EJ. From the archives of the AFIP: central nervous system infections associated with human immunodeficiency virus infection: radiologic–pathologic correlation. *Radiographics* 2008;**28**:2033–58.

2. Buckle C, Castillo M. Use of diffusion-weighted imaging to evaluate the initial response of progressive multifocal leukoencephalopathy to highly active antiretroviral therapy: early experience. *AJNR* 2010;**31**:1031–5.

3. Gray F, Bazille C, Adle-Biassette H, *et al.* Central nervous system immune reconstitution disease in acquired immunodeficiency syndrome patients receiving highly active antiretroviral treatment. *J Neurovirol* 2005;**11**(Suppl 3):16–22.

4. Rushing EJ, Liappis A, Smirniotopoulos JD, *et al.* Immune reconstitution inflammatory syndrome of the brain: case illustrations of a challenging entity. *J Neuropathol Exp Neurol* 2008;**67**:819–27.

5. Miravalle A, Jensen R, Kinkel RP. Immune reconstitution inflammatory syndrome in patients with multiple sclerosis following cessation of natalizumab therapy. *Arch Neurol* 2011;**68**:186–91.

Brain Imaging with MRI and CT, ed. Zoran Rumboldt *et al.* Published by Cambridge University Press. © Cambridge University Press 2012.

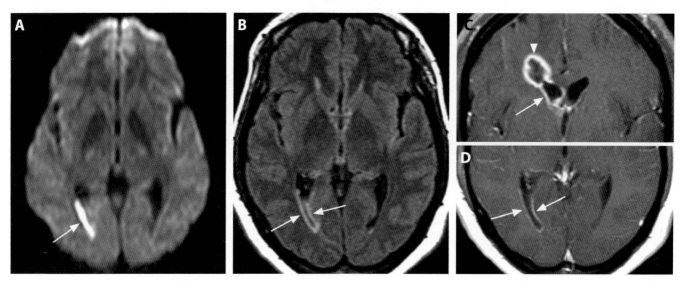

Figure 1. Axial DWI (A) shows a very bright collection (arrow) within the occipital horn of the right lateral ventricle. Corresponding FLAIR image (B) reveals adjacent hyperintensity (arrows) along the ventricular walls. The collection is of higher signal intensity than the CSF. (C) Coronal post-contrast T1WI with fat saturation shows enhancement along the frontal horn of the right lateral ventricle (arrow), contiguous with a parenchymal rim-enhancing lesion (arrowhead) that ruptured into the ventricles. (D) Axial post-contrast T1WI demonstrates linear ependymal enhancement (arrows) corresponding to the hyperintensity on FLAIR.

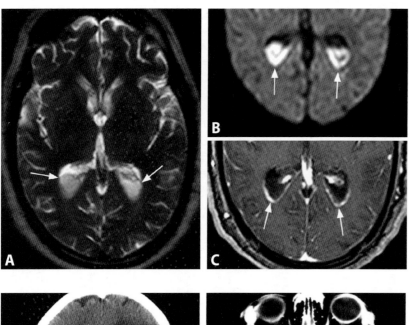

Figure 2. Axial single shot T2WI (A) in a patient with meningitis shows dependent intraventricular layering of material that is of lower signal than the CSF. Note the arched instead of a straight line at the interface with the CSF (arrows). Matching DWI (B) reveals marked bright signal (arrows) of the dependent intraventricular material. There is linear ependymal enhancement (arrows) on corresponding post-contrast T1WI (C).

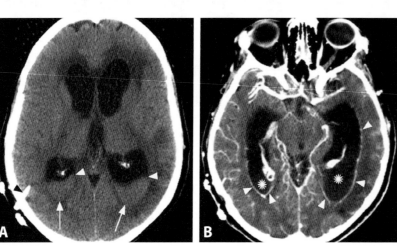

Figure 3. Axial non-enhanced CT image (A) following a neurosurgical procedure shows hydrocephalus with dense collections (arrows). Note their dependent location and undulating contours (white arrowheads). Ventricular drainage catheter is present (black arrowhead). Follow-up post-contrast CT (B) reveals decrease in attenuation of the material (*) and ependymal enhancement (arrowheads).

Ventriculitis

ZORAN RUMBOLDT AND MAJDA THURNHER

Specific Imaging Findings

In patients with ventriculitis CT may show hydrocephalus, while characteristic dependent layering of debris is seen with pyogenic ventriculitis. The debris is of higher attenuation than the CSF and its margin may be indistinct and irregular. Post-contrast CT images may show linear enhancement along the ventricular walls. Ventricular debris, ventriculomegaly, periventricular T2 hyperintensity, and ependymal contrast enhancement are the signs of ventriculitis on MR imaging. Similar to CT, the ventricular debris is seen as dependent layering material with higher signal intensity than the CSF on FLAIR and T1WI. The material characteristically shows irregular and undulating interface with the CSF, unlike the typical straight horizontal fluid–fluid levels. The purulent intraventricular material is very bright on DWI with corresponding low ADC values. Ependymal and periventricular edema is best seen on FLAIR images as linear hyperintensity lining the affected ventricles. DWI/ADC and FLAIR images are more sensitive for detection of pyogenic ventriculitis than post-contrast T1WI. However, in cases of non-pyogenic ventriculitis, there is usually no ventricular debris so that ependymal enhancement and hyperintensity on FLAIR images may be the only imaging findings.

Pertinent Clinical Information

Pyogenic ventriculitis is an uncommon but often severe and life-threatening intracranial infection. It is a relatively frequent complication of neonatal meningitis, but rare with adult purulent meningitis, most commonly occuring when an abscess ruptures into the ventricles. Clinical features of ventriculitis are often obscure and nonspecific as it typically occurs in already critically ill patients. Early detection is essential for prompt treatment, which is crucial for these patients, as devastating neurological damage can occur with delayed treatment, even if the infection is ultimately eradicated. High doses of systemic antibiotics may be combined with ventricular drainage and intraventricular administration of antibiotics.

Differential Diagnosis

Intraventricular Hemorrhage (99, 177)

- absence of periventricular hyperintensity on FLAIR images
- absence of ependymal contrast enhancement
- high density consistent with blood clot on CT in the acute phase
- MRI signal intensity pattern consistent with blood products
- straight level of acute blood or the casting configuration of clotted blood

CNS Lymphoma (usually PCNSL) (158)

- periventricular enhancement is frequently nodular
- additional leptomeningeal and/or intra-axial lesions are frequently present
- very low ADC values

Subependymal Tumor Spread

- presence of the primary neoplasm (such as medulloblastoma or ependymoma)
- enhancement is frequently nodular

Background

Ventriculitis is an uncommon CNS infection that has been described using a variety of terms including ependymitis, intraventricular abscess, ventricular empyema, and pyocephalus. Gram-negative bacteria and *Staphylococcus* species are the most common agents causing pyogenic ventriculitis. In immunocompromised individuals fungal, viral, and toxoplasma ventriculitis may occur. Cytomegalovirus (CMV) is the most common infectious agent responsible for ventriculitis in patients with AIDS. The possible routes of infection are hematogenous spread to the choroid plexus, contiguous extension from a brain abscess, and direct implantation secondary to trauma or surgery, such as with ventricular catheter placement. Sonography is the initial imaging method for evaluating ventriculitis in the newborn. Ultrasound findings include ventricular dilatation with irregularity of the ventricular margins and increased periventricular echogenicity. The choroid plexus margins also appear poorly defined with loss of the normally smooth contour. Echogenic material is seen within the lateral ventricles, and intraventricular septa formation results in ventricular compartmentalization. ADC values are negatively correlated with pleocytosis and the protein content of CSF, indicating that ADC value may be a useful non-invasive method for the follow-up evaluation of ventriculitis as well as the diagnosis.

REFERENCES

1. Fukui MB, Williams RL, Mudigonda S. CT and MR imaging features of pyogenic ventriculitis. *AJNR* 2001;**22**:1510–6.
2. Fujikawa A, Tsuchiya K, Honya K, Nitatori T. Comparison of MRI sequences to detect ventriculitis. *AJR* 2006;**187**:1048–53.
3. Pezzullo JA, Tung GA, Mudigonda S, Rogg JM. Diffusion-weighted MR imaging of pyogenic ventriculitis. *AJR* 2003;**180**:71–5.
4. Hong JT, Son BC, Sung JH, *et al.* Significance of diffusion-weighted imaging and apparent diffusion coefficient maps for the evaluation of pyogenic ventriculitis. *Clin Neurol Neurosurg* 2008;**110**:137–44.
5. Reeder JD, Sanders RC. Ventriculitis in the neonate: recognition by sonography. *AJNR* 1983;**4**:37–41.

SECTION 5

Primarily Extra-Axial Focal Space-Occupying Lesions

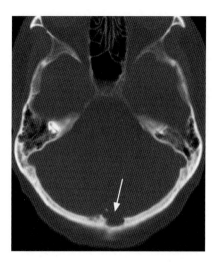

Figure 1. Axial CT with bone algorithm and window shows a smooth lobulated oval defect (arrow) of the inner table in the region of the torcular.

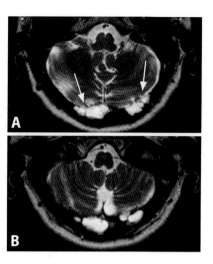

Figure 2. Axial T2WIs (A, B) show bilateral CSF-like lobulated extra-axial collections (arrows) at the location of the proximal transverse sinuses.

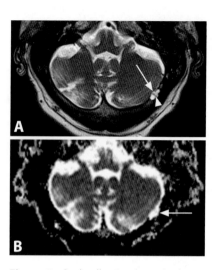

Figure 3. Oval collection (arrow) adjacent to the transverse sinus is CSF-like on both T2WI (A) and ADC map (B) and contains a linear band (arrowhead).

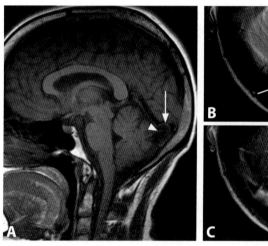

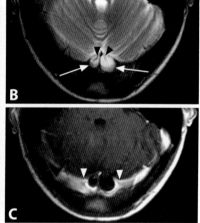

Figure 4. Midsagittal T1WI (A) shows a rounded subarachnoid space extension (arrow) into the confluence of venous sinuses, containing a linear band (arrowhead). Axial T2WI (B) reveals two oval structures with predominant CSF signal intensity (arrows) and internal bands (arrowheads). Post-contrast T1WI (C) reveals normal enhancement of the adjacent transverse sinuses (arrowheads) and no enhancement of the oval structures.

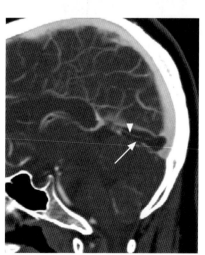

Figure 5. Sagittal MIP of a CT angiogram reveals a small vein (arrowhead) within an oval filling defect (arrow) of the straight sinus and torcular.

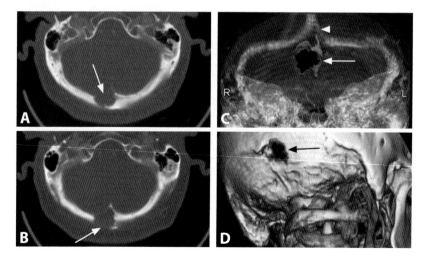

Figure 6. Axial post-contrast CT with bone algorithm and window demonstrates a lobulated smooth calvarial defect (arrow). Another image (B) reveals extension through the outer table (arrow). 3D reconstructions (C, D) show smooth margins of the lesion (arrow), located just inferior to the torcular (arrowhead).

Arachnoid Granulations

ZORAN RUMBOLDT

Specific Imaging Findings

Arachnoid granulations (AGs, Pacchionian bodies or granulations) are protrusions of subarachnoid space into the cerebral venous sinus lumen. On dedicated imaging, AGs may be found in 60–90% of individuals, most commonly adjacent and/or within the superior sagittal, transverse, and straight sinuses. The detection rate primarily depends on image quality/resolution and active search for AGs – they are present in at least 20% of modern routine head CT or MRI scans, most commonly within the lateral transverse sinuses adjacent to venous entrance sites. They may be single or multiple, oval or smoothly lobulated structures that follow the CSF density and signal intensities. Internal septa and vessels may lead to linear areas of different appearance and AGs may also contain calcifications. On post-contrast images they are well-defined, filling defects wholly or partly within a venous sinus. A majority of AGs, based on their location and size, produce smooth calvarial remodeling. On MR or CT venography, displacement, distortion, and narrowing of the sinus lumen may be seen. With high-resolution post-contrast imaging one or more veins are seen to enter AGs in almost all cases. On DWI, AGs are iso-intense to normal brain tissue, while they are CSF-like on ADC maps. Large AGs, over 1 cm in size, may lead to punched out calvarial defects from the inner into the outer table on CT images. Nonfluid signal intensity is present on at least some, most commonly FLAIR, images in the vast majority of these AGs and varies from absent/hypointense (flow-voids) to gray matter iso-intense (stromal tissue).

Pertinent Clinical Information

AGs are incidentally discovered on imaging studies and are typically asymptomatic. Rare cases of benign intracranial hypertension from venous sinus compression have been described. However, large AGs in patients with headache are usually unrelated. A significant pressure gradient across the AG confirms it as the cause of symptoms on invasive dural sinus measurement. When harvesting cranial bone grafts, there is a risk of entering the intracranial venous system through the calvarial foveolae for AGs.

Differential Diagnosis

Venous Sinus Thrombosis (97)
- typically T1 bright and dark on T2*-weighted images
- thick defects with irregular margins (especially recanalized)

Metastatic Neoplasms
- bone erosions, irregular margins
- enhancement with contrast

Epidermoid (143)
- characteristically "light bulb" bright on DWI

Dermoid (75)
- characteristic T1 hyperintensity of fat

Meningioma (138)
- dense contrast enhancement

Endolymphatic Sac Tumor
- retrocochlear location with spiculated erosions of the temporal bone
- characteristic T1 and T2 hyperintensity

Arachnoid Cyst (142)
- usually a single large cyst
- frequently between the posterior aspect of the cerebellar hemispheres

Infectious Cysts (Hydatid Disease, Cysticercosis) (145, 167)
- bone involvement is rare, extremely unusual along dural sinuses
- may contain sediment of various signal intensity
- abnormal peaks on MR spectroscopy

Background

AGs are anatomic variants that were initially described by Pacchioni more than 300 years ago. Histologically, they are bulbous aggregates of fibroelastic tissue that are continuous with the subarachnoid space and can be divided into single and lobulated types. CSF circulates through AGs and thereby enters the venous system. Major calvarial foveolae for arachnoid granulations are located within 2.5 cm of the coronal and 1.5 cm of the sagittal suture. In cadavers, AGs are also commonly found in the middle cranial fossa along the middle meningeal and sphenoparietal sinuses, as well as foramen rotundum and cavernous sinus, which are rarely identified on routine clinical imaging studies.

REFERENCES

1. Leach JL, Jones BV, Tomsick TA, *et al.* Normal appearance of arachnoid granulations on contrast-enhanced CT and MR of the brain: differentiation from dural sinus disease. *AJNR* 1996;**17**:1523–32.

2. Liang L, Korogi Y, Sugahara T, *et al.* Normal structures in the intracranial dural sinuses: delineation with 3D contrast-enhanced magnetization prepared rapid acquisition gradient-echo imaging sequence. *AJNR* 2002;**23**:1739–46.

3. Trimble CR, Harnsberger HR, Castillo M, *et al.* "Giant" arachnoid granulations just like CSF?: NOT!! *AJNR* 2010;**31**:1724–8.

4. Kiroglu Y, Yaqci B, Cirak B, Karabulut N. Giant arachnoid granulation in a patient with benign intracranial hypertension. *Eur Radiol* 2008;**18**:2329–32.

5. Sweeney WM, Afifi AM, Zor F, *et al.* Anatomic survey of arachnoid foveolae and the clinical correlation to cranial bone grafting. *J Craniofac Surg* 2011;**22**:118–21.

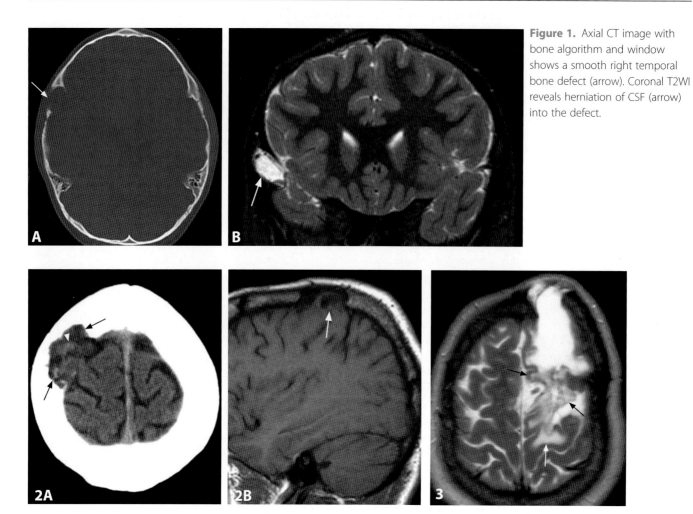

Figure 1. Axial CT image with bone algorithm and window shows a smooth right temporal bone defect (arrow). Coronal T2WI reveals herniation of CSF (arrow) into the defect.

Figure 2. CT (A) shows a smoothly marginated right parietal bone lesion (arrows) containing both brain parenchyma (arrowhead) and CSF. Sagittal T1WI (B) shows brain herniating through the defect (arrow).

Figure 3. Axial T2WI shows a left frontal bone defect with extrusion of CSF-containing porencephalic cyst. Note underlying encephalomalacia (arrows) in left frontal lobe. This was a consequence of a previous craniotomy.

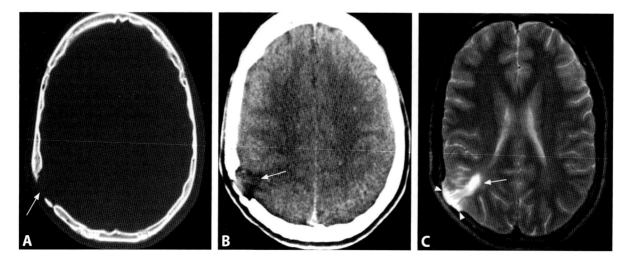

Figure 4. A smooth, well-defined bony defect (A) is present in the right parietal bone on CT image with bone window (A). Corresponding soft tissue window CT shows abnormal hypodensity (arrow) of the underlying brain. Axial T2WI at a similar level (C) reveals hyperintensity of the brain (arrow), consistent with encephalomalacia and gliosis. There is mild herniation of both CSF and brain into the bony defect. This patient presented with seizures 23 years after a head trauma sustained in infancy.

Leptomeningeal Cyst

BENJAMIN HUANG

Specific Imaging Findings

Skull radiographs show a "growing" or expanding fracture accompanied by a soft tissue subcutaneous mass. CT shows a defect in calvarium that is filled with a cyst of CSF density and may also contain brain tissue. MRI shows the cyst to be isointense to CSF in all sequences, while the contained brain is usually of bright T2 signal due to encephalomalacia and gliosis. The adjacent brain may be atrophic and the ventricles dilated. There is no abnormal contrast enhancement. In the past, a follow-up skull radiograph was obtained in all young children to exclude this complication; however, nowadays this complication is known to be so rare that this is no longer indicated.

Pertinent Clinical Information

Leptomeningeal cysts present as slowly growing, soft calvarial subcutaneous masses at the site of known (and sometimes unknown) fractures or craniotomy defects. On physical examination, patients classically demonstrate a cranial defect with a bulging and pulsatile center. Because there generally is underlying malacia of the brain, seizures may accompany the cyst. The cyst will grow up to a size and then remain stable for years, but it generally becomes apparent within one year of the initial trauma. However, onset of seizures has been described even more than two decades after the initial trauma. Thin bones, such as those surrounding the orbits, are preferentially involved. If the cyst projects into an orbit, proptosis ensues. If the cyst projects into the nasal cavities, CSF leak may be the initial presentation with or without meningitis. Surgical treatment involves resection of the cyst and dural repair. If the cyst contains malacic brain, this too can be resected.

Differential Diagnosis

Arachnoid Cyst (142)
- may show some bone scalloping, but no associated skull defect
- no brain parenchyma within the cyst

Background

Leptomeningeal cysts are also called "growing fractures". They are a complication of a fracture in which a piece of arachnoid gets trapped or insinuates itself into the site of the fracture. These meninges accumulate CSF (possibly trapping and/or secreting it) and cause a "cyst" to form. Presumably, the pulsation of CSF and/or the brain cause the bone defect to enlarge, via a ball-valve mechanism. This is the typical scenario in young (almost never more than 8 years of age) patients, with the majority of reported cases occuring in infants under the age of 1. These cysts may also occur following craniosynostosis surgery and after delivery with forceps or vacuum extraction. They may develop in as little as two months and typically will present within 3 years of the initial traumatic event. In adults the cysts are generally the result of a previous craniotomy, they may also harbor brain within them and are better categorized as meningoencephaloceles. A three-type classification has been proposed for growing skull fractures, based on the type of tissue extending through the bony defect. Type I fractures contain CSF lined by arachnoid tissue only. Type II fractures contain brain tissue. In type III fractures, a porencephalic cyst develops which extends into the skull defect. Leptomeningeal cysts are rare, probably seen in less than 1% of fractures or surgical defects. It is said that a bone diastasis of over 4 mm is needed for these cysts to form, but that fact has never been proven.

REFERENCES

1. Muhonen MG, Piper JG, Menezes AH. Pathogenesis and treatment of growing skull fractures. *Surg Neurol* 1995;**43**:367–73.
2. Naim-Ur-Rahman, Jamjoom Z, Jamjoom A, Murshid WR. Growing skull fractures: classification and management. *Br J Neurosurg* 1994; **8**:667–79.
3. Moses CK, Rumboldt Z. Neuroradiology: Brain. In *Aunt Minnie's Atlas and Imaging Specific Diagnosis*, 3rd edn, Pope TL, ed. Lippincott Williams and Wilkins, Philadelphia, PA, 2009;248–308.
4. Suri A, Mahapatra AK. Growing fractures of the orbital roof. A report of two cases and a review. *Pediatr Neurosurg* 2002;**36**:96–100.
5. Meier JD, Dublin AB, Strong EB. Leptomeningeal cyst of the orbital roof in an adult: case report and literature review. *Skull Base* 2009;**19**:231–5.

Brain Imaging with MRI and CT, ed. Zoran Rumboldt *et al.* Published by Cambridge University Press. © Cambridge University Press 2012.

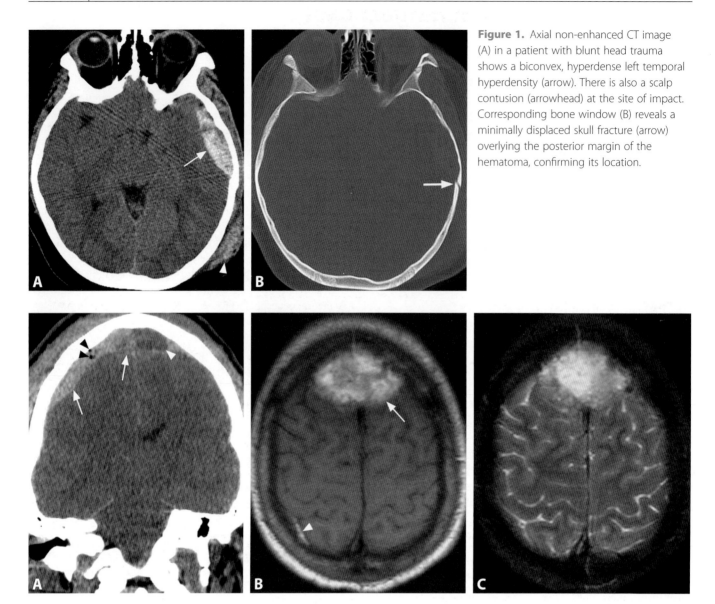

Figure 1. Axial non-enhanced CT image (A) in a patient with blunt head trauma shows a biconvex, hyperdense left temporal hyperdensity (arrow). There is also a scalp contusion (arrowhead) at the site of impact. Corresponding bone window (B) reveals a minimally displaced skull fracture (arrow) overlying the posterior margin of the hematoma, confirming its location.

Figure 2. Reformatted coronal CT image shows a hyperdense vertex hematoma (arrows) crossing the midline. Its isodense portion (white arrowhead) is consistent with hyperacute blood, while the gas bubbles (black arrowhead) indicate skull fracture. Axial T1WI (B) and T2WI (C) show heterogenous predominantly hyperintense signal of the bifrontal hematoma. A small additional extra-axial bleed (arrowhead) is seen on B.

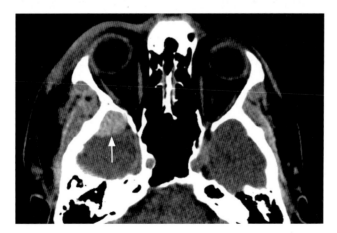

Figure 3. CT image shows a characteristic anterior temporal biconvex collection of venous origin (arrow).

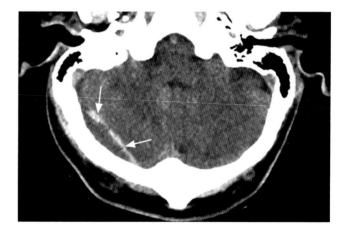

Figure 4. Non-enhanced CT image reveals a right posterior fossa collection with hyperdense rim (arrows).

Epidural Hematoma

BENJAMIN HUANG

Specific Imaging Findings

Epidural (or extradural) hematomas (EDH) appear as well-defined, frequently biconvex extra-axial collections, associated with skull fractures in the vast majority of cases. Acute EDHs are hyperdense on CT. EDHs may be isodense to gray matter if they are imaged in the hyperacute stage before a clot has formed. The presence of a swirled appearance formed by alternating crescentic regions of varying densities generally indicates active hemorrhage, which may be confirmed by post-contrast enhancement within a hematoma. The MRI signal intensities will vary depending on the age of blood products similar to other intracranial hemorrhages; however, this occurs much more rapidly so that most EDHs are bright on all sequences. Unlike subdural hematomas, EDHs can cross the midline but usually respect suture lines (unless the fracture line crosses the suture). In some cases the acute blood products may be resorbed into the exposed bone marrow of the adjacent fracture, leading to rapid (within hours) decrease in size or even complete disappearance of the hematoma.

Pertinent Clinical Information

Head trauma due to traffic accidents, falls, and assaults accounts for over 90% of EDHs. Non-traumatic (spontaneous) EDHs are rare and associated with infections, coagulation disorders, vascular malformations, and neoplasms involving the dura or skull. Approximately half of patients with EDH are comatose on admission or immediately before surgery, and roughly half of patients may have the classic "lucid interval" characterized by a patient who is initially unconscious, wakes up, and secondarily deteriorates. Because arterial EDHs can rapidly enlarge and cause prominent mass effect, they often present as surgical emergencies requiring urgent evacuation. Hematoma volume, presence of midline shift, and mixed clot density appear to portend a poorer outcome. Smaller EDHs in conscious patients without neurologic defects may be managed nonoperatively. In these patients a follow-up CT scan performed within 6–8 h is recommended to ensure that no growth occurs. Approximately a quarter of EDHs initially managed conservatively show growth, which typically occurs within the first 36 h.

Differential Diagnosis

Subdural Hematoma (133)
- may cross sutures, does not cross midline
- may be located along the falx or tentorium
- usually crescentic

Dural Neoplasms (Meningioma, Lymphoma, Metastases) (135, 138)
- enhance avidly following contrast administration
- reactive or erosive changes may be present in the adjacent bone
- usually not as dense as acute EDH on CT

Epidural Empyema (134)
- peripheral enhancement usually prominent
- adjacent inflammatory changes (bone marrow signal, paranasal sinuses)
- characteristic reduced diffusion (may be present with hyperacute and late subacute hematoma)

Background

EDHs are located in the potential space between the calvarium and the dura, which essentially represents the periosteum of the inner table of the skull. These hematomas dissect the dura from the inner table. Because the dura is tightly adherent to the inner table at cranial suture lines, EDHs typically do not cross sutures. Up to 85% of epidural hematomas have an arterial source, and the majority are associated with a skull fracture. A common site for epidural hematomas is beneath the temporal squama, where a fracture may disrupt the underlying middle meningeal artery. Venous epidural hematomas tend to occur in three typical locations: the posterior fossa (due to rupture of the torcula Herophili or transverse sinus), anteriorly in the middle cranial fossa (due to disruption of the sphenoparietal sinus), and at the vertex (due to superior sagittal sinus injury). Venous EDHs rarely grow and are managed conservatively. The mechanism of the occasional spontaneous rapid resolution of the hematoma adjacent to a skull fracture may be related to the concomitant acute brain swelling.

REFERENCES

1. Gean AD, Fischbein NJ, Purcell DD, *et al*. Benign anterior temporal epidural hematoma: indolent lesion with a characteristic CT imaging appearance after blunt head trauma. *Radiology* 2010;**257**:212–8.

2. Hassan MD, Dhamija B, Palmer JD, *et al*. Spontaneous cranial extradural hematoma: case report and review of the literature. *Neuropathology* 2009;**29**:480–4.

3. Ugarriza LF, Cabezudo JM, Fernandez-Portales I. Rapid spontaneous resolution of an acute extradural haematoma: case report. *Br J Neurosurg* 1999;**13**:604–5.

4. Provenzale J. CT and MR imaging of acute cranial trauma. *Emerg Radiol* 2007;**14**:1–12.

5. Sullivan TP, Jarvik JG, Cohen WA. Follow-up of conservatively managed epidural hematomas: implications for timing of repeat CT. *AJNR* 1999;**20**:107–13.

Brain Imaging with MRI and CT, ed. Zoran Rumboldt *et al*. Published by Cambridge University Press. © Cambridge University Press 2012.

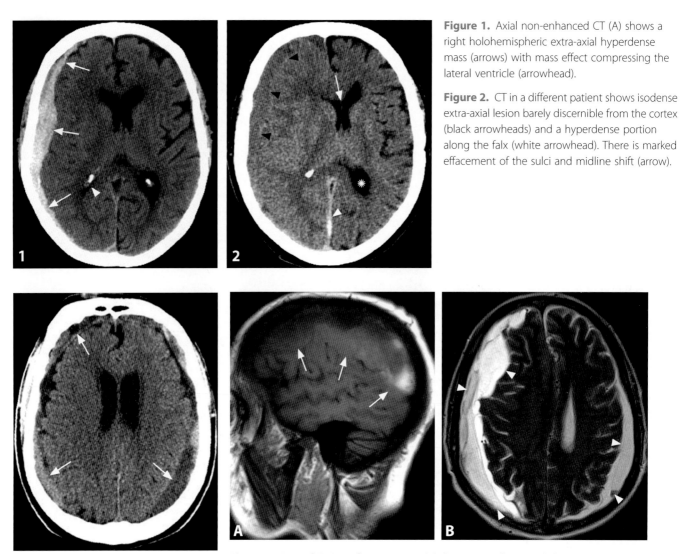

Figure 1. Axial non-enhanced CT (A) shows a right holohemispheric extra-axial hyperdense mass (arrows) with mass effect compressing the lateral ventricle (arrowhead).

Figure 2. CT in a different patient shows isodense extra-axial lesion barely discernible from the cortex (black arrowheads) and a hyperdense portion along the falx (white arrowhead). There is marked effacement of the sulci and midline shift (arrow).

Figure 3. Non-enhanced CT reveals bilateral extra-axial collections with compartments of various densities (arrows).

Figure 4. Sagittal T1WI without contrast (A) shows a predominantly hyperintense extra-axial collection (arrows). Axial T2WI (B) shows bilateral bright lesions (arrowheads) containing membranes and compartments with various signal intensities.

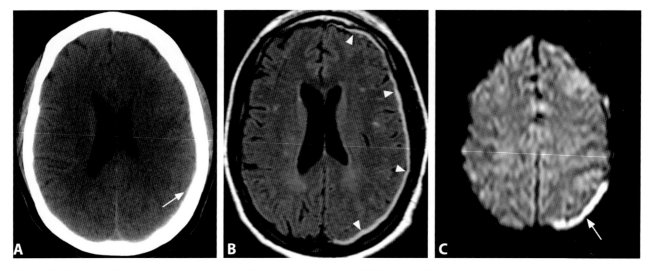

Figure 5. CT image (A) shows a questionable small hyperdensity (arrow). FLAIR image (B) reveals a holohemispheric subdural collection (arrowheads), which is also predominantly bright (arrow) on DWI (C).

Subdural Hematoma

DONNA ROBERTS

Specific Imaging Findings

Acute subdural hematoma (SDH) is usually a hyperdense mass located along the brain surface on CT. It may displace and compress the adjacent brain, but it does not extend into the cortical sulci. SDH has a characteristic concave interface with the underlying parenchyma, although it may also present with a lenticular shape, particularly in the hyperacute setting. Hyperacute SDH can also be of mixed density (due to active bleeding, unclotted blood and admixture of CSF), sometimes with a characteristic "swirling" pattern. SDH can spread along an entire hemisphere as it is located underneath the dura and not limited by dural attachments at the cranial sutures; however, it may not cross the falx and the tentorium. MRI reveals small SDHs that may be inconspicuous on CT. The evolution of MRI signal characteristics of SDHs differs from the intraparenchymal hematomas and they are most commonly bright on all sequences, including DWI, with a frequent relative hypointensity on T2* images. On post-contrast images, SDH shows peripheral enhancement of the dura, which may also be thickened, especially with chronic SDH. Chronic SDH may also show calcification of the thickened dura, best seen on CT.

Pertinent Clinical Information

SDHs occur with various types of injury, including motor vehicle collisions, falls, and non-accidental trauma; they may also occur spontaneously (as with coagulopathies). SDH may resolve or develop into chronic collections. Re-bleeding can occur within an existing SDH following only minor injury, often not even noticed by the patient. Surgical management of an acute SDH is based on the patient's clinical status, size of the collection, and associated mass affect; rapid treatment is the goal as the chance of survival falls off steeply if elevated intracranial pressure is not relieved within the first 60 min, known as the "golden hour".

Differential Diagnosis

Epidural Hematoma (132)
- limited by the cranial sutures and not by the falx cerebri and the tentorium cerebelli
- associated with a fracture in almost all cases
- characteristic lenticular shape

Subarachnoid Hemorrhage (99)
- extends deep into the cortical sulci
- cortical vessels course through the collection

Subdural Hygroma
- CSF density/signal characteristics
- can also be associated with trauma, even in an acute setting

Cortical Atrophy or Benign Extra-axial Collections of Infancy (87, 89)
- cortical vessels course through the collection
- the collection follows CSF intensity on all MR sequences

Dural Mass (Meningioma, Lymphoma, Metastasis, Granuloma) (135, 138)
- diffuse post-contrast enhancement
- additional changes may be present in the adjacent bone and/or brain

Background

SDH is a collection of blood between the inner (meningeal) layer of the dura and the arachnoid membrane. SDHs are usually venous in origin, resulting from stretching or tearing of cortical veins as they course towards the dural-based venous sinuses. Elderly patients with coagulopathies or who are on anti-coagulation therapy are at increased risk for developing an SDH, even following only minor trauma such as a fall from standing. A mixed-density SDH in an infant is more commonly found with non-accidental trauma. However, birth-related subdural bleeds are much more frequent than previously thought and SDHs can occur spontaneously, especially in children with benign extra-axial collections of infancy. SDHs can also occur in the setting of intracranial hypotension. Significant coagulopathy should be reversed expeditiously in patients with chronic SDH. Twist-drill craniostomy drainage at the bedside is recommended for high-risk surgical candidates with non-septated chronic SDH, while craniotomy is the evacuation technique for SDH with significant membranes.

REFERENCES

1. Gean AD, Fischbein NJ. Head trauma. *Neuroimaging Clin N Am* 2010;**20**:527–56.

2. Reed D, Robertson WD, Graeb DA, *et al.* Acute subdural hematomas: atypical CT findings. *AJNR* 1986;**7**:417–21.

3. Tung GA, Kumar M, Richardson RC, *et al.* Comparison of accidental and nonaccidental traumatic head injury in children on noncontrast computed tomography. *Pediatrics* 2006;**118**:626–33.

4. McNeely PD, Atkinson JD, Saigal G, *et al.* Subdural hematomas in infants with benign enlargement of the subarachnoid spaces are not pathognomonic for child abuse. *AJNR* 2006;**27**:1725–8.

5. Ducruet AF, Grobelny BT, Zacharia BE, *et al.* The surgical management of chronic subdural hematoma. *Neurosurg Rev* 2012;**35**:155–69.

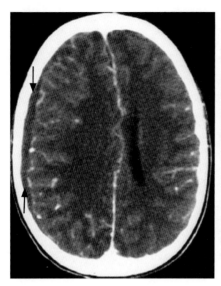
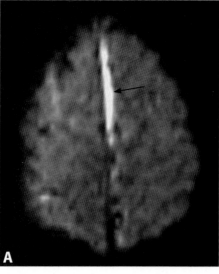
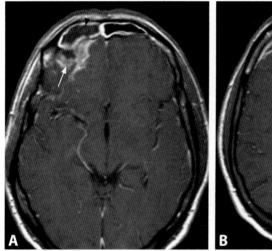

Figure 1. Post-contrast CT shows a non-specific right-sided subdural collection (arrows) in a child with *Haemophilus influenza* meningitis.

Figure 2. Axial DWI (A) shows bright left parafalcine subdural collection (arrow). Coronal post-contrast T1WI (B) shows parafalcine (arrow) and left frontal (arrowheads) peripheral enhancement of the multi-loculated lesions. Note left frontal scalp defect (surgical bur hole).

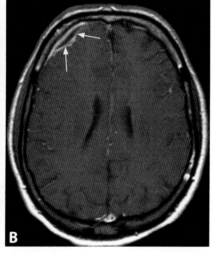

Figure 3. Axial post-contrast T1WI (A) shows right-sided frontal sinusitis (arrowhead). The adjacent brain in the right frontal lobe posterior to the infected sinus is displaced by an enhancing mass (arrow). Axial post-contrast image at a more cephalad level (B) demonstrates marginal enhancement of the right frontal subdural collection (arrows).

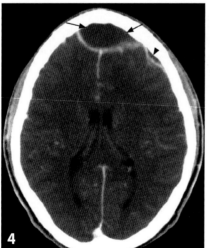
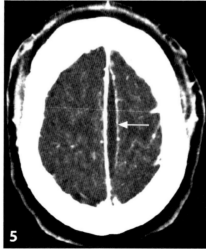

Figure 4. Axial post-contrast CT shows a rim-enhancing extra-axial frontal hypodense mass that is crossing the midline (arrows), consistent with an epidural location. A smaller left frontal abnormality (arrowhead) is also present.

Figure 5. Axial post-contrast CT demonstrates an elongated left parafalcine hypodense mass with peripheral enhancement (arrow).

Empyema

MAURICIO CASTILLO

Specific Imaging Findings

On CT, there are no specific findings to distinguish between sterile and infected intracranial extra-axial fluid collections. Both may show peripheral contrast enhancement, although underlying brain edema is more common in infected ones. Sterile fluid collections nearly follow the CSF signal intensity on all MRI sequences. They may be slightly T1 bright depending on their protein contents. Both sterile and infected collections are of high signal on T2-weighted and FLAIR images and both may show peripheral contrast enhancement. DWIs are critical in reaching the correct diagnosis. Infected collections behave similar to brain abscesses with reduced diffusion (bright on DWI, signal lower than brain parenchyma on ADC maps). Occasionally, infected collections have a "dirty" appearance on T1- and T2-weighted sequences. It has been reported that DWI for the diagnosis of pyogenic infection following craniotomy is associated with a high false-negative and false-positive rate, especially within the epidural space. The absence of reduced diffusivity within a postoperative collection is therefore not sufficient to exclude infection.

Pertinent Clinical Information

Subdural empyemas are rare and generally found in young children who have underlying bacterial meningitis. In older children, most subdural empyemas (and epidural ones) are secondary to infections in the sinonasal and temporal bone cavities. In adults, the causes are similar but they may also be iatrogenic in nature. Extra-axial empyemas may irritate the cortex and produce seizures. Other complications include venous thrombosis (veins and sinuses) and arteritis leading to infarctions. Empyemas may spread to the brain and result in abscesses or vice versa. During the acute period, subdural collections may produce neurological symptoms including seizures, but if they remain sterile and resolve, no chronic sequela should develop. For the majority of these sterile collections, no specific treatment is needed but if significant mass effect ensues, drainage may be indicated (which in itself increases the risk of infection). For subdural and epidural empyemas, aggressive antibiotic treatment is needed and surgical drainage is indicated. Subdural empyemas tend to be notoriously difficult to drain and the prognosis is poor in many instances.

Differential Diagnosis

Subdural and Epidural Hematomas (132, 133)
- follow blood degradation sequence, bright on T1 images, history of trauma

Dural Tumors such as "En Plaque" Meningiomas and Metastases (138)
- mass-like contrast enhancement, not peripheral

Dural Thickening (Fibrosis, Pachymeningitis) (136)
- isointense to brain in most MRI sequences
- absence of focal masses

Background

Empyemas may involve the subdural space and less commonly the epidural space. The subdural space is a virtual compartment (not normally present) between the dura and the arachnoid membrane that contains only some bridging cortical veins on their way to dural sinuses. The epidural space is located between the dura and the outer layer of the periosteum and in the cranial cavity contains blood vessels (such as the meningeal artery and veins). Adjacent inflammatory conditions such as meningitis can cause fluid leakage into these spaces which may remain sterile (e.g. subdural effusion) or become infected (e.g. subdural empyema).

REFERENCES

1. Wong AM, Zimmerman RA, Simon EM, *et al*. Diffusion-weighted MR imaging of subdural empyemas in children. *AJNR* 2004;**25**:1016–21.
2. Tsuchiya K, Osawa A, Katase S, *et al*. Diffusion-weighted MRI of subdural and epidural empyemas. *Neuroradiology* 2003;**45**:220–3.
3. Sadhu VK, Handel SF, Pinto RS, Glass TF. Neuroradiologic diagnosis of subdural empyema and CT limitations. *AJNR* 1980;**1**:39–44.
4. Farrell CJ, Hoh BL, Pisculli ML, *et al*. Limitations of diffusion-weighted imaging in the diagnosis of postoperative infections. *Neurosurgery* 2008;**62**:577–83.
5. Blumfield E, Misra M. Pott's puffy tumor, intracranial, and orbital complications as the initial presentation of sinusitis in healthy adolescents, a case series. *Emerg Radiol* 2011;**18**:203–10.

Brain Imaging with MRI and CT, ed. Zoran Rumboldt *et al*. Published by Cambridge University Press. © Cambridge University Press 2012.

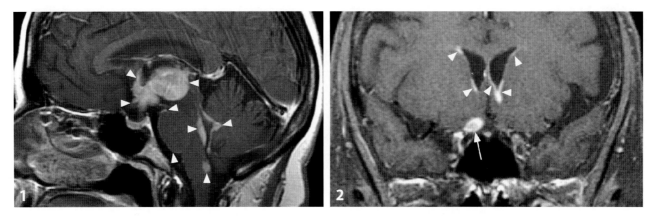

Figure 1. Midsagittal T1WI post-contrast (A) reveals multiple smooth enhancing lesions along the brain surface (arrowheads).

Figure 2. Coronal post-contrast T1WI with fat saturation shows linear enhancement along the ependyma (arrowheads) and surrounding the right optic nerve (arrow).

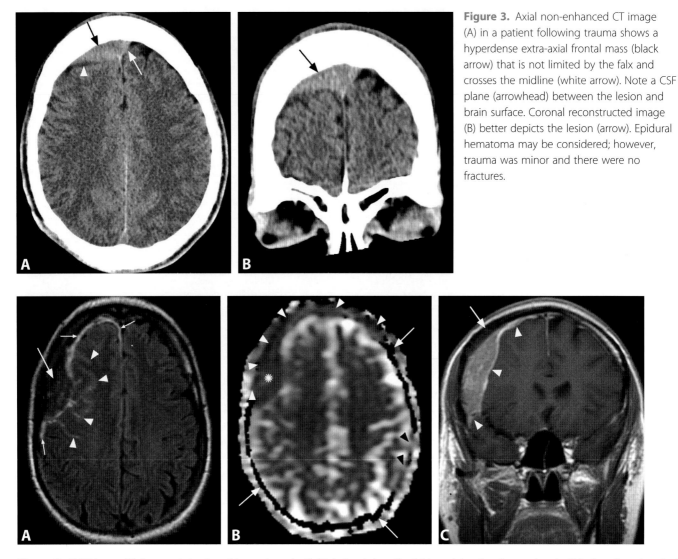

Figure 3. Axial non-enhanced CT image (A) in a patient following trauma shows a hyperdense extra-axial frontal mass (black arrow) that is not limited by the falx and crosses the midline (white arrow). Note a CSF plane (arrowhead) between the lesion and brain surface. Coronal reconstructed image (B) better depicts the lesion (arrow). Epidural hematoma may be considered; however, trauma was minor and there were no fractures.

Figure 4. FLAIR image (A) shows a dark extra-axial mass (arrow) with high signal along the thickened dura (small arrows) and within the adjacent cortical sulci (arrowheads). ADC map (B) reveals abnormal signal of the adjacent bone marrow (white arrowheads) extending from the mass (*). Compare to the expected signal loss of the intact marrow (arrows). An additional area of abnormal marrow (black arrowheads) is also present. Coronal post-contrast T1WI (C) shows homogenous enhancement of the dural-based mass (arrowheads). Note the abnormal low signal of the adjacent marrow (arrow).

Secondary (Systemic) Lymphoma

ZORAN RUMBOLDT

Specific Imaging Findings

Systemic lymphoma with intracranial spread (metastatic lymphoma, secondary CNS lymphoma – SCNSL) is characteristically extra-axial in location, typically with thin, smooth enhancement that may extend along the surface of the brain, the cranial nerves and the subependyma, which is best seen on post-contrast MR images. In addition to this leptomeningeal spread, the dura is also frequently involved with larger masses and because it is hyperdense on non-enhanced CT scans, it may mimic extra-axial hematomas and meningiomas. SCNSL avidly enhances with contrast and shows similar MR signal characteristics as the primary CNS lymphoma (PCNSL) – relatively low T2 signal and reduced diffusion on ADC maps. It frequently invades the adjacent bone, usually without destruction, so that it may not be appreciated on CT images. However, bone marrow infiltration is well seen on MRI as decreased T1 signal and brain-like intensity on DWI and ADC, along with contrast enhancement. SCNSL may extend into the brain showing intra-axial spread of enhancement that is usually accompanied with surrounding T2 hyperintense edema. Although intra-axial enhancing lesions are characteristic of PCNSL, a minority of SCNSL also present in this fashion and they show the same patterns of avid homogenous nodular and infiltrative/perivenular enhancement. Intra-axial SCNSL are usually limited to the supratentorial white matter. Perfusion studies typically reveal a relatively mild increase in cerebral blood volume in both secondary and primary CNS lymphomas.

Pertinent Clinical Information

CNS involvement in aggressive lymphoma, usually non-Hodgkin lymphoma (NHL), tends to occur early at around 6 months after the primary diagnosis. Headache is present in around a third of patients, which may be due to increased intracranial pressure caused by metastatic obstruction of CSF flow and absorption. SCNSL has an even worse prognosis than PCNSL, with a median survival of only months and very few long-term survivors. Lumbar puncture may induce dural enhancement in the cranial or spinal space, which may be falsely interpreted as CNS spread of lymphoma and should be avoided before neuroimaging.

Differential Diagnosis

Neurosarcoidosis, TB and Other Granulomas (118, 160)
- extension into the adjacent bone is rare with dural lesions
- additional leptomeningeal and/or parenchymal lesions frequently present
- leptomeningeal enhancement is usually nodular, not smooth and thin

Metastatic Neoplasms
- frequently heterogenous and necrotic

- additional parenchymal lesions may be present
- invasion into the adjacent bone is frequently destructive
- may be indistinguishable, especially leptomeningeal carcinomatosis

Subdural or Epidural Hematoma (132, 133)
- enhancement with contrast is absent or peripheral, which may be difficult to appreciate and may be indistinguishable on CT
- MRI signal characteristics are consistent with blood products, contrast enhancement is absent or peripheral

Meningioma (138, 203)
- extension into the adjacent bone is rare
- CT may show periosteal reaction with subtle spiculations in the adjacent bone

Primary CNS Lymphoma (158)
- typically intra-axial masses
- may arise from leptomeninges but dural involvement is very rare
- may arise infra-tentorially and within the deep gray matter
- may be indistinguishable

Background

Lymphoma of the CNS consists of two major subtypes: secondary CNS involvement by systemic lymphoma (the most common) and primary CNS lymphoma. A small proportion of CNS lymphomas belong to a third type – primary dural lymphomas. Distinguishing among types of CNS lymphoma can be difficult, and the distinction is sometimes obscured in the literature due to lumping of all meningeal lymphomas together. Aggressive treatment of SCNSL can improve neurologic outcome, but as it is often associated with contemporaneous systemic relapse, it rarely leads to a long-term survival. Preventing occurrence of SCNSL therefore remains an important goal of the initial lymphoma treatment.

REFERENCES

1. Haldorsen IS, Espeland A, Larsson E. Central nervous system lymphoma: characteristic findings on traditional and advanced imaging. *AJNR* 2011;**32**:984–92.

2. Senocak E, Oguz KK, Ozgen B, et al. Parenchymal lymphoma of the brain on initial MR imaging: a comparative study between primary and secondary brain lymphoma. *Eur J Radiol* 2011;**79**:288–94.

3. Lee IH, Kim ST, Kim HJ, et al. Analysis of perfusion weighted image of CNS lymphoma. *Eur J Radiol* 2010;**76**:48–51.

4. Nagpal S, Glantz MJ, Recht L. Treatment and prevention of secondary CNS lymphoma. *Semin Neurol* 2010;**30**:263–72.

5. Iwamoto FM, Abrey LE. Primary dural lymphomas: a review. *Neurosurg Focus* 2006;**21**:E5.

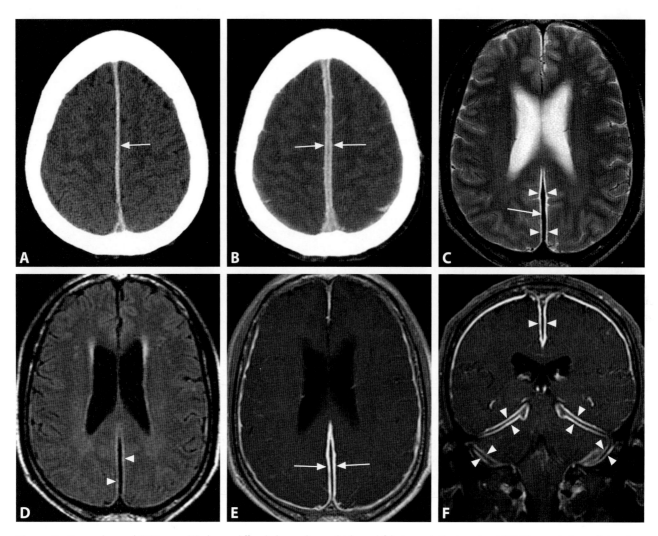

Figure 1. Non-enhanced CT image (A) shows diffusely hyperdense thickened falx (arrow). Post-contrast CT (B) reveals its peripheral enhancement (arrows) along the central non-enhancing stripe. T2WI at a lower level (C) shows very low signal of the thickened posterior falx (arrow) with peripheral hyperintensity (arrowheads), better seen on FLAIR (D). Post-contrast T1WI (E) reveals peripheral enhancement around the central non-enhancing portion (arrows). Coronal post-contrast T1WI with fat saturation (F) shows the triple layer pattern of enhancement along the falx, tentorium, and skull base (arrowheads).

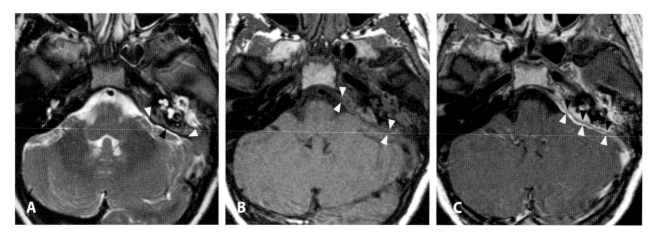

Figure 2. Axial T2WI (A) in a patient with headache and left-sided hearing loss reveals thickened centrally hypointense dura (arrowheads). There is effusion in the middle ear and mastoid. Pre-contrast T1WI (B) shows central low signal and peripheral isointensity (arrowheads) of the thickened dura. Post-contrast T1WI (C) best shows the triple layer appearance of the thickened peripherally enhancing dura (arrowheads).

Idiopathic Hypertrophic Pachymeningitis

ZORAN RUMBOLDT

Specific Imaging Findings

Idiopathic hypertrophic pachymeningitis (IHP) presents with isolated dural thickening, which may be focal or extend over large portions of the intracranial dura mater, most commonly along the falx and tentorium. The thickened dura is hyperdense on CT and demonstrates peripheral enhancement on post-contrast images. MRI is the imaging modality of choice and it shows very low T2 signal intensity of the thickened dura with peripheral high T2 signal and contrast enhancement. The central pachymeningeal layer does not enhance, which is responsible for the characteristic triple layer appearance on post-contrast T1WI. The thickened dura is isointense on pre-contrast T1WI, sometimes with a central dark stripe. Spinal involvement may occur either with cranial IHP or as an isolated finding. Nodular masses may sometimes be encountered, while associated cranial hyperostosis is rarely present. Secondary brain edema, venous congestion, cavernous sinus thrombosis, hydrocephalus, and intracranial hemorrhages may sometimes be found.

Pertinent Clinical Information

The most common presenting symptoms of intracranial IHP are chronic daily headaches and cranial nerve palsies, followed by cerebellar dysfunction and seizures. Laboratory findings include mild elevation of C-reactive protein (CRP) and erythrocyte sedimentation rate (ESR). CSF studies usually show aseptic inflammatory changes. Left untreated, the clinical course is usually marked by severe headaches, progressive neurologic deterioration, and visual loss. High-dose corticosteroid therapy results in improved symptoms and shrinkage of the lesions and methotrexate is an effective therapeutical option. Surgical decompression may provide symptomatic relief. Even with treatment, the disease may be recurrent and chronically progressive.

Differential Diagnosis

Subdural Hematoma (133)

- typically more focal masses, density/signal intensity changes over time
- mild peripheral linear contrast enhancement is thinner than the hematoma
- typically bright on T1WI and other MR sequences

Spontaneous Intracranial Hypotension (37)

- diffuse and symmetrical dural thickening and enhancement
- homogenous enhancement without the triple layer appearance
- "sagging brain" with effaced suprasellar cisterns

Granulomatous Infectious and Inflammatory Processes (TB, Fungal, Sarcoid) (118, 160)

- dural thickening is frequently nodular
- typically homogenous enhancement without the triple layer appearance

- additional intra- and extra-axial granulomas are commonly present

(Secondary) Lymphoma (135)

- homogenous enhancement without the triple layer appearance
- abnormal signal in the underlying bone marrow is common
- extension into the cortical sulci may be present

Meningioma (138, 203)

- a more focal mass with homogenous enhancement, without the triple layer appearance
- adjacent periosteal reaction is frequently present on CT

Background

IHP is a chronic progressive diffuse inflammatory fibrosis of the dura mater for which the etiology remains unknown. This rare disorder is usually found intracranially and is a diagnosis of exclusion because meningioma, lymphoma, tuberculosis, sarcoidosis and other diseases may present in a very similar fashion. Most frequently, IHP affects the tentorium and falx, followed by the cavernous sinus. There are also spinal and craniospinal forms of the disease. It is probable that IHP is an isolated intracranial localization of multifocal fibrosis, and Tolosa–Hunt syndrome may represent a focal manifestation of IHP. Headache presumably reflects inflammation of the meninges or increased intracranial pressure and progressive multiple nerve palsies are due to fibrous entrapment or ischemic damage. Histology shows central fibrosis of the meninges along with inflammatory cell infiltration, which is composed mainly of lymphocytes and plasma cells, especially at the surface of the dura mater. The peripheral enhancement pattern on MRI likely corresponds to the zone of active inflammation along the lesion periphery, in contrast to the fibrosis throughout the central portions. Thallium-201 SPECT shows a remarkable accumulation in the affected dura matter, which may also correlate with fluctuation of symptoms while the MRI findings remain stable. The linear enhancement pattern appears to show better therapeutic response than the nodular form, possibly related to less fibrosis and more vascularity.

REFERENCES

1. Friedman D, Flanders A, Tartaglino L. Contrast-enhanced MR imaging of idiopathic hypertrophic craniospinal pachymeningitis. *AJR* 1993;**160**:900–1.
2. Goyal M, Malik A, Mishra NK, Gaikwad SB. Idiopathic hypertrophic pachymeningitis: spectrum of the disease. *Neuroradiology* 1997;**39**:619–23.
3. Kupersmith MJ, Martin V, Heller G, *et al.* Idiopathic hypertrophic pachymeningitis. *Neurology* 2004;**62**:686–94.
4. Riku S, Kato S. Idiopathic hypertrophic pachymeningitis. *Neuropathology* 2003;**23**:335–44.
5. Pai S, Welsh CT, Patel S, Rumboldt Z. Idiopathic hypertrophic spinal pachymeningitis: report of two cases with typical MR imaging findings. *AJNR* 2007;**28**:590–2.

Brain Imaging with MRI and CT, ed. Zoran Rumboldt *et al.* Published by Cambridge University Press. © Cambridge University Press 2012.

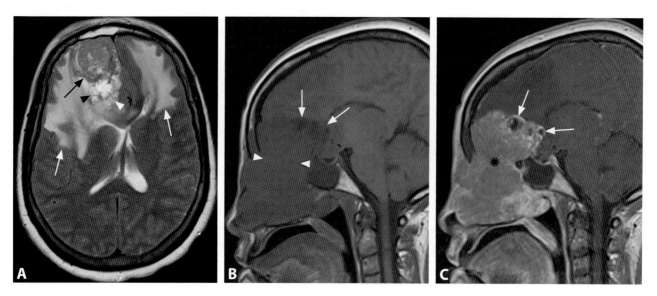

Figure 1. Axial T2WI (A) shows a right frontal extra-axial mass (black arrow) with peripheral hyperintense areas (arrowheads) and prominent bilateral vasogenic edema (white arrows). Sagittal T1WI pre- (B) and post-contrast (C) reveal that the waist of the lesion (*) is located at the cribriform plate (arrowheads). Peripheral cysts are again seen (arrows).

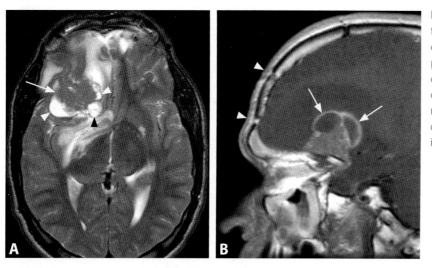

Figure 2. Axial T2WI (A) shows recurrent right frontal mass (arrow) with peripheral very bright oval to round portions (arrowheads) in another patient following previous resection. Sagittal post-contrast T1WI clearly demonstrates enhancement of the recurrent lesion with non-enhancing marginal cysts (arrows). Postoperative craniotomy changes (arrowheads) are better appreciated than in (A).

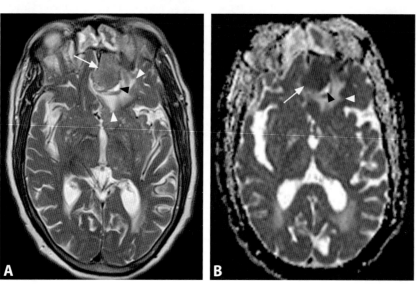

Figure 3. Axial T2WI (A) demonstrates a left frontal extra-axial mass (arrow) containing a peripheral cyst (black arrowhead) and inducing vasogenic edema (white arrowheads). Corresponding ADC map (B) reveals dark signal (arrow) consistent with very low diffusivity within the lesion. Vasogenic edema (white arrowhead) has increased diffusivity, and the marginal cyst (black arrowhead) is even brighter, similar to the CSF.

Specific Imaging Findings

Olfactory neuroblastoma (ONB, also known as esthesioneuroblastoma – ENB) typically arises in the roof of the nasal cavity and from there it characteristically grows in both superior and inferior directions with intracranial extension and spread through the nasal cavity, paranasal sinuses, and orbits. The tumors are T1 and T2 iso- to hypointense compared to the gray matter and usually exhibit prominent contrast enhancement. Diffusion of water in ONBs is lower compared to the brain, seen as dark signal intensity on ADC maps. In the periphery of the intracranial lesions, adjacent to the brain parenchyma, MRI may show well-defined ovoid to round cysts with T1, T2, and diffusion signal characteristics similar to the CSF. These peripheral or marginal cysts are a very characteristic and specific feature of ONB; however, in many cases they are not present, especially with smaller tumors. Large ONBs may be heterogenous with irregular necrotic areas and create a significant mass effect with surrounding vasogenic edema in the brain parenchyma. On CT the tumors tend to be iso- to slightly hyperdense. MRI is the imaging modality of choice as a small intracranial extension of the lesion may not be appreciated on CT. Dural masses in a distant non-contiguous location are a feature of recurrent ONBs.

Pertinent Clinical Information

ONB most commonly presents with nonspecific symptoms of nasal obstruction and epistaxis, followed by headache, visual disturbances and anosmia. There is a bimodal age distribution with the tumors primarily involving patients in their second and sixth decades of life. Overall 5-year survival is approximately 65%.

Differential Diagnosis

Other Sinonasal Malignancies with Intracranial Extension
- absence of peripheral tumor cysts
- may be indistinguishable

Allergic Fungal Sinusistis
- characteristic hyperdense appearance on CT
- lack of internal contrast enhancement
- history of chronic inflammatory sinus disease in a teenage patient

Meningioma (138, 203)
- extension into the nasal cavity is extremely rare
- peripheral intratumoral cysts are very unusual; however, trapped CSF may simulate this finding

Metastatic Tumors
- cribriform plate is a very unusual location
- additional parenchymal lesions may be present

Background

ONB is an uncommon neuroendocrine malignancy of the olfactory epithelium typically arising from the cribriform plate and extending into the adjacent structures. In addition to sinonasal, intracranial, and intraorbital spread, the tumors may metastasize to the retropharyngeal and neck lymph nodes. Treatment with craniofacial surgery and adjuvant radiotherapy offers best outcomes. Neck dissection is performed for nodal disease, while preoperative chemotherapy is considered for large tumors. Local recurrence is not uncommon and there is a propensity for (sub) dural spread. Distant metastases may present at any time during the course of the disease, generally within 3 years, and may respond to radiation or chemotherapy. ONBs may be limited to the nasal cavity without any intracranial extension, but tumors arising intracranially away from the cribriform plate have also been reported, primarily within sella turcica.

REFERENCES
1. Yu T, Xu YK, Li L, *et al.* Esthesioneuroblastoma methods of intracranial extension: CT and MR imaging findings. *Neuroradiology* 2009;**51**:841–50.
2. Bradley PJ, Jones NS, Robertson I. Diagnosis and management of esthesioneuroblastoma. *Curr Opin Otolaryngol Head Neck Surg* 2003;**11**:112–8.
3. Zollinger LV, Wiggins RH 3rd, Cornelius RS, Phillips CD. Retropharyngeal lymph node metastasis from esthesioneuroblastoma: a review of the therapeutic and prognostic implications. *AJNR* 2008;**29**:1561–3.
4. Platek ME, Merzianu M, Mashtare TL, *et al.* Improved survival following surgery and radiation therapy for olfactory neuroblastoma: analysis of the SEER database. *Radiat Oncol* 2011;**6**:41.
5. Capelle L, Krawitz H. Esthesioneuroblastoma: a case report of diffuse subdural recurrence and review of recently published studies. *J Med Imaging Radiat Oncol* 2008;**52**:85–90.

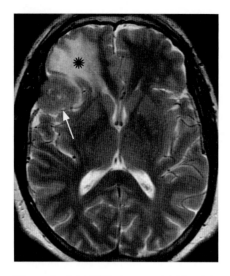

Figure 1. Axial T2WI shows a right frontal isointense extra-axial mass (arrow) and adjacent vasogenic edema (*).

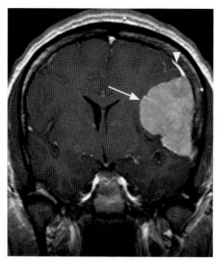

Figure 2. Coronal post-contrast T1WI shows avidly enhancing left frontal mass (arrow) with a "dural tail" (arrowhead).

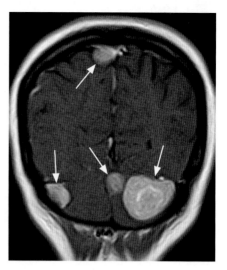

Figure 3. Coronal post-contrast T1WI reveals multiple enhancing dural-based masses (arrows).

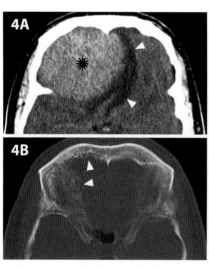

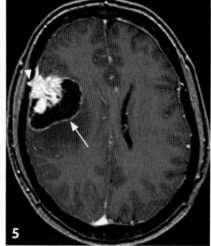

Figure 4. Axial non-enhanced CT (A) shows a hyperdense mass (*) with vasogenic edema (arrowheads). Bone algorithm and window CT at a more caudal level (B) reveals adjacent reactive hyperostosis (arrowheads).

Figure 5. Axial post-contrast T1WI shows a dural-based lesion with peripherally enhancing cystic component (arrow) and calvarial extension (arrowhead).

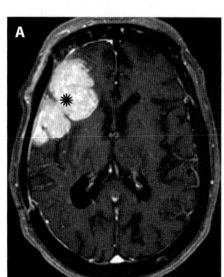

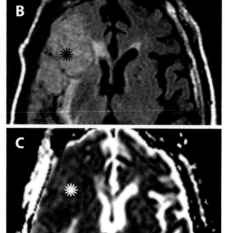

Figure 6. Axial post-contrast T1WI (A) demonstrates a lobulated dural-based mass with marked and homogenous enhancement (*). Corresponding FLAIR image (B) reveals hyperintensity of the lesion (*) compared to the brain parenchyma. The mass (*) is also slightly darker than the brain on ADC map (C), consistent with low diffusivity within the lesion.

Meningioma

ALESSANDRO CIANFONI AND ZORAN RUMBOLDT

Specific Imaging Findings

Meningioma is the prototype extra-axial dural-based mass. Its extra-axial location is ascertained by a large dural base, obtuse angles at dural margins, CSF clefts, buckling of the adjacent cortex, and vessels between the tumor and brain. The mass is isodense to slightly hyperdense, with possible calcifications and hyperostotic changes of the adjacent bone on CT. The T2 signal usually ranges from slightly hypointense to mildly hyperintense, T1signal is isointense to the cortex, with dense and homogenous contrast enhancement on both MRI and CT. Calcifications may lead to heterogeneous MRI appearance, while true cystic and necrotic changes are rare. These tumors frequently show adjacent dural thickening, the so-called "dural tail", a nonspecific sign. Perfusion MR imaging shows high rCBV and incomplete T2* signal drop recovery to baseline, typical for non-glial neoplasms. A characteristic but not very frequent alanine peak at 1.3–1.5 ppm is found on MRS. CTV and MRV are helpful in assessing dural sinus invasion and patency. These neoplasms may also have a flat appearance along the thickened dura ("en-plaque" meningioma), or grow exclusively within the diploic space with very high CT density and low MRI signal (intra-osseous meningioma). Vasogenic edema in the adjacent compressed brain, and peritumoral collections of trapped CSF may be present. Tumors can also extend extracranially through the skull base foramina. T2 hyperintensity suggests a more rapid tumor growth. Atypical and malignant meningiomas tend to exhibit a combination of T2 hyperintensity and low ADC values, as well as an irregular "mushrooming" border, and can invade the adjacent brain and bone.

Pertinent Clinical Information

Meningiomas are the most frequent adult intracranial neoplasms with a predilection for women and African ethnicity. They can be clinically silent incidental findings (90%), or can cause variable signs and symptoms depending on their size and location. Most meningiomas are benign and slow-growing; some grow rapidly, which is not limited to higher-grade tumors. DSA demonstrates a characteristic early contrast blush and delayed wash out. Meningiomas in children are rare, but usually large and rapidly growing. These tumors may also be induced by radiation therapy.

Differential Diagnosis

Dural Lymphoma (135)
- infiltrative changes of the calvarium frequently present
- possible leptomeningeal extension
- may be indistinguishable

Dural Metastasis
- common lytic changes of the calvarium
- frequently multifocal
- may be heterogenous
- most common with prostate cancer, olfactory neuroblastoma

Hemangiopericytoma (140)
- characteristic prominent intratumoral flow voids
- heterogenous and infiltrative

Neurosarcoidosis (118)
- more commonly leptomeningeal
- infiltration into the brain parenchyma

Idiopathic Hypertrophic Pachymeningitis (136)
- smooth dural thickening and enhancement, without a focal mass
- characteristic "split dura" sign – a central non-enhancing area within the thickened dura

Solitary Fibrous Tumor of the CNS
- rare, indistinguishable by imaging

(Vestibular) Schwannoma (141)
- arises from the internal auditory canal, which may be expanded
- heterogenous and high T2 signal in larger tumors
- increased diffusion on ADC maps

Background

The vast majority of meningiomas are WHO grade I tumors and they can be multiple in about 10% of patients. Atypical (grade II) and malignant (grade III) meningiomas are rare. Nonskull-base location, male sex, and prior surgery impart increased risk for higher grade. Different histologic subtypes have no clinical significance. Vascular supply is via the meningeal external carotid artery branches, and pial vessels may be parasitized. Dural origin and high vascularization are responsible for the rapid contrast enhancement and high rCBV. Treatment, when necessary, is primarily surgical, with possible preoperative embolization; radiation is usually reserved for atypical and malignant tumors.

REFERENCES

1. Maiuri F, Iaconetta G, de Divitiis O, et al. Intracranial meningiomas: correlations between MR imaging and histology. Eur J Radiol 1999;31:69–75.
2. Nagar VA, Ye JR, Ng WH, et al. Diffusion-weighted MR imaging: diagnosing atypical or malignant meningiomas and detecting tumor dedifferentiation. AJNR 2008;29:1147–52.
3. Kaplan RD, Coons S, Drayer BP, et al. MR characteristics of meningioma subtypes at 1.5 tesla. J Comput Assist Tomogr 1992;16:366–71.
4. Kane AJ, Sughrue ME, Rutkowski MJ, et al. Anatomic location is a risk factor for atypical and malignant meningiomas. Cancer 2011;117:1272–8.
5. Gao X, Zhang R, Mao Y, Wang Y. Childhood and juvenile meningiomas. Childs Nerv Syst 2009;25:1571–80.

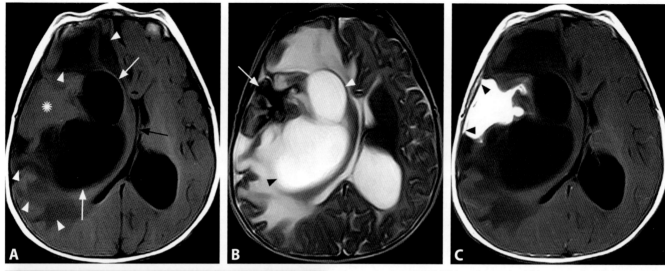

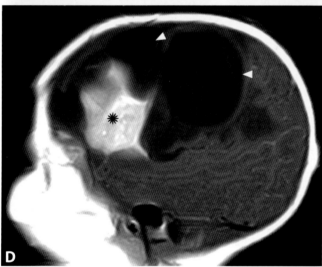

Figure 1. Axial T1WI (A) in a 6-month-old boy reveals a large, rounded, hypointense right fronto-parietal mass (white arrows) with a superficial isointense portion (*). There is marked vasogenic edema (arrowheads) and mass effect with leftward midline shift (black arrow). Matching T2WI (B) shows a predominantly very dark signal of the superficial portion (arrow) and large areas of very high signal (arrowheads). Post-contrast T1WI (C) reveals dense enhancement of the superficial portion, which has a wide dural base (arrowheads). There is no enhancement in the rest of the mass. Post-contrast sagittal (D) T1WI again shows enhancing solid portion (*) and non-enhancing cysts (arrowheads).

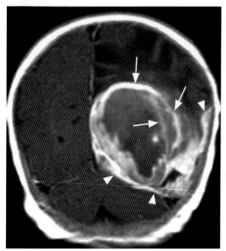

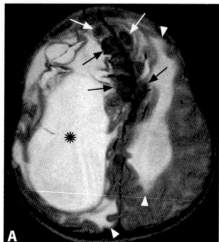

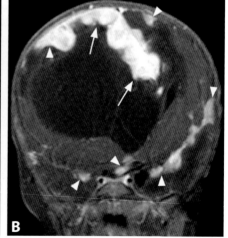

Figure 2. Coronal post-contrast T1WI in an infant reveals a cystic enhancing mass, which is dural-based (arrowheads) and shows enhancement of the cyst walls (arrows).

Figure 3. Axial T2WI (A) in a 1-year-old boy shows a hypointense nodular mass (arrows) arising from the falx and associated large cyst (*). There is also prominent vasogenic edema (arrowheads). Coronal post-contrast T1WI with fat saturation (B) reveals dense avid enhancement of the parafalcine nodular masses (arrows), as well as multiple additional extra-axial enhancing masses (arrowheads).

Desmoplastic Infantile Ganglioglioma

GIOVANNI MORANA

Specific Imaging Findings

Desmoplastic infantile ganglioglioma (DIG) is an extra-axial mass consisting of a large cyst with a solid superficial component. The cystic portion is hypodense on CT, T1 hypointense and T2 hyperintense, with variable signal intensity on FLAIR images (isointense or slightly hyperintense to CSF). The cystic component is invariably associated with a mural, meningeal-based mass or plaque, which is iso- to slightly hyperdense on CT, isointense to gray matter on T1, with a typical very low signal intensity on T2-weighted images (due to its fiber-rich content). Post-contrast images show marked enhancement of the solid portion along with enhancement extending to the adjacent leptomeninges and dura. Typically it shows non-enhancing walls and may appear multilobulated due to the presence of septations; areas of enhancement may at times be present within the cystic septa. Calcification and hemorrhagic foci are usually absent whereas perifocal edema is variable and often very prominent. Diffusion imaging can demonstrate reduced diffusivity in the solid portion whereas MR spectroscopy shows elevated choline and reduced NAA peaks with near-normal *myo*-inositol levels. In rare cases, diffuse dissemination may be present at the time of diagnosis.

Pertinent Clinical Information

Affected infants present with asymmetric macrocrania, bulging of the fontanels and other nonspecific symptoms such as seizures and vomiting. DIG typically has a favorable prognosis, confirmed by absence of recurrence following surgical removal. However, incomplete excision occurs in about 30% of cases due to the lack of a definite cleavage between the tumor and the surrounding brain and sometimes due to infiltration of eloquent CNS structures.

Differential Diagnosis

Ganglioglioma (166)
- usually located within the temporal lobe
- calcifications are common
- usually a much smaller lesion at diagnosis
- intra-axial mass, not involving the dura

Pilocytic Astrocytoma (173)
- solid portion is very bright on ADC maps
- solid nodule is T2 hyperintense
- hemispheric location extremely uncommon
- intra-axial mass without dural involvement

Pleomorphic Xanthoastrocytoma (165)
- same superficial location with meningeal involvement
- intra-axial mass
- occurs in older children

PNET, Anaplastic Ependymoma and ATRT (172, 174)
- the solid component is usually intra-axial, less peripheral in location
- rarely as hypointense on T2-weighted images
- more heterogeneous contrast enhancement of the solid portion
- necrotic and hemorrhagic component often present

Meningioma (138)
- may be very large in children but typically a solid mass, cysts are rare

Background

DIGs are rare benign neoplasms occurring mostly in infants in the first 2 years of life, with a male predilection; nevertheless, these tumors are not exclusively seen in early childhood and may be diagnosed in older patients. The lesion is usually massive and replaces large portions of the affected hemisphere. Most tumors are located in the frontal and parietal lobes. The superficial solid portion primarily involves the leptomeninges and superficial cortex, and is commonly attached to the dura. Histologically, it is characterized by the presence of a prominent desmoplastic stroma, a variable amount of neuroepithelial and neuronal cells, and aggregates of poorly differentiated cells. The presence of desmoplasia (dense fibrocollagenous bands) represents a distinctive feature of these tumors and accounts for the very low signal intensity on T2-weighted images. Knowledge and recognition of DIG is very important in order to avoid misinterpretation of its benign nature, which may lead to inappropriate management of the patient.

REFERENCES

1. Rypens F, Esteban MJ, Lellouch-Tubiana A, *et al*. Desmoplastic supratentorial neuroepithelial tumours of childhood: imaging in 5 patients. *Neuroradiology* 1996;**38**:S165–8.
2. Tenreiro-Picon OR, Kamath SV, Knorr JR, *et al*. Desmoplastic infantile ganglioglioma: CT and MRI features. *Pediatr Radiol* 1995;**25**:540–3.
3. Trehan G, Bruge H, Vinchon M, *et al*. MR imaging in the diagnosis of desmoplastic infantile tumor: retrospective study of six cases. *AJNR* 2004;**25**:1028–33.
4. Balaji R, Ramachandran K. Imaging of desmoplastic infantile ganglioglioma: a spectroscopic viewpoint. *Childs Nerv Syst* 2009;**25**:497–501.
5. Gelabert-Gonzalez M, Serramito-García R, Arcos-Algaba A. Desmoplastic infantile and non-infantile ganglioglioma. Review of the literature. *Neurosurg Rev* 2010;**34**:151–8.

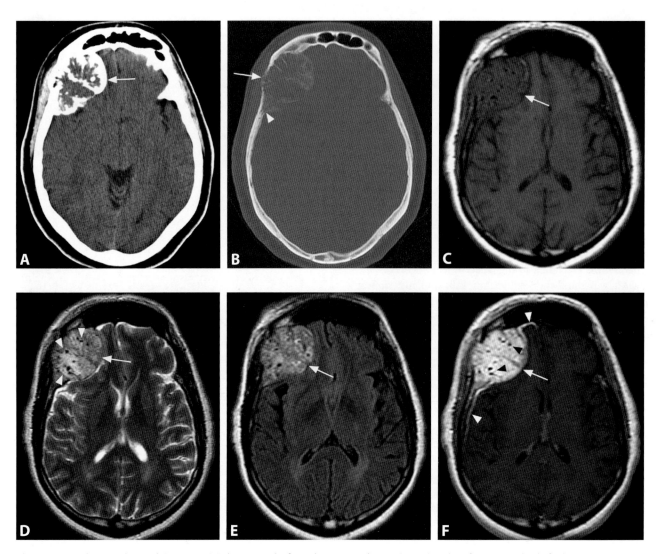

Figure 1. Axial non-enhanced CT image (A) shows a right frontal intracranial mass (arrow) with soft tissue and calcified/osseus components. CT image with bone algorithm and window (B) at a slightly higher level reveals calcified septations within the lesion, which is eroding into the bone (arrowhead) and exhibits osteolytic behavior (arrow). T1WI without contrast (C) shows predominantly hypointense signal of the mass (arrow), which is of high signal on T2WI (D) and contains flow-voids (arrowheads). The lesion (arrow) is hyperintense on FLAIR image (E) and demonstrates avid enhancement on post-contrast T1WI (F), along with dural tails (white arrowheads) and flow-voids (black arrowheads).

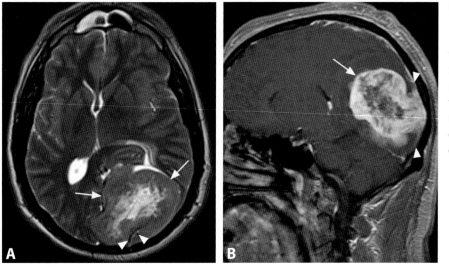

Figure 2. Axial T2WI (A) in another patient shows a centrally hyperintense right parieto-occipital extra-axial mass (arrows) with internal flow-voids (arrowheads). Sagittal post-contrast T1WI (B) reveals dense, predominantly peripheral enhancement of the lesion (arrow), along with its dural tails (arrowheads). Central high T2 signal and decreased enhancement are suggestive of degenerated/necrotic areas.

Specific Imaging Findings

Cranial nerve (CN) schwannoma (neuroma, neurinoma, Schwann cell tumor, neurolemmoma, neurilemmoma) is typically well-delineated, hypodense on CT and T1 hypointense to isointense to the pons on pre-contrast images and with avid post-contrast enhancement. Schwannomas can arise along any cranial nerve, most commonly the vestibular nerve in the internal auditory canal (IAC), followed by the trigeminal nerve (including Meckel's cave), facial nerve, glossopharyngeal, vagus, and spinal accessory nerve. Schwannomas involving oculomotor, trochlear, abducens, and hypoglossal nerves are rare. Enhancement may be homogenous or heterogenous, based on the absence or presence of necrosis and/or intramural cysts. Calcifications are not present. Smaller tumors are usually round, ovoid-shaped or less frequently poly-lobular, T2 iso- to hypointense. Larger tumors are typically of high T2 signal and heterogenous with internal cystic areas. Schwannomas exhibit increased diffusion and are hyperintense on ADC maps. Eighty-five percent of vestibular schwannomas are centered at the IAC meatus. Larger tumors show the typical "ice cream on cone" appearance and usually lead to smooth widening of the internal auditory canal. Arachnoid cysts/trapped CSF are found around the tumor in a minority of cases, while increased signal within the ipsilateral inner ear structures is frequently present on FLAIR images.

Pertinent Clinical Information

CN schwannoma may be an incidental finding; however, they usually present with loss of function of the affected nerve. The goal of treatment is to eradicate the tumor while preserving existing (residual) nerve function, primarily hearing with vestibular neoplasms. Late hearing loss is infrequent after initially successful hearing preservation. When hearing degradation occurs, it is suggestive of tumor recurrence. Stereotactic radiosurgery is now an accepted and possibly preferred treatment option for patients with vestibular schwannomas providing high rates of long-term tumor control and nerve preservation. Mild transient increase in tumor size is frequently observed in the early post-treatment period. DTI appears to allow early detection of radiation-induced effects.

Differential Diagnosis

Meningioma (138, 203)
- usually homogenous, with low T2 signal, without increased diffusion
- "dural tail" is frequently present
- calcifications may be present
- rarely arises within the IAC

Epidermoid (143)
- CSF-like on T1WI and T2WI
- absence of calcifications
- characteristically very bright on DWI

Dermoid (75)
- bright fat-like T1 signal
- no enhancement
- calcifications are common
- chemical shift artifact around the edges on T2WI (bright and dark lines along the frequency encoding direction)

Arachnoid Cyst (142)
- follows CSF on CT and all MR pulse sequences, without enhancement

Metastasis
- usually multifocal meningeal involvement
- adjacent bone erosion/marrow invasion may be present

Aneurysm (144, 192)
- presence of flow-void, contiguous with an artery
- possible T1 bright thrombus, "onion-skin" appearance

Background

CN schwannoma accounts for approximately 8% of brain tumors. Vestibular schwannoma represents the most common tumor in the cerebellopontine angle-internal auditory canal region (85–90%). The majority of vestibular schwannomas develop from the vestibular portion of the vestibulocochlear nerve. Less than 5% arise from the cochlear nerve. Two histologic types have been identified: Antoni A tissue consists of "palisading pattern" elongated spindle cells, while Antoni B tissue shows a markedly reduced cellularity and a loose spongy texture. Antoni A and B tissues frequently coexist in the same neoplasm. Besides morphologic differences, type B cells may display a distinct biologic behavior as vestibular paresis appears to be more frequently associated with this type. Presence of bilateral vestibular schwannomas implies the diagnosis of neurofibromatosis type 2.

REFERENCES

1. Mulkens TH, Parizel PM, Martin JJ, et al. Acoustic schwannoma: MR findings in 84 tumors. *AJR* 1993;**160**:395–8.
2. Bonneville F, Sarrazin JL, Marsot-Dupuch K, et al. Unusual lesions of the cerebellopontine angle: a segmental approach. *Radiographics* 2001;**21**:419–38.
3. Lee IH, Kim HJ, Chung WH, et al. Signal intensity change of the labyrinth in patients with surgically confirmed or radiologically diagnosed vestibular schwannoma on isotropic 3D fluid-attenuated inversion recovery MR imaging at 3 T. *Eur Radiol* 2010;**20**:949–57.
4. Lin YC, Wang CC, Wai YY, et al. Significant temporal evolution of diffusion anisotropy for evaluating early response to radiosurgery in patients with vestibular schwannoma: findings from functional diffusion maps. *AJNR* 2010;**31**:269–74.
5. Stipkovits EM, Graamans K, Jansen GH, Velthof MA. Acoustic neuroma: predominance of Antoni type B cells in tumors of patients with vestibular paresis. *Otol Neurotol* 2001;**22**:215–7.

Brain Imaging with MRI and CT, ed. Zoran Rumboldt et al. Published by Cambridge University Press. © Cambridge University Press 2012.

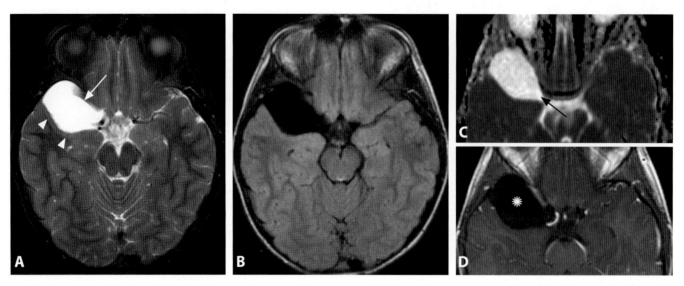

Figure 1. Axial T2WI (A) shows right anterior temporal extra-axial hyperintense mass (arrow). Note buckling of the adjacent preserved cortex (arrowheads). FLAIR image (B) shows very low, and ADC map (C) very bright signal (arrow) of the mass, comparable to the CSF. There is no enhancement of the hypointense lesion (*) on post-contrast T1WI (D).

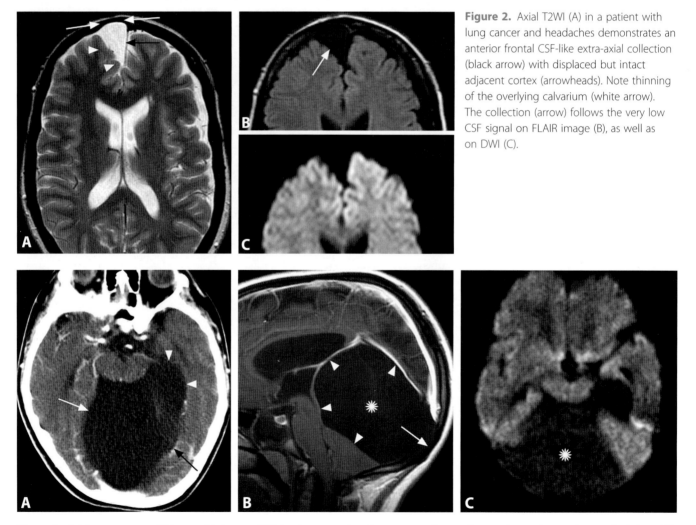

Figure 2. Axial T2WI (A) in a patient with lung cancer and headaches demonstrates an anterior frontal CSF-like extra-axial collection (black arrow) with displaced but intact adjacent cortex (arrowheads). Note thinning of the overlying calvarium (white arrow). The collection (arrow) follows the very low CSF signal on FLAIR image (B), as well as on DWI (C).

Figure 3. Axial post-contrast CT image (A) shows a CSF density non-enhancing posterior fossa collection (arrows) extending to the left middle fossa (arrowheads). Sagittal post-contrast T1WI (B) reveals the compression of the CSF-like non-enhancing mass (*) on the adjacent structures (arrowheads) and bone remodeling (arrow). Axial DWI (C) shows internal low signal (*), similar to the CSF.

Arachnoid Cyst

MARIA GISELE MATHEUS

Specific Imaging Findings

Arachnoid cyst (AC) is an extra-axial mass that follows the CSF appearance on all imaging modalities. It is sharply demarcated and displaces brain parenchyma with buckling of the adjacent intact cortex. It also displaces arteries and cranial nerves and frequently leads to thinning and remodeling of the overlying bone. AC is T1 hypointense, hyperintense on T2WI and ADC maps, dark on FLAIR and DWI and does not enhance with contrast. Arachnoid cysts are also CSF-like hypodense on CT. Hemorrhage may rarely occur within the cyst which changes the imaging appearance, depending on the blood products degradation state and protein-aceous contents. AC has a predilection for the middle cranial fossa followed by the suprasellar cisterns, cerebellopontine angle, convexities and quadrigeminal plate region.

Pertinent Clinical Information

AC is typically an incidental imaging finding, but it has been sporadically associated with headache, dizziness, sensorineural hearing loss and hemifacial spasm, depending on its location. There is increased prevalence of subdural hematomas in patients with middle cranial fossa AC. Mass effect from midline and posterior fossa ACs may lead to obstructive hydrocephalus and suprasellar AC may also cause endocrine symptoms, such as hyperprolactinemia and precocious puberty. Treatment is usually not necessary and ACs may recur following surgery. When needed, fenestration, endoscopic resection and cystoperitoneal shunt are possible options.

Differential Diagnosis

Epidermoid Cyst (143)
- engulfs vessels and cranial nerves with insinuating growth pattern
- usually heterogenous and brighter than the CSF on FLAIR images
- characteristically very bright on DWI (and signal similar to brain on ADC maps)

Porencephalic Cyst (83)
- surrounded by abnormal gliotic parenchyma instead of buckled normal cortex

Neurenteric Cyst
- intra-axial location
- usually hyperintense on T1WI and FLAIR due to high protein-aceous contents
- usually hyperdense on CT

Racemose Neurocysticercosis (145)
- typically multiseptated cysts
- insinuating growth pattern along the subarachnoid spaces
- enhancement of the cyst wall may be present
- remain dark while the CSF becomes bright on FLAIR images obtained during 100% O_2 inhalation

Background

ACs account for about 1% of all intracranial space-occupying lesions and can be congenital (true AC) or acquired. Congenital AC is related to primary developmental abnormalities of the meninges. An incomplete breakdown of the primitive mesen-chymal meshwork, which will form the arachnoid, results in splitting or duplication of the arachnoid membrane with accumulation of the CSF between the two arachnoid layers. It appears separated from the arachnoid space and is completely isolated from the ventricles. Acquired ACs are arachnoid loculations occurring as a consequence of prior trauma, hemorrhage, infection or inflammation. ACs are typically stable, but they may sometimes decrease or increase in size. Spontaneous reduction of ACs is usually observed in the middle cranial fossa. The proposed mechanisms for AC growth include pulsation and ball-valve effect, production of CSF by the cyst walls, and ectopic choroid plexus located within the cysts. Minimally invasive neuroendoscopic surgery is becoming the treatment of choice for symptomatic or growing ACs, due to a high likelihood of clinical improvement and low rates of complications. Visualization of anatomical landmarks is essential in achieving successful endoscopic fenestration, for which preoperative assessment with high-resolution 3D T2WI is very helpful.

REFERENCES

1. Awaji M, Okamoto K, Nishiyama K. Magnetic resonance cysternography for preoperative evaluation of arachnoid cysts. *Neuroradiology* 2007;**49**:721–6.

2. Bergui M, Zhong J, Bradac GB, Sales S. Diffusion-weighted images of intracranial cyst-like lesions *Neuroradiology* 2001;**43**:824–9.

3. Al-Holou WN, Yew AY, Boomsaad ZE, *et al.* Prevalence and natural history of arachnoid cysts in children. *J Neurosurg Pediatr* 2010;**5**:578–85.

4. Cincu R, Agrawal A, Eiras J. Intracranial arachnoid cysts: current concepts and treatment alternatives. *Clin Neurol Neurosurg* 2007;**109**:837–43.

5. Russo N, Domenicucci M, Beccaglia MR, Santoro A. Spontaneous reduction of intracranial arachnoid cysts: a complete review. *Br J Neurosurg* 2008;**22**:626–9.

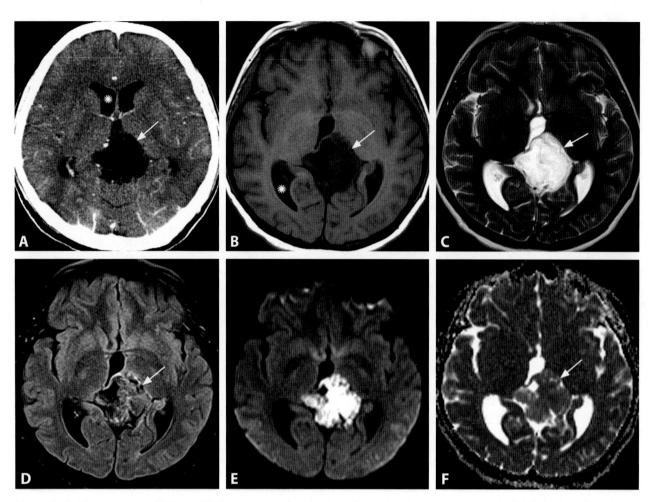

Figure 1. Axial post-contrast CT image (A) shows a non-enhancing hypodense pineal region mass (arrow), slightly brighter than the CSF (*). Axial T1WI (B) shows slightly increased signal of the lesion (arrow) compared to the CSF (*). Corresponding T2WI (C) shows lesion hyperintensity and subtle linear internal structures. FLAIR (D) reveals lesion heterogeneity (arrow) with higher signal intensity than the CSF. The mass is extremely bright on DWI (E). The ADC map (F) shows that the diffusivity of the lesion (arrow) is similar to slightly higher compared to the brain.

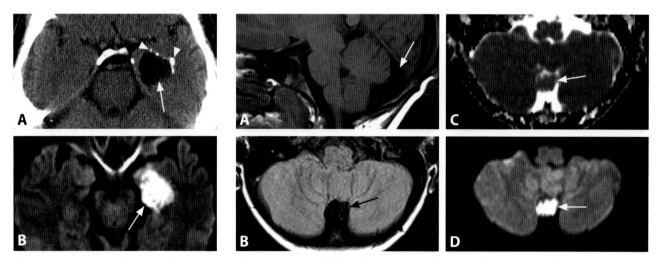

Figure 2. Axial non-enhanced CT image (A) shows a left temporal hypodense CSF-like collection (arrow) with marginal calcifications (arrowheads). DWI (B) reveals its marked hyperintensity (arrow).

Figure 3. Sagittal T1WI without contrast (A) in a child shows a CSF-like collection (arrow) posterior to the vermis. The collection is slightly heterogenous (arrow) on axial FLAIR image (B). Matching ADC map (C) shows that the lesion's (arrow) diffusivity is very similar to the brain parenchyma. DWI (D) demonstrates the characteristic "light bulb" brightness of the extra-axial mass (arrow).

Epidermoid

MARIA GISELE MATHEUS

Specific Imaging Findings

Epidermoid (epidermoid cyst, cholesteatoma) is typically a non-enhancing extra-axial intradural mass. Epidermoids are lobulated space-occupying lesions that insinuate through subarachnoid spaces displacing and engulfing adjacent structures, primarily cranial nerves and arteries. They are typically iso-dense to slightly hyperdense to the CSF on CT. Rare variants may show calcifications and/or hyperdense contents ("dense epidermoid"). Epidermoids are iso- to slightly hyperintense to CSF on T1WI and with CSF-like hyperintensity on T2WI. These neoplasms do not enhance with contrast. FLAIR and especially DWI are the imaging techniques of choice. FLAIR images show internal "dirty" heterogeneity with signal intensity generally similar to the brain parenchyma. DWI reveals their striking hyperintensity, while the ADC values are similar to the brain. A small number of epidermoids may show high T1 and even low T2 signal, due to proteinaceous contents. This T1 hyperintensity is not suppressed on images with fat saturation pulse. Intra-axial and intradiploic skull lesions are much less frequent. The most common locations are cerebellopontine angle, pineal region, parasellar areas, and middle cranial fossa.

Pertinent Clinical Information

Epidermoids are usually silent until the third or fourth decade of life. Clinical presentation depends on the location and includes cranial nerve deficits, hydrocephalus, neuroendocrine symptoms, and seizures (with middle cranial fossa tumors). Surgical resection is curative. Chemical meningitis caused by cyst rupture is a possible complication, which very rarely follows dissemination of the cyst contents.

Differential Diagnosis

Arachnoid Cyst (142)
- signal intensity follows CSF on all imaging techniques and modalities

Racemose Neurocysticercosis (145)
- variable signal intensity on DWI, rarely very bright
- may show post-contrast enhancement of the cyst wall and adjacent meninges
- typically multiloculated septated cysts
- cysts remain dark on FLAIR images obtained while the patient is inhaling 100% oxygen

Abscess (156)
- intra-axial masses
- the capsule is T1 bright and T2 dark, with marked contrast enhancement
- central very low diffusivity with dark signal on ADC maps

Background

Epidermoids and dermoids are benign neoplasms formed by inclusion of epithelial elements. In contrast to dermoids, epidermoids arise from ectoderm-derived epidermis only and do not contain dermal appendages (hair, sebaceous glands, and sweat glands). Their capsule has a characteristic shiny glistening "mother of pearl" appearance. The internal layers consist of stratified squamous epithelium mounted on collagenous connective tissue. Progressive tumor enlargement is related to otherwise normal epithelial desquamation and accumulation of keratin, cholesterol and other debris within the cavity. These contents are soft and waxy allowing the typical insinuating growth pattern. The combination of their very high T2 signal and diffusivity that is similar to brain parenchyma is responsible for the extreme hyperintensity of epidermoids on DWI (which is formed by a combination of diffusion and T2-weighting). Two types of atypical appearance on T1WI have been described: "white epidermoid" with high signal due to triglycerides and unsaturated fatty acids; and "black epidermoid" caused by cholesterol and keratin crystals. Transformation of intracranial epidermoid cysts to squamous cell carcinoma can occur in rare cases, presenting as rapid neurological deterioration and with contrast enhancement on imaging studies.

REFERENCES

1. Chen S, Ikawa F, Kurisu K, et al. Quantitative MR evaluation of intracranial epidermoid tumor by fast fluid-attenuated inversion recovery imaging and echo-planar diffusion-weighted imaging. AJNR 2001;22:1089–96.
2. Kallmes DF, Provenzale JM, Cloft HJ, McClendon RE. Typical and atypical MR imaging features of intracranial epidermoid tumors. AJR 1997;169:883–7.
3. Li F, Zhu S, Liu Y, et al. Hyperdense intracranial epidermoid cysts: a study of 15 cases. Acta Neurochir 2007;149:31–9.
4. Nagasawa D, Yew A, Safaee M, et al. Clinical characteristics and diagnostic imaging of epidermoid tumors. J Clin Neurosci 2011;18:1158–62.
5. Agarwal S, Rishi A, Suri V, et al. Primary intracranial squamous cell carcinoma arising in an epidermoid cyst – a case report and review of the literature. Clin Neurol Neurosurg 2007;109:888–91.

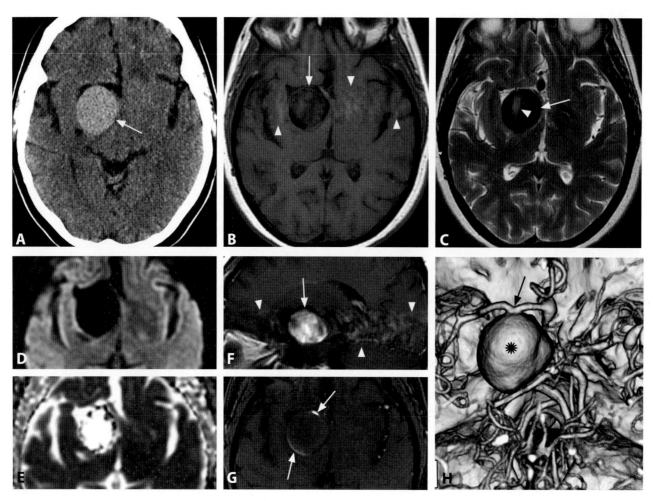

Figure 1. Axial non-enhanced CT image (A) shows an oval homogenously hyperdense mass (arrow) that appears extra-axial in location. T1WI without contrast (B) reveals low signal of the lesion (arrow) and an artifact propagating along the phase-encoding direction (arrowheads). The mass (arrow) is very dark on T2WI (C), except for a brighter linear area (arrowhead). DWI (D) shows its very low signal, which blends in with the adjacent CSF. ADC map (E) shows its CSF-like diffusivity. Peripheral very dark areas (arrows) may correspond to calcifications. The lesion (arrow) enhances on sagittal post-contrast T1WI (F) and the artifact is accentuated (arrowheads). A source 3D-TOF image (G) shows only peripheral high signal (arrows). CTA volume rendering (H) clearly shows the lesion (*) and its parent artery (arrow). Additional fusiform aneurysms.

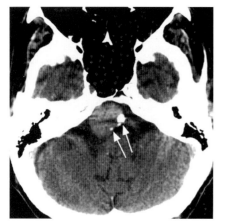

Figure 2. Non-enhanced CT reveals an oval hyperdense mass in the prepontine cistern with rim calcifications (arrows) and associated streak artifact.

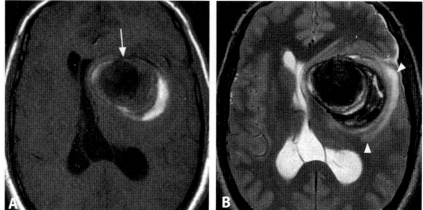

Figure 3. T1WI without contrast (A) shows an oval lesion (arrow) with notable mass effect. Note laminated structure with eccentric intervening bands of low signal, isointensity, and bright signal. T2WI (B) shows the layered structure with different signals. There is surrounding edema (arrowheads). Incidental cavum verge.

Aneurysm

ZORAN RUMBOLDT

Specific Imaging Findings

Small aneurysms arising from intracranial arteries are rarely seen on routine CT or MR brain imaging, however CTA and MRA are reliable modalities for detection and evaluation of these lesions. Aneurysms without intraluminal thrombus are round to oval structures that are slightly hyperdense on CT and flow-void dark on T2WI, contiguous with the parent artery, and densely enhancing with contrast. Large (> 1 cm) and giant (> 2.5 cm) aneurysms are characteristically round, densely enhancing extra-axial masses hyperdense on CT and flow-void dark on MRI. Additional flow effects include a bright linear "jet" of flow within the dark signal void and a band of pulsation artifact radiating along the phase-encoding direction, accentuated on post-contrast images. Common peripheral calcifications are reliably detected with CT but may not be identified on MRI. Endoluminal turbulent flow is responsible for frequent lack of flow-related hyperintensity and hence decreased conspicuity on MRA without contrast. Aneurysms with intraluminal thrombus are characteristically laminated with bands of varying signal intensities, frequently with "onion skin" appearance. The bands correspond to thrombus and are usually eccentric, with signal intensities depending on the stage of hemoglobin degradation products – typically at least a portion is T1 bright and T2 dark. The thrombosed parts do not enhance with contrast. Complete thrombosis is identified as high T1 and T2 signal filling the lumen without any flow effects. Presence of either flow-void on pre-contrast T1WI, contrast enhancement, or pulsation artifact provides a definite confirmation of patency. Giant aneurysms may be surrounded by vasogenic edema in the adjacent brain. Rarely associated aneurysms and arachnoid cysts appear as cystic masses with mural nodules.

Pertinent Clinical Information

A majority of patients with very large aneurysms present with neurological deficits from the mass effect, which depend on the lesion location. Hemorrhage, typically subarachnoid and/or parenchymal, may be the initial presentation. Some patients suffer from transient ischemic attacks or infarcts caused by dislodged intra-luminal thrombus occluding distal branches. Aneurysms may also be incidentally discovered. Subarachnoid hemorrhage is the most common cause of death if giant aneurysms are not treated.

Differential Diagnosis

Meningioma (138, 203)
- dural based or intraventricular
- absence of flow effects and laminated appearance

Schwannoma (141)
- occurs along the nerves
- absence of flow effects and laminated appearance
- calcifications are very unusual

Cavernous Hemangioma (183, 193)
- characteristic dark hemosiderin ring, frequently with internal bright "popcorn" contents
- absence of flow effects and laminated appearance
- may be indistinguishable from a small aneurysm

Craniopharyngioma (44, 202)
- cystic areas do not enhance with contrast
- absence of flow effects

Background

Giant aneurysms are believed to develop from progressive complex changes of small aneurysms, due to hemodynamic stress and secondary healing response. They include saccular (from small berry aneurysm), fusiform (from angioectasia due to atherosclerosis or connective tissue disorder), and serpentine (presumed thrombosis and recanalisation of fusiform aneurysm) forms. Partial thrombosis is very common but complete obliteration occurs in less than 20% of cases. The propensity for spontaneous thrombosis is attributed to the ratio between the aneurysm volume and neck size. A small orifice and a large lumen result in slow flow, propagating spontaneous clotting. A growing thrombus then reduces the patent volume, which leads to increasing velocity of the intra-aneurysmal blood flow and prevents total thrombosis. Although most of the wall may be fibrocalcific, small vulnerable areas remain unprotected – more than 50% of giant aneurysms rupture and mortality is > 60% in 2 years. In partially thrombosed aneurysms with mass effect, the results of parent vessel occlusion appear to be much better than those of selective coiling.

REFERENCES

1. Choi IS, David C. Giant intracranial aneurysms: development, clinical presentation and treatment. *Eur J Radiol* 2003;**46**:178–94.
2. Teng MM, Nasir Qadri SM, Luo CB, et al. MR imaging of giant intracranial aneurysm. *J Clin Neurosci* 2003;**10**:460–4.
3. Sari A, Kandemir S, Kuzeyli K, Dinc H. Giant serpentine aneurysm with acute spontaneous complete thrombosis. *AJNR* 2006;**27**:766–8.
4. de Oliveira JG, Giudicissi-Filho M, Rassi-Neto A, et al. Intracranial aneurysm and arachnoid cyst: a rare association between two cerebral malformations. *Br J Neurosurg* 2007;**21**:406–10.
5. Ferns SP, van Rooij WJ, Sluzewski M, et al. Partially thrombosed intracranial aneurysms presenting with mass effect: long-term clinical and imaging follow-up after endovascular treatment. *AJNR* 2010;**31**:1197–205.

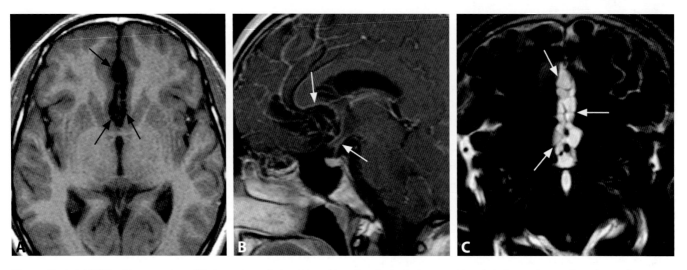

Figure 1. Axial T1WI without contrast (A) shows irregularly widened interhemispheric fissure with subtle internal septations (arrows). Post-contrast sagittal T1WI (B) reveals enhancement along the brain surface (arrows) adjacent to the CSF-like anterior interhemispheric area. Axial 3D high-resolution T2WI (C) clearly demonstrates multicystic abnormality (arrows) in the interhemispheric fissure.

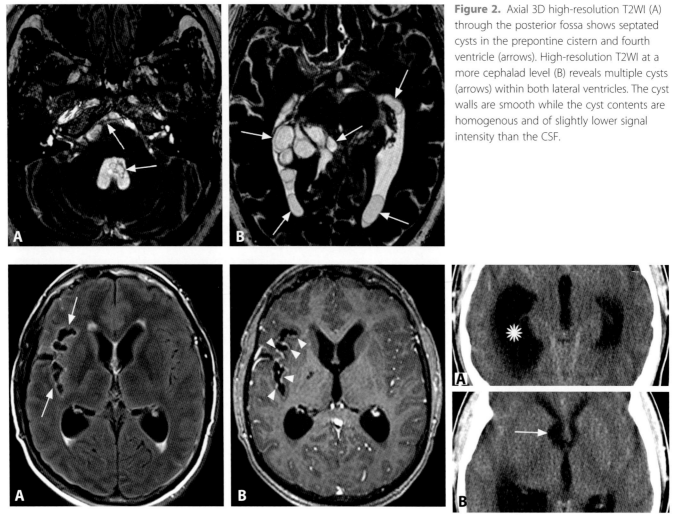

Figure 2. Axial 3D high-resolution T2WI (A) through the posterior fossa shows septated cysts in the prepontine cistern and fourth ventricle (arrows). High-resolution T2WI at a more cephalad level (B) reveals multiple cysts (arrows) within both lateral ventricles. The cyst walls are smooth while the cyst contents are homogenous and of slightly lower signal intensity than the CSF.

Figure 3. Axial FLAIR image (A) shows irregular dilation of the right sylvian fissure with subtle adjacent cortical hyperintensity (arrows).The lateral ventricles are enlarged. Corresponding post-contrast T1WI (B) demonstrates linear enhancement (arrowheads) along the dilated fissure, of varying thickness.

Figure 4. Non-enhanced CT (A, B) shows right greater than left hydrocephalus (*) with a subtle bulging adjacent to the right foramen of Monro (arrow).

Racemose Neurocysticercosis

ZORAN RUMBOLDT AND MAURICIO CASTILLO

Specific Imaging Findings

The vesicles in this racemose type of neurocysticercosis (NCC) are extra-axial and may be located throughout the CSF-containing spaces. Fluid in racemose cysts has CT attenuation values and MR signal properties closely paralleling CSF. Intraventricular cysticerci can cause rapidly progressive and potentially fatal non-communicating hydrocephalus but are typically not seen on standard CT and MR imaging studies. Racemose cysts lack the usual scolex and are seen as single or, more commonly, multilobulated cystic masses, best depicted on 3D high-resolution heavily T2-weighted images (CISS, DRIVE, FIESTA, etc.). FLAIR images obtained following continuous inhalation of 100% oxygen show increased signal intensity of the CSF, leading to much better conspicuity of cyst walls, because the cyst contents do not increase in signal. A thin subependymal or subpial rim of high T2 signal due to inflammatory tissue reaction may be present along with a thin peripheral contrast enhancement. The subarachnoid cysts may also lead to vasculitis of the adjacent arteries and associated infarcts. MR spectroscopy demonstrates presence of lactate and a large resonance at 2.4 ppm corresponding to pyruvate within racemose NCC cysts.

Pertinent Clinical Information

In around 10–15% of the individuals affected with NCC the parasites are extra-axial, located in the subarachnoid spaces. The patients present with headaches and transient disorders of consciousness. This racemose NCC may result in ventriculitis and meningitis, with hydrocephalus and raised intracranial pressure as a common complication. High intracranial pressure may be a contraindication to antiparasite treatment. High-dose albendazole combined with corticosteroids is an effective treatment for subarachnoid and intraventricular cysticercosis, leading to decreasing volume of the lesions.

Differential Diagnosis

Arachnoid Cyst (142)
- usually a single cyst, frequently large
- no pyruvate peak (at 2.4 ppm) on MR spectroscopy

Ependymal Cyst (146)
- typically a single large cyst
- intraventricular, most commonly located in the atria
- sometimes slightly increased signal of the cyst contents

Choroid Plexus Cyst (147)
- enclosed within choroid plexus glomus
- usually hyperintense to CSF on FLAIR and T1WI, very bright on DWI
- frequently bilateral

Cystic Neoplasms (148, 150, 172, 173, 175)
- often have solid components, may enhance and are rarely iso-intense with CSF

Other Infectious Cysts (Hydatid Disease)
- single to a few in number, tend to be large in size
- cysts may contain sediment of various signal intensity
- acetate peak (at 1.92 ppm) may be present on MR spectroscopy
- may be indistinguishable from racemose cysticercosis

Colloid Cyst (54)
- characteristic midline location at the foramina of Monro
- typically bright on CT, density/signal intensity is different from the CSF

Asymmetric CSF-containing Spaces
- no evidence of the cyst wall even with high-resolution 3D heavily T2-weighted sequences

Background

Parasitic CNS diseases frequently present as cystic lesions on imaging studies and cysticercosis is a typical example. This most common parasitic disease of the immunocompetent population is caused by the pork tapeworm (*Taenia solium*). Humans become the definitive host when ingesting larvae, which then grow in the small bowel and cause intestinal disease. However, if the eggs are ingested, humans become the intermediate host and when the eggs mature larvae are released into the bloodstream. Once this occurs, the incidence of CNS involvement is nearly 100%. The complication rate of ventricular shunting in patients with racemose NCC is high due to obstruction or material infection, which may justify endoscopic third ventriculostomy. The endoscopic view of the intraventricular cysts has been described as a "full moon", which appears to be a pathognomonic intraoperative finding.

REFERENCES

1. Braga F, Rocha AJ, Gomes HR, et al. Noninvasive MR cisternography with fluid-attenuated inversion recovery and 100% supplemental O₂ in the evaluation of neurocysticercosis. *AJNR* 2004;**25**:295–7.
2. Barinagarrementeria F, Cantu C. Frequency of cerebral arteritis in subarachnoid cysticercosis: an angiographic study. *Stroke* 1998;**29**:123–5.
3. Jayakumar PN, Srikanth SG, Chandrashekar HS, et al. Pyruvate: an in vivo marker of cestodal infestation of the human brain on proton MR spectroscopy. *J Magn Reson Imaging* 2003;**18**:675–80.
4. Göngora-Rivera F, Soto-Hernández JL, González Esquivel D, et al. Albendazole trial at 15 or 30 mg/kg/day for subarachnoid and intraventricular cysticercosis. *Neurology* 2006;**66**:436–8.
5. Rumboldt Z, Thurnher M, Gupta RK. Imaging of CNS infections. *Semin Roentgenol* 2007;**42**:62–91.

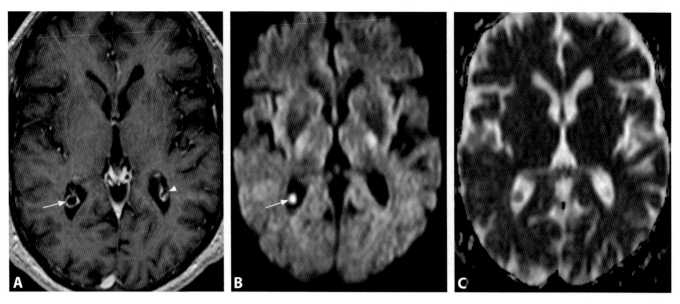

Figure 1. Axial post-contrast T1WI (A) shows a peripherally enhancing, ovoid, low signal intensity area (arrow) in the atrium of the right lateral ventricle located at the choroid plexus. Contralateral choroid plexus (arrowhead) is also seen. Corresponding DWI (B) shows hyperintensity of the cyst (arrow), while the corresponding ADC map (C) reveals diffusivity similar to the brain.

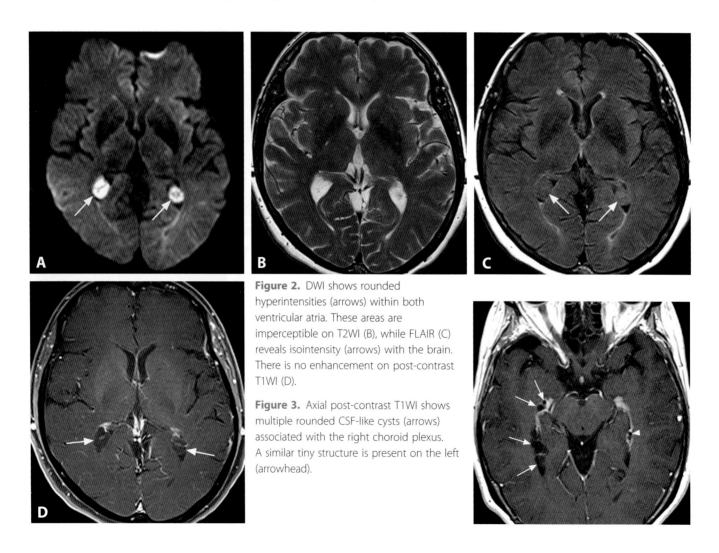

Figure 2. DWI shows rounded hyperintensities (arrows) within both ventricular atria. These areas are imperceptible on T2WI (B), while FLAIR (C) reveals isointensity (arrows) with the brain. There is no enhancement on post-contrast T1WI (D).

Figure 3. Axial post-contrast T1WI shows multiple rounded CSF-like cysts (arrows) associated with the right choroid plexus. A similar tiny structure is present on the left (arrowhead).

Choroid Plexus Cyst

BENJAMIN HUANG

Specific Imaging Findings

Choroid plexus cysts are most frequently located in the trigones of the lateral ventricles, but can occur throughout the ventricular system. They are typically less than 1 cm in diameter and are round or ovoid in shape. On CT, choroid plexus cysts usually demonstrate CSF density but can occasionally appear hyperdense relative to the CSF. The rims of the cysts may contain calcification. On T1- and T2-weighted images, choroid plexus cysts usually exhibit signal similar to that of CSF and may be difficult to identify. Post-contrast imaging may show a sharply marginated rim of peripheral enhancement, particularly in adults. On FLAIR images, cyst contents are often hyperintense relative to the CSF. Around two-thirds of choroid plexus cysts will be very bright on DWI and hence much easier to detect. Choroid plexus cysts are also seen in approximately 1% of fetal ultrasounds in the second trimester and some may persist into the neonatal period.

Pertinent Clinical Information

Choroid plexus cysts are extremely common, occuring in over half of individuals in serial autopsy studies with a similar incidence across all age groups. Most choroid plexus cysts are completely asymptomatic; however, in rare instances, when large or strategically located in the third ventricle they can cause symptoms of acute hydrocephalus due to obstruction. The prevalence of choroid plexus cysts on prenatal ultrasound is increased in fetuses with trisomy 18 (and with some other abnormalities). It has been suggested that identification of cysts which are > 1 cm in size, irregular, bilateral, or in mothers of advanced age should trigger a careful search for additional structural abnormalities. However, the incidence of trisomy 18 in fetuses with choroid plexus cysts but no other abnormalities on fetal ultrasound is exceedingly low, and this isolated finding is of little clinical significance.

Differential Diagnosis

Ependymal Cyst (146)
- closely attached to ventricular lining, wall very thin to imperceptible

Intraventricular Meningioma (149)
- typically homogenous mass with isointense to hypointense T2 signal
- avid contrast enhancement

Xanthogranuloma
- high T1 signal
- may enhance
- may contain stromal calcifications

Choroid Plexitis
- dense contrast enhancement

Choroid Plexus Hemorrhage
- acutely hyperdense on CT, follows signal intensity of blood products on MRI

Racemose Neurocysticercosis (145)
- scolex within the cyst may be present
- usually multiple cysts, not isolated to the choroid plexus

Colloid Cyst (54)
- located in the third ventricle near the foramina of Monro
- characteristically hyperdense on CT

Background

Fetal and neonatal choroid plexus cysts are most likely of different origins than choroid plexus cysts found in adults. In utero, choroid plexus cysts are believed to be the result of altered histogenesis of the plexus in the form of neuroepithelial folds that fill with cerebrospinal fluid and cellular debris. These cysts have an inner neuroepithelial lining. In older patients, choroid plexus cysts are likely caused by regressive changes of the plexus related to normal aging, and are lined with connective tissue. Peripheral enhancement of these cysts may be due to the presence of blood vessels within the thickened fibrous walls. Increased signal on DWI and FLAIR probably reflects increased protein content compared to the CSF, and can be seen in all age groups.

REFERENCES

1. Cakir B, Karakas HM, Unlu E, et al. Asymptomatic choroid plexus cysts in the lateral ventricles: an incidental finding on diffusion-weighted MRI. Neuroradiology 2002;44:830–3.
2. Kinoshita T, Moritani T, Hiwatashi A, et al. Clinically silent choroid plexus cyst: evaluation by diffusion-weighted MRI. Neuroradiology 2005;47:251–5.
3. Bethune M. Time to reconsider our approach to echogenic intracardiac focus and choroid plexus cysts. Aust N Z J Obstet Gynaecol 2008;48:137–41.
4. Chitkara U, Cogswell C, Norton K, et al. Choroid plexus cysts in the fetus: a benign anatomic variant or pathologic entity? Report of 41 cases and review of the literature. Obstet Gynecol 1988;72:185–9.
5. Kariyattil R, Panikar D. Choroid plexus cyst of the third ventricle presenting as acute triventriculomegaly. Childs Nerv Syst 2008;24:875–7.

Brain Imaging with MRI and CT, ed. Zoran Rumboldt et al. Published by Cambridge University Press. © Cambridge University Press 2012.

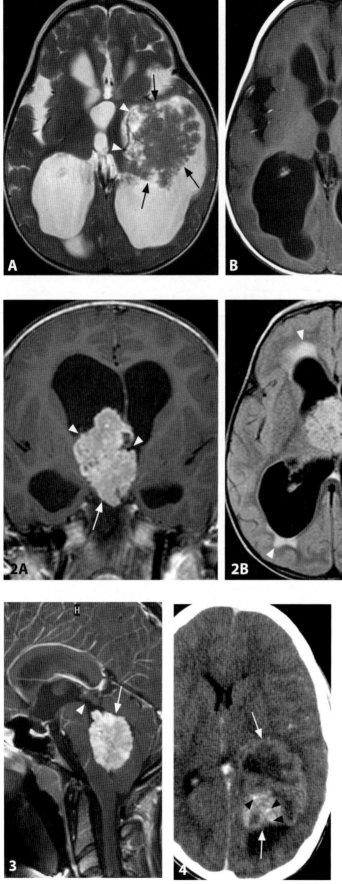

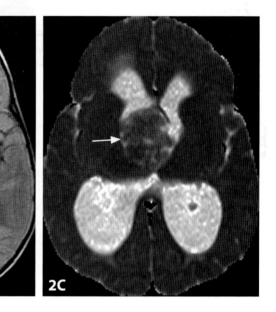

Figure 1. Axial T2WI (A) in a17-month-old boy shows an isointense mass (arrows) within the left ventricular atrium. The mass is composed of multiple strands of tissue and has a cauliflower-like shape. A large choroidal vessel (arrowheads) is also visible. Corresponding post-contrast T1WI (B) shows enhancement of the lesion. Note chronic ventriculomegaly with wavy ventricular contours and without periventricular edema.

Figure 2. Post-contrast coronal (A) T1WI in a 21-month-old shows lobulated enhancing mass (arrow) filling the third ventricle and extending through the right foramen of Monro (arrowheads). Axial FLAIR image (B) reveals uncompensated hydrocephalus with periventricular edema (arrowheads). The intralesional (arrow) diffusion is slightly increased compared to the brain on ADC map (C).

Figure 3. Midsagittal post-contrast T1WI in a young adult shows a multilobulated enhancing mass (arrow) filling the fourth ventricle. Note dilated cerebral aqueduct (arrowhead).

Figure 4. Enhanced axial CT image in another patient shows a heterogenous lobulated right lateral ventricle mass (arrows) with internal calcifications (arrowheads).

Choroid Plexus Papilloma

ANDREA ROSSI

Specific Imaging Findings

Choroid plexus papilloma (CPP) is seen on imaging studies as a large, intraventricular cauliflower-like mass that may adhere to the ventricular wall but is usually separated from brain tissue. The tumor is typically T1 iso- to hypointense and iso- to hyperintense to gray matter on T2WI. Diffusion is slightly increased with respect to the brain parenchyma. Presence of calcifications and/or hemorrhages may locally modify the signal of the tumor and may also be seen on CT scans. CT otherwise shows an iso- to hypodense mass consistent with low tumor cellularity. Intense and homogeneous contrast enhancement is due to rich vascularity. Enlarged feeding arteries may be identified on both MRI and MR angiography. In supratentorial CPP, the blood supply is provided by the anterior, posterolateral and posteromedial choroidal arteries, whose tumoral branches are constantly hypertrophied, tortuous, and elongated. Albeit rarely, benign CPP may spread cells into the CSF; thus, contrast-enhanced MRI of the entire neuraxis is warranted for correct disease staging.

Pertinent Clinical Information

Raised intracranial pressure secondary to hydrocephalus is the most frequent presentation of children with CPP regardless of location. The hydrocephalus is caused by either CSF overproduction by the tumor, obstruction of CSF flow, or both. Newborns or small infants may present with macrocrania and a progressive increase of head circumference prior to developing neurological signs.

Differential Diagnosis

Choroid Plexus Carcinoma
- usually reduced diffusion on ADC maps and CT hyperdensity due to hypercellularity
- possible invasion into adjacent brain parenchyma

Choroid Plexus Hyperplasia
- may not be distinguishable from CPP on imaging

Choroid Plexus Cyst (147)
- usually an incidental finding
- bilateral or unilateral, rounded cystic lesion of the choroid plexus glomus in the ventricular trigone
- iso- to hyperintense on FLAIR, peripheral enhancement due to surrounding choroid plexus

Choroid Plexitis
- enhancing choroid plexus with mild enlargement
- *Cryptococcus neoformans* is the typical causative agent
- may be indistinguishable on imaging

Subependymal Giant Cell Astrocytoma (170)
- located at the foramen of Monro
- often bilateral
- additional tuberous sclerosis complex lesions (cortical tubers, subependymal nodules)

Sturge–Weber Syndrome (86)
- hypertrophied choroid plexus ipsilateral to pial angioma and port-wine stain
- ipsilateral brain atrophy

Background

CPPs are highly vascular tumors composed of mature epithelial cells, histologically closely resembling non-neoplastic choroid plexus and corresponding to WHO grade I. CPP are relatively very common in fetal life. While they account for just 0.5–3% of intracranial tumors in children, they represent 5–20% of all perinatal brain neoplasms. Although male predilection is widely reported, a high female incidence is found in girls with Aicardi syndrome, an X-linked dominant condition defined by the triad of total or partial agenesis of the corpus callosum, chorioretinal lacunae, and infantile spasms; the morphology of the corpus callosum should therefore be evaluated carefully in all girls with CPP. A few cases of choroid plexus tumors have occurred in patients with Li–Fraumeni syndrome, a cancer-predisposing syndrome caused by the mutation of the *TP53* gene. CPP may arise wherever choroid plexus is found within the ventricular system, but there is a strong age-location correlation in that greater than 80% of infantile CPPs arise in the lateral ventricle; only very rarely are they located in the third ventricle (4% of pediatric cases), whereas the fourth ventricle (16% of pediatric cases) and the cerebellopontine angle cisterns are more typical adult locations.

REFERENCES

1. Severino M, Schwartz ES, Thurnher MM, *et al.* Congenital tumors of the central nervous system. *Neuroradiology* 2010;**52**:531–48.

2. Jinhu Y, Jianping D, Jun M, *et al.* Metastasis of a histologically benign choroid plexus papilloma: case report and review of the literature. *J Neurooncol* 2007;**83**:47–52.

3. Schijman E, Monges J, Raimondi AJ, *et al.* Choroid plexus papillomas of the IIIrd ventricle in childhood. Their diagnosis and surgical management. *Childs Nerv Syst* 1990;**6**:331–4.

4. Buxton N, Punt J. Choroid plexus papilloma producing symptoms by secretion of cerebro-spinal fluid. *Pediatr Neurosurg* 1997;**27**:108–11.

5. Wagle V, Melanson D, Ethier R, *et al.* Choroid plexus papilloma: magnetic resonance, computed tomography, and angiographic observations. *Surg Neurol* 1987;**27**:466–8.

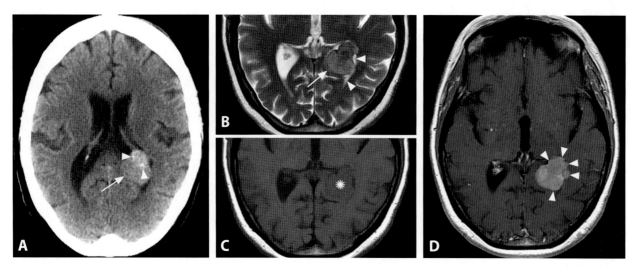

Figure 1. Axial non-enhanced CT (A) shows a hyperdense mass (arrow) in the trigone of the left lateral ventricle containing internal calcifications (arrowheads). The mass (arrow) is iso- to slightly hyperintense on T2WI (B) and slightly hypointense (*) on T1WI (C). Post-contrast T1WI (D) reveals homogenous enhancement of the lobulated lesion (arrowheads).

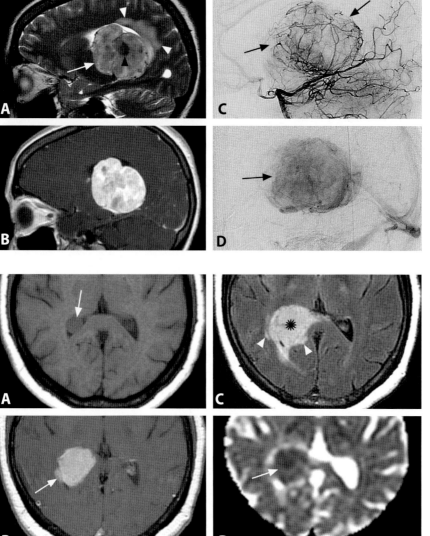

Figure 2. Sagittal T2WI (A) shows a large intraventricular mass (arrow) with internal focal low signal (black arrowhead), likely calcification. There is edema (white arrowheads) in the adjacent brain. Matching T1WI (B) shows marked enhancement of the lesion. Lateral view of a vertebral artery injection DSA shows early tumor blush (arrows) in the arterial phase (C), which is still clearly present (arrow) in the venous phase (D).

Figure 3. Axial T1WI without contrast (A) shows a questionable small, rounded lesion (arrow) in the atrium of the right lateral ventricle. Matching follow-up post-contrast T1WI (B) reveals substantial interval growth of the lobulated homogenously enhancing mass (arrow). The mass (*) is very bright on corresponding FLAIR image (C). There is also edema in the adjacent brain (arrowheads). The lesion is dark (arrow) on ADC map (D).

Intraventricular Meningioma

ZORAN RUMBOLDT

Specific Imaging Findings

Intraventricular meningiomas typically arise from the trigone in the posterior aspect of the lateral ventricles, more commonly on the left side, characteristically with a lobulated contour. Similar to meningiomas in other locations, the masses are hyperdense to calcified on non-enhanced CT. The tumors are usually homogenous with dense contrast enhancement. On MR imaging they show iso- to hyperintensity compared to the brain gray matter and are usually of low T1 and T2 signal intensity. Similar to meningiomas in other locations, very high cerebral blood volume is found on perfusion studies and MR spectroscopy may show the presence of alanine. These neoplasms may also arise around the foramina of Monro as well as within the third and fourth ventricles. Irregular lobulations, necrotic (nonenhancing) portions, and a combination of high T2 signal (bright on FLAIR images) and low diffusion values (dark on ADC maps) suggest higher-grade (atypical or malignant) subtypes, which are relatively common in intraventricular meningiomas.

Pertinent Clinical Information

The tumors often grow slowly to a substantial size before they become symptomatic. The most common presenting symptoms and signs are headache, mental change, hemianopsia, and vertigo. Total surgical removal can be achieved in most cases.

Differential Diagnosis

Choroid Plexus Papilloma (148)

- heterogenous with prominent vascular structures (flow-voids)
- characteristically arise at the trigone of lateral ventricles in children and in the fourth ventricle in adults

Metastatic Tumors

- frequently heterogenous and necrotic
- additional parenchymal lesions may be present
- no alanine peak on MR spectroscopy
- may be indistinguishable

Central Neurocytoma (150)

- characteristically at the midline, around the septum pellucidum
- multicystic appearance

Subpendymoma (171)

- enhancement usually minimal to absent; inhomogenous if more prominent
- within the fourth ventricle and around the foramina of Monro
- low cerebral blood volume on perfusion studies

Subependymal Giant Cell Astrocytoma (SEGA) (170)

- occurs exclusively in patients with tuberous sclerosis
- almost always arises at the foramen of Monro

Ependymoma (172, 200)

- more heterogenous and ill-defined, calcifications and hemorrhage are common
- prominent vasculature (flow-voids) is frequently present within the tumor
- supratentorial are typically extraventricular (anaplastic)

Hemangioblastoma (175)

- characteristic prominent vessels (flow-voids) within the tumor
- may contain a large cystic portion
- solid portion avidly enhances with contrast and is very bright on ADC maps
- very rare outside the cerebellum except in the setting of von Hippel–Lindau disease (VHL)

Background

Intraventricular meningiomas are rare tumors comprising only about 0.5–3% of all intracranial meningiomas; however, they are relatively common among intraventricular masses. Catheter angiography may show typical early and prolonged tumor blush, with preoperative embolization frequently performed. Gamma knife radiosurgery may be an additional minimally invasive management option for small intraventricular meningiomas in patients who either fail or are unsuitable for resection.

REFERENCES

1. Kim EY, Kim ST, Kim HJ, et al. Intraventricular meningiomas: radiological findings and clinical features in 12 patients. *Clin Imaging* 2009;**33**:175–80.

2. Koeller KK, Sandberg GD. From the archives of the AFIP. Cerebral intraventricular neoplasms: radiologic–pathologic correlation. *Radiographics* 2002;**22**:1473–505.

3. Zimny A, Sasiadek M. Contribution of perfusion-weighted magnetic resonance imaging in the differentiation of meningiomas and other extra-axial tumors: case reports and literature review. *J Neurooncol* 2011;**103**:777–83.

4. McDermott MW. Intraventricular meningiomas. *Neurosurg Clin N Am* 2003;**14**:559–69.

5. Kim IY, Kondziolka D, Niranjan A, et al. Gamma knife radiosurgery for intraventricular meningiomas. *Acta Neurochir (Wien)* 2009;**151**:447–52.

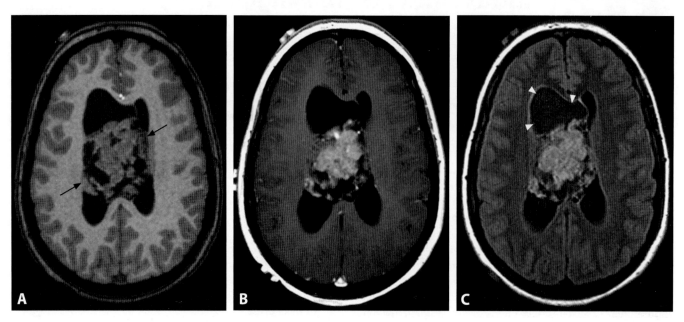

Figure 1. Axial non-contrast T1WI (A) shows a midline "bubbly" mass (arrows) in the lateral ventricles and hydrocephalus. Post-contrast T1WI at a slightly lower level (B) shows marked lesion enhancement. Corresponding FLAIR image (C) shows the lesion to be hyperintense with respect to the brain. A large loculated cyst (arrowheads) is well seen anterior to the mass.

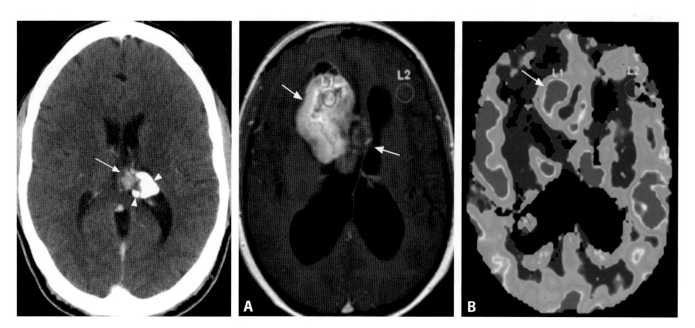

Figure 2. Enhanced CT image shows an enhancing midline mass (arrow) that extends into the left lateral ventricle and contains prominent calcifications (arrowheads).

Figure 3. Axial post-contrast T1WI (A) in another patient shows a heterogenous enhancing mass (arrows) extending from the midline into the right lateral ventricle. The ventricles are dilated. Corresponding dynamic susceptibility MR perfusion rCBV map (B) shows increased vascularity of this lesion (arrow).

Central Neurocytoma

MAURICIO CASTILLO

Specific Imaging Findings

Central neurocytomas are typically located in the frontal horn and corpus of the lateral ventricles. They are isodense to brain on CT and contain multiple cysts, generally small ones. Up to two-thirds of them contain calcifications and nearly all show some contrast enhancement. Intraventricular blood is not uncommon. On MR imaging, T1 and T2 sequences typically demonstrate heterogeneous signal intensity with cysts, hemorrhage and large flow-voids. Central neurocytomas are hyperintense on FLAIR images and commonly show reduced diffusion on ADC maps. Associated hydrocephalus is very frequent. Perfusion studies show increased relative cerebral blood volume of the tumor. MR spectroscopy shows high choline and low *n*-acetyl aspartate, while the presence of a high glycine peak (at 3.55 ppm) appears to be a characteristic feature. Rare extraventricular neurocytomas arise in frontal and parietal lobes and exhibit the same imaging features – intratumoral cysts, calcifications and/or blood products.

Pertinent Clinical Information

Although central neurocytoma may occur at any age and equally in both genders, it tends to be found in younger individuals (20–40 years of age). They may be incidentally discovered or produce signs of increased intracranial pressure or intraventricular (with extension into the subarachnoid spaces) hemorrhage. Large tumors may compress the hypothalamus and produce hormonal and visual changes. As it is a localized tumor, complete resection is frequently curative and survival rates even after incomplete resection are over 80% at 5 years. Recently, neurocytomas have been found to recur more often after surgery than previously thought. Radiosurgery is an effective treatment for residual and/or recurrent tumors.

Differential Diagnosis

Subependymoma (171)
* solid and not bubbly like central neurocytoma
* generally does not enhance, no high perfusion
* most commonly found in the fourth ventricle

Subependymal Giant Cell Astrocytoma (170)
* almost exclusively in patients with tuberous sclerosis complex

Choroid Plexus Tumors (148)
* in adults they are more often in the fourth ventricle
* in children typically in the atria of the lateral ventricles

Intraventricular Meningioma (149)
* solid, homogenous enhancement
* usually at the atrium of the lateral ventricles, more commonly on the left

Ependymoma (172, 200)
* most supratentorial ependymomas are outside of the ventricles, usually anaplastic

Metastatic Neoplasm
* isolated intraventricular lesions are very rare
* look for primary and metastases elsewhere

Background

This neuroepithelial tumor with neuronal differentiation was, in the past, believed to be an intraventricular oligodendroglioma. Today it is recognized as a distinct entity that nearly always occurs in the lateral ventricles adjacent to the septum pellucidum and the foramen of Monro. Rare locations include: third and fourth ventricles and the brain parenchyma. It is a WHO grade II tumor comprising less than 1% of all intracranial neoplasias and about 10% of intraventricular ones. As it is a vascular tumor it may have increased perfusion and bleed easily into the ventricular system. In addition to perfusion, its MR diffusion and spectroscopy features also resemble high-grade gliomas and may be misleading. Occasionally, central neurocytoma may have a malignant behavior.

REFERENCES

1. Zhang D, Wen L, Henning TD, *et al*. Central neurocytoma: clinical, pathological and neuroradiological findings. *Clin Radiol* 2006;**61**:348–57.
2. Koeller KK, Sandberg GD. From the archives of the AFIP. Cerebral intraventricular neoplasms: radiologic–pathologic correlation. *Radiographics* 2002;**22**:1473–505.
3. Choudhari KA, Kaliaperumal C, Jain A, *et al*. Central neurocytoma: a multi-disciplinary review. *Br J Neurosurg* 2009;**23**:585–95.
4. Shah T, Jayasundar R, Singh VP, Sarkar C. MRS characterization of central neurocytomas using glycine. *NMR Biomed* 2011;**24**:1408–13.
5. Yang G-F, Wu S-Y, Zhang L-J, *et al*. Imaging findings of extraventricular neurocytoma: report of 3 cases and review of the literature. *AJNR* 2009;**30**:581–5.

Brain Imaging with MRI and CT, ed. Zoran Rumboldt *et al*. Published by Cambridge University Press. © Cambridge University Press 2012.

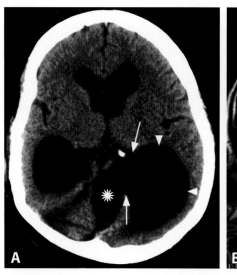 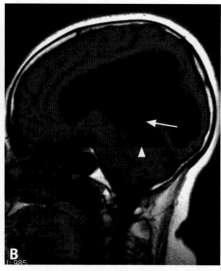

Figure 1. Non-enhanced axial CT (A) in a patient with long-standing hydrocephalus shows dilated ventricular system, especially the atrium of left lateral ventricle (arrowheads). There is a paramedial CSF collection (*) that widely communicates (arrows) with the left atrium. Sagittal T1WI (B) reveals infratentorial extension of the collection through the tentorial incisura (arrow) compressing the cerebellum (arrowhead).

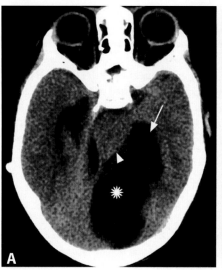 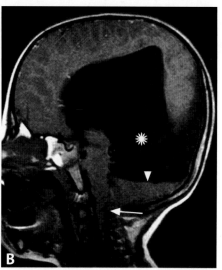

Figure 2. Non-enhanced axial CT image (A) in another patient shows enlarged left lateral ventricle (arrow). The dilated ventricle extends postero-medially (*), displacing and flattening the brainstem (arrowhead). Sagittal T1WI (B) shows a wide communication (*) between the dilated lateral ventricle and an infratentorial CSF collection that is compressing the cerebellum (arrowhead) with subsequent small tonsillar herniation (arrow).

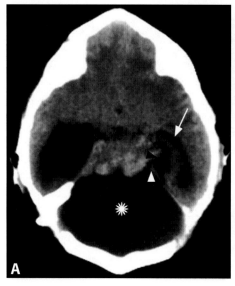 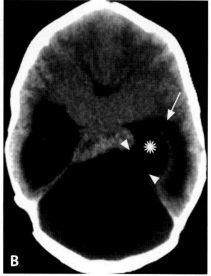

Figure 3. Non-enhanced CT (A) in a child with CNS malformations shows enlarged ventricles, primarily the fourth ventricle (*), which appears to communicate with a CSF collection (black arrowhead) close to the temporal horn (arrow), around the tentorial edge (white arrowhead). A more cephalad image (B) reveals a wide communication (arrowheads) between the fourth ventricle and this collection (*), separate from the temporal horn (arrow).

Ventricular Diverticula

ZORAN RUMBOLDT

Specific Imaging Findings

Ventricular diverticula are focal dilations of the ventricular system resulting from severe chronic obstructive hydrocephalus. Despite their different origins, they are typically unilateral and similarly located in the quadrigeminal and superior cerebellar cisterns. Most of them arise from the inferomedial atrium of the lateral ventricles and frequently extend into the posterior fossa through the tentorial incisura, displacing the brain stem, vermis, and fourth ventricle. Detection of an ostium of a diverticulum or a communication between the cyst and the ventricular system is the key for diagnosis and is usually best seen on sagittal or coronal MRI. The communication may be confirmed with a phase-contrast study demonstrating uninterrupted CSF flow. Lateral ventricular diverticula may be identified and distinguished from other cystic lesions when all of the following signs are present on CT: (1) marked unilateral atrial dilation; (2) focal dehiscence of the medial atrial wall; (3) ipsilateral shortening of the tentorial band on axial images; (4) focal defect in the tentorial band in coronal section; (5) draping of the medial atrial wall over the free margin of tentorium, with continuity of CSF density around the edge of tentorium; (6) bowing of the crus of fornix; (7) separation of fornix from splenium, with visualization of the hernia ostium; (8) asymmetrical position of the choroid plexi (which attach to and define the lateral borders of the fornices); (9) contralateral displacement of the internal cerebral veins; and (10) septa separating diverticulum from the third ventricle. In patients with Chiari II malformations, the small third ventricle may occasionally exhibit diverticula, usually posterior. Diverticula of the fourth ventricle are uncommon and usually extend superiorly through the tentorial hiatus. Ventriculography (contrast injection through the ventricular drain) can also be used to differentiate diverticula from other lesions.

Pertinent Clinical Information

The underlying cause for ventricular diverticula is typically congenital (aqueductal stenosis), neoplastic (intra/paraventricular slow growing tumors), or a colloid cyst. Patients present with symptoms of chronic increased intracranial pressure, such as headaches and forgetfulness, and macrocephaly in infants. Large infra-tentorial diverticula may lead to cerebellar ataxia. Rarity of these pouches, along with variability in their extent and location, make them difficult to diagnose on imaging. Correct identification is, however, of significant importance as it prevents unnecessary surgery. Progressive collapse of diverticula along with resolution of symptoms occurs after ventricular decompression, either by shunting or removal of the obstructing lesion.

Differential Diagnosis

Ependymal Cyst (146)
- expands the ventricle without a focal herniation

Choroid Plexus Cyst (147)
- arises from the choroid plexus, herniation is extremely rare

Arachnoid Cyst (142)
- no communication with ventricles

Epidermoid (143)
- no communication with ventricles
- characteristically very bright on DWI

Background

Chronically increased intraventricular pressure raises wall tension, causing shearing of the ependymal lining and focal weakening of the ventricular surface. If increased pressure is sustained, the affected area stretches and herniates into the subarachnoid space, forming a diverticulum. This is thought to occur in up to 25% of patients with severe long-standing obstructive hydrocephalus. These pouches histologically consist of only two layers, pia and arachnoid, without ependymal lining. Diverticula may rupture creating communication with the external surface of the brain, referred to as spontaneous ventriculostomy. Because wall tension is proportional to cavity size and inversely proportional to wall thickness, diverticula are expected to occur at points where the lumen is wide and the distance between the ependyma and pia is the shortest. The choroidal fissure and the rostral portion of the superior medullary velum may be the origins of diverticula from the atrium and the superior fourth ventricle.

REFERENCES
1. Naidich TP, McLone DG, Hahn YS, Hanaway J. Atrial diverticula in severe hydrocephalus. *AJNR* 1982;**3**:257–66.
2. Huh JS, Hwang YS, Yoon SH, *et al.* Lateral ventricular diverticulum extending into supracerebellar cistern from unilateral obstruction of the foramen of Monro in a neonate. *Pediatr Neurosurg* 2007;**43**:115–20.
3. Wakai S, Nagai M. Ventricular diverticulum. *J Neurol Neurosurg Psychiatry* 1984;**47**:514–7.
4. Abe M, Uchino A, Tsuji T, Tabuchi K. Ventricular diverticula in obstructive hydrocephalus secondary to tumor growth. *Neurosurgery* 2003;**52**:65–70.
5. Jabaudon D, Charest D, Porchet F. Pathogenesis and diagnostic pitfalls of ventricular diverticula: case report and review of the literature. *Neurosurgery* 2003;**52**:209–12.

Brain Imaging with MRI and CT, ed. Zoran Rumboldt *et al.* Published by Cambridge University Press. © Cambridge University Press 2012.

SECTION 6

Primarily Intra-Axial Masses

Cases

A. Typically Without Blood Products

Other Relevant Cases

B. Typically With Blood Products

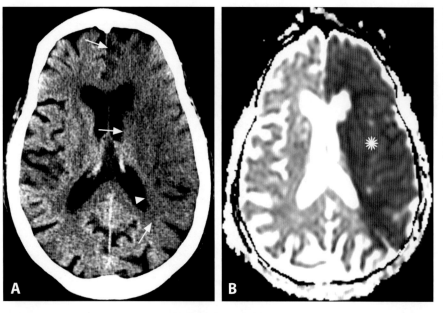

Figure 1. Axial CT image (A) at the level of the lateral ventricles shows hypodensity in the anterior three quarters of the left cerebral hemisphere with effacement of the cortical sulci and loss of contrast between the gray and white matter (arrows). There is minimal associated mass effect on the lateral ventricle (arrowhead). ADC map at a similar level (B) reveals reduced diffusion (*) in the entire left anterior circulation.

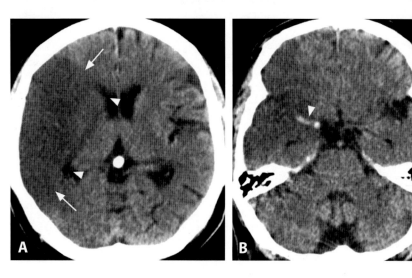

Figure 2. Non-enhanced CT image (A) shows a hypodensity (arrows) in the right middle cerebral artery (MCA) territory with effacement of the cortical sulci and subtle mass effect on the right lateral ventricle (arrowheads). CT image at a lower level (B) reveals hyperdense right MCA (arrowhead), in addition to the hypodense lesion.

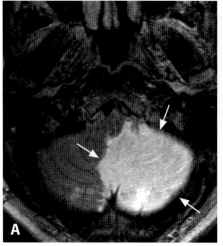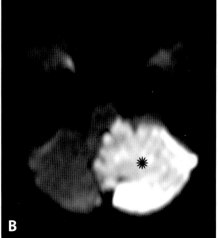

Figure 3. Axial T2WI (A) shows hyperintensity and mild swelling of the inferior left cerebellar hemisphere (arrows). The lesion is very bright (*) on DWI at a similar level (B).

Acute Infarction

MAJDA THURNHER

Specific Imaging Findings

On non-enhanced CT scan acute infarction will be recognized as a hypoattenuating area of the brain parenchyma in a typical vascular distribution, involving both the gray and white matter with loss of contrast between the two and effacement of the cortical sulci. In larger infarcts a more prominent mass effect such as compression of the ventricular system or even herniations may be observed. Increased T2 signal intensity with cortical swelling and mild mass effect is observed on MRI, along with gyral effacement and T1 hypointensity. FLAIR images may show hyperintensity along the occluded vessels (comparable to the CT "hyperdense vessel" sign). Acute ischemic lesions are characterized by a very bright signal on DWI and low ADC values. ADC gradually normalizes over time, but remains decreased for the first 5–10 days. Contrast enhancement may be present in the acute phase, which is usually gyriform along the cortex. However, smaller infarcts (especially in the brainstem and basal ganglia) may show ring-like or patchy enhancement, mimicking neoplasms. T2* MR images are highly susceptible to the paramagnetic effect of the blood products, and thus highly specific for identifying areas of microscopic and macroscopic hemorrhage. Extremely low rCBV and rCBF values are present in infarcted areas on perfusion imaging.

Pertinent Clinical Information

Stroke is characterized with sudden onset of symptoms, depending on the area of the brain affected. Most common clinical signs are sudden onset of face weakness, unilateral hemiplegia and abnormal speech. Brain stem infarction will present with ptosis (or other muscle weakness), altered breathing, decreased reflexes, and nystagmus. If the cerebellum is affected, patients will have gait difficulties, vertigo, altered movement coordination. Memory deficits will suggest infarction in the temporal lobe. Headache, loss of consciousness, and vomiting are common with hemorrhagic infarcts (due to increased intracranial pressure). Asymptomatic silent infarcts are more frequent in the right hemisphere and cerebellum.

Differential Diagnosis

Cerebral Hyperperfusion Syndrome (CHS)
- elevated CBF
- following surgical treatment of carotid stenosis, or carotid stenting
- high or low signal on DWI in the brain hemisphere ipsilateral to the treated carotid stenosis

Low-Grade Glioma (162)
- typically increased diffusion – lesions are bright on ADC maps
- does not follow vascular territory
- rCBV slightly lower to slightly higher compared to the normal brain on perfusion studies

- choline levels may be increased compared to the normal brain on MR spectroscopy

Herpes Simplex Encephalitis (HSE) (20)
- rCBV is slightly decreased to normal, and not extremely low on perfusion studies
- typically involves the anterior temporal lobe
- frequently bilateral
- lesions are sharply marginating the lateral border of the putamen

Progressive Multifocal Leukoencephalopathy (PML) (116)
- lesions isolated to the white matter (vasogenic edema appearance with sparing of cortical ribbon)
- bright on ADC maps centrally with low ADC at the periphery
- rCBV slightly lower to slightly higher compared to the normal brain on perfusion studies

Posterior Reversible Encephalopathy Syndrome (PRES) (32)
- bilateral and primarily involving the white matter
- bright on ADC maps (vasogenic edema); however, low ADC when infarcted

Background

CT of the brain enables rapid assessment of patients with acute ischemia. MRI defines early ischemic changes with greater conspicuity, especially in posterior circulation infarcts. DWI and perfusion MR are useful in differentiating ischemic lesions from neoplastic or inflammatory conditions, as the combination of very bright DWI/very low ADC signal with extremely low to non-existent rCBV is pathognomonic for acute infarction. Assessment of intracranial and extracranial vasculature can be perfomed using CTA or MRA.

REFERENCES

1. Kunst MM, Schaefer PW. Ischemic stroke. *Radiol Clin North Am* 2011;**49**:1–26.
2. Misra V, Fadil H, Hoque R, et al. Clinically presenting acute/subacute ischemic stroke: differential diagnosis of the non-enhanced CT hypodensity by advanced neuroimaging. *Neurol Res* 2009;**31**:816–23.
3. Cunlife CH, Fischer I, Monoky D, et al. Intracranial lesions mimicking neoplasms. *Arch Pathol Lab Med* 2009;**133**:101–23.
4. Tanaka Y, Uematsu Y, Owai Y, Itakura T. Two cases of ringlike enhancement on MRI mimicking malignant brain tumors. *Brain Tumor Pathol* 2006;**23**:107–11.
5. Hirooka R, Ogasawara K, Sasaki M, et al. Magnetic resonance imaging in patients with cerebral hyperperfusion and cognitive impairment after carotid endarterectomy. *J Neurosurg* 2008;**108**:1178–83.

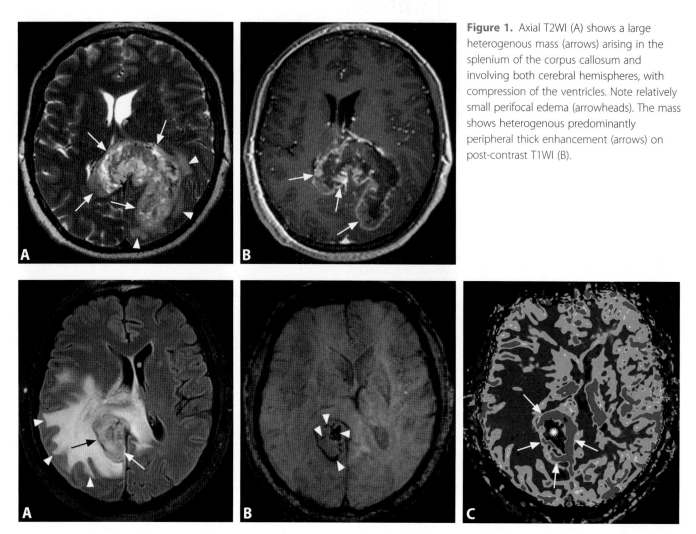

Figure 1. Axial T2WI (A) shows a large heterogenous mass (arrows) arising in the splenium of the corpus callosum and involving both cerebral hemispheres, with compression of the ventricles. Note relatively small perifocal edema (arrowheads). The mass shows heterogenous predominantly peripheral thick enhancement (arrows) on post-contrast T1WI (B).

Figure 2. FLAIR image (A) shows an intra-axial mass (black arrow) with vasogenic edema (arrowheads). There is also infiltrative edema with involvement of the cortex (white arrow). Areas of internal signal loss (arrowheads) are present on T2* SWI (B). The rCBV is high along the lesion periphery (arrows) while low in the central necrotic region (*) on perfusion MRI (C).

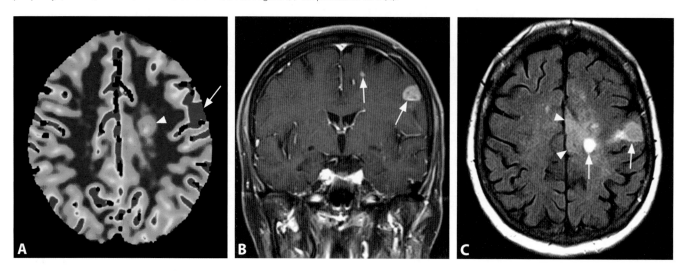

Figure 3. CT perfusion CBV image (A) in a patient with right hemiparesis and dysphasia (suspected acute infarct) shows a left frontal cortico-subcortical area of very high CBV (arrow) and a focal white matter hyperperfusion (arrowhead). Coronal post-contrast T1WI reveals enhancement of both lesions (arrows). FLAIR image (C) at a similar level as A shows hyperintensity of the masses (arrows). The abnormal increased signal extends to involve the cortex (arrowheads), consistent with infiltrative edema.

Glioblastoma Multiforme

ZORAN RUMBOLDT AND MAJDA THURNHER

Specific Imaging Findings

Glioblastoma multiforme (GBM) usually presents as a heterogenous enhancing mass. It is frequently hypodense on CT and with high T2 signal on MRI. The T2 hyperintense/CT hypodense area with the appearance of vasogenic edema surrounding the enhancing lesion is almost always present, but its size varies. A characteristic of gliomas is the infiltrative edema with signal abnormality not being limited to the white matter but extending to involve the cortex and/or deep gray matter. This feature is almost always present along at least a portion of the abnormality. Although frank intratumoral hematomas are not common, multiple areas of signal loss caused by susceptibility effects from small amounts of blood products are almost always detected on T2* MR imaging. Gadolinium-enhanced T1WI most commonly demonstrates a necrotic mass with thick, irregular predominantly peripheral enhancement. Nodular or ring-like enhancement may also be present, and enhancement is absent in rare cases. Solid portions of the neoplasm commonly show low diffusion with reduced ADC values, while necrotic areas are bright on ADC maps. Increased choline, decreased NAA and elevated lactate/lipid peak will be detected on MRS. Very high rCBV of solid tumor areas is a hallmark of GBM on perfusion studies. Analysis of the signal intensity curve on susceptibility-weighted post-contrast perfusion studies shows return to the baseline value following the first pass of contrast medium. In around 10% of cases GBM presents as multifocal lesions on initial imaging studies.

Pertinent Clinical Information

Patients may present with focal neurological deficits or signs of increased intracranial pressure. Seizures are less common at presentation compared to low-grade gliomas. GBM usually arises in the cerebral hemispheres and the peak age of onset is the sixth or seventh decade.

Differential Diagnosis

Metastatic Tumor (155)
- prominent vasogenic edema, absence of infiltrative edema
- normal findings on spectroscopy outside of the enhancing area
- on perfusion studies the signal does not return to baseline
- areas of signal loss due to susceptibility effects on T2* imaging are subtle and few

Primary CNS Lymphoma (158)
- homogenous lesion without necrosis, except in HIV-positive patients
- very low diffusion, dark on ADC maps
- no areas of signal loss due to susceptibility effects on T2* imaging
- prominent vasogenic edema

Tumefactive Demyelinating Lesion (TDL) (159)
- characteristic incomplete ring of enhancement is frequently present
- low rCBV on perfusion imaging

Abscess (156)
- reduced diffusion in the necrotic core with bright DWI signal and low ADC values

Subacute Infarction (124)
- common gyriform enhancement
- follows a vascular territory
- very low rCBV on perfusion imaging
- usually homogenous signal intensity throughout the lesion, unless hemorrhagic

Background

GBM is the most common malignant glioma in adults. According to the WHO classification of the CNS tumors, it presents in two additional variants: giant cell glioblastoma and gliosarcoma, and all are grade IV neoplasm. Tumor is found outside the signal abnormalities on MRI, as the peritumoral region is infiltrated with malignant cells. There is also evidence that neoplastic infiltration is present in the contralateral hemisphere even with newly diagnosed tumors in untreated patients and GBM should be considered a disease of the entire brain.

REFERENCES

1. Park SM, Kim HS, Jahng GH, et al. Combination of high-resolution susceptibility-weighted imaging and the apparent diffusion coefficient: added value to brain tumour imaging and clinical feasibility on non-contrast MRI at 3 T. Br J Radiol 2010;**83**:466–75.

2. Bohman LE, Swanson KR, Moore JL, et al. Magnetic resonance imaging characteristics of glioblastoma multiforme: implications for understanding glioma ontogeny. Neurosurgery 2010;**67**:1319–27.

3. Cha S, Lupo JM, Chen MH, et al. Differentiation of glioblastoma multiforme and single brain metastasis by peak height and percentage of signal intensity recovery derived from dynamic susceptibility-weighted contrast-enhanced perfusion MR imaging. AJNR 2007;**28**:1078–84.

4. Toh CH, Castillo M, Wong AM, et al. Primary cerebral lymphoma and glioblastoma multiforme: differences in diffusion characteristics evaluated with diffusion tensor imaging. AJNR 2008;**29**:471–5.

5. Kallenberg K, Bock HC, Helms G, et al. Untreated glioblastoma multiforme: increased myo-inositol and glutamine levels in the contralateral cerebral hemisphere at proton MR spectroscopy. Radiology 2009;**253**:805–12.

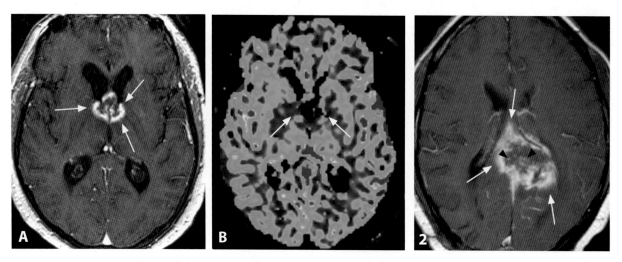

Figure 1. Post-contrast T1WI (A) following high-grade glioma therapy shows an enhancing mass with internal specks of contrast and ill-defined rim (arrows). Corresponding MR perfusion (B) does not reveal any increased rCBV (arrows).

Figure 2. Post-contrast T1WI for a treated meningioma shows an intra-axial lesion crossing the midline with enhancing internal foci (arrowheads) and feathery ill-defined outer margin (arrows).

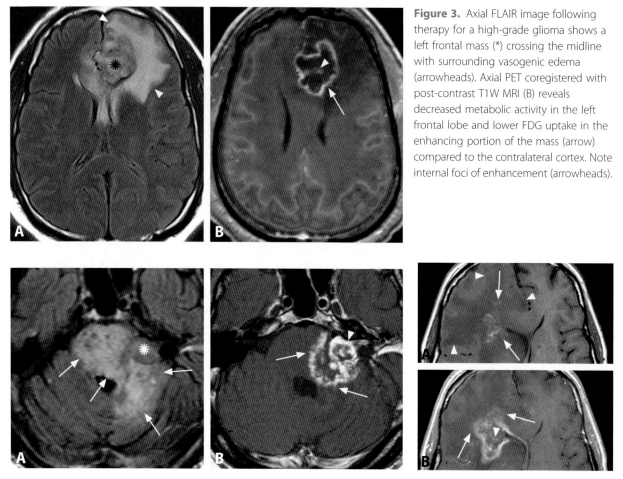

Figure 3. Axial FLAIR image following therapy for a high-grade glioma shows a left frontal mass (*) crossing the midline with surrounding vasogenic edema (arrowheads). Axial PET coregistered with post-contrast T1W MRI (B) reveals decreased metabolic activity in the left frontal lobe and lower FDG uptake in the enhancing portion of the mass (arrow) compared to the contralateral cortex. Note internal foci of enhancement (arrowheads).

Figure 4. Axial FLAIR image (A) of a vestibular schwannoma (*) treated with surgery and radiosurgery shows a surrounding hyperintensity and mass effect (arrows). Post-contrast T1WI (B) reveals central speckled and peripheral feathery enhancement (arrows) around the tumor (arrowhead). Note similar internal enhancement pattern within the treated tumor.

Figure 5. Right frontal mass effect and edema (arrowheads) surround an irregular T1 hyperintensity (arrows) (A), which shows ill-defined peripheral (arrows) and scattered internal (arrowhead) contrast enhancement (B).

Therapy-Induced Cerebral Necrosis (Radiation Necrosis)

MARIA VITTORIA SPAMPINATO AND ZORAN RUMBOLDT

Specific Imaging Findings

Therapy-induced (radiation) cerebral necrosis (TCN) cannot be reliably differentiated from residual/progressive malignancy on CT or conventional MR imaging. TCN appears as an enhancing mass with surrounding vasogenic edema, frequently increasing in size on serial examinations. Internal irregular linear areas of high T1 signal may be found. Typical patterns of contrast enhancement include internal localized specks of bright signal within necrotic areas ("Swiss cheese/soap bubble" – presumably due to contrast leakage into the cavity) and ill-defined feathery peripheral enhancement ("spreading wavefront"). Edema is limited to the white matter without infiltrative gray matter involvement. On perfusion imaging TCN characteristically shows very low relative cerebral blood volume (rCBV), in contrast to malignant neoplasms. The perfusion signal intensity–time curve shows substantially lower signal recovery than in gliomas, reflecting the high degree of contrast leakage within TCN. Necrosis shows higher signal on ADC maps, compared to relatively low ADC values of viable neoplasms. TCN is characterized by decrease of all metabolites on MR spectroscopy and a dominant very high level of lipids, known as "death peak".

Pertinent Clinical Information

TCN is a serious complication of radiation therapy for intracranial tumors and non-neoplastic conditions. It also occurs following treatment of extracranial diseases, most notably nasopharyngeal carcinoma. Development of TCN is related to the method of radiation delivery, total dose, fraction size, treatment volume, patient age, and administration of chemotherapy. The changes occur from several months to years after treatment, more frequently following high-dose local radiation, such as radiosurgery or brachytherapy. Radiation therapy with concomitant temozolomide, especially within the first 3 months, frequently leads to TCN in patients with primary brain tumors, known as pseudoprogression. Standard treatment includes surgical resection, which also establishes the diagnosis, and corticosteroids. Antiangiogenic therapy with bevazucimab has recently shown excellent results in patients with TCN.

Differential Diagnosis

Progressive High-Grade Glioma (153)
- increased cerebral blood volume on perfusion studies
- elevated Cho/NAA and Cho/Cr ratios on MRS
- low ADC of solid component

Abscess (156)
- smooth rim of enhancement without internal enhancing foci
- central non-enhancing portion is extremely DWI bright/ADC dark
- peripheral rim is T2 hypointense and T1 hyperintense

Metastatic Neoplasm (155)
- increased cerebral blood volume on perfusion studies
- increased Cho, no evidence of NAA on MRS
- usually rounded and well-defined

Background

TCN has been traditionally called radiation necrosis; however, additional antineoplastic therapies frequently contribute to the radiation tissue injury. Several mechanisms may be involved in pathogenesis; however, damage to the brain microvasculature is likely the primary event in the development of brain injury. Endothelial cell death results in breakdown of the blood–brain barrier, edema, and hypoxia. Hypoxia is thought to cause upregulation of vascular endothelial growth factor, which causes increased permeability of the vasculature, vasogenic edema, vessel thrombosis, and tissue necrosis. Histologically, focal necrotic lesions show typical vascular changes consisting of hyalinization, fibrinoid necrosis of the blood vessel wall, and a narrowed lumen. White matter at the margin of lesions may show myelin loss and astrocytic gliosis, while coagulative necrosis is present in the central regions. Glioma progression and radiation treatment necrosis frequently coexist, and residual tumor foci are often present even in the so-called pure radiation necrosis. Recent studies show that a very reliable differentiation of necrosis from viable metastatic tumors may be achieved with dual phase FDG-PET/CT by using the change of lesion to gray matter SUVmax ratio as a function of time.

REFERENCES

1. Rogers LR, Gutierrez J, Scarpace L, et al. Morphologic magnetic resonance imaging features of therapy-induced cerebral necrosis. J Neurooncol 2011;101:25–32.
2. Barajas RF Jr, Chang JS, Segal MR, et al. Differentiation of recurrent glioblastoma multiforme from radiation necrosis after external beam radiation therapy with dynamic susceptibility-weighted contrast-enhanced perfusion MR imaging. Radiology 2009;253:486–96.
3. Pruzincova L, Steno J, Srbecky M, et al. MR imaging of late radiation therapy- and chemotherapy-induced injury: a pictorial essay. Eur Radiol 2009;19:2716–27.
4. Alexiou GA, Tsiouris S, Kyritsis AP, et al. Glioma recurrence versus radiation necrosis: accuracy of current imaging modalities. J Neurooncol 2009;95:1–11.
5. Horky LL, Hsiao EM, Weiss SE, et al. Dual phase FDG-PET imaging of brain metastases provides superior assessment of recurrence versus post-treatment necrosis. J Neurooncol 2011;103:137–46.

Brain Imaging with MRI and CT, ed. Zoran Rumboldt et al. Published by Cambridge University Press. © Cambridge University Press 2012.

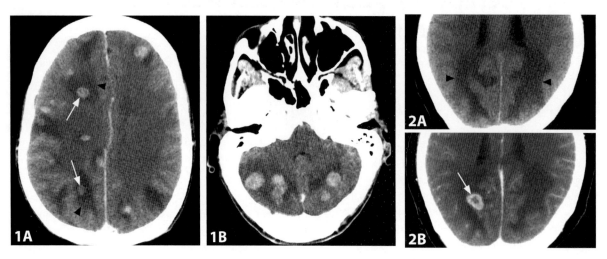

Figure 1. Post-contrast CT image (A) shows multiple enhancing cerebral lesions (arrows) with surrounding hypodense vasogenic edema (arrowheads). There are additional bilateral cerebellar masses (B).

Figure 2. Non-enhanced CT (A) shows bilateral symmetric vasogenic edema (arrowheads) in the posterior cerebral hemispheres. Post-contrast image (B) reveals an oval lesion (arrow) with irregular enhancing rim.

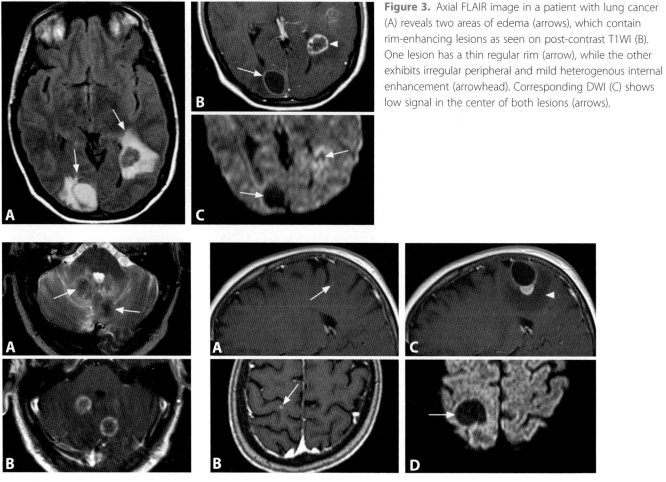

Figure 3. Axial FLAIR image in a patient with lung cancer (A) reveals two areas of edema (arrows), which contain rim-enhancing lesions as seen on post-contrast T1WI (B). One lesion has a thin regular rim (arrow), while the other exhibits irregular peripheral and mild heterogenous internal enhancement (arrowhead). Corresponding DWI (C) shows low signal in the center of both lesions (arrows).

Figure 4. T2WI (A) in a patient with breast cancer shows hypointense masses (arrows) with surrounding edema. Predominantly peripheral lesion enhancement is seen on post-contrast T1WI (B).

Figure 5. Sagittal post-contrast T1WI (A) shows an initially overlooked punctuate enhancement (arrow) in the right post-central gyrus, also seen on axial image (B). Follow-up sagittal post-contrast image (C) reveals substantial increase in lesion size. Partly nodular rim enhancement is surrounded by vasogenic edema (arrowhead). Very low signal is present in the non-enhancing central portion (arrow) on DWI (D).

Non-Hemorrhagic Metastases

MARIA GISELE MATHEUS

Specific Imaging Finding

Metastatic neoplasms to the brain can occur anywhere; however, most are found at the supratentorial peripheral gray–white matter junction, followed by the cerebellum and basal ganglia. They are discrete, multiple or solitary masses, with variable degree of vasogenic edema in the surrounding white matter. The edema and mass effect are often very prominent and out of proportion to the lesion size except with cortical and very small metastases, where edema may be minimal. A majority are hypodense on CT and of low T1 signal. Tumors with high nuclear/cytoplasm ratios or mucinous contents, such as adenocarcinomas, are CT hyperdense. Necrotic and cystic tumors are T2 hyperintense. Highly cellular tumors show iso- to hypointense signal, while mucinous contents and calcifications lead to very low T2 signal, typically seen with adenocarcinomas. Non-hemorrhagic metastases always enhance with contrast, either in a nodular or ring-like pattern, typically with irregular but sharp margins. Volumetric T1WI improves detection of punctate deposits without edema. Metastatic tumors show variable MRI diffusivity characteristics. However, the center of ring-enhancing lesions is characteristically dark on DWI and bright on ADC maps, consistent with high diffusivity, with very rare exceptions. Perfusion studies reveal increased rCBV of the enhancing tumor, with delayed signal recovery on the signal intensity–time curve, in contrast to normal brain and gliomas. MRS shows nonspecific increased choline and decreased NAA levels. Both the MRS spectra and rCBV are essentially normal in the adjacent non-enhancing edema.

Pertinent Clinical Information

Symptoms are nonspecific and progressive, including headaches, focal neurological deficits, seizures, nausea, vomiting, and alteration of consciousness. Treatment consists of symptomatic management and whole-brain radiation (WBRT), along with surgery (for one to a few lesions) or radiosurgery (for smaller lesions). Systemic tumor control, number and location of brain lesions, along with patient's age and performance status, are important prognostic factors.

Differential Diagnosis

High-Grade Glioma (153)

- poorly demarcated contrast enhancement, non-enhancing solid portions may be present
- infiltrative edema around the enhancement extends into the gray matter
- non-enhancing edema shows increased rCBV on perfusion studies
- non-enhancing edema shows high choline and low NAA on MRS
- typically deep white matter lesion

Abscess (156)

- central bright "light bulb" appearance on DWI
- contrast enhancement of the rim is thin and regular
- lesion rim is T2 dark and T1 hyperintense
- rCBV is not increased on perfusion studies

Tumefactive Demyelination (159)

- absent to mild vasogenic edema and minimal mass effect
- chracteristic incomplete ring enhancement of large lesions
- rCBV is not increased on perfusion studies
- non-enhancing lesions are very common

Primary CNS Lymphoma (158)

- usually deep and not peripheral lesions
- homogenous low signal on ADC maps
- typical dense homogenous enhancement

Background

Approximately 10% of patients with cancer develop brain metastases and in some cases they cause the initial symptoms. The incidence of brain metastases is apparently rising, threatening to limit the gains that have been made by new systemic treatments. The brain is considered a "sanctuary site" as the blood–tumor barrier limits the ability of drugs to enter and kill malignant cells. Severe WBRT side-effects coupled with recent improvements in local control and survival have led to a reconsideration of the WBRT role, which may not be beneficial for all patients.

REFERENCES

1. Fertikh D, Krejza J, Cunqueiro A, et al. Discrimination of capsular stage brain abscesses from necrotic or cystic neoplasms using diffusion-weighted magnetic resonance imaging. J Neurosurg 2007;**106**:76–81.
2. Toh CH, Wei KC, Ng SH, et al. Differentiation of brain abscesses from necrotic glioblastoma and cystic metastatic brain tumors with diffusion tensor imaging. AJNR 2011;**32**:1646–51.
3. Server A, Orheim TE, Graff BA, et al. Diagnostic examination performance by using microvascular leakage, cerebral blood volume, and blood flow derived from 3-T dynamic susceptibility-weighted contrast-enhanced perfusion MR imaging in the differentiation of glioblastoma multiforme and brain metastasis. Neuroradiology 2011;**53**:319–30.
4. Gaspar LE, Mehta MP, Patchell RA, et al. The role of whole-brain radiation therapy in the management of newly diagnosed brain metastases: a systematic review and evidence-based clinical practice guideline. J Neurooncol 2010;**96**:17–32.
5. Steeg PS, Camphausen KA, Smith QR. Brain metastases as preventive and therapeutic targets. Nat Rev Cancer 2011;**11**:352–63.

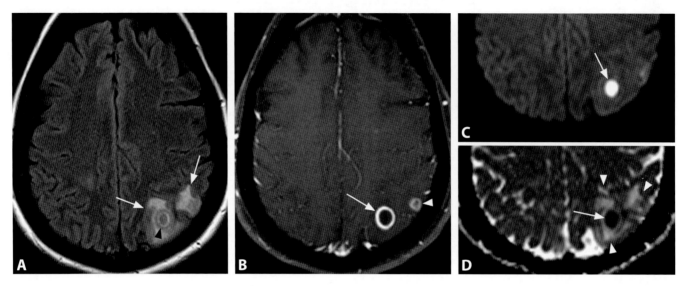

Figure 1. Axial FLAIR (A) shows a patchy area of hyperintense signal (arrows) in the left parietal subcortical area with an internal oval lesion demarcated by a sharp hypointense rim (arrowhead). Matching post-contrast T1WI (B) shows marked ring-like enhancement of the lesion rim (arrow) and another enhancing lesion (arrowhead). DWI (C) shows very bright (arrow) and ADC map (D) very dark (arrow) internal contents consistent with reduced diffusivity. Associated vasogenic edema is of increased diffusivity (arrowheads).

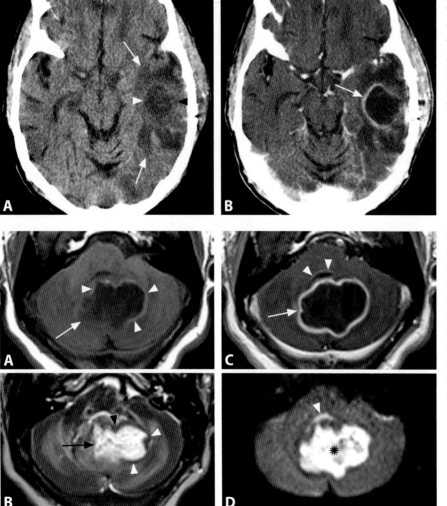

Figure 2. Axial non-enhanced CT image in a patient with headaches, seizures, and fever following recent left-sided temporal craniotomy shows low attenuation (arrows) vasogenic edema in the underlying brain, with a central rounded hypodensity (arrowheads). Post-contrast CT image (B) shows thin and smooth peripheral enhancement (arrow) of the rounded lesion.

Figure 3. Axial T1WI (A) shows a hypointense cerebellar lesion (arrow) with peripheral linear hyperintensity (arrowheads). The rim of the hyperintense mass (arrow) is dark (arrowheads) on T2WI (B). Post-contrast T1WI (C) shows enhancement of the lesion rim (arrow) and along the fourth ventricle (arrowhead), indicating intraventricular extension. The lesion (*) is extremely bright on DWI (D), with similar high signal within the ventricle (arrowhead).

Cerebral Abscess

MARIA GISELE MATHEUS

Specific Imaging Findings

Cerebral abscess can occur in any part of the brain, but has a predilection for the supratentorial gray–white matter junction of the frontal and parietal lobes. On CT it typically presents as a subcortical area of prominent hypodense vasogenic edema with mass effect and a central rounded lesion of even lower attenuation, at times with a thin isodense rim, which shows enhancement on post-contrast images. The central portion of an abscess is of low T1 and high T2 signal (slightly brighter than the CSF). The capsule is characteristically T1 hyperintense and T2 hypointense with marked contrast enhancement. The rim enhancement is generally thin and smooth, especially on the outer side. Abscesses tend to expand medially becoming oval in shape, the capsule may accordingly be thinner toward the ventricles and thicker toward the cortex. Diffusion MR imaging is the most accurate imaging technique to differentiate bacterial abscess from other intracranial cystic/necrotic masses. In addition to hyperintensity on FLAIR and T1WI, the abscess center is very bright on DWI and dark on ADC, reflecting reduced diffusivity within the purulent material. Fungal abscesses may be more heterogenous, show higher ADC values, and involve the deep gray matter. MR spectroscopy shows complex spectra within abscesses with multiple abnormal peaks including lactate and lipids, as well as acetate, succinate, and amino acids. Perfusion studies, similar to other inflammatory and infectious processes, typically show decreased to normal cerebral blood volume.

Pertinent Clinical Information

Abscess is a potentially fatal but readily treatable disease. The most common clinical symptom is headache followed by fever, altered mental status, focal neurological deficits, and seizures. Prognosis depends on the size and location of the abscess, virulence of the organism, and immune status of the patient. Complications include rupture into the ventricles with ventriculitis, which has high mortality, and herniation from mass effect. Treatment includes surgical drainage or excision and intravenous antibiotics.

Differential Diagnosis

Necrotic Neoplasm (primary or, more commonly, metastatic) (153, 155)
- the central portion of rim-enhancing lesions is dark on DWI and bright on ADC maps
- rim enhancement is frequently irregular and thick with nodular contours
- T2 hypointensity of the rim is rare

Tumefactive Demyelinating Lesion (159)
- minimal to absent vasogenic edema and mass effect
- characteristic incomplete ring of peripheral enhancement

Subacute Hematoma (177)
- presence of blood products
- thin irregular/lobulated peripheral enhancement

Neurocysticercosis (colloidal and granular phase) (167)
- usually not bright on DWI
- vasogenic edema is usually mild
- calcified lesions may be present

Background

Abscess is caused by pathogens entering the CNS by hematogenous spread in sepsis or from distant infection, contiguous extension of infection, or traumatic (including surgery) implantation. Overall the most common organism is *Streptococcus*; however, multiple other bacteria may be involved, and the causative agent is strongly related to the patient's age and systemic conditions. Abscess evolves from cerebritis to mature abscess usually over 2–3 weeks. Injury to the microvasculature by bacterial seeding leads to local inflammation, petechial hemorrhage, perivascular fibrinous exudates, edema, and parenchymal necrosis. Over time, purulent material coalesces and is confined by inflammatory granulation tissue and collagenous capsule. MR spectroscopy may help differentiate aerobic, anaerobic, fungal, and TB abscesses. While residual contrast enhancement may persist for months following successful therapy, decreasing T2 hypointensity of the capsule and shrinkage of the necrotic center occur earlier and are more reliable signs of healing. Persistent or reappearing DWI hyperintensity and low ADC values are indicative of treatment failure.

REFERENCES

1. Falcone S, Post MJ. Encephalitis, cerebritis and brain abscess: pathophysiology and imaging findings. *Neuroimag Clin N Am* 2000;**10**:333–53.
2. Rumboldt Z, Thurnher M, Gupta RK. Imaging of CNS infections. *Semin Roentgenol* 2007;**42**:62–91.
3. Mueller-Mang C, Castillo M, Mang TG, *et al.* Fungal versus bacterial brain abscesses: is diffusion-weighted MR imaging a useful tool in the differential diagnosis? *Neuroradiology* 2007;**49**:651–7.
4. Chiang IC, Hsieh TJ, Chiu ML, *et al.* Distinction between pyogenic brain abscess and necrotic brain tumour using 3-tesla MR spectroscopy, diffusion and perfusion imaging. *Br J Radiol* 2009;**82**:813–20.
5. Pal D, Bhattacharyya A, Husain M, *et al.* In vivo proton MR spectroscopy evaluation of pyogenic brain abscesses: a report of 194 cases. *AJNR* 2010;**31**:1355–62.

Brain Imaging with MRI and CT, ed. Zoran Rumboldt *et al.* Published by Cambridge University Press. © Cambridge University Press 2012.

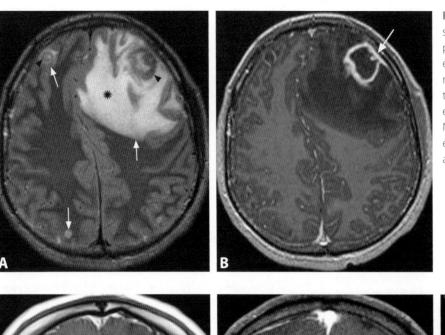

Figure 1. Axial T2WI (A) demonstrates high signal in multiple regions (arrows) with prominent vasogenic edema (*) and mass effect in the left frontal lobe. There is also ring-like hypointensity (arrowheads) within the areas of edema. These lesions show ring enhancement on the post-contrast T1WI (B). Note the small peripheral nodule of enhancement of the left frontal lesion (arrow), an example of the "eccentric target sign".

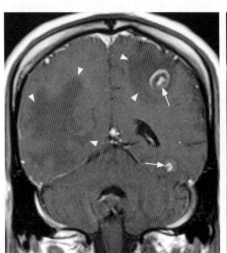

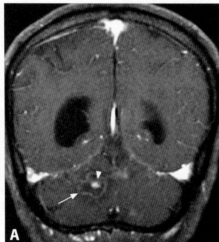

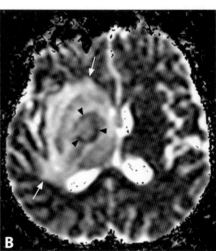

Figure 2. Coronal post-contrast T1WI shows ring-enhancing lesions with eccentric nodules (arrows). There is bilateral vasogenic edema (arrowheads).

Figure 3. Coronal fat-saturated post-contrast T1WI (A) in a patient with AIDS shows a cerebellar peripherally enhancing lesion (arrow) with an eccentric nodule (arrowhead). Axial ADC map (B) shows a large bright area with mass effect centered at the right basal ganglia (arrows), consistent with vasogenic edema. There is an internal dark ring (arrowheads), with centrally increased diffusion.

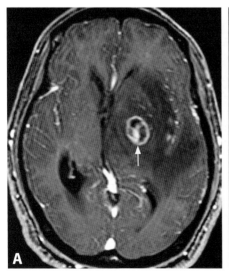

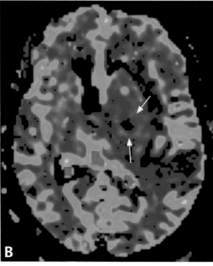

Figure 4. Axial post-contrast T1WI from a volumetric GRE acquisition (A) shows a right basal ganglia mass (arrow) with peripheral and internal nodular enhancement. There is prominent surrounding hypointense vasogenic edema and associated mass effect. Corresponding DSC MR perfusion image (B) reveals relatively low cerebral blood volume of the lesion (arrows).

Cerebral Toxoplasmosis

BENJAMIN HUANG

Specific Imaging Findings

In immunocompromised hosts, lesions due to cerebral toxoplasmosis will appear on unenhanced CT as multiple areas of low attenuation, most commonly in the deep gray matter and at the corticomedullary junction. Lesions exhibit nodular or ring enhancement on post-contrast CT and T1-weighted images. Ring-enhancing lesions in about one-third of cases show an internal eccentric nodule, referred to as the "eccentric target sign", which is considered highly specific for toxoplasmosis. The enhancing portions of the lesions will typically show iso- to hypointense T2 signal with surrounding hyperintense vasogenic edema. Hemorrhage is occasionally present. Butterfly lesions crossing the corpus callosum have also been described. The lesions of toxoplasmosis demonstrate central high signal intensity on ADC maps, consistent with increased diffusivity, and decreased rCBV on perfusion imaging. MR spectroscopy tends to show moderately reduced choline peaks.

Pertinent Clinical Information

Cerebral toxoplasmosis is the most common opportunistic CNS infection in AIDS patients, who are most susceptible to develop an active disease when their CD4 count falls below 100 cells/μl. The most common presenting symptom is headache, frequently accompanied by fever and altered mental status. Seizures, visual field defects, cranial neuropathies, and other focal neurologic deficits may also be present. Diagnosis usually relies on direct detection of the organism (usually through PCR amplification) in CSF, blood, or urine. Thallium-201 SPECT and FDG-PET may reliably differentiate CNS lymphoma from toxoplasmosis in lesions over 2 cm in size, as toxoplasmosis is not radiotracer-avid. Current treatment regimens do not completely eradicate the organism; therefore, AIDS patients with toxoplasmosis require lifelong maintenance therapy to prevent relapses of active infection.

Differential Diagnosis

Primary CNS Lymphoma (158)
- dark on ADC maps
- elevated rCBV on perfusion imaging
- elevated choline on MRS
- hot on thallium-201 SPECT and FDG-PET

Metastatic Neoplasms (155)
- high rCBV on perfusion imaging
- elevated choline on MR spectroscopy

Pyogenic Abscess (156)
- the core is characteristically very bright on DWI

Background

Toxoplasmosis is a parasitic infection caused by the intracellular protozoan *Toxoplasma gondii*. The organism is transmitted to humans primarily through ingestion of oocysts contained in undercooked meats or contaminated vegetables, or through contact with cat feces. In immunocompetent hosts, infection with *T. gondii* usually causes no symptoms or results in only mild, self-limited flu-like symptoms. The infection then often enters an asymptomatic latent phase characterized by persistence of the organisms in the form of tissue cysts (bradyzoites) in brain and muscle tissue. It is estimated that up to 75% of the population are seropositive for *T. gondii*. Cerebral toxoplasmosis in immunocompromised patients usually results from reactivation of a latent infection; it used to occur in up to a half of patients with AIDS, but the incidence has declined since the advent of HAART regimens. Toxoplasmosis causes necrotizing encephalitis, pathologically characterized by multiple foci of necrosis and microglia nodules, without abscess formation. Numerous intra- and extracellular *Toxoplasma* tachyzoites (the rapidly multiplying form of the organism) and cysts are seen in and adjacent to the necrotic foci and in cerebral tissue uninvolved by the inflammatory change. Identification of tachyzoites is pathognomonic of active infection.

REFERENCES

1. Camacho DL, Smith JK, Castillo M. Differentiation of toxoplasmosis and lymphoma in AIDS patients by using apparent diffusion coefficients. *AJNR* 2003;**24**:633–7.
2. Chaudhari VV, Yim CM, Hathout H, *et al.* Atypical imaging appearance of toxoplasmosis in an HIV patient as a butterfly lesion. *J Magn Reson Imaging* 2009;**30**:873–5.
3. Montoya JG, Liesenfeld O. Toxoplasmosis. *Lancet* 2004;**363**: 1965–76.
4. Smith AB, Smirniotopoulos JG, Rushing EJ. From the archives of the AFIP: central nervous system infections associated with human immunodeficiency virus infection: radiologic–pathologic correlation. *Radiographics* 2008;**28**:2033–58.
5. Rumboldt Z. Brain lesions in AIDS. In: *Neuroradiology* (Third Series) Test and Syllabus. Castillo M, ed. American College of Radiology, Reston, VA, 2006;142–56.

Brain Imaging with MRI and CT, ed. Zoran Rumboldt *et al.* Published by Cambridge University Press. © Cambridge University Press 2012.

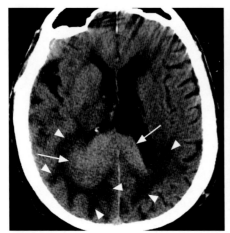

Figure 1. Non-enhanced CT shows a hyperdense splenium mass (arrows) with vasogenic edema (arrowheads).

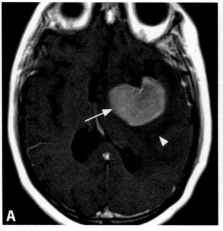

Figure 2. Post-contrast T1WI (A) shows a homogenous enhancing lesion (arrow) deep in the left hemisphere with mass effect and vasogenic edema (arrowhead). Diffusion is low within the mass (arrow) and high in the edema (arrowheads) on ADC map (B).

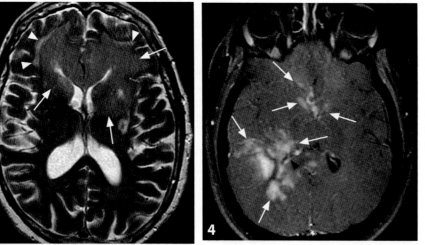

Figure 3. Axial T2WI shows a homogenous infiltrative lesion (arrows) extending from the genu of corpus callosum with a "butterfly" appearance. The mass is slightly hyperintense with minimal edema.

Figure 4. Post-contrast fat-saturated T1WI shows ill-defined patchy areas of enhancement (arrows) and mass effect on the right lateral ventricle (arrowhead).

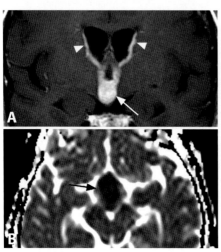

Figure 5. An enhancing third ventricle mass (arrow) tracks along the subependyma of the lateral ventricles (arrowheads) on coronal post-contrast T1WI (A). Axial ADC map (B) reveals its low diffusion (arrow).

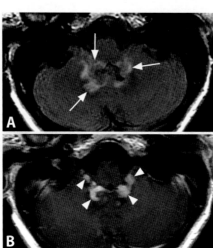

Figure 6. Axial FLAIR image (A) shows hyperintensity (arrows) around the fourth ventricle. Post-contrast T1WI (B) reveals subependymal and leptomeningeal enhancement (arrowheads).

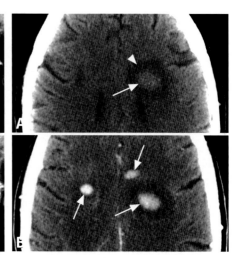

Figure 7. Non-enhanced CT (A) shows a periventricular hyperdense mass (arrow) with edema (arrowhead). Post-contrast image (B) reveals multiple densely enhancing lesions (arrows).

Primary CNS Lymphoma

ALESSANDRO CIANFONI AND ZORAN RUMBOLDT

Specific Imaging Findings

Primary CNS lymphoma (PCNSL) most commonly presents as a homogenous, well-defined intra-axial mass, hyperdense on non-enhanced CT and of low to isointense T2 signal (primarily due to high cellularity). The typical lesions show dense homogenous enhancement and very low diffusion with characteristic dark appearance on ADC maps. PCNSL may also manifest with a predominantly perivascular, ill-defined infiltrative spread pattern. Associated vasogenic edema and mass effect are usually present. PCNSL primarily involves the deep brain structures, periventricular regions, corpus callosum and septum pellucidum with tendency to spread along the subependymal white matter. Lesions may be multiple and leptomeningeal spread can be observed. However, PCNSL may also present with necrotic and even hemorrhagic lesions, primarily in immunocompromised, usually HIV-positive patients. Contrast enhancement can also vary and, in very rare cases, it may even be completely absent, more frequently after steroid treatment. Vasogenic edema and mass effect can sometimes also be minimal. Perfusion imaging shows increased rCBV; however, lower than with high-grade gliomas or metastases. FDG PET and SPECT reveal high metabolic activity of PCNSL. Rare spontaneously fluctuating lesions with changes of shape, size and location have been reported.

Pertinent Clinical Information

Clinical presentation is nonspecific, related to infiltration of brain structures or mass effect, frequently with relatively minor symptoms considering the size of the lesion. Prognosis is generally poor and disease rapidly progressing, especially in HIV-positive patients. Due to its infiltrative characteristics, MRI tends to underestimate the burden of disease. Body FDG PET may disclose a systemic site of malignancy in some patients. Lesions respond dramatically and temporarily to steroid treatment. Stereotactic biopsy is followed by high-dose chemotherapy with methotrexate or other agents capable of penetrating the blood–brain barrier, frequently together with whole-brain radiation therapy. Recurrences are common and long-term survival is the exception.

Differential Diagnosis

Glioblastoma Multiforme (153)
- usually necrotic and heterogeneous with irregular enhancement pattern
- very high rCBV on perfusion studies
- ADC values of the solid enhancing tumor are not as low as with PCNSL

Tumefactive Demyelination (159)
- incomplete ring contrast enhancement pattern
- usually absent to minimal edema
- low rCBV on perfusion studies

Toxoplasmosis (157)
- no subependymal spread
- low rCBV on perfusion studies
- high ADC values
- hypometabolism on PET and SPECT

Metastatic Neoplasm (155)
- very high rCBV on perfusion studies

Abscess (156)
- low ADC of pus in the necrotic non-enhancing core
- low rCBV on perfusion studies
- smooth ring-enhancing capsule
- MR spectroscopy shows amino acid peaks

Background
Initially thought to be characteristically associated with immuno-suppression and with a high prevalence in HIV-positive individuals, PCNSL is now also recognized with increasing frequency in immunocompetent individuals, usually in the sixth and seventh decades of life. It comprises 4–5% of all primary brain tumors, the vast majority of which are diffuse large B-cell non-Hodgkin lymphoma. Single or multiple periventricular or superficial enhancing lesions are characteristic of parenchymal CNS lymphoma, representing one-third of secondary CNS lymphomas and almost 100% of PCNSLs. In very rare cases the lesions may not be detectable on imaging studies. Low ADC values and high FDG uptake suggest shorter progression-free and overall survival, while patients with improved clinical outcome may exhibit a decrease in ADC measurements following methotrexate. High response rates and improved survival with chemotherapy has led to treatment strategies that defer or eliminate radiation, reducing the risk of neurotoxicity; however, with a higher rate of relapse.

REFERENCES

1. Haldorsen IS, Espeland A, Larsson E. Central nervous system lymphoma: characteristic findings on traditional and advanced imaging. AJNR 2011;32:984–92.
2. Thurnher MM, Rieger A, Kleibl-Popov C, et al. Primary central nervous system lymphoma in AIDS: a wider spectrum of CT and MRI findings. Neuroradiology 2001;43:29–35.
3. Barajas RF Jr, Rubenstein JL, Chang JS, et al. Diffusion-weighted MR imaging derived apparent diffusion coefficient is predictive of clinical outcome in primary central nervous system lymphoma. AJNR 2010;31:60–6.
4. Kawai N, Zhen HN, Miyake K, et al. Prognostic value of pretreatment 18F-FDG PET in patients with primary central nervous system lymphoma: SUV-based assessment. J Neurooncol 2010;100:225–32.
5. Schultz CJ, Bovi J. Current management of primary central nervous system lymphoma. Int J Radiat Oncol Biol Phys 2010;76:666–78.

Brain Imaging with MRI and CT, ed. Zoran Rumboldt et al. Published by Cambridge University Press. © Cambridge University Press 2012.

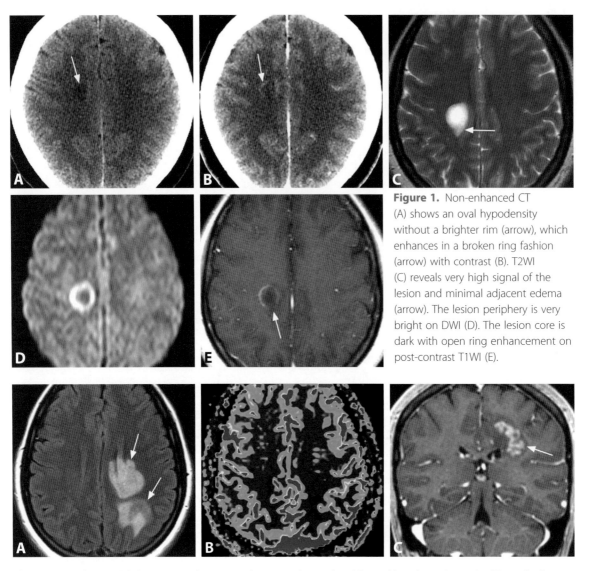

Figure 1. Non-enhanced CT (A) shows an oval hypodensity without a brighter rim (arrow), which enhances in a broken ring fashion (arrow) with contrast (B). T2WI (C) reveals very high signal of the lesion and minimal adjacent edema (arrow). The lesion periphery is very bright on DWI (D). The lesion core is dark with open ring enhancement on post-contrast T1WI (E).

Figure 2. Axial FLAIR (A) shows two white matter lesions with peripheral finger-like edema (arrows). rCBV in the lesions is similar to the contralateral white matter on corresponding perfusion MRI (B). There is patchy and nodular arc-like lesion enhancement (arrow) around the ventricle on post-contrast coronal T1WI (C).

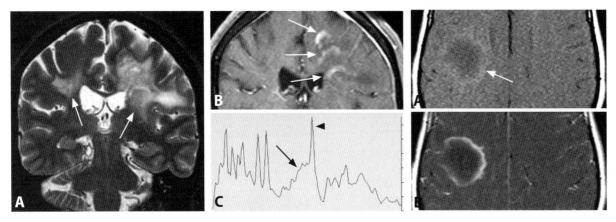

Figure 3. Coronal T2WI (A) shows bilateral white matter abnormalities (arrows) with heterogenous internal structure and mild mass effect. Post-contrast T1WI (B) reveals layers of patchy arc-like enhancement (arrows). MRS with TE 30 ms shows a prominent Glx peak (arrow), to the left of NAA (arrowhead).

Figure 4. Magnetization transfer T1WI (A) shows a round dark lesion with brighter rim (arrow), which demonstrates open ring enhancement post-contrast (B).

Tumefactive Demyelinating Lesion

ZORAN RUMBOLDT

Specific Imaging Findings

Mass-like features of multiple sclerosis and other demyelinating processes are referred to as tumefactive demyelinating lesions (TDLs). TDLs are typically located in the cerebral white matter ranging from 1 to over 10 cm in size. They may be unifocal; however, additional lesions are usually either present or occur over time. Edema surrounds most TDLs, but is usually very mild, and mass effect is typically even less prominent. The lesions are T1 hypointense in the center and their periphery may be brighter on magnetization transfer imaging. Almost all TDLs enhance with contrast, which may co-localize with a T2 hypointense rim. Incomplete rim enhancement ("open ring"), along with mixed T2 iso- and hyperintensity of the enhancing components, absence of cortical involvement, and absence of mass effect are highly specific for TDL, but not always present. Vessel-like structures, presumably veins, running through the lesion are typical but only occasionally seen. Other characteristic features are bright peripheral rim on DWI (dark on ADC maps) and relatively low rCBV on perfusion studies. CT hypodensity of the enhanced regions on MRI (the MRI enhancing rim is not discernible on non-enhanced CT) is also very specific. Marked elevation of glutamate and glutamine (Glx, at 2.1–2.5 ppm) are characteristically present on short echo time (TE around 30 ms) MR spectroscopy. Nonspecific findings are commonly observed with intermediate echo times.

Pertinent Clinical Information

TDL may affect all age groups, most commonly young adults, usually as the initial presentation of multiple sclerosis. Presentation is typically polysymptomatic, including aphasia, agnosia, seizures, and visual disturbances. TDL may show delayed or absent response to steroids and progressive lesion growth over several weeks. Using the imaging characteristics of the lesions, the diagnosis should be made in the vast majority of cases, obviating the need for brain biopsy, which, apart from morbidity, is frequently nondiagnostic.

Differential Diagnosis

Primary Brain Neoplasms (High-Grade Gliomas) (153)
- enhancing portions are not CT hypodense
- infiltrative edema with cortical and/or deep gray matter involvement
- very high rCBV on perfusion studies
- do not show incomplete ring enhancement pattern
- Glx peak (glutamine and glutamate, "shoulder" of the NAA peak) not increased on MRS

Lymphoma (PCNSL) (158)
- hyperdense on non-enhanced CT
- typically dense homogenous enhancement, not incomplete ring enhancement pattern

- characteristic diffusely very low ADC values
- typically increased rCBV on perfusion studies
- Glx peak not increased on MRS

Metastatic Neoplasms (155)
- complete ring or nodular enhancement
- characteristic cortico-subcortical location
- increased rCBV on perfusion studies
- Glx peak not increased on MRS

Abscess (156)
- central core is DWI bright/ADC dark
- complete and smooth ring enhancement
- typically prominent edema

Background

Common pathological findings in TDL include hypercellular lesions with confluent demyelination, abundant foamy macrophages containing myelin debris, reactive astrogliosis, relative axonal preservation and variable perivascular and parenchymal lymphocytic inflammation. Infiltrating macrophages and reactive astrocytes are commonly closely intermingled. Histologic features may mimic tumour including hypercellularity, astrocytic pleomorphism, variable nuclear atypia, a rare mitotic figure and occasional necrosis or cystic changes. The pathologic diagnosis may be challenging, especially on the initial frozen-section specimen when the primary suspicion is malignancy. Additional histologic features that point toward a demyelinating process are absence of coagulative necrosis, rather evenly distributed plump, reactive astrocytes, some with multiple micronuclei (Creutzfeldt cells), and absence of microvascular proliferation.

Tumefactive demyelination has also been described with HIV infection and as an uncommon form of tacrolimus neurotoxicity.

REFERENCES

1. Kim DS, Na DG, Kim HK, *et al*. Distinguishing tumefactive demyelination lesions from glioma or central nervous system lymphoma: added value of unenhanced CT compared with conventional contrast-enhanced MR imaging. *Radiology* 2009;**251**:467–75.
2. Lucchinetti CF, Gavrilova RH, Metz I, *et al*. Clinical and radiographic spectrum of pathologically confirmed tumefactive multiple sclerosis. *Brain* 2008;**131**:1759–75.
3. Jain R, Ellika S, Lehman NL, *et al*. Can permeability measurements add to blood volume measurements in differentiating tumefactive demyelinating lesions from high grade gliomas using perfusion CT? *J Neurooncol* 2010;**97**:383–8.
4. Cianfoni A, Niku S, Imbesi SG. Metabolite findings in tumefactive demyelinating lesions utilizing short echo time proton magnetic resonance spectroscopy. *AJNR* 2007;**28**:272–7.
5. Given CA 2nd, Stevens BS, Lee C. The MRI appearance of tumefactive demyelinating lesions. *AJR* 2004;**182**:195–9.

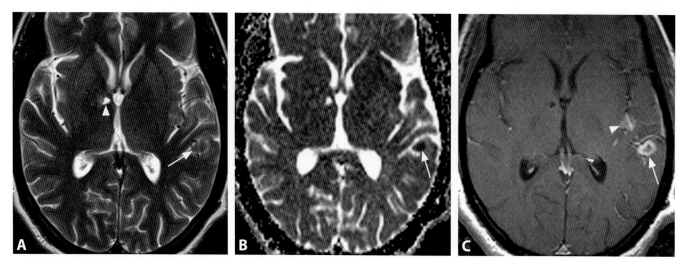

Figure 1. Axial T2WI (A) in a patient with seizures shows a small slightly hypointense oval cortico-subcortical left temporal lesion (arrow) with a small amount of surrounding hyperintensity. There is also a chronic lacunar infarct (arrowhead) in the ventral right thalamus. Corresponding ADC map (B) reveals dark signal of the lesion (arrow) consistent with low diffusivity, while post-contrast T1WI (C) demonstrates rim enhancement (arrow). There is additional enhancement along the sylvian fissure (arrowhead).

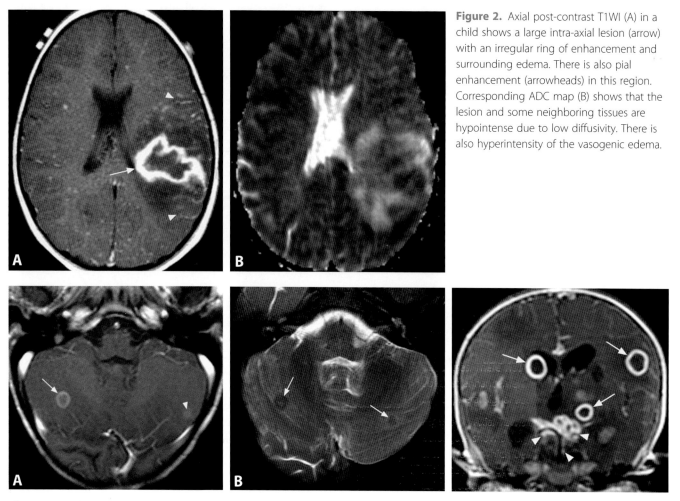

Figure 2. Axial post-contrast T1WI (A) in a child shows a large intra-axial lesion (arrow) with an irregular ring of enhancement and surrounding edema. There is also pial enhancement (arrowheads) in this region. Corresponding ADC map (B) shows that the lesion and some neighboring tissues are hypointense due to low diffusivity. There is also hyperintensity of the vasogenic edema.

Figure 3. Axial post-contrast T1WI (A) shows a ring-enhancing lesion (arrow) in the right cerebellar hemisphere. A faintly enhancing lesion is present in the left hemisphere (arrowhead). T2WI (B) shows bilateral low-intensity masses (arrows) corresponding to the enhancing lesions.

Figure 4. Coronal post-contrast T1WI shows ring-enhancing lesions (arrows) and diffuse leptomeningeal enhancement most prominent at the basal cisterns (arrowheads).

Tuberculoma

MAURICIO CASTILLO

Specific Imaging Findings

Tuberculomas are ring-enhancing lesions that vary in size significantly from less than a centimeter to several centimeters in size. Although they are commonly found in the cerebral hemispheres, they may occur anywhere in the brain including the cerebellum and brainstem. On CT the lesion density varies and is surrounded by variable degrees of vasogenic edema. There is contrast enhancement of the capsule, while calcifications are seen in about 20% of tuberculomas. Occasionally the central aspect of the lesion contains an enhancing nodule or calcification giving rise to the so-called "target" sign, which is highly suggestive of tuberculoma. On MRI, tuberculomas with a necrotic center show low T1 and high T2 signal intensities, while those with a solid center show intermediate T1 and low T2 signal, along with low ADC values. Thick adjacent meningeal enhancement suggests the diagnosis. Thus an abscess-like lesion with low T2 centrally suggests tuberculosis or fungus. On magnetization transfer T1-weighted images the capsule is characteristically hyperintense. MRS findings show increased levels of lipids and lactate, low NAA and creatine with variable levels of choline, but no amino acids that are present in pyogenic abscess. Perfusion studies show low rCBV. Infarcts are common, especially in the "tubercular zone" – caudate nucleus, anterior thalamus, and anterior internal capsule.

Pertinent Clinical Information

Most patients with tuberculomas will have underlying tuberculous meningitis. Clinical findings are insidious and non-specific with seizures being relatively common. CSF shows high proteins, pleocytosis, low glucose and the microorganisms may be difficult to find. CSF cultures are positive in less than 50% of patients and take long (4–8 weeks) to grow the microorganism. PPD skin test is often negatives; complicating the initial diagnosis. PCR for tuberculosis is positive and very helpful in establishing the correct diagnosis. Most patients are young and there is no gender predilection. Morbidity is significant and includes chronic seizures, paralysis, mental retardation, hydrocephalus, and stroke. Even with appropriate treatment, tuberculomas take years to resolve and may need surgical resection. Untreated CNS tuberculosis is fatal and patients may die as a result of the primary infection or as a result of hydrocephalus.

Differential Diagnosis

Pyogenic Abscess (156)
- central high T2 signal intensity
- MRS shows multiple amino acids (such as succinate and acetate)

Neoplasm (Primary or Secondary) (153, 155)
- central necrotic regions show high and not low diffusion
- MRS shows high choline

Fungal Infection; Sarcoidosis Granuloma
- may be indistinguishable

Primary CNS Lymphoma (158)
- typically homogenous contrast enhancement
- elevated rCBV on perfusion studies

Background

Worldwide, there are over 10 million documented cases of tuberculosis annually and its prevalence is increasing due to migration trends. Tuberculosis is also more common in immunosuppressed patients such as those with AIDS. About 10% of tuberculosis patients have CNS involvement. Tuberculoma is the local manifestation of tuberculous infection and may occur intra- or extra-axially. They are typically intra-axial and arise from hematogeneous dissemination, generally from a lung primary infection. Tuberculomas are second to meningitis as the most common manifestation of CNS tuberculosis. The microorganism penetrates the walls of veins and arteries lodging itself in the brain generally at the gray–white matter junction. The result is a caseating or non-caseating granuloma with a necrotic center. Initially there is diffuse inflammation, but eventually a thick collagen capsule develops.

REFERENCES

1. Kim TK, Chang KH, Kim CJ, Goo JM, et al. Intracranial tuberculoma: comparison of MR with pathologic findings. AJNR 1995;**16**:1903–8.
2. Gupta RK, Vatsal DK, Husain N, Chawla S, et al. Differentiation of tuberculous from pyogenic brain abscesses with in vivo proton MR spectroscopy and magnetization transfer MR imaging. AJNR 2001;**22**:1503–9.
3. Saxena S, Prakash M, Kumar S, Gupta RK. Comparative evaluation of magnetization transfer contrast and fluid attenuated inversion recovery sequences in brain tuberculoma. Clin Radiol 2005;**60**:787–93.
4. Gupta RK, Husain M, Vatsal DK, et al. Comparative evaluation of magnetization transfer MR imaging and in-vivo proton MR spectroscopy in brain tuberculomas. Magn Reson Imaging 2002;**20**:375–81.
5. Haris M, Gupta RK, Husain M, et al. Assessment of therapeutic response in brain tuberculomas using serial dynamic contrast-enhanced MRI. Clin Radiol 2008;**63**:562–74.

Brain Imaging with MRI and CT, ed. Zoran Rumboldt *et al.* Published by Cambridge University Press. © Cambridge University Press 2012.

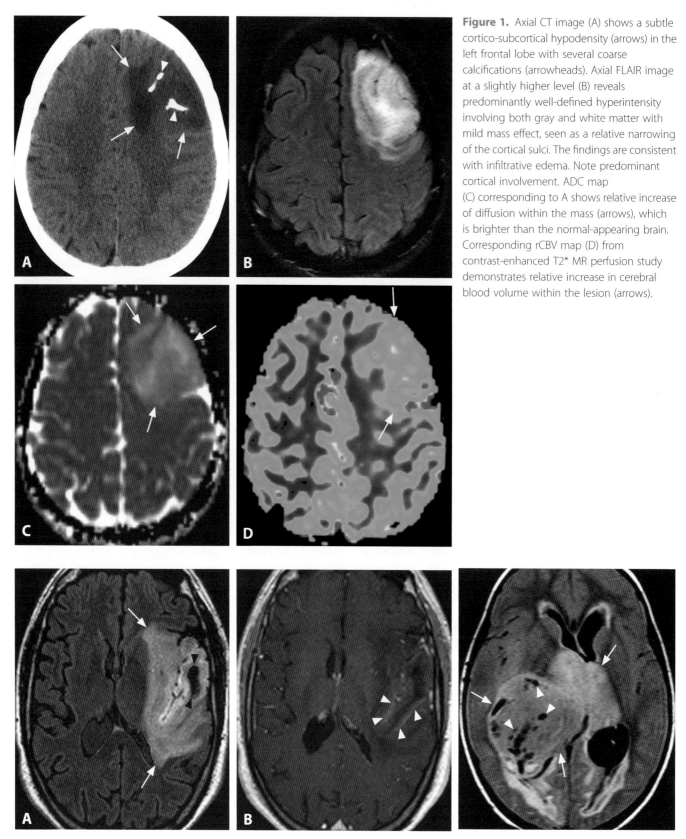

Figure 1. Axial CT image (A) shows a subtle cortico-subcortical hypodensity (arrows) in the left frontal lobe with several coarse calcifications (arrowheads). Axial FLAIR image at a slightly higher level (B) reveals predominantly well-defined hyperintensity involving both gray and white matter with mild mass effect, seen as a relative narrowing of the cortical sulci. The findings are consistent with infiltrative edema. Note predominant cortical involvement. ADC map (C) corresponding to A shows relative increase of diffusion within the mass (arrows), which is brighter than the normal-appearing brain. Corresponding rCBV map (D) from contrast-enhanced T2* MR perfusion study demonstrates relative increase in cerebral blood volume within the lesion (arrows).

Figure 2. Axial FLAIR image (A) shows a cortico-subcortical hyperintense lesion (arrows) primarily involving the left insula and temporal lobe with mild mass effect and an internal cystic area (arrowheads). Corresponding post-contrast T1WI (B) reveals subtle linear areas of cortical enhancement (arrowheads) within the lesion.

Figure 3. FLAIR image shows an intraventricular mass involving the thalami (arrows). Multiple areas of very low signal (arrowheads) represent vessels and calcifications.

Oligodendroglioma

MARIA VITTORIA SPAMPINATO

Specific Imaging Findings

Oligodendrogliomas are usually well-demarcated supratentorial lesions that arise from the gray matter, most commonly in the frontal lobes. The typical CT findings include the presence of clumped and nodular calcification within a hypodense to isodense mass involving the cortex. Cystic changes commonly occur, while intratumoral hemorrhages are rare. Oligodendrogliomas are usually T1 hypointense and T2 hyperintense cortical-based lesions with mild mass effect, and areas of signal loss/susceptibility artifact on T2* sequences, caused by calcifications, may be found. Development of new areas of contrast enhancement and edema have been traditionally considered signs of anaplastic transformation in gliomas; however, contrast enhancement has shown very poor accuracy in differentiating anaplastic from low-grade oligodendroglial tumors. Also, increased relative cerebral blood volume (rCBV) on contrast-enhanced T2* MR perfusion studies, a marker for rapid progression and poor outcome in patients with gliomas, may be found in some low-grade oligodendrogliomas. Increase in tumor size within 6 months appears to be the best prognosticator of rapid tumor progression and poor outcome, better than the high initial tumor volume or high rCBV. Signal heterogeneity, irregular borders, and high rCBV of the tumors are suggestive of the 1p/19q deletion, which is associated with a better treatment response.

Pertinent Clinical Information

The most common clinical presentation of oligodendroglial tumors is seizures, often of several years' duration. Peak incidences are around the fifth decade and they are slightly more common in males. Serial longitudinal multimodality MR imaging, including conventional MRI, MR spectroscopy, MR perfusion and diffusion imaging, has been used to detect the conversion from low- to high-grade neoplasms.

Differential Diagnosis

Astrocytoma (162)
- calcifications uncommon
- primarily involving the white matter

Ganglioglioma (166, 196)
- most commonly temporal lobe location
- cystic component is very common

Dysembryoplastic Neuroepithelial Tumor (DNET) (108)
- cortical-based lesion with "bubbly" appearance, may be wedge-shaped
- absence of mass effect and enhancement

Pleomorphic Xanthoastrocytoma (165)
- typically large cystic component with the solid portion abutting the pial surface
- "dural tail" is frequently present
- possible scalloping of the adjacent inner table of the skull

Cerebritis
- cortical/subcortical T2 hyperintensity and gyriform enhancement
- reduced diffusion on ADC maps

Acute to Subacute Infarct (152, 124)
- commonly wedge-shaped cortical/subcortical signal abnormality
- respects vascular territories
- reduced diffusion in the acute phase
- enhancement, when present, is usually gyriform

Background

Oligodendroglial tumors, encompassing pure oligodendroglioma and mixed oligoastrocytoma, represent the second most common glioma in adults after glioblastoma. Pure oligodendrogliomas have a better treatment outcome and longer survival than astrocytomas and oligoastrocytomas. The expected median survival is estimated at about 10 years for low-grade and 4 years for anaplastic oligodendrogliomas. Loss of heterozygosity/deletions at chromosomes 1p and 19q found in some tumors is associated with both an improved treatment response and longer survival. Oligodendrogliomas arise from neoplastic transformation of oligodendrocytes or immature glial precursors. The natural history of low-grade oligodendroglioma is to evolve to high-grade gliomas with a variable interval between the diagnosis and anaplastic conversion. Anaplastic oligodendrogliomas are also often diagnosed de novo. Low-grade oligodendrogliomas are characterized histologically by presence of a network of branching capillaries within their stroma described as having the appearance of "chicken wire", explaining the typical finding of increased rCBV in these neoplasms. Anaplastic transformation is characterized by increased cellularity, marked atypia and high mitotic activity, endothelial hyperplasia, and tumoral microvascular proliferation. These tumors may rarely metastasize outside the CNS.

REFERENCES

1. Koeller KK, Rushing EJ. From the archives of the AFIP: Oligodendroglioma and its variants: radiologic–pathologic correlation. *Radiographics* 2005;**25**:1669–88.
2. Cha S, Tihan T, Crawford F, *et al.* Differentiation of low-grade oligodendrogliomas from low-grade astrocytomas by using quantitative blood-volume measurements derived from dynamic susceptibility contrast-enhanced MR imaging. *AJNR* 2005;**26**:266–73.
3. Lev MH, Ozsunar Y, Henson JW, *et al.* Glial tumor grading and outcome prediction using dynamic spin-echo MR susceptibility mapping compared with conventional contrast-enhanced MR: confounding effect of elevated rCBV of oligodendrogliomas [corrected]. *AJNR* 2004; **25**:214–21.
4. Jenkinson MD, Smith TS, Joyce KA, *et al.* Cerebral blood volume, genotype and chemosensitivity in oligodendroglial tumours. *Neuroradiology* 2006;**48**:703–13.
5. Brasil Caseiras G, Ciccarelli O, Altmann DR, *et al.* Low-grade gliomas: six-month tumor growth predicts patient outcome better than admission tumor volume, relative cerebral blood volume, and apparent diffusion coefficient. *Radiology* 2009;**253**:505–12.

Brain Imaging with MRI and CT, ed. Zoran Rumboldt *et al.* Published by Cambridge University Press. © Cambridge University Press 2012.

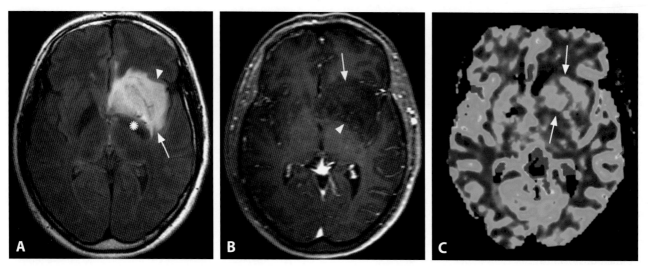

Figure 1. Axial FLAIR image (A) shows a deep hyperintense lesion (arrow) centered at the left insula with mild mass effect, displacing globus pallidus (*), and with mostly preserved overlying cortex (arrowhead). The lesion (arrow) has a relatively sharp margin and is hypointense on corresponding post-contrast T1WI (B) with some minimal questionable enhancement (arrowhead). rCBV MR perfusion map (C) reveals similar values in the lesion (arrows) and normal contralateral brain.

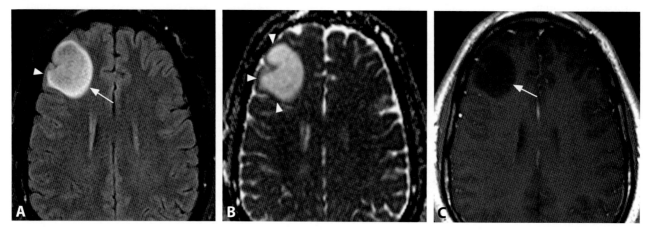

Figure 2. FLAIR image (A) in a 34-year-old patient with seizures shows a well-defined hyperintense lesion (arrow) with mild mass effect arising in the right frontal white matter. The overlying cortex appears preserved (arrowhead). The lesion is homogenously bright on corresponding ADC map (B). Lower signal intensity of the relatively intact cortex (arrowheads). There is no enhancement on post-contrast T1WI (C).

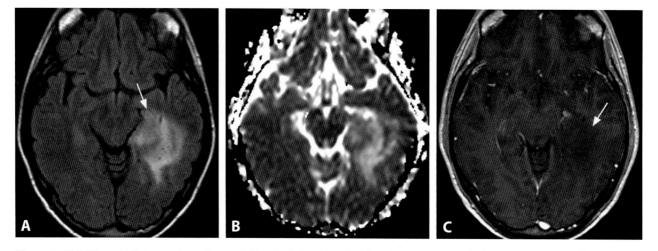

Figure 3. FLAIR image (A) shows a hyperintense infiltrative lesion (arrow) with indistinct margins. The lesion shows high diffusivity on ADC map (B) and hypointensity without enhancement on post-contrast T1WI (C).

Specific Imaging Findings

MRI is the imaging modality of choice for low-grade diffuse astrocytomas and the extent of the lesion is best defined on FLAIR images. They are typically homogenous intra-axial masses with the epicenter within the white matter and minimal to mild associated mass effect. They can be found in all parts of the supratentorial brain, more commonly in the insula. The tumors are usually well-delineated with high T2 signal and iso- to hypointense on T1WI, infiltrating and expanding the underlying brain; the margins are in some cases poorly defined. Diffuse low-grade astrocytomas are typically bright on ADC maps, consistent with increased diffusivity, and usually do not enhance with contrast. On perfusion studies they show relatively low cerebral blood volume, on average only slightly higher compared to the normal brain. MR spectroscopy usually shows decreased NAA levels with slightly elevated choline and without lactate. Low-grade diffuse astrocytomas are typically slightly hypodense to normal brain on CT.

Pertinent Clinical Information

The patients are typically young adults presenting with seizures without other symptoms, or even asymptomatic with the lesion found incidentally on imaging studies. These tumors undergo malignant transformation portended by clinical decline and radiographic progression. There is no consensus on the best management of adults with presumed low-grade glioma; it usually includes surgical resection, which may be followed by chemotherapy. Alternatively, the tumors can be followed with imaging after the initial biopsy, as patients may prefer to defer surgery until there is progression or a change in quality of life.

Differential Diagnosis

Focal Cortical Dysplasia (106)
- presence of gray matter thickening
- associated homogeneous subcortical hyperintensity may taper toward the ventricle
- absence of mass effect
- more frequent frontal lobe location

Oligodendroglioma (161, 197)
- peripherally based with extensive cortical involvement in frontal or temporal lobes
- calcifications are common
- may have increased rCBV on perfusion studies
- may be indistinguishable

Pilocytic Astrocytoma (173)
- almost always located in the posterior fossa or hypothalamic region
- typically avidly enhancing, at least a portion

- may present as a cyst with an enhancing mural nodule
- usually found in children

Glioblastoma Multiforme (153)
- typically a very heterogenous mass
- almost always avid and heterogenous enhancement
- necrotic portions are very common
- prominent mass effect and edema

Background

Diffuse low-grade astrocytomas are slow-growing, infiltrative primary brain tumors that according to the 2007 WHO classification include fibrillary, gemistocytic, and protoplasmic variants. They are considered grade II, in contrast to grade I focal localized gliomas, such as pilocytic astrocytoma and pleomorphic xanthoastrocytoma. Grading of astrocytic tumors is based on cytological atypia which is considered grade II, while tumors with anaplasia and mitotic activity are considered grade III. WHO Grade II tumors also include oligodendrogliomas and oligoastrocytomas. They transform to a higher grade over time with a median survival of 5–10 years. p53 mutations are the first detectable alteration in a majority of astrocytomas that go on to transformation. Relative cerebral blood volume (rCBV) measurements on perfusion MRI correlate well with time to progression or death and high rCBV seems to predict rapid progression in low-grade diffuse astrocytomas. Conventional MR imaging underestimates the extent of disease and an extended "supratotal" resection with a margin beyond MRI-defined abnormality might improve the outcome.

REFERENCES

1. Cha S. Update on brain tumor imaging: from anatomy to physiology. *AJNR* 2006;**27**:475–87.
2. Caseiras GB, Chheang S, Babb J, *et al.* Relative cerebral blood volume measurements of low-grade gliomas predict patient outcome in a multi-institution setting. *Eur J Radiol* 2010;**73**:215–20.
3. Cha S, Tihan T, Crawford F, *et al.* Differentiation of low-grade oligodendrogliomas from low-grade astrocytomas by using quantitative blood-volume measurements derived from dynamic susceptibility contrast-enhanced MR imaging. *AJNR* 2005;**26**:266–73.
4. Sanai N, Chang S, Berger MS, *et al.* Low-grade gliomas in adults. *J Neurosurg* 2011;**115**:948–65.
5. van den Bent MJ, Wefel JS, Schiff D, *et al.* Response assessment in neuro-oncology (a report of the RANO group): assessment of outcome in trials of diffuse low-grade gliomas. *Lancet Oncol* 2011;**12**:583–93.

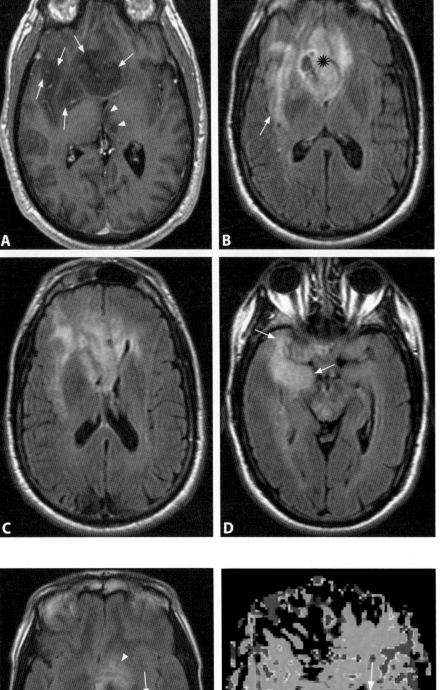

Figure 1. Axial post-contrast T1WI (A) shows a non-enhancing hypointense lesion with mild mass effect infiltrating the right temporal lobe, insula and basal ganglia as well as both frontal lobes (arrows). Also note involvement of the left thalamus (arrowheads). Axial FLAIR image (B) at a similar level shows the lesion to be of high signal intensity and to affect the genu of the corpus callosum (*) crossing the midline. Note involvement of the insular cortex (arrow). FLAIR image at a more cephalad level (C) shows the abnormality in the anterior corpus callosum, both frontal lobes and right insula. FLAIR image at a lower level (D) shows involvement of the right mesial and anterior temporal lobe (arrows). Hyperintense infiltration of the cortical gray matter is clearly visible.

Figure 2. Axial FLAIR image (A) shows hyperintensity with mass effect involving the white and gray matter of the left occipital and posterior temporal lobes (arrows) and also around the anterior commissure on the left (arrowhead). Corresponding cerebral blood volume map (B) from the dynamic post-contrast T2* MR perfusion study shows low rCBV throughout the lesion (arrows).

Gliomatosis Cerebri

MAURICIO CASTILLO

Specific Imaging Findings

The main feature of gliomatosis cerebri (GC) is diffuse infiltration with involvement of three or more contiguous cerebral lobes with preserved architecture. The tumor is of low density by CT and may result in thickening of the white matter particularly the corpus callosum. Enhancement on CT and hemorrhage are rare. CT may occasionally be normal and MR is the imaging method of choice. The tumor is T1 hypointense and bright on T2-weighted sequences. The cortex is characteristically involved and brainstem may be affected. Contrast enhancement is rare and may be patchy in distribution. MR spectroscopic patterns vary with zones showing normal or even low choline, low n-acetyl aspartate (NAA), along with high myo-inositol and, possibly, creatine. Other zones may show increased choline levels. Perfusion studies show either normal or slightly decreased cerebral blood volume. Diffusion within the lesion is usually increased and DTI studies may show preservation of directionality but decreased fractional anisotropy. Subpial extension of GC is very rare.

Pertinent Clinical Information

This is a tumor of adults with most cases found between 40 and 50 years of age, but it may occur at any age. The presentation is nonspecific and includes long tract symptoms, dementia, headaches (generally due to underlying hydrocephalus) and seizures (implying infiltration of the cerebral cortex). Brainstem involvement may result in multiple cranial nerve deficits and corpus callosum infiltration may lead to personality changes. It is a rare process whose exact incidence is not known and the diagnosis is frequently missed initially. The definitive diagnosis used to be made at autopsy, while a biopsy showing astrocytoma and infiltration of three or more cerebral lobes on imaging studies is now diagnostic. GC is a progressive process leading to death in over 50% of patients at one year. Recent chemotherapy and chemo-radiotherapy protocols appear to be effective in patients with GC. Absence of bilateral symmetric infiltration and certain gene mutations (IDH1) are associated with prolonged survival.

Differential Diagnosis

Herpes Encephalitis (20)
- involved areas show reduced diffusion: bright on DWI and dark on ADC maps
- involvement is frequently bilateral but separate, without continuous extension
- enhancement and hemorrhage may be present
- presentation is typically acute to subacute, fever may be present

Limbic Encephalitis (21)
- mass effect minimal or absent
- frequently bilateral but without continuous extension
- enhancement and reduced diffusivity may be present
- systemic malignancy may be known

Low-Grade Diffuse Astrocytoma (162)
- does not extend into three cerebral lobes
- histologically indistinguishable

Lymphoma (PCNSL) (158)
- avid contrast enhancement
- characteristically hyperdense on CT and dark on ADC maps

Rasmussen Encephalitis (79)
- progressive atrophy after possible initial swelling
- characteristically unilateral
- usually in children

Background

GC is a process of glial origin considered as a part of the astrocytoma line of tumors by the WHO. It affects three or more cerebral lobes and imaging criteria are crucial for correct diagnosis as the histology is nonspecific, usually showing infiltrative astrocytoma (WHO grade II). There is extensive tumor infiltration with preservation of the underlying anatomy leading to enlargement of the affected parts of the brain. There is no necrosis or neovascularity at diagnosis in the classical form (type I), which is a WHO grade III tumor, reflected in absence of contrast enhancement and decreased perfusion. Focal enhancement and increased rCBV are observed in the focal mass of type II GC. Leptomeningeal gliomatosis is even less common and presents with diffuse leptomeningeal enhancement of the brain and spinal cord, followed by development of intraparenchymal lesions with widespread diffuse infiltration.

REFERENCES

1. Desclée P, Rommel D, Hernalsteen D, et al. Gliomatosis cerebri, imaging findings of 12 cases. J Neuroradiol 2010;37:148–58.
2. Yang S, Wetzel S, Law M, et al. Dynamic contrast-enhanced T2*-weighted MR imaging of gliomatosis cerebri. AJNR 2002;23:350–5.
3. Guzmán-de-Villoria JA, Sánchez-González J, Muñoz L, et al. 1H MR spectroscopy in the assessment of gliomatosis cerebri. AJR 2007;188:710–4.
4. Knox MK, Ménard C, Mason WP. Leptomeningeal gliomatosis as the initial presentation of gliomatosis cerebri. J Neurooncol 2010;100:145–9.
5. Glas M, Bähr O, Felsberg J, et al. NOA-05 phase 2 trial of procarbazine and lomustine therapy in gliomatosis cerebri. Ann Neurol 2011;70:445–53.

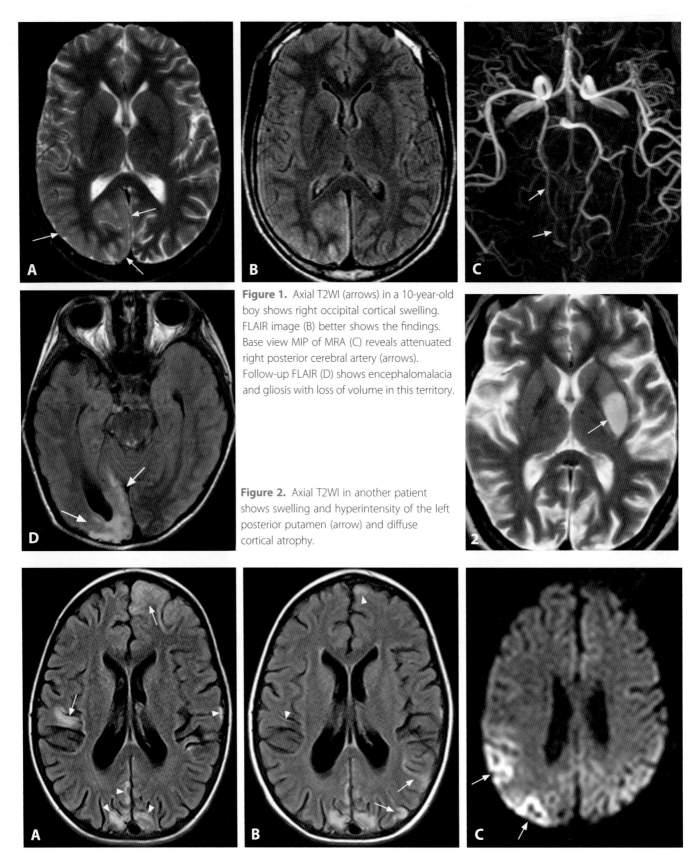

Figure 1. Axial T2WI (arrows) in a 10-year-old boy shows right occipital cortical swelling. FLAIR image (B) better shows the findings. Base view MIP of MRA (C) reveals attenuated right posterior cerebral artery (arrows). Follow-up FLAIR (D) shows encephalomalacia and gliosis with loss of volume in this territory.

Figure 2. Axial T2WI in another patient shows swelling and hyperintensity of the left posterior putamen (arrow) and diffuse cortical atrophy.

Figure 3. Axial FLAIR image (A) shows old cortical lesions (arrowheads) with mild volume loss as well as acute lesions (arrows) with cortical swelling. Corresponding FLAIR image a year later reveals near-complete resolution of the previous acute cortical hyperintensities (arrowheads) with minimal volume loss. There are new cortical abnormalities in the left parietal lobe (arrows). Axial DWI 6 months later (C) shows right parietal areas of cortical hyperintensity (arrows).

Mitochondrial Myopathy, Encephalopathy, Lactic Acidosis, and Stroke-Like Episodes (Melas)

MAURICIO CASTILLO

Specific Imaging Findings

The typical finding is that of cerebral infarct-like lesions, both territorial and crossing territories. The posterior temporal lobes and the parietal and occipital lobes are most frequently involved. Involvement of the cortex and deep gray matter nuclei with a swollen appearance is typical. Diffusion MR imaging may show increased or reduced ADC values. Hemorrhage does not occur and MRA shows the large and medium-size arteries to be normal. MR spectroscopy shows low *n*-acetyl aspartate and lactate in the regions of infarctions and even more typically in those areas of the brain which are normal on MRI. Selective involvement of the cortex with laminar necrosis is frequently present. Some of the cortical lesions may almost completely resolve after the acute phase. Severe cortical atrophy is found in the chronic stage.

Pertinent Clinical Information

Mitochondrial myopathy, encephalopathy, lactic acidosis, and stroke-like episodes (MELAS) is an uncommon disorder but needs to be considered in the differential diagnosis of children with cerebral infarctions, particularly those with more than one. The overall incidence of mitochondriopathies is about 1 in 20 000 persons. Most patients are diagnosed before reaching 15 years of age and MELAS is more common in males. Acute symptoms include stroke-like episodes, headaches, seizures, hearing loss and visual deficits. Chronic symptoms are generalized weakness, cognitive impairment and, lastly, dementia.

Differential Diagnosis

Infarction (80, 124, 152)
- frequently involves the underlying white matter, not limited to gray matter
- lesions do not resolve after the acute phase

Background

MELAS is probably a group of disorders and not just one. It is transmitted through maternal mitochondrial DNA. These genetic aberrations give rise to faulty encoding of at least 13 proteins involved in the respiratory cycle. The genetic defect in mitochondrial protein synthesis that causes impairment of oxidative phosphorylation subsequently leads to insufficient energy production within the cell. The end result is a shift from aerobic to anaerobic metabolism leading to production of pyruvate and lactate and failure of cellular energy. Neurons are more vulnerable to energy depletion than glial cells and vascular elements. This process affects muscle cells and also those in the walls of arteries, particularly endothelial ones. Apart from the muscle weakness and cardiomyopathy, the morbidity of the disease is strongly related to cerebral infarctions and the prognosis is poor. Acute laminar cortical necrosis is seen as swelling of the cortex with cortical hyperintensity on T2-weighted images. The subacute stage is displayed as T1 hyperintensity and T2 hypointensity of the gyral surface, with T2 hyperintensity and swelling of the rest of the cortex and underlying white matter. As with all other means used to diagnose mitochondrial disorders, MR spectroscopy does not depict elevated lactate in all cases. Abnormal CNS concentrations of lactate may be undetected because of differences in the type of mitochondrial disorder, timing, severity, or location of the affected tissues.

REFERENCES

1. Castillo M, Kwock L, Green C. MELAS syndrome: imaging and proton MR spectroscopic findings. *AJNR* 1995;**16**:233–9.
2. Valanne L, Ketonen L, Majander A, *et al.* Neuroradiologic findings in children with mitochondrial disorders. *AJNR* 1998;**19**:369–77.
3. Lin DD, Crawford TO, Barker PB. Proton MR spectroscopy in the diagnostic evaluation of suspected mitochondrial disease. *AJNR* 2003;**24**:33–41.
4. Ito H, Mori K, Kagami S. Neuroimaging of stroke-like episodes in MELAS. *Brain Dev* 2011;**33**:283–8.
5. Ikawa M, Okazawa H, Arakawa K, *et al.* PET imaging of redox and energy states in stroke-like episodes of MELAS. *Mitochondrion* 2009;**9**:144–8.

Brain Imaging with MRI and CT, ed. Zoran Rumboldt *et al.* Published by Cambridge University Press. © Cambridge University Press 2012.

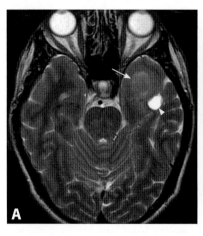 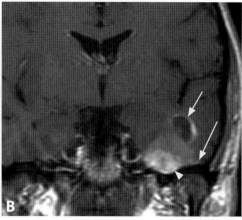

Figure 1. Axial T2WI shows a left temporal mildy hyperintense mass (arrow) with associated very bright area (arrowhead), likely cystic. Coronal post-contrast T1WI (B) reveals enhancement of the solid portion (short arrow) and the wall of the cyst (arrowhead). There is also enhancing "dural tail" (long arrow).

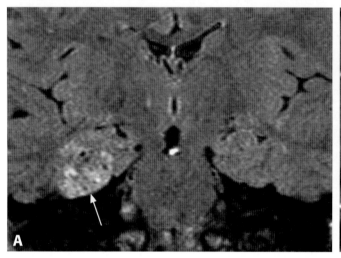 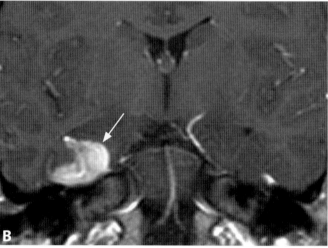

Figure 2. Coronal FLAIR image (A) in a young adult with seizures shows a slightly hyperintense heterogenous mass (arrow), which involves both gray and white matter in the mesial right temporal lobe, and extends to the brain surface. Post-contrast T1WI at a similar level (B) shows avid enhancement of the lesion (arrow), particularly along its peripheral aspects.

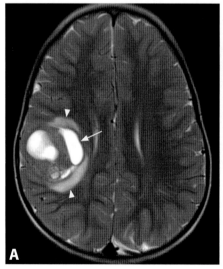 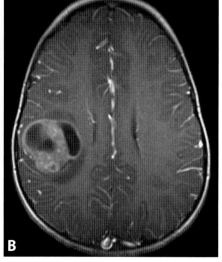

Figure 3. A large right fronto-parietal mass (arrow) with probable cystic portions is demonstrated in this axial T2WI (A) at the level of corona radiata. The lesion is well-delineated with a small amount of surrounding vasogenic edema (arrowheads). Corresponding post-contrast T1WI (B) shows enhancement of the solid portions in this partially cystic mass.

Pleomorphic Xanthoastrocytoma (PXA)

MAURICIO CASTILLO

Specific Imaging Findings

Pleomorphic xanthoastrocytomas (PXAs) generally present as supratentorial hemispheric peripherally located cystic masses (60%) with a solid portion that abuts the meninges. The solid nodule enhances with contrast and may result in enhancement of a "dural tail" (70%) or scalloping of the adjacent inner table of the skull. They are most commonly found in the temporal, frontal, and parietal lobes but may occur anywhere in the cerebral hemispheres and even within the ventricles. Their size and degree of contrast enhancement are variable and calcifications and hemorrhage are rare. On MRI, the signal intensity of the solid tumor is variable but the cyst is nearly always of signal intensity similar to CSF on all sequences. Rarely, brain invasion, metastases, and/or necrosis are seen.

Pertinent Clinical Information

PXAs are tumors of young adults (with about 60% found below 18 years of age) without gender predilection. These are slow growing tumors which most commonly present with chronic seizures, headaches, and dizziness. Survival rates are better than 70% at 10 years after the initial diagnosis, however they may degenerate into higher grades. Surgery is the treatment of choice with gross total resection giving the best results, and re-resection is done for recurrences. Chemotherapy and radiation may be used for unresectable tumors as well as for primary and recurrent anaplastic PXAs, but their role is not clearly established. The only features that correlate with survival are the extent of initial resection and mitotic rate.

Differential Diagnosis

Ganglioglioma (166, 196)
- calcification in 50%
- no dural tail
- enhancement usually less prominent
- may be indistinguishable (tumors with components of both have been described)

DNET (Dysembryoplastic Neuroepithelial Tumor) (108)
- multicystic "bubbly" appearance
- no dominant nodule
- absent to minimal mass effect
- contrast enhancement is very rare

Pilocytic Astrocytoma (173)
- more common in cerebellum or hypothalamic/suprasellar region
- no dural tail
- very bright on ADC maps

Oligodendroglioma (161,197)
- mostly cortical tumor
- calcifications are common

Desmoplastic Infantile Ganglioglioma (139)
- prominent dural involvement, very large, extra-axial
- multiple lesions common
- younger children

Background

PXAs represent less than 1% of all intracranial primary tumors. Histologically they contain many pleomorphic giant cells, spindle cells, and foamy cells that express glial fibrillary acidic protein and are located in a network of reticulin and eosinophilic granular bodies. They are superficial in location with involvement of the meninges and they probably originate from subpial astrocytes. Rarely, they occur in the cerebellum, spinal cord, and retina but most are found in the cerebral hemispheres. There is no specific etiology or genetic aberrations. PXAs are WHO grade II tumors, considered "localized" and thus entirely resectable. Occasionally they invade the brain and may be considered grade III. More importantly, up to 20% of them degenerate into higher grades. High mitotic activity (five or more mitoses per ten high power fields) is the main anaplastic/high-grade feature.

REFERENCES

1. Lipper MH, Eberhard DA, Phillips CD, *et al.* Pleomorphic xanthoastrocytoma, a distinctive astroglial tumor: neuroradiologic and pathologic features. *AJNR* 1993;**14**:1397–404.

2. Yu S, He L, Zhuang X, Luo B. Pleomorphic xanthoastrocytoma: MR imaging findings in 19 patients. *Acta Radiol* 2011;**52**:223–8.

3. Levy RA, Allen R, McKeever P. Pleomorphic xanthoastrocytoma presenting with massive intracranial hemorrhage. *AJNR* 1996;**17**:154–6.

4. Rao AA, Laack NN, Giannini C, Wetmore C. Pleomorphic xanthoastrocytoma in children and adolescents. *Pediatr Blood Cancer* 2010;**55**:290–4.

5. Sugita Y, Irie K, Ohshima K, *et al.* Pleomorphic xanthoastrocytoma as a component of a temporal lobe cystic ganglioglioma: a case report. *Brain Tumor Pathol* 2009;**26**:31–6.

Brain Imaging with MRI and CT, ed. Zoran Rumboldt *et al.* Published by Cambridge University Press. © Cambridge University Press 2012.

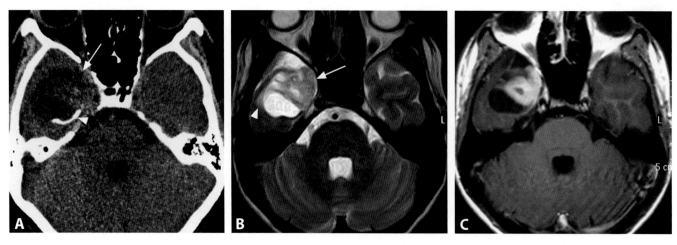

Figure 1. Axial non-enhanced CT (A) in a teenage boy with seizures shows a heterogenous prevailingly hypodense mass (arrow) with peripheral, shell-like calcification (arrowhead) in the right temporal pole. Cortical involvement and different components of the lesion are seen on T2WI (B). The solid component is mildly hyperintense (arrow), while the perifocal edema is minimal (arrowhead). There is marked enhancement of the solid portion on post-contrast T1WI (C).

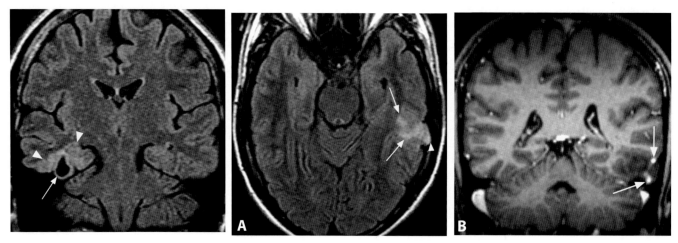

Figure 2. Coronal FLAIR shows a hypointense right temporal cortical mass (arrow) with peripheral hyperintensity (arrowheads). The lesion did not enhance with contrast.

Figure 3. Axial FLAIR image (A) shows a left temporal, cortical area of high signal intensity extending into the underlying white matter (arrows). The lesion expands the cortex and slightly remodels the overlying inner skull (arrowhead). Reformatted coronal post-contrast T1WI (B) shows minimal enhancement in the superficial aspects of the mass (arrows).

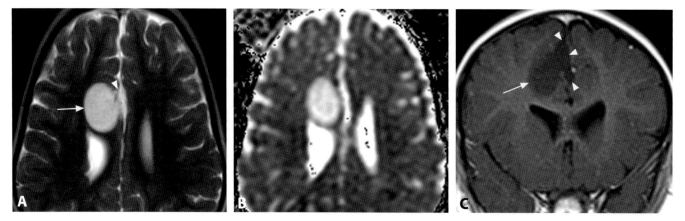

Figure 4. Axial T2WI (A) shows a right frontal well-delineated homogenously hyperintense oval mass (arrow). The lesion involves the cortex (arrowhead). ADC map (B) reveals very high diffusion within the mass. Post-contrast T1WI (C) shows no lesion (arrow) enhancement. Cortical involvement is clearly visible (arrowheads).

Ganglioglioma

GIOVANNI MORANA AND MAURICIO CASTILLO

Specific Imaging Findings

The classic imaging appearance of ganglioglioma (GG) is a cystic mass with a solid tumor nodule which may or may not enhance after contrast administration (about 50% show some enhancement on CT and MRI). This appearance probably occurs in only one-half of the tumors, more commonly in children. Another characteristic feature is the presence of calcifications, which are typically peripheral and shell-like; this is again found in about half of cases. Most GGs occur in the temporal lobes and involve the cortex (and thereby cause seizures). Unfortunately, most GGs have nonspecific imaging features and may be found anywhere in the brain, more likely in the cerebellum, brainstem, spinal cord, optic chiasm, pineal gland, and inside the ventricular system. The lesion size is usually between 3 and 6 cm at the time of discovery. Other imaging appearances include a solid mass (without or with contrast enhancement) and an infiltrating lesion. GGs do show relatively high diffusion, being bright on ADC maps, reflecting their low cellularity. Superficially located tumors tend to expand the overlying cortex and at times MRI may show a discreet cortical dysplasia associated with the tumor. Because they are longstanding, the overlying skull may demonstrate remodeling of its inner table. On nuclear medicine studies with both FDG and thallium, GGs show increased uptake. On MRS they demonstrate nonspecific findings with low *n*-acetyl aspartate, mildly elevated choline, normal creatine and high *myo*-inositol on short echo time studies. Lactate may be present, often related to recent seizure activity.

Pertinent Clinical Information

GGs are a common cause of intractable epilepsy. GGs are the most common tumor to be associated with chronic temporal lobe seizures (90%), mostly of the partial complex type. The tumors grow very slowly which explains the longstanding nature of the symptoms. Following surgical resection, 80% of patients are seizure-free. Patients with Turcot's syndrome have an increased incidence of cerebral GGs.

Differential Diagnosis

Pleomorphic Xanthoastrocytoma (PXA) (165)
- adjacent meninges frequently enhance with contrast
- no associated cortical dysplasia
- tumors may be much larger
- calcifications are rare

DNET (Dysembryoplastic Neuroepithelial Tumor) (108)
- typical bubbly appearance with multiple small cysts
- absence of mass effect and perifocal edema
- enhancement is very rare
- may be indistinguishable

Pilocytic Astrocytoma (173)
- a vast majority arise in the posterior fossa or hypothalamic region
- no associated cortical dysplasia
- seizures are extremely rare

Low-Grade Infiltrative Astrocytoma (Grade II) (162)
- may show a more infiltrative appearance and relatively lower ADC values
- no contrast enhancement
- may be indistinguishable

Oligodendroglioma (161, 197)
- may show a more infiltrative appearance and relatively lower ADC values
- may enhance with contrast and show increased rCBV on perfusion studies
- may be indistinguishable

Background

GGs are rare, well-differentiated, slow-growing tumors composed of neoplastic glial and ganglion cells. Associated cortical dysplasias may be present. They probably represent about 1% of all primary intracerebral tumors in adults and about 5% of those found in children. They can be found at any age, but tend to occur in children and young adults. GGs are generally WHO grades I and II but malignancy or malignant transformation is seen in about 5–10% of cases. The first method of treatment is surgical resection with radiation therapy and chemotherapy reserved for the malignant or recurrent tumors.

REFERENCES

1. Castillo M, Davis PC, Takei Y, Hoffman JC. Intracranial ganglioglioma: MR, CT, and clinical findings in 18 patients. *AJNR* 1990;**11**:109–14.

2. Adachi Y, Yagishita A. Gangliogliomas: characteristic imaging findings and role in the temporal lobe epilepsy. *Neuroradiology* 2008;**50**:829–34.

3. Zhang D, Henning TD, Zou LG, *et al*. Intracranial ganglioglioma: clinicopathological and MRI findings in 16 patients. *Clin Radiol* 2008;**63**:80–91.

4. Kikuchi T, Kumabe T, Higano S, *et al*. Minimum apparent diffusion coefficient for the differential diagnosis of ganglioglioma. *Neurol Res* 2009;**31**:1102–7.

5. Kincaid OK, El-Saden SM, Park SH, Goy BW. Cerebral gangliogliomas: preoperative grading using FDG-PET and 201Tl-SPECT. *AJNR* 1990;**19**:801–6.

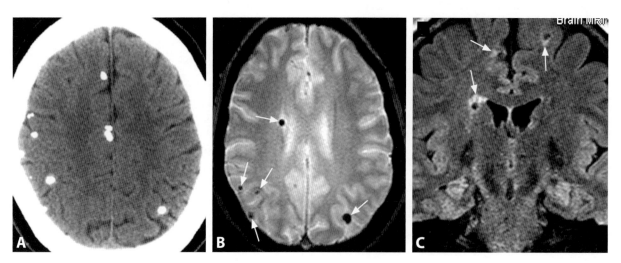

Figure 1. Non-enhanced axial CT image (A) in a young man with headache and seizures shows multifocal cortico-subcortical calcifications. T2*WI at a lower level (B) shows parenchymal foci of signal loss (arrows). Coronal FLAIR image (C) reveals a rim of peripheral high signal intensity around the lesions (arrows).

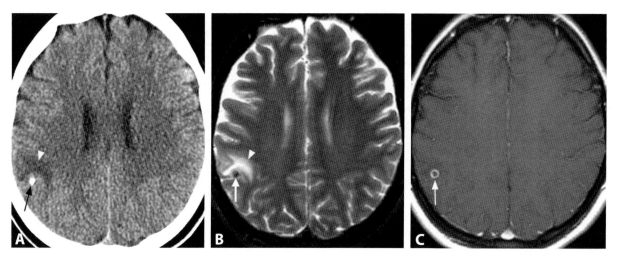

Figure 2. Non-enhanced CT (A) shows a peripheral right hemisphere calcification (arrow) and adjacent hypodensity (arrowhead). There is corresponding cortical hypointensity (arrow) with vasogenic edema (arrowhead) on T2WI (B). Post-contrast T1WI (C) shows ring enhancement of the lesion (arrow).

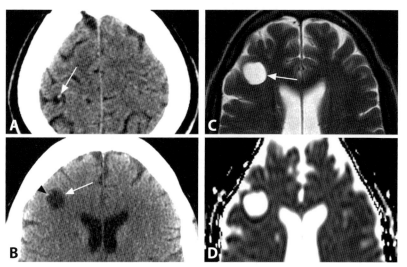

Figure 3. Axial non-enhanced CT image (A) shows a round cortical hypodensity with a punctuate wall calcification (arrow) along the right postcentral sulcus. CT image at the level of the lateral ventricles (B) reveals an additional similar hypodense lesion (arrow) with a peripheral calcification (arrowhead). T2WI (C) reveals CSF-like signal of the cystic lesion (arrow), which also has CSF-like diffusivity and a thin dark rim on ADC map (D).

Neurocysticercosis – Parenchymal

MATTHEW OMOJOLA

Specific Imaging Findings

Brain parenchymal cysticercosis (CC) usually manifests with multiple lesions. The lesions are commonly located at the junction of gray and white matter, reflecting hematogenous disease spread. The early (vesicular) infection stage is seen as CSF density/intensity cysts with a tiny eccentric calcification representing the scolex, usually without surrounding edema and with possible minimal peripheral enhancement. The scolex is best seen as a bright dot on FLAIR images. The colloidal stage is usually a cyst with ring contrast enhancement and surrounding edema. The cyst density/intensity may be slightly different from CSF. The granular stage shows a contracted nodular or ring enhancement without a cystic component. There may be a thin rim of surrounding edema. The final nodular stage is seen as a calcified lesion which may show a rim of high T1 signal, contrast enhancement, and surrounding edema. Most patients harbor parasites in all phases of their evolution, leading to frequent heterogenous imaging appearance. Delayed post-contrast T1WI identifies the highest number of CC lesions.

Pertinent Clinical Information

Neurocysticercosis is a major cause of acquired epilepsy in most low-income countries and it is becoming more common in high-income countries because of increased migration and travel. The most common clinical presentation is seizures (over 70%) and headache. Calcified CC lesions may be incidentally seen in patients investigated for other disease processes.

Differential Diagnosis

Tuberculoma (160)
- increased choline and lactate on MRS
- tuberculomas are bright on images with magnetization transfer (low MT ratio)

Cystic Tumors (Ganglioglioma, Pleomorphic Xanthoastrocytoma) (165, 166)
- tend to be larger
- multifocality of lesions is extremely unusual
- different calcification pattern

Dystrophic Calcifications (191)
- usually single and irregular
- no surrounding edema

Microhemorrhages (on MRI) (177, 178)
- will not show calcification on CT
- no cystic portions

Cavernoma (183, 193)
- usually not cystic
- characteristic "popcorn" appearance with central lobulated T2 hyperintensity

Congenital Toxoplasmosis (185)
- random frequently white matter calcifications
- associated posterior ventriculomegaly, abnormal white matter
- occurs in infants

Background

CC is the most common parasitic infection of the brain caused by *Taenia solium* (pork tapeworm). Humans become the definitive host when ingesting larvae, which then grow in the small bowel and cause intestinal disease. However, if the eggs are ingested, humans become the intermediate host and when the eggs mature, larvae are released into the bloodstream. Once this occurs, the incidence of CNS involvement is nearly 100%. There are four stages of the disease in the brain parenchyma. The first is the vesicular (larval) active stage. As the larva dies, it triggers inflammation resulting in edema in the colloidal stage. This is followed by the contraction of the dying larva and granuloma formation in the granular stage. The lesions may resemble granulomas of other etiology and the surrounding edema recedes. Calcification occurs in the final nodular stage. The edema and enhancement are indicative of inflammatory reaction due to CC antigen leakage, which is responsible for seizures and most commonly occurs when the parasites die. Contrast enhancement may be an indication of a resolving lesion or persistent inflammation. It has been suggested that persistent enhancement may increase the likelihood of seizures in patients with calcified lesions. CT and T2* images have similar sensitivity for visualization of calcified CC lesions. Cysticidal drugs, albendazole and praziquantel, are effective against parenchymal parasites. Therapy may hasten resolution of active cysts and perilesional inflammation but does not affect the later stages.

REFERENCES

1. Lucato LT, Guedes MS, Sato JR, *et al.* The role of conventional MR imaging sequences in the evaluation of neurocysticercosis: impact on characterization of the scolex and lesion burden. *AJNR* 2007;**28**:1501–4.

2. Kimura-Hayama ET, Higuera JA, Corona-Cedillo R, *et al.* Neurocysticercosis: radiologic–pathologic correlation. *Radiographics* 2010;**30**:1705–19.

3. Sheth TN, Pilon L, Keystone J, Kucharczyk W. Persistent MR contrast enhancement of calcified neurocysticercosis lesions. *AJNR* 1998;**19**:79–82.

4. Carpio A, Kelvin EA, Bagiella E, *et al.* Effects of albendazole treatment on neurocysticercosis: a randomised controlled trial. *J Neurol Neurosurg Psychiatry* 2008;**79**:1050–5.

5. Pretell EJ, Martinot C Jr, Garcia HH, *et al.* Differential diagnosis between cerebral tuberculosis and neurocysticercosis by magnetic resonance spectroscopy. *J Comput Assist Tomogr* 2005;**29**:112–4.

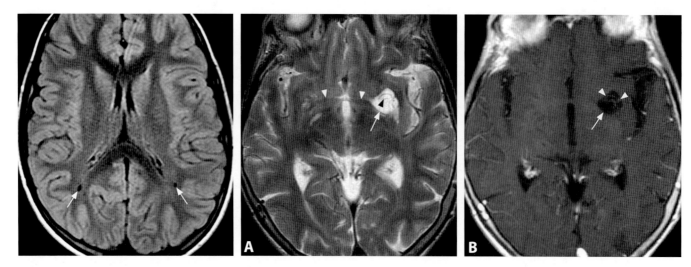

Figure 1. Axial FLAIR in a child shows bilateral CSF-like oval areas (arrows) in the posterior deep white matter with a radial orientation, without mass effect or adjacent signal abnormality.

Figure 2. T2WI (A) shows a CSF-like mass (arrow) adjacent to the anterior commisure (white arrowheads), with internal linear dark structures (black arrowheads). A smaller elongated area is present on the right. Post-contrast T1WI (B) shows smooth margins of the cyst (arrow) without enhancement. Enhancing linear structures (arrowheads) represent blood vessels.

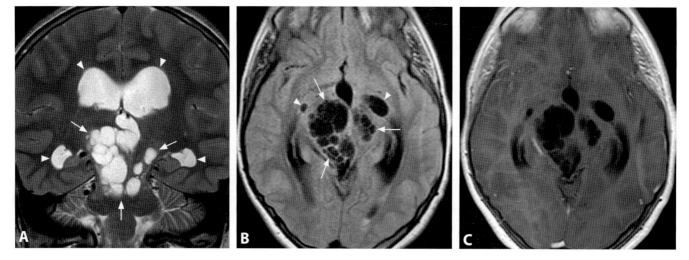

Figure 3. Coronal T2WI (A) shows a multicystic lesion (arrows) in the mesencephalo-thalamic region with CSF-like signal and ventriculomegaly (arrowheads). FLAIR (B) shows the multiseptated lesion (arrows) without any surrounding signal abnormality. Note bilateral cystic areas adjacent to the anterior commissure (arrowheads). The sylvian aqueduct is obstructed. Post-contrast T1WI (C) shows no lesion enhancement.

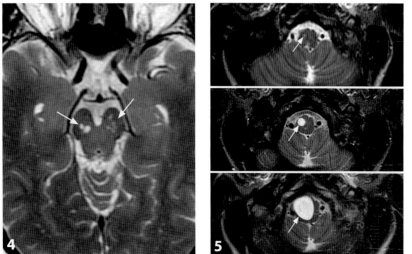

Figure 4. Axial T2WI through the midbrain reveals small cystic structures at the cerebral peduncles. There was no associated contrast enhancement or peripheral signal abnormality on other images.

Figure 5. Axial T2WIs at the medulla oblongata show a very small hyperintense area (arrow), which demonstrates continuous increase in size over 14 years. Note no adjacent signal abnormality.

Dilated Perivascular Spaces

GIOVANNI MORANA

Specific Imaging Findings

Perivascular spaces (PVS) show a well-defined oval, rounded, or tubular configuration with smooth margins and are commonly seen bilaterally in the supratentorial white matter with a radial orientation and in the basal nuclei (around the anterior commissure and in the midbrain). PVS appear on CT as hypodense areas, with similar attenuation as CSF. Calcifications or other associated abnormalities are not present. On MRI, their signal intensity also follows the CSF, being hypointense on FLAIR images, typically without any bright rim. Contrast enhancement is absent and there is water-like diffusivity on ADC maps. MR spectroscopy around dilated PVS shows normal spectra. In rare cases PVS may continuously enlarge to over 2 cm in size, frequently containing internal septations. The surrounding brain parenchyma generally has normal signal intensity; however, adjacent to dilated and enlarging PVS, hyperintense signal on FLAIR images may be present, likely representing reactive gliosis or spongiosis.

Pertinent Clinical Information

Small PVS ($\leq$ 5 mm) are seen on high-resolution MRI in all age groups. Dilatation of PVS has been associated with aging. In healthy children, they are present in 25–30% of cases and must be considered a benign normal variant. They are usually asymptomatic and discovered incidentally. However, in the pediatric age group, prominent PVS are also well-known findings of mucopolysaccharidoses (types I and II). In those cases, PVS dilation specifically involves the corpus callosum, in addition to the periventricular white matter. Therefore, the presence of multiple callosal PVS, in the appropriate clinical context, should prompt metabolic investigations.

Differential Diagnosis

Chronic Lacunar Infarct
- commonly located within the deep gray and white matter
- characteristic bright rim on FLAIR images

Neuroglial Cysts (169)
- usually solitary, non-enhancing CSF-like parenchymal cyst
- absence of radial distribution
- may be indistinguishable

Cystic Neoplasms (165, 166, 172, 173, 175)
- often have solid components and may enhance
- at least a portion is different from the CSF on one or more imaging techniques
- purely cystic gangliogliomas may be indistinguishable

Infectious Cysts (167, 194)
- variable signal depending on the stage of evolution of the infection
- cyst wall may enhance, may show calcifications
- usually at least a small area of different signal on at least one MR sequence
- hydatid cysts may be isointense to CSF on all imaging studies and indistinguishable

Background

PVS, also known as Virchow–Robin spaces (V–R spaces), are tiny, fluid-filled spaces that surround the arteries, arterioles, veins, and venules as they penetrate the brain parenchyma. Electron microscopy studies have demonstrated that the pia mater separates the PVS from the subarachnoid spaces; therefore, PVS are not in direct communication with the CSF in the subarachnoid space. They are not filled with CSF but, rather, with interstitial fluid, and measurements using quantitative MRI have shown that they have a slightly different MR signal intensity than the CSF-containing structures within and around the brain. The mechanisms underlying expanding PVS are still unknown. Dilated PVS spaces typically occur around the anterior commissure and in the periventricular regions, particularly posteriorly and around the atria; they may also appear in the subinsular cortex and in the midbrain. Occasionally, PVS show frank dilation, may cause mass effect, and assume bizarre cystic configurations. In the mesencephalothalamic region they may appear as clusters of variably sized cysts and can cause hydrocephalus by compression of the third ventricle or the sylvian aqueduct, therefore requiring surgical intervention.

REFERENCES

1. Kwee RM, Kwee TC. Virchow–Robin spaces at MR imaging. *Radiographics* 2007;**27**:1071–86.

2. Groeschel S, Chong WK, Surtees R, Hanefeld F. Virchow–Robin spaces on magnetic resonance images: normative data, their dilatation, and a review of the literature. *Neuroradiology* 2006;**48**: 745–54.

3. Mathias J, Koessler L, Brissart H, *et al.* Giant cystic widening of Virchow–Robin spaces: an anatomofunctional study. *AJNR* 2007;**28**:1523–5.

4. Salzman KL, Osborn AG, House P, *et al.* Giant tumefactive perivascular spaces. *AJNR* 2005;**26**:298–305.

5. Ozturk MH, Aydingoz U. Comparison of MR signal intensities of cerebral perivascular (Virchow–Robin) and subarachnoid spaces. *J Comput Assist Tomogr* 2002;**26**:902–4.

Brain Imaging with MRI and CT, ed. Zoran Rumboldt *et al.* Published by Cambridge University Press. © Cambridge University Press 2012.

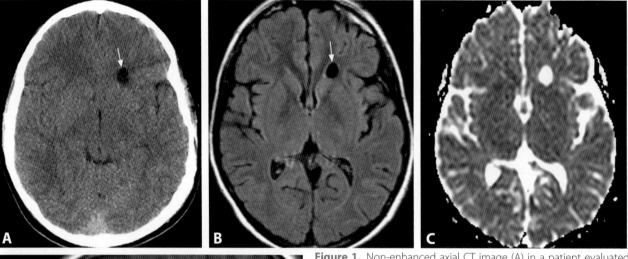

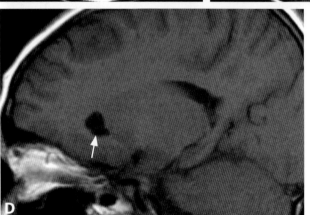

Figure 1. Non-enhanced axial CT image (A) in a patient evaluated for head trauma demonstrates a left frontal oval hypodensity (arrow) with attenuation similar to the CSF. FLAIR image (B) obtained for follow-up of this lesion reveals a well-defined area (arrow) that is isointense with the CSF and with only minimal and partial peripheral signal abnormality. Corresponding ADC map (C) shows very high diffusion within the cyst that equals the CSF. Sagittal T1WI without contrast (D) reveals lobulated nature of the cyst (arrow).

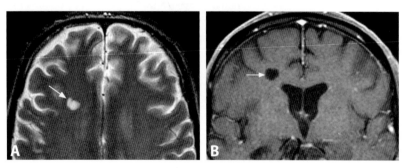

Figure 2. Axial T2WI (A) shows a well-demarcated and lobulated deep right frontal lesion (arrow) with CSF-like signal intensity, without edema or mass effect. Post-contrast coronal T1WI (B) shows no enhancement of this CSF-like area (arrow).

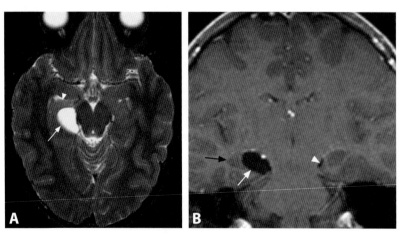

Figure 3. Fat-saturated T2WI (A) shows a CSF-like oval mass (arrow) arising adjacent to or from the hippocampus (arrowhead). The pathognomonic location of the cyst (white arrow) medial to the hippocampus (black arrow) is well portrayed on coronal post-contrast T1WI (B). Note contralateral choroidal fissure (arrowhead).

Neuroepithelial Cyst

ZORAN RUMBOLDT AND BENJAMIN HUANG

Specific Imaging Findings

Neuroepithelial cysts appear as well-circumscribed, ovoid, non-enhancing masses that follow CSF density/signal intensity. They can be of variable size and occur virtually anywhere, sometimes with a multiloculated appearance. No surrounding hyperintense gliosis is observed on FLAIR images. In the supra-tentorial compartment, they are usually in the cerebral white matter, with the frontal lobe being the most typical location. Another common location is adjacent to the hippocampus, referred to as a choroidal fissure cyst.

Pertinent Clinical Information

Neuroglial cysts are usually asymptomatic and incidentally noted. Symptomatic ones present in the fourth or fifth decades of life related to their mass effect. Cysts in the posterior fossa have been reported to cause cranial nerve palsies, focal brainstem dysfunction, and hydrocephalus. Supratentorial cysts may rarely cause seizures or focal motor and/or sensory deficits. Small, incidentally detected neuroepithelial cysts require no follow-up; large cysts may warrant serial imaging to ensure the lack of growth.

Differential Diagnosis

Enlarged Perivascular (Virchow–Robin) Space (168)
- usually multiple
- typically at basal ganglia, white matter of the convexities, and midbrain
- may be indistinguishable from neuroepithelial cysts

Neurocysticercosis (167, 194)
- often demonstrates a mural nodule (the scolex)
- may partially enhance or show surrounding edema
- calcification very common

Neurenteric Cyst
- hyperintense to CSF on FLAIR, variable density on CT

Lacunar Infarct
- characteristic bright rim on FLAIR images corresponding to surrounding gliosis

Porencephalic Cyst (83)
- communicates with the lateral ventricle
- may show surrounding gliosis

Arachnoid Cyst (142)
- extra-axial location

Background

Also referred to as glioependymal cysts, epithelial cysts, or neuroglial cysts, they are congenital benign cysts defined by the presence of epithelial lining. Choroidal fissure cysts and ependymal cysts are considered types of neuroepithelial cysts, and even choroid plexus cysts may be included in this group. Several theories have been proposed to explain their etiology – a leading theory proposes their origin from the embryonic neural tube elements that become sequestered in the developing white matter. The cyst wall usually consists of one or more layers of columnar epithelium (presumably of ependymal origin) or cuboidal epithelium (choroid plexus origin) which rest on a bed of GFAP-positive neuroglial tissue. A layer of connective tissue may also be present. Definitive diagnosis requires histopathologic examination, but this is rarely clinically indicated. Complete surgical removal is the preferred treatment for symptomatic cysts, as they can recur following an incomplete resection.

REFERENCES

1. Sherman JL, Camponovo E, Citrin CM. MR imaging of CSF-like choroidal fissure and parenchymal cysts of the brain. *AJNR* 1990;**11**:939–45.
2. Osborn AG, Preece MT. Intracranial cysts: radiologic–pathologic correlation and imaging approach. *Radiology* 2006;**239**:650–64.
3. Lustgarten L, Papanastassiou V, McDonald B, Kerr RSC. Benign intracerebral cysts with ependymal lining: pathological and radiological features. *Br J Neurosurg* 1997;**11**:393–7.
4. Morioka T, Nishio S, Suzuki S, *et al.* Choroidal fissure cyst in the temporal horn associated with complex partial seizure. *Clin Neurol Neurosurg* 1994;**96**:164–7.
5. Preece MT, Osborn AG, Chin SS, Smirniotopoulos JG. Intracranial neurenteric cysts: imaging and pathology spectrum. *AJNR* 2006;**27**:1211–6.

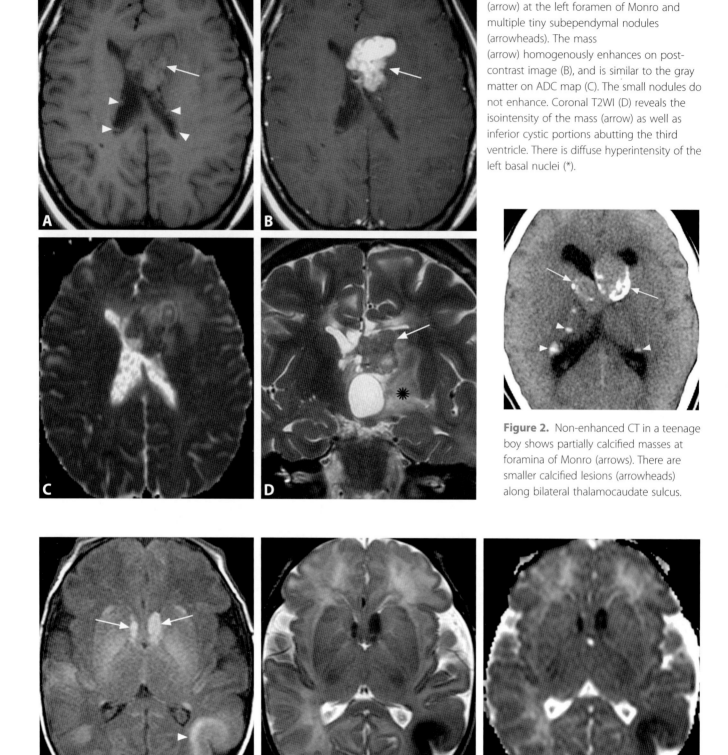

Figure 1. Axial T1WI (A) in a 9-year-old girl shows an isointense multilobulated mass (arrow) at the left foramen of Monro and multiple tiny subependymal nodules (arrowheads). The mass (arrow) homogenously enhances on post-contrast image (B), and is similar to the gray matter on ADC map (C). The small nodules do not enhance. Coronal T2WI (D) reveals the isointensity of the mass (arrow) as well as inferior cystic portions abutting the third ventricle. There is diffuse hyperintensity of the left basal nuclei (*).

Figure 2. Non-enhanced CT in a teenage boy shows partially calcified masses at foramina of Monro (arrows). There are smaller calcified lesions (arrowheads) along bilateral thalamocaudate sulcus.

Figure 3. MRI in a newborn shows typical neonatal characteristics of bilateral lesions (arrows) at the foramina of Monro: hyperintense on T1WI (A), hypointense on T2WI (B), and with low ADC values (D). This signal pattern is similar to that of a left parietal tuber (arrowhead) and is consistent with hypermyelination.

Subependymal Giant Cell Astrocytoma (SEGA)

ANDREA ROSSI

Specific Imaging Findings

Subependymal giant cell astrocytomas (SEGAs) almost exclusively originate from the subependymal surface of the caudate nucleus, near the foramen of Monro, in patients with tuberous sclerosis complex (TSC). Bilateral lesions are common; they are often asymmetric both in size and growth rate. SEGAs are prevailingly solid, although cystic components may be present, especially in large masses. Lesions may show lobulated margins and resemble a conglomeration of nodules. Calcification is common, and is best seen on CT. The solid component is isointense with gray matter on all MR imaging sequences, and enhances homogeneously with gadolinium administration. The lesions are similar to the brain on diffusion imaging. Diameter over 12 mm, or a lesion more than 5 mm in size with growth on serial imaging are the characteristics indicative of SEGA. All lesions at the foramen of Monro in TSC patients should be presumed to be SEGA until proven otherwise. Contrast enhancement was considered a differentiating feature of SEGA on CT; however, many subependymal nodules enhance on MRI.

Pertinent Clinical Information

SEGA is found predominantly during the first and second decades of life, sometimes even in utero. The lesion may be asymptomatic per se; however, when sufficiently large it may obstruct CSF flow at the foramen of Monro, leading to elevated intracranial pressure and hydrocephalus. Worsening of epilepsy may lead to neuroimaging and diagnosis of SEGA. Neurosurgical resection is an effective standard treatment and may be performed before the lesions become symptomatic; however, SEGAs frequently recur. Everolimus selectively inhibits an underlying molecular abnormality of SEGAs and is a particularly attractive therapeutic option for patients with inoperable or recurrent tumors. Radiosurgery is another option.

Differential Diagnosis

Subependymal Nodules (SEN) (107, 199)
- location not at the foramen of Monro, size < 12 mm and no growth on serial imaging
- enhancement (on MRI) is not a differential feature because it may occur in SEN

Choroid Plexus Papilloma (148)
- lobulated, grape-like appearance may simulate choroid plexus papilloma
- foramen of Monro is an unlikely location for papillomas, extension to frontal horns is not a feature

Central Neurocytoma (150)
- originates from septum pellucidum
- in older patients (generally young adults)
- not associated with TSC features

Background

SEGA is a WHO grade I slow-growing tumor that typically arises in the wall of the lateral ventricles and very rarely undergoes anaplastic degeneration. SEGA is one of the major diagnostic criteria for TSC, and it occurs almost exclusively in patients harboring this genetic disease, with incidence ranging from 5 to 20%. Retinal giant cell astrocytomas are present in 50% of TSC patients. Typical histopathological findings of SEGA are solid sheets and perivascular pseudorosettes of large, gemistocytic, polygonal and occasionally ganglion-like cells within a fibrillated background, which are accompanied by spindle-shaped cells creating broad fascicles. Rich vascular stroma and numerous calcifications are common. Mutations in *TSC1* (hamartin) or *TSC2* (tuberin) are found in over 85% of TSC patients. The proteins encoded by these genes form a tumor-suppressor complex acting through the Ras homolog enriched in brain protein (RHEB) to limit activation of the mammalian target of rapamycin (mTOR) complex 1. When either *TSC1* or *TSC2* is deficient, mTOR complex 1 is upregulated, leading to abnormal cellular growth, proliferation, and protein synthesis. Everolimus inhibits mTOR complex 1 and leads to marked reduction in the size of SEGAs. Additional benefits of everolimus therapy may include a decrease in seizure burden as well as shrinkage of other sytemic tumors (angiofibromas and angiomyolipomas) in TSC patients. On the other hand, SEGAs have been reported to regrow if mTOR inhibitor therapy is stopped.

REFERENCES

1. Baron Y, Barkovich AJ. MR Imaging of tuberous sclerosis in neonates and young infants. *AJNR* 1999;**20**:907–16.

2. Raju GP, Urion DK, Sahin M. Neonatal subependymal giant cell astrocytoma: new case and review of literature. *Pediatr Neurol* 2007;**36**:128–31.

3. Grajkowska W, Kotulska K, Jurkiewicz E, et al. Subependymal giant cell astrocytomas with atypical histological features mimicking malignant gliomas. *Folia Neuropathol* 2011;**49**:39–46.

4. Campen CJ, Porter BE. Subependymal Giant Cell Astrocytoma (SEGA) treatment update. *Curr Treat Options Neurol* 2011;**13**:380–5.

5. Krueger DA, Care MM, Holland K, et al. Everolimus for subependymal giant-cell astrocytomas in tuberous sclerosis. *N Engl J Med* 2010;**363**:1801–11.

Brain Imaging with MRI and CT, ed. Zoran Rumboldt *et al.* Published by Cambridge University Press. © Cambridge University Press 2012.

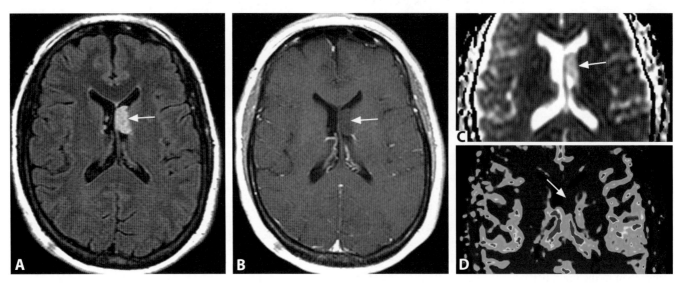

Figure 1. Axial FLAIR image (A) shows a very bright lesion (arrow) in the left lateral ventricle, just above the foramen of Monro, without mass effect or surrounding edema. The mass (arrow) is slightly hypointense and shows no enhancement on corresponding post-contrast T1WI (B). ADC map (C) reveals increased intralesional diffusivity (arrow). The mass (arrow) exhibits very low blood volume on perfusion MRI (D).

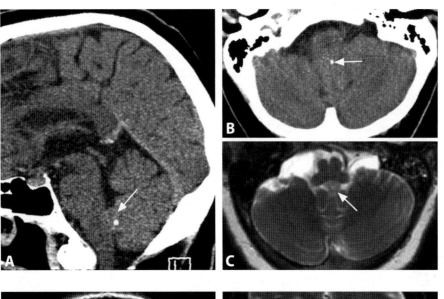

Figure 2. Non-enhanced CT image reconstructed in the sagittal plane (A) shows a small isodense lesion (arrow) in the inferior aspect of the fourth ventricle. Axial CT image (B) shows a small internal calcification (arrow) to a better advantage. The oval mass (arrow) is mildly hyperintense and heterogenous on T2WI (C). There was no lesion enhancement on post-contrast images (not shown).

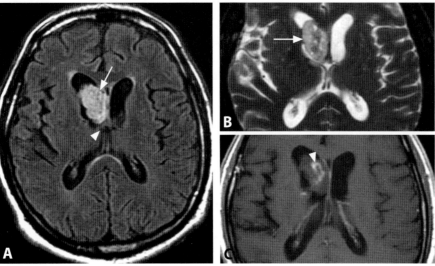

Figure 3. FLAIR image (A) reveals a very bright intraventricular lesion (arrow) adjacent to the right foramen of Monro (arrowhead). The mass (arrow) is overall hyperintense and mildly heterogenous on corresponding T2WI (B), with small bright and dark areas. The lesion shows a focal area of internal enhancement (arrowhead) on post-contrast T1WI (C).

Subependymoma

ZORAN RUMBOLDT

Specific Imaging Findings

Subependymomas are well-defined round to oval masses usually not exceeding 2 cm in greatest diameter that occur around the foramen of Monro and in the fourth ventricle. These neoplasms are hypodense on CT, of low to mildly increased T1 signal, and hyperintense on T2-weighted sequences, with characteristically very bright signal on FLAIR images. They are generally homogenous with absent or minimal focal contrast enhancement, although lobulated contours and intratumoral cysts may be encountered. Heterogenous signal intensities and/or internal calcifications are not unusual and some tumors may sho3w moderate to prominent enhancement on MR imaging. Diffusion of water molecules is higher than in the brain parenchyma resulting in high signal on ADC maps. Perfusion studies show very low blood volume. Subependymomas may very rarely arise in an intra-axial location, and even in those cases the presence of surrounding edema is an exception. MR spectroscopy shows normal choline peak and depressed NAA. Rare cases of recurrent subependymoma may demonstrate increased choline to creatine (Cho/Cr) ratio on MRS.

Pertinent Clinical Information

Subependymomas are rare, slow-growing, low-grade gliomas, the majority of which are asymptomatic and found incidentally at postmortem examination. They are typically associated with the ventricular system and become apparent clinically only when symptoms of hydrocephalus or mass effect develop. Their clinical features may vary widely, most commonly presenting with headache and vomiting in older adult patients.

Differential Diagnosis

Hemangioblastoma (175)
- characteristic prominent vessels (flow-voids) within the tumor
- may contain a large cystic portion
- solid portion avidly enhances and shows high perfusion (CBV)
- very rare outside the cerebellum except in the setting of VHL

Ependymoma (172)
- more heterogenous, calcifications and hemorrhage are common
- ill-defined, extends through the foramina of Luschka and Magendie when in the fourth ventricle
- supratentorial are typically extraventricular (anaplastic)

Choroid Plexus Papilloma (148)
- avid contrast enhancement
- heterogenous with prominent vascular structures
- origin at the trigone of lateral ventricles in children; fourth ventricle in adults

Pilocytic Astrocytoma (173)
- usually found in children
- may contain a large cyst/cystic portion
- solid portion of the tumor avidly enhances with contrast

Subependymal Giant Cell Astrocytoma (SEGA) (170, 199)
- occurs exclusively in patients with tuberous sclerosis
- almost always arises at the foramen of Monro

Central Neurocytoma (150)
- characteristically supratentorial paramedian location, around the septum pellucidum
- multicystic appearance
- majority occur in patients under 40 years of age

Intraventricular Meningioma (149)
- densely and homogenously enhancing mass
- when intraventricular, almost always at the trigone of lateral ventricle

Metastatic Neoplasms
- frequently heterogenous and necrotic
- additional parenchymal lesions may be present

Background

Subependymomas are rare, representing less than 1% of all CNS tumors. Macroscopically these are characteristically rubbery and white, well-demarcated masses. Histologically, they are characterized by clustering of isomorphic cells arranged against a dense fibrillary matrix of glial cell processes. Focal cystic degeneration may be present.

Following surgical resection, the patients are typically symptom-free with no evidence of recurrence. Some subependymomas show progressive biological behavior, especially the markedly enhancing, irregularly contoured large lesions located in the trigone. It is not clear whether the risk of recurrence is correlated with Ki-67 labeling index. Overall, the histopathological examination is of little help in determining tumor aggressiveness. In rare cases the tumors may even lead to subependymal seeding. Radiation does not appear to be an effective treatment for subependymomas.

REFERENCES

1. Ragel BT, Osborn AG, Whang K, et al. Subependymomas: an analysis of clinical and imaging features. *Neurosurgery* 2006;**58**:881–90.
2. Hoeffel C, Boukobza M, Polivka M, et al. MR manifestations of subependymomas. *AJNR* 1995;**16**:2121–9.
3. Im SH, Paek SH, Choi YL, et al. Clinicopathological study of seven cases of symptomatic supratentorial subependymoma. *J Neurooncol* 2003;**61**:57–67.
4. Fujisawa H, Hasegawa M, Ueno M. Clinical features and management of five patients with supratentorial subependymoma. *J Clin Neurosci* 2010;**17**:201–4.
5. Koeller KK, Sandberg GD. From the archives of the AFIP. Cerebral intraventricular neoplasms: radiologic–pathologic correlation. *Radiographics* 2002;**22**:1473–505.

Brain Imaging with MRI and CT, ed. Zoran Rumboldt *et al.* Published by Cambridge University Press. © Cambridge University Press 2012.

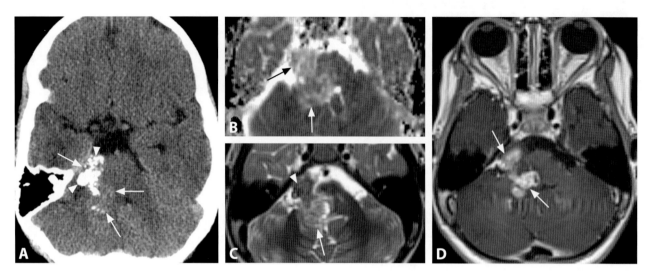

Figure 1. Non-enhanced axial CT image (A) shows a posterior fossa mass (arrows) with dense calcifications (arrowheads). ADC map obtained at a different angle (B) reveals mildly increased diffusion of the lesion (arrows). The mass (arrow) is heterogenous on T2WI (C) and its hypointense portion (arrowhead) extends through the foramen of Luschka. There is avid lesion enhancement (arrow) on post-contrast T1WI (D).

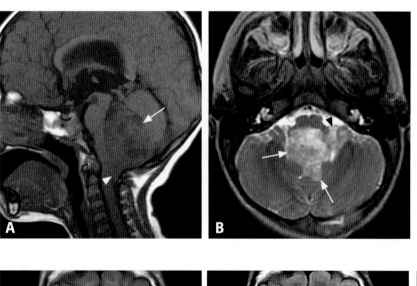

Figure 2. Sagittal T1WI without contrast (A) shows a heterogenous hypointense mass (arrow) filling the fourth ventricle and extending inferiorly through the foramen of Magendie (arrowhead). Axial T2WI (B) shows the heterogenously hyperintense mass (arrows) expanding the fourth ventricle and extending through the left foramen of Luschka (arrowhead).

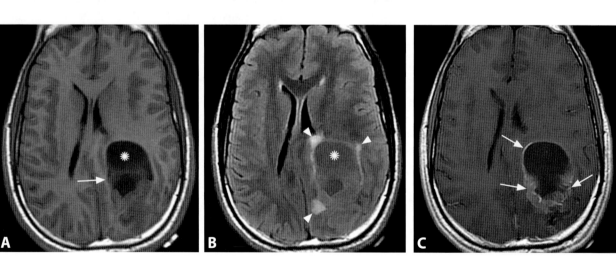

Figure 3. Axial T1WI without contrast (A) shows a heterogenous mass (arrow) along the margin of the left lateral ventricle with a presumed large cystic portion (*). The cystic area (*) is hyperintense to the CSF on FLAIR (B) indicating proteinaceous contents. There is mild surrounding edema (arrowheads). Post-contrast T1WI (C) reveals heterogenous enhancement (arrows) of the solid portions.

Specific Imaging Findings

On CT, ependymomas are usually iso- to hypodense compared with normal brain. Approximately 50% contain internal calcifications and hemorrhage can also be seen in approximately 10% of tumors. The tumor is heterogenous, T1 iso- to hypointense, and hyperintense on T2-weighted imaging. T1 hyperintense and T2 hypointense areas may be found, representing calcifications and sometimes blood products. The lesions are frequently heterogenous on ADC maps, the more solid portion of the tumor is generally slightly brighter than the normal brain; anaplastic (higher grade) ependymomas may contain dark areas of very low diffusion. Following contrast, ependymomas show some degree of usually heterogenous enhancement, although non-enhancing tumors can occasionally be seen, especially with recurrent disease. Perfusion studies demonstrate markedly elevated cerebral blood volume (but, unlike other glial neoplasms, poor return to baseline). Due to the propensity for leptomeningeal disease and drop metastases, imaging of the entire neural axis is required. A fourth ventricle mass that extends through the foramina of Luschka and Magendie into the cerebellopontine angle and cisterna magna is a characteristic appearance of the infra-tentorial ependymomas. Supratentorial ependymomas are commonly extraventricular, located along or near the ventricular margin within the cerebral hemispheres; they also tend to be larger and more heterogenous and are frequently anaplastic.

Pertinent Clinical Information

Intracranial ependymomas typically occur in childhood. Infratentorial tumors tend to present earlier due to their intraventricular location with resultant hydrocephalus and increased intracranial pressure. Supratentorial ependymomas typically present with neurological deficits and seizures. Dissemination at the time of diagnosis is not very common (3–11%), but is a poor prognostic sign. MRI is overall more sensitive for the leptomeningeal disease than CSF cytology. Complete resection at initial surgery is of critical importance, followed by irradiation of the primary site. Five-year progression-free survival is approximately 50–60%.

Differential Diagnosis

Pilocytic Astrocytoma (173)
- typically well-delineated
- hypodense on CT
- T2 hyperintense and very bright on ADC maps
- may present as a cystic lesion with an enhancing mural nodule

Medulloblastoma (174)
- hyperdense on CT
- typically of low T2 signal

- very dark on ADC maps
- may contain cysts, but is generally a well-defined mass
- extension along the foramina of Luschka and Magendie is unusual

Hemangioblastoma (175)
- presence of flow-voids
- solid portion is very bright on ADC maps
- may present as a cystic lesion with an enhancing mural nodule
- exceedingly rare in children

Background

Intracranial ependymomas account for 6–12% of all pediatric brain tumors and almost one-third of brain neoplasms in children under 3 years of age. Ependymomas arise from differentiated ependymal cells lining the ventricles and the central canal of the spinal cord. Supratentorial tumors located away from the ventricular surface are thought to arise from ependymal rests that become trapped during embryonic development. Approximately 60–70% of intracranial ependymomas arise in the posterior fossa and 30–40% in the supratentorial brain. Posterior fossa tumors occur more commonly in infants and young children whereas supratentorial tumors occur more often in older children and young adults. There are three grades of ependymal tumors, including grade I (subependymoma, myxopapillary ependymoma), grade II (ependymoma), and grade III (anaplastic ependymoma). Four histological subtypes are also recognized: cellular, papillary, clear cell and tanycytic ependymomas. Because 25–40% of ependymomas are diagnosed in children less than 3 years of age, the neurocognitive sequelae of irradiation are a major concern. New radiotherapeutic regimes have shown promising results, and postoperative chemotherapy may avoid or delay radiotherapy in a substantial proportion of these patients without compromising survival.

REFERENCES

1. Yuh EL, Barkovich AJ, Gupta N. Imaging of ependymomas: MRI and CT. *Childs Nerv Syst* 2009;**25**:1203–13.

2. Chen CJ, Tseng YC, Hsu HL, Jung SM. Imaging predictors of intracranial ependymomas. *J Comput Assist Tomogr* 2004;**28**:407–13.

3. Boop FA, Sgouros S. Intracranial ependymoma in children: current status and future trends on diagnosis and management. *Childs Nerv Syst* 2009;**25**:1163–5.

4. Godfraind C. Classification and controversies in pathology of ependymomas. *Childs Nerv Syst* 2009;**25**:1185–93.

5. Merchant TE, Li C, Xiong X, *et al*. Conformal radiotherapy after surgery for paediatric ependymoma: a prospective study. *Lancet Oncol* 2009;**10**:258–66.

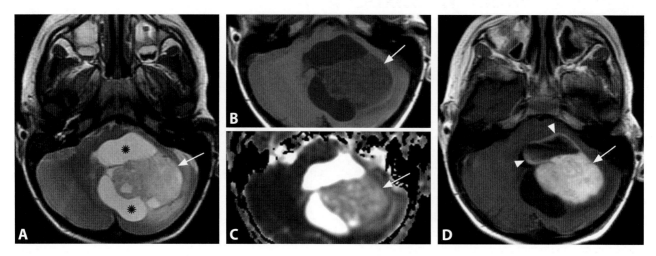

Figure 1. Axial T2WI (A) shows a well-defined cerebellar mass (arrow) with hyperintense solid and cystic (*) components. Corresponding pre-contrast T1WI (B) shows low signal of the solid component (arrow). ADC map (D) reveals increased diffusion within the solid portion (arrow) compared to the normal brain. Post-contrast T1WI (C) shows intense enhancement of the solid component (arrow) and cyst wall (arrowheads).

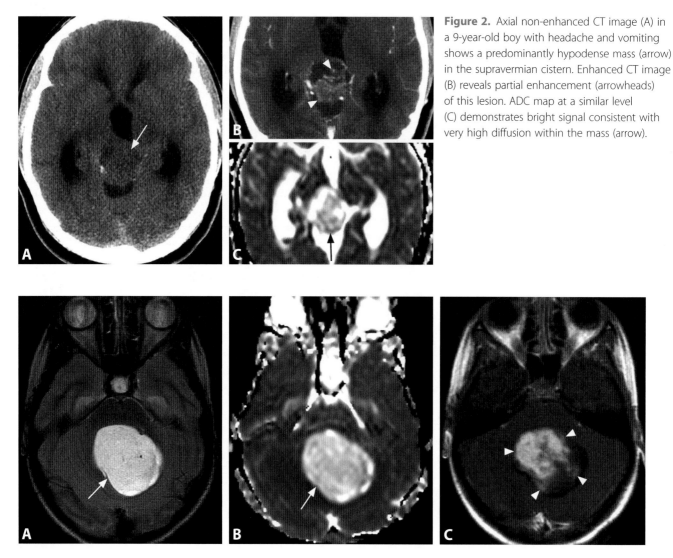

Figure 2. Axial non-enhanced CT image (A) in a 9-year-old boy with headache and vomiting shows a predominantly hypodense mass (arrow) in the supravermian cistern. Enhanced CT image (B) reveals partial enhancement (arrowheads) of this lesion. ADC map at a similar level (C) demonstrates bright signal consistent with very high diffusion within the mass (arrow).

Figure 3. Axial T2WI (A) shows a bright posterior fossa mass (arrow) centered at the fourth ventricle. The lesion (arrow) is also very bright on ADC map (B), while post-contrast T1WI (C) reveals partial and heterogenous enhancement (arrowheads).

Pilocytic Astrocytoma

DONNA ROBERTS

Specific Imaging Findings

The classic imaging appearance of a pilocytic astrocytoma (PA) is a well circumscribed cerebellar/fourth ventricle mass composed of a cyst and intensely enhancing mural nodule. This appearance is, however, absent in many cases of PA and is common with other neoplasms in this location and age group. The cysts are frequently absent, but the solid portions are characteristically hypodense on CT, T1 hypointense and of very high T2 signal. PAs typically exhibit avid contrast enhancement, which may be partial and patchy, and non-enhancing solid portions may also be present. The tumors ar3e bright on ADC maps, approaching the CSF signal. This very high diffusion is essentially pathognomonic for pediatric posterior fossa PA. Peritumoral edema is typically minimal or absent. PAs also occur in the brainstem, usually as well circumscribed, exophytic lesions. Supratentorial PAs commonly involve the optic pathways and hypothalamus. Perfusion imaging reveals relative cerebral blood volume to be only mildly elevated or similar to the normal brain. PAs are also found in adults and these tumors show the same imaging characteristics as in the pediatric population.

Pertinent Clinical Information

Patients with cerebellar lesions can present with headache, nausea and vomiting, and gait disturbance. Children with optic pathway gliomas can present with visual changes, proptosis, and precocious puberty. If location allows it, treatment is surgical with survival rates of 90% at 10 years with gross total resection. If surgery is not possible, chemotherapy and radiation therapy can be offered. In the setting of neurofibromatosis type I, patients are often followed by observation only due to the indolent course of their optic pathway gliomas. PAs may even spontaneously regress, sometimes following partial resection.

Differential Diagnosis

Medulloblastoma (174)
- very low ADC values, may be T2 hypointense
- hyperdense on CT

Ependymoma (172, 200)
- usually very heterogenous appearance, possible calcifications and hemorrhage

- lower ADC values, diffusion similar to brain parenchyma
- extension through the fourth ventricle foramina into the spinal canal

Hemangioblastoma (175)
- presence of flow-voids
- extremely rare in children
- very high CBV on perfusion studies

Background

Gliomas account for approximately 40% of childhood CNS tumors and PAs are the most common histological subtype. They usually present within the first two decades of life and have a typically benign course. Prognosis is thought to be even better in children with neurofibromatosis type I, an autosomal dominant disorder which accounts for between 50 and 70% of optic pathway gliomas with the vast majority being pilocytic astrocytomas. In the setting of neurofibromatosis type I, only 35–50% of cases found at imaging progress and there are documented cases of spontaneous tumor regression. A recently described neoplasm similar to PA is the pilomyxoid astrocytoma, which more commonly arises in the hypothalamic–chiasmatic area, behaves more aggressively and tends to present with early leptomeningeal spread of disease.

REFERENCES

1. Rumboldt Z, Camacho DLA, Lake D, *et al*. Apparent diffusion coefficients for differentiation of cerebellar tumors in children. *AJNR* 2006;**27**:1362–9.
2. Koeller KK, Rushing EJ. From the archives of the AFIP: pilocytic astrocytoma: radiologic–pathologic correlation. *Radiographics* 2004;**24**:1693–708.
3. Kumar VA, Knopp EA, Zagzag D. Magnetic resonance dynamic susceptibility-weighted contrast-enhanced perfusion imaging in the diagnosis of posterior fossa hemangioblastomas and pilocytic astrocytomas: initial results. *J Comput Assist Tomogr* 2010;**34**:825–9.
4. Foroughi M, Hendson G, Sargent MA, Steinbok P. Spontaneous regression of septum pellucidum/forniceal pilocytic astrocytomas – possible role of cannabis inhalation. *Childs Nerv Syst* 2011;**27**:671–9.
5. Linscott LL, Osborn AG, Blaser S, *et al*. Pilomyxoid astrocytoma: expanding the imaging spectrum. *AJNR* 2008;**29**:1861–6.

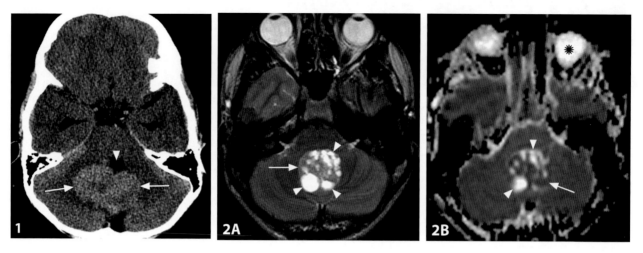

Figure 1. Axial non-enhanced CT image in a 5-year-old child shows a hyperdense midline cerebellar mass (arrow) located adjacent to the fourth ventricle (arrowhead).

Figure 2. On axial T2WI (A) in another patient, the fourth ventricle is filled with a mass that consists of slightly hyperintense strands (arrow) and bright oval portions (arrowheads). The strands (arrow) are darker than the brain on ADC map (B), consistent with solid tissue. The very bright components (arrowheads) are similar to the CSF and globes (*) and consistent with cysts.

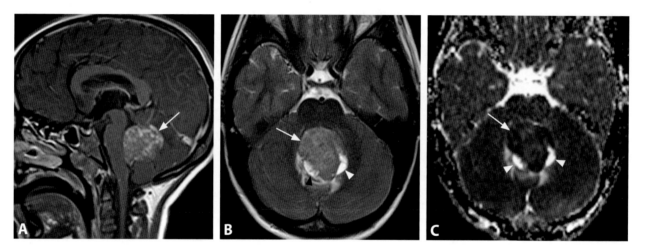

Figure 3. Midsagittal post-contrast T1WI (A) shows mild to moderate primarily linear enhancement of the fourth ventricle mass (arrow). Axial T2WI (B) reveals mild hyperintensity of the lesion (arrow) and apparent cystic components (arrowheads). Corresponding ADC map (C) shows low diffusivity within the solid portion of the mass (arrow). Diffusivity within the cysts (arrowheads) is similar to that of the CSF.

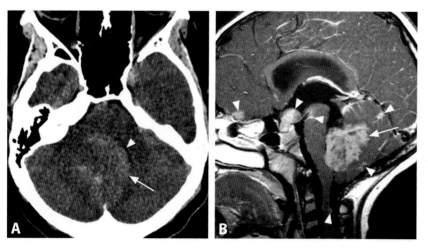

Figure 4. Non-enhanced axial CT image (A) shows a hyperdense mass (arrow) almost completely filling the fourth ventricle (arrowhead). Post-contrast sagittal T1WI (B) shows heterogenous enhancement of the mass (arrow). There are multiple additional enhancing lesions (arrowheads) along the surface of the brain and spinal cord, consistent with leptomeningeal spread.

Medulloblastoma

DONNA ROBERTS AND ZORAN RUMBOLDT

Specific Imaging Findings

Medulloblastomas typically arise in the midline of the posterior fossa, but may occur more laterally and sometimes extend through the fourth ventricle foramina. They are characteristically hyperdense on CT and with very low signal on ADC maps, typically darker than the normal brain. Cystic components are present in a majority of cases and the tumors are hypo- to iso-intense on T1WI. The appearance on post-contrast images is variable, ranging from marked and solid to only subtle marginal or linear enhancement. Calcification and hemorrhage may occasionally be observed, while surrounding edema is rarely prominent. Medulloblastomas have a high rate of early leptomeningeal disease and drop metastases, requiring MR imaging of the entire neural axis (head and spine). There are notable differences between the classic medulloblastoma (CMB) and some of the recently defined variants. CMB is T2 hyperintense, whereas desmoplastic/nodular (DMB) and medulloblastoma with extensive nodularity (MB-EN) are usually isointense; these two variants are also frequently located off-midline. MB-EN may show a characteristic gyriform pattern. In contrast to CMB, all medulloblastoma variants show marked contrast enhancement.

Pertinent Clinical Information

Patients with medulloblastoma are typically children, and increased intracranial pressure is responsible for common presentation with nausea, vomiting, and hydrocephalus. Due to the propensity for early leptomeningeal spread, the initial presentation may also be caused by metastatic disease, such as seizures or spinal cord compression. Extra-CNS spread may rarely occur, usually to the bone. Although the tumor remains incurable in about a third of patients, current treatment regimens have substantially improved survival rates. Risk stratification is currently based on the patient's age, histopathology, presence or absence of metastatic disease at presentation, and the amount of postoperative residual tumor.

Differential Diagnosis

Pilocytic Astrocytoma (173)
- hypodense on CT
- the solid portion is very bright on ADC maps and T2WI
- may present as a cyst with an enhancing mural nodule

Ependymoma (172, 200)
- heterogenous mass, frequently contains calcifications
- typical extension through the CSF outflow foramina

Hemangioblastoma (175)
- presence of vascular flow-voids best seen on T2WI
- the solid portion is very bright on ADC maps
- may present as a cyst with an enhancing mural nodule
- exceedingly rare in children

Atypical Teratoid–Rhabdoid Tumor (ATRT)
- presents at a younger age
- hemorrhage is common
- frequently involves cerebellopontine angle, may extend into the internal auditory canal

Background

Medulloblastoma is the most common pediatric malignant brain tumor and one of the two most common primary tumors of the posterior fossa in children (the other being pilocytic astrocytoma). These neoplasms are thought to arise from progenitor cells in the superior medullary velum along the roof of the fourth ventricle, which is a cerebellar germinal matrix zone early in life. The tumor is composed of sheets of highly packed, small, round cells. Medulloblastomas are classified into CMB and four variants: DMB, MB-EN, large cell medulloblastoma, and anaplastic medulloblastoma. Although all medulloblastomas are classified as grade IV lesions, the wide histological and molecular variation among these tumors means that the risk and prognosis also vary widely. While radiotherapy has significantly improved survival, its neurocognitive effects can be devastating. Patients are also at a high risk of developing postoperative cerebellar mutism. Efforts are underway to stratify medulloblastomas into subgroups with different levels of risk based on molecular profiling.

REFERENCES

1. Fruehwald-Pallamar J, Puchner SB, Rossi A, et al. Magnetic resonance imaging spectrum of medulloblastoma. *Neuroradiology* 2011;**53**:387–96.
2. Koral K, Gargan L, Bowers DC, et al. Imaging characteristics of atypical teratoid–rhabdoid tumor in children compared with medulloblastoma. *AJR* 2008;**190**:809–14.
3. Rumboldt Z, Camacho DL, Lake D, et al. Apparent diffusion coefficients for differentiation of cerebellar tumors in children. *AJNR* 2006;**27**:1362–9.
4. Mulhern RK, Merchant TE, Gajjar A, et al. Late neurocognitive sequelae in survivors of brain tumours in childhood. *Lancet Oncol* 2004;**5**:399–408.
5. Ellison DW. Childhood medulloblastoma: novel approaches to the classification of a heterogeneous disease. *Acta Neuropathol* 2010;**120**:305–16.

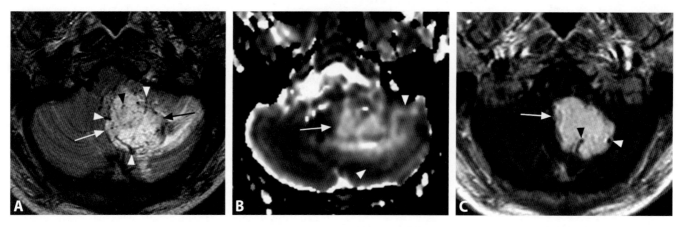

Figure 1. Axial T2WI (A) shows a very bright cerebellar mass (arrows) and multiple flow-voids (arrowheads) located within and along the edges of the lesion. Surrounding edema is also seen. Corresponding ADC map (B) reveals very high signal of the lesion (arrows), consistent with high diffusivity, similar to the signal of the surrounding edema (arrowheads). Matching post-contrast T1WI (C) demonstrates marked homogenous enhancement of the mass (arrow). Some internal flow-voids are still visible (arrowheads).

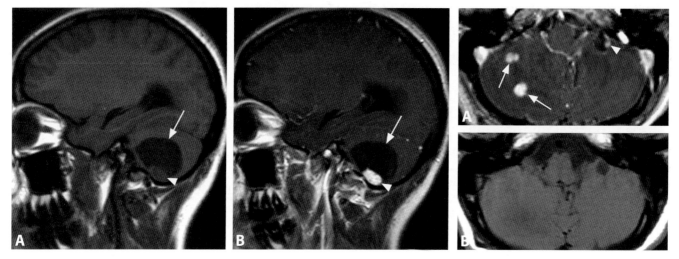

Figure 2. Sagittal pre-contrast T1WI (A) in a 41-year-old patient with headache and dizziness shows a CSF-like hypointense cerebellar mass (arrow) with an eccentric isointense nodule (arrowhead). Matching post-contrast T1WI (B) shows marked enhancement of the mural nodule (arrowhead), which has a large base at the cerebellar surface. The rest of the mass remains CSF-like, consistent with a cyst. The cyst wall does not enhance.

Figure 3. Axial post-contrast T1WI (A) shows two enhancing lesions (arrows) and a cyst with enhancing mural nodule (arrowhead). Small solid cerebellar tumors are not conspicuous on pre-contrast T1WI (B).

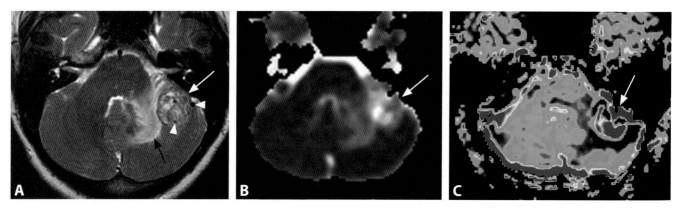

Figure 4. T2WI (A) shows a left cerebellar mass (white arrow) with flow-voids (arrowheads) and adjacent edema (black arrow). The mass (arrow) is bright on ADC map (B) and has high CBV on perfusion MRI (C).

Hemangioblastoma

ZORAN RUMBOLDT AND MARIA GISELE MATHEUS

Specific Imaging Findings

Hemangioblastomas are typically located along the cerebellar surface and their classic appearance is a cystic mass with a mural nodule; however, solid masses with or without internal cysts are frequently encountered. The lesions are spherical and sharply demarcated, with the cystic component being usually CT hypodense, of very low T1 and high T2 signal. The signal of the cyst may vary, based on the protein content, and hemorrhage may be present. The solid tumor is T2 hyperintense and typically abuts the surface of the cerebellum and markedly enhances with contrast, whereas the cystic wall does not enhance. There is moderate to marked surrounding edema. Characteristic vascular flow-voids on MRI are present within larger lesions and best seen on T2WI. Solid portions have high diffusivity and are very bright on ADC maps. Perfusion studies reveal extremely high relative cerebral blood volume. While sporadic hemangioblastomas are found almost exclusively in the cerebellum, these tumors may occur anywhere throughout the CNS in patients with von Hippel–Lindau disease (VHL). The size of the lesion varies from punctate to several centimeters and post-contrast MR images are needed to detect small lesions. Catheter angiography of some hemangioblastomas shows characteristic tightly packed wide vessels and a nodule in the early arterial phase, resembling a "cherry attached to its stalk". The constellation of MRI findings including intralesional flow-voids, contrast enhancement, increased diffusivity, and very high perfusion are diagnostic in most cases.

Pertinent Clinical Information

Familial forms, associated with VHL, often show ocular hemorrhage as the first manifestation. The symptoms are otherwise nonspecific and usually include headache and dizziness. Mean age of presentation is 30 years for familial forms and 40 for sporadic forms. Erythrocytosis and increased erythropoietin levels may be found. Resection and radiosurgery are the treatment options, depending on lesion location, multiplicity and vascularity. Preoperative embolization is a helpful adjuvant procedure for spinal hemangioblastomas, while severe complications (cerebellar infarct, tumor swelling and massive hemorrhage) may occur with cerebellar tumors.

Differential diagnosis

Metastatic Neoplasm (155)
• intralesional flow-voids are exceptionally rare
• solid portions are not bright on ADC maps

Pilocytic Astrocytoma (173)
• absence of flow-voids
• surrounding edema is absent or minimal
• usually affects children
• rCBV may be only mildly increased on perfusion studies

Schwannoma (141)
• absence of flow-voids
• extra-axial mass located along cranial nerves
• rCBV is not elevated on perfusion studies

Arteriovenous Malformation (AVM) (182, 193)
• entangled multiple flow voids without associated solid mass or cyst
• calcifications may be present

Background

Hemangioblastomas are highly vascular benign tumors of uncertain histogenesis, with ultrastructural studies indicating an angioblastic origin. They are characterized by a dense capillary network with intermingled stromal cells. Macroscopically hemangioblastomas can be classified in four subtypes: type 1 presents as a cystic tumor without macroscopic nodule (5%); type 2 as a cyst and mural nodule (60%); type 3 a solid tumor (26%); and type 4 as a solid tumor with small internal cysts (9%). The stromal component of the tumor produces erythropoietin and leads to consequent erythrocytosis.

Of these neoplasms, 20–30% are associated with VHL, an autosomal-dominant disorder characterized by multiple benign and malignant tumors mostly seen in the retina, kidney, adrenal gland, pancreas, epididymis, and endolymphatic sac. Tumors in VHL patients may be found in multiple various supra- and infra-tentorial locations. In a small percentage of patients, hemangioblastomas recur following apparently total surgical excision.

REFERENCES

1. Lee SR, Sanches J, Mark AS, et al. Posterior fossa hemangioblastomas: MR imaging. *Radiology* 1989;**171**:463–8.
2. Quadery FA, Okamoto K. Diffusion-weighted MRI of haemangioblastomas and other cerebellar tumours. *Neuroradiology* 2003;**45**:212–9.
3. Kumar VA, Knopp EA, Zagzag D. Magnetic resonance dynamic susceptibility-weighted contrast-enhanced perfusion imaging in the diagnosis of posterior fossa hemangioblastomas and pilocytic astrocytomas: initial results. *J Comput Assist Tomogr* 2010;**34**:825–9.
4. Butman J, Linehan WM, Russell RL. Neurological manifestations of von Hippel–Lindau disease. *JAMA* 2008;**300**:1334–42.
5. Karabagli H, Genc Ali, Karabagli P, et al. Outcomes of gamma knife treatment for solid intracranial hemangioblastomas. *J Clin Neurosci* 2010;**17**:706–10.

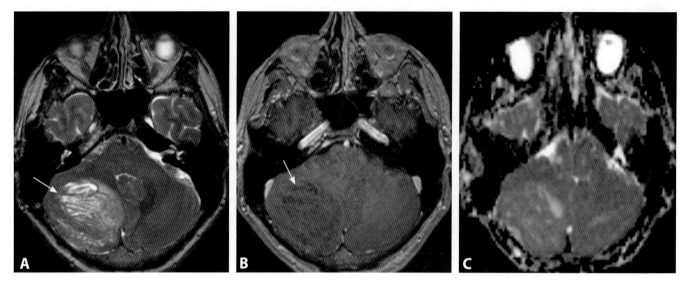

Figure 1. Axial T2WI (A) in a young adult patient with ataxia shows a large right cerebellar hemisphere mass (arrow) with only mild compression of the fourth ventricle. The lesion is of predominantly striated appearance. Post-contrast T1WI (B) shows no enhancement in the slightly hypointense mass (arrow). Corresponding ADC map (C) shows normal to slightly increased diffusivity of the lesion.

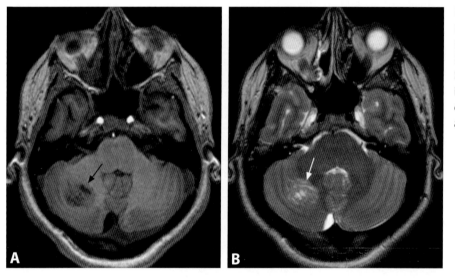

Figure 2. Axial T1WI (A) in a 36-year-old patient with gastrointestinal polyps and oral papillomas demonstrates a right cerebellar lesion (arrow) with internal striations. The lesion exhibits minimal mass effect and there is no surrounding edema. The characteristic corduroy appearance of the mass (arrow) is also seen on axial T2WI at a similar level (B).

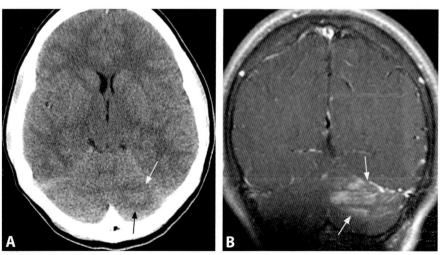

Figure 3. Non-enhanced axial CT image (A) in a patient with headaches shows a subtle abnormality in the superior portion of the left cerebellar hemisphere that has a slightly striped appearance (arrows). Post-contrast T1WI (B) demonstrates "tiger striping" pattern of enhancement (arrows), without notable mass effect of the abnormality.

Lhermitte–Duclos (Cowden Syndrome)

MAURICIO CASTILLO

Specific Imaging Findings

Lhermitte–Duclos disease (LDD) is hypodense on CT and contains slightly hyperdense striations, referred to as "corduroy" or "tiger striping" patterns. It is relatively well-defined and has no surrounding edema. The lesion produces relatively little mass effect for its size but compression on the fourth ventricle may lead to obstructive hydrocephalus. On MRI, the mass is T1 hypointense with striations and its bulk is T2 hyperintense. The characteristic striations tend to have signal intensity similar to the gray matter. The lesions are bright on DWI but without reduced diffusion on ADC maps. Contrast enhancement is rare, has no clinical significance and usually follows the striated appearance. Susceptibility-weighted imaging (SWI) demonstrates large veins and perfusion studies may show elevated relative cerebral blood volume. On MR spectroscopy, choline is normal, creatine and *myo*-inositol levels are increased, *n*-acetyl aspartate is low, and lactate may be present.

Pertinent Clinical Information

All patients with LDD have Cowden syndrome. Other manifestations of this syndrome include: facial trichilemmomas, oral papillomatosis, palmar and plantar keratosis, gastrointestinal polyps, genitourinary malignancies, and hamartomas in the breast and thyroid gland. Most patients are male and although the disease may manifest itself at any age, Lhermitte–Duclos is generally encountered in young adults between 30 and 40 years old. Neurological symptoms may include hydrocephalus, ataxia, and brainstem findings such as multiple cranial nerve problems. The lesions grow very slowly or not at all and when indicated, surgical resection is the treatment of choice. Recurrence is possible after incomplete surgical resection.

Differential Diagnosis

Desmoplastic Medulloblastoma (174)
- nearly all enhance with contrast
- dark on ADC map
- absence of striations

Ganglioglioma (166, 196)
- 50% have calcifications and/or show contrast enhancement
- absence of striations

Background

Lhermitte–Duclos disease is also referred to as dysplastic gangliocytoma of the cerebellum and is the CNS hallmark of Cowden syndrome. Overall, this lesion is very rare and occurs exclusively in the cerebellum. Histologically it is benign (WHO grade I) and composed of abnormal ganglion cells and hypertrophy of the granular cell layer of the cerebellar cortex. Some authors consider it to be a hamartoma that produces mass effect. Parallel linear striations on the surface of the lesion on imaging studies represent dysplastic cerebellar folia. The syndrome is autosomal dominant and due to an abnormality in chromosome 10 that leads to mutation of the *PTEN* gene. Increased uptake of FDG and 201-thallium may be seen on nuclear medicine studies; however, no malignant transformation of LDD has been reported.

REFERENCES

1. Thomas B, Krishnamoorthy T, Radhakrishnan VV, Kesavadas C. Advanced MR imaging in Lhermitte–Duclos disease: moving closer to pathology and pathophysiology. *Neuroradiology* 2007; **49**:733–8.

2. Klisch J, Juengling F, Spreer J, et al. Lhermitte–Duclos disease: assessment with MR imaging, positron emission tomography, single-photon emission CT, and MR spectroscopy. *AJNR* 2001; **22**:824–30.

3. Awwad EE, Levy E, Martin DS, Merenda GO. Atypical MR appearance of Lhermitte–Duclos disease with contrast enhancement. *AJNR* 1995;**16**:1719–20.

4. Williams DW 3rd, Elster AD, Ginsberg LE, Stanton C. Recurrent Lhermitte–Duclos disease: report of two cases and association with Cowden's disease. *AJNR* 1992;**13**:287–90.

5. Hayasaka K, Nihashi T, Takebayashi S, Bundoh M. FDG PET in Lhermitte–Duclos disease. *Clin Nucl Med* 2008;**33**:52–4.

Brain Imaging with MRI and CT, ed. Zoran Rumboldt *et al.* Published by Cambridge University Press. © Cambridge University Press 2012.

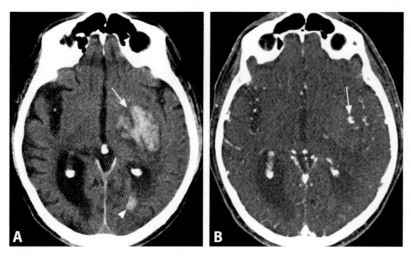

Figure 1. Non-enhanced axial CT image (A) shows an irregular hyperdense mass (arrow) in the left basal ganglia with thin surrounding hypodensity. There is also intraventricular hyperdense material (arrowhead). Source CTA image (B) reveals the "spot sign" of contrast extravasation (arrow).

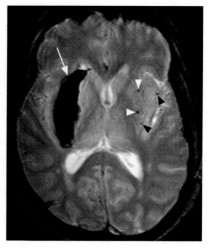

Figure 2. T2*WI in another patient shows right putaminal hematoma (arrow) and contralateral punctate areas of signal loss (arrowheads), consistent with microhemorrhages.

Figure 3. Axial T2WI (A) shows a right thalamic hypointense acute hematoma within a hyperintense ring (arrow), corresponding to extruded serum and edema. There is a characteristic bright artifactual ring (arrow) on matching DWI (B). Coronal post-contrast T1WI (C) reveals subtle hypointensity of the hematoma (arrow) with linear areas of peripheral enhancement (arrowheads).

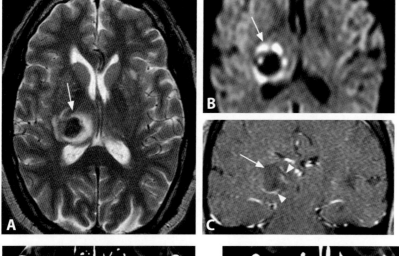

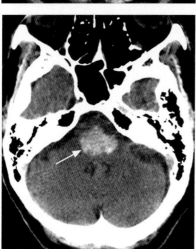

Figure 4. Non-enhanced CT shows pontine hyperdense lesion (arrow) consistent with acute hematoma.

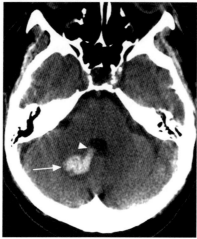

Figure 5. Cerebellar white matter hematoma (arrow) extends into the fourth ventricle (arrowhead) on non-enhanced CT.

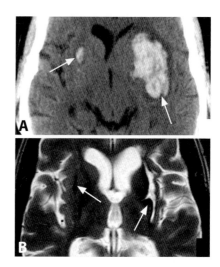

Figure 6. Bilateral putaminal hematomas (arrows): acute on CT (A), chronic slit-like lesions with dark rim on T2WI (B).

Hypertensive Hematoma

ZORAN RUMBOLDT

Specific Imaging Findings

The imaging modality in the acute setting is usually CT, which reveals hyperdense mass typically in one of the following locations: basal ganglia, thalamus, central pons, and medial cerebellum. It is primarily the location that allows for hypertensive hematoma characterization on imaging, as blood products have the same appearance irrespective of the etiology. A clot forms after the extravasation of blood, with progressively increasing density over the first 3 days, caused by clot retraction with extrusion of the hypodense serum. This low attenuation surrounding the clot increases in size with development of vasogenic edema. Ring contrast enhancement may be observed around the hematoma. Hypertensive hematomas typically dissect the brain without a considerable amount of associated tissue necrosis, so that chronic lesions are transformed into slit-like hypodense cavities, with a rim of very low T2 signal caused by hemosiderin deposition. MRI is more sensitive than CT for parenchymal hemorrhage, primarily with T2*-weighted images, which frequently demonstrate additional multifocal small hypointensities, corresponding to hemosiderin from previous microhemorrhages. Contrast extravasation on CTA, known as spot sign, predicts hematoma expansion.

Pertinent Clinical Information

Hypertensive bleeds more commonly occur in males, on average at around 55 years of age. Rapid elevation of blood pressure is the main predisposing factor, and drugs such as cocaine and amphetamine are commonly responsible in younger individuals. The presenting symptoms depend on the location: confusion and hemiparesis in basal ganglia and thalamus, cranial nerve deficits and coma in pons, and nausea and vomiting in cerebellum. Prognosis is highly variable and depends on the size and location of the bleed. Overall mortality is in the range of 20–70% and can be predicted by contrast extravasation on CT. Dissection of hematoma into the ventricular system may lead to hydrocephalus and is associated with poor prognosis. Recombinant activated factor VII is beneficial for large hematomas, while surgical evacuation is considered if brain herniation occurs.

Differential Diagnosis

Amyloid Hemorrhage (178)
- elderly patients
- usually large hemorrhages with relatively small mass effect
- lobar location
- fluid level may be present in the hemorrhage within 24 h

Ischemic Infarct with Hemorrhagic Transformation
- shows a vascular distribution
- typically involves an area of both the cortex and white matter
- round or oval shape is very unusual

Arteriovenous Malformation (AVM) (182, 193)
- presence of calcifications/hyperdensities on CT
- abnormal vascular flow-voids on T2WI
- large draining veins and arterial feeders may be seen

Hemorrhagic Neoplasm (Metastatic) (180)
- typically prominent large surrounding edema
- areas of nodular contrast enhancement are frequently present

Deep Venous Thrombosis (11)
- typically bilateral thalamic hemorrhages
- thrombosed veins are seen

Cortical Contusion (179)
- characteristically superficial in the anterior basal frontal and temporal lobes
- following trauma

Background

Intraparenchymal hemorrhage accounts for approximately 10–15% of all strokes and hypertension is the presumed cause in a majority of cases. Systemic hypertension weakens the vessel walls, which then become prone to rupture in the setting of an acute elevation of the blood pressure. Hypertensive hemorrhages typically occur in areas supplied by penetrating vessels with the most common locations being lentiform nucleus (especially putamen, around 65%), thalamus (about 20%), pons (5–10%), and medial cerebellum (around 5%). Subcortical cerebral white matter is an atypical site, encountered in about 1% of cases. Microaneurysms of small perforating arteries, known as Charcot–Bouchard aneurysms, have been traditionally implicated in genesis of these hematomas. Re-evaluation with modern histopathologic techniques showed that these microaneurysms are distinctly uncommon and probably only rarely responsible for hypertensive hemorrhages.

REFERENCES

1. Kim J, Smith A, Hemphill JC 3rd, *et al*. Contrast extravasation on CT predicts mortality in primary intracerebral hemorrhage. *AJNR* 2008;**29**:520–5.
2. Smith EE, Nandigam KR, Chen YW, *et al*. MRI markers of small vessel disease in lobar and deep hemispheric intracerebral hemorrhage. *Stroke* 2010;**41**:1933–8.
3. Greer DM, Koroshetz WJ, Cullen S, *et al*. Magnetic resonance imaging improves detection of intracerebral hemorrhage over computed tomography after intra-arterial thrombolysis. *Stroke* 2004;**35**:491–5.
4. Challa VR, Moody DM, Bell MA. The Charcot–Bouchard aneurysm controversy: impact of a new histologic technique. *J Neuropathol Exp Neurol* 1992;**51**:264–71.
5. Rumboldt Z. Intracranial hemorrhages. In: *Neuroradiology* (Third Series) Test and Syllabus. Castillo M, ed. American College of Radiology, Reston, VA, 2006;158–80.

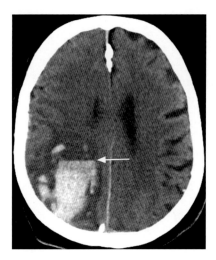

Figure 1. Non-enhanced CT shows a right parietal hyperdense mass consistent with acute hemorrhage with a small surrounding hypodensity. Note fluid level (arrow) and a relatively mild mass effect.

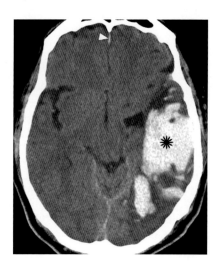

Figure 2. Non-enhanced CT in a 72-year-old woman with sudden neurologic deficit shows a large left temporo-parietal hemorrhage (*) with subdural extension (arrowhead) and relatively minimal mass effect.

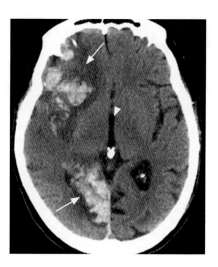

Figure 3. CT without contrast in another patient reveals two lobar hemorrhages (arrows) in the right cerebral hemisphere with mild mass effect. There is minimal displacement of the third ventricle (arrowheads).

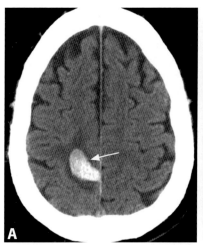

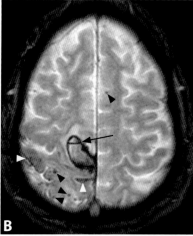

Figure 4. Non-enhanced axial CT image (A) shows an acute superficial right fronto-parietal hemorrhage (arrow) with a small amount of surrounding edema. Corresponding gradient echo T2*WI (B) better shows a fluid level (arrow) within the hemorrhage. There are also dark punctate cortico-subcortical microhemorrhages (black arrowheads) and superficial siderosis (white arrowheads).

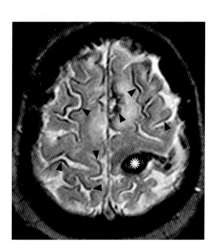

Figure 5. T2*WI reveals low signal of diffuse superficial siderosis (arrowheads) and a small hematoma in the left post-central gyrus (*).

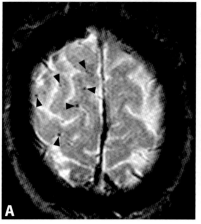

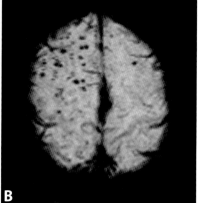

Figure 6. Axial T2*WI with gradient echo sequence (A) shows multiple cortico-subcortical punctate hypointensities (arrowheads). Susceptibility-weighted T2*WI (SWI; B) demonstrates greater conspicuity of the lesions with increased number and size of the microbleeds.

Amyloid Hemorrhage – Cerebral Amyloid Angiopathy

ZORAN RUMBOLDT

Specific Imaging Findings

Cerebral amyloid angiopathy (CAA) typically presents in patients over 60 years of age with hemorrhages that are characteristically superficial, large, and lobar. They usually involve the cortex and subjacent white matter of the frontal and parietal lobes, with relatively minimal associated mass effect. The hemorrhage often extends to the subarachnoid and subdural spaces. Multiple hemorrhages of different ages and even multiple simultaneous bleeds may be seen. The blood products within the hematoma tend to sediment posteriorly, frequently giving the appearance of fluid levels. All these acute findings are well seen on CT images. The other characteristic feature of CAA are punctuate cortico-subcortical hypointensities on T2*-weighted images that correspond to chronic microhemorrhages. The sensitivity for microbleeds can be further increased with thin sections and susceptibility-weighted imaging (SWI). Superficial siderosis also occurs with high prevalence, and CAA is one of the most common causes of non-traumatic cortical subarachnoid hemorrhage. MRI is best suited for identification of small or chronic hemorrhages, exclusion of other causes, and assessment of disease progression.

Pertinent Clinical Information

CAA is probably the most common cause of spontaneous intracerebral hemorrhage after 70 years of age, and may be responsible for up to 10% of all nontraumatic intraparenchymal hemorrhages, with female predominance. There is a propensity for multiple and recurrent hemorrhages, and mortality is relatively low. However, many cases of CAA are asymptomatic. The diagnosis is established according to Boston criteria, with probable CAA defined as multiple T2*WI microbleeds restricted to lobar cortico-subcortical regions in patients ≥ 55 years old. Dementia, primarily Alzheimer's disease, and Down's syndrome are associated with CAA.

Differential Diagnosis

Hypertensive Hematoma (177)
- characteristically arising within putamen, thalamus, pons, and cerebellar white matter
- microbleeds typically in the deep gray and white matter

Ischemic Infarct with Hemorrhagic Transformation
- shows a vascular distribution
- more prominent mass effect

Arteriovenous Malformation (AVM) (182, 193)
- presence of calcifications/hyperdensities on CT
- abnormal vascular flow-voids on T2WI
- large draining veins and arterial feeders may be seen

Hemorrhagic Neoplasm (Metastatic) (180)
- typically prominent large surrounding edema
- areas of nodular contrast enhancement are frequently present

Cortical Contusion (179)
- characteristically superficial in the anterior basal frontal and temporal lobes
- following trauma

Cortical Vein Thrombosis (181)
- edema or hemorrhage usually subcortical
- thrombosed cortical vein or dural venous thrombosis may be seen

Cavernous Hemangiomas (183, 193)
- characteristic central "popcorn" T2 and T1 hyperintensity with T2 dark rim
- tiny ones show only signal loss on T2*WI and may be indistinguishable from microhemorrhages

Diffuse Axonal Injury (114)
- signal loss on T2*WI is in a characteristic distribution (corpus callosum, paramedian gray–white matter junction, dorsolateral brainstem), frequently linear
- chronic hemorrhagic injuries may be indistinguishable from other microhemorrhages

Background

CAA results from deposition of beta-amyloid, an insoluble extracellular protein, within the media and adventitia of small and medium-sized vessels of the cerebral cortex and leptomeninges. It has no association with systemic amyloidosis. Fibrinoid degeneration and microaneurysms are revealed on histologic examination. These changes lead to loss of elasticity and increased fragility of the affected vessels. Amyloid is detected with Congored stain by apple-green birefringence under polarized light. Amyloid deposition increases with age and is associated with microbleeds on T2*WI, but has no correlation with hypertension.

CAA may very rarely form white matter masses, known as amyloidomas, which tend to be CT hyperdense and enhance with contrast. MRI appearances are variable, from hyper- to hypointense on both T1- and T2-weighted images.

REFERENCES

1. Chao CP, Kotsenas AL, Broderick DF. Cerebral amyloid angiopathy: CT and MR imaging findings. *Radiographics* 2006;**26**:1517–31.
2. Miller JH, Wardlaw JM, Lammie GA. Intracerebral haemorrhage and cerebral amyloid angiopathy: CT features with pathological correlation. *Clin Radiol* 1999;**54**:422–9.
3. Linn J, Halpin A, Demaerel P, *et al*. Prevalence of superficial siderosis in patients with cerebral amyloid angiopathy. *Neurology* 2010;**74**:1346–50.
4. Dierksen GA, Skehan ME, Khan MA, *et al*. Spatial relation between microbleeds and amyloid deposits in amyloid angiopathy. *Ann Neurol* 2010;**68**:545–8.
5. Rumboldt Z. Intracranial hemorrhages. In: *Neuroradiology (Third Series) Test and Syllabus.* Castillo M, ed. American College of Radiology, Reston, VA, 2006;158–80.

Brain Imaging with MRI and CT, ed. Zoran Rumboldt *et al.* Published by Cambridge University Press. © Cambridge University Press 2012.

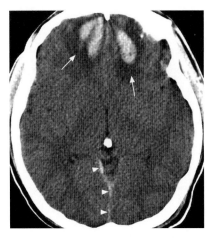

Figure 1. Non-enhanced CT shows bifrontal peripheral hemorrhages with surrounding edema (arrows), and subdural hematoma along the falx and tentorium (arrowheads).

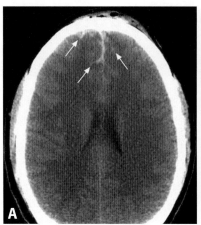
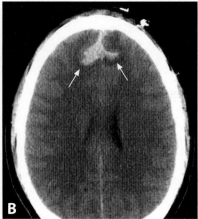

Figure 2. Initial non-enhanced CT image (A) in a different patient shows subtle anterior bifrontal hyperdensities (arrows), consistent with blood products, likely a combination of subarachnoid, subdural and cortical hemorrhages. Corresponding CT image obtained on the next day (B) reveals now prominent bilateral parafalcine hemorrhages with surrounding edema (arrows).

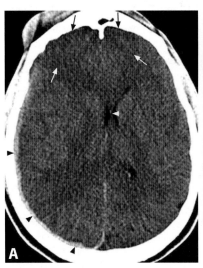
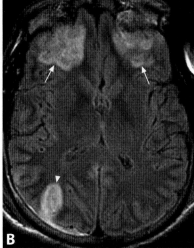

Figure 3. Non-enhanced CT (A) shows very subtle bilateral frontal hypodensity with loss of normal gray–white matter distinction (arrows). There is a right subdural hematoma (black arrowheads) and associated leftward midline shift with displaced septum pellucidum (white arrowhead). On FLAIR image (B) the nonhemorrhagic bifrontal lesions (arrows) are much more conspicuous, as is a right parieto-occipital lesion (arrowhead) just beneath the subdural hematoma.

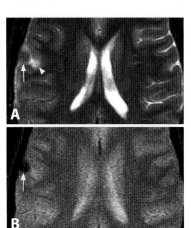

Figure 4. T2WI (A) shows subtle peripheral hypointensity (arrow) with surrounding edema (arrowhead). T2*WI (B) reveals signal loss (arrow) from blood products.

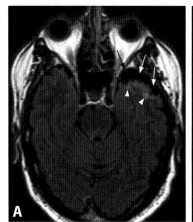
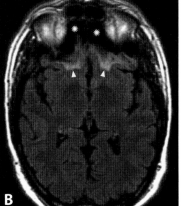

Figure 5. Chronic lesion years after trauma is depicted on axial FLAIR image (A) as left anterior temporal CSF-like encephalomalacia (arrows) with adjacent hyperintense gliosis (arrowheads). A more cranial image (B) shows additional bifrontal encephalomalacia (*) and surrounding gliosis (arrowheads).

Cortical Contusion

BENJAMIN HUANG

Specific Imaging Findings

Hemorrhagic cortical contusions on CT appear as ovoid hyperdensities centered at a gyral surface, characteristically located in the antero-inferior frontal and temporal lobes. It may be quite difficult to differentiate small contusions from streak artifacts and multiplanar reconstructions from spiral acquisitions can be very helpful. Early nonhemorrhagic contusions appear as very subtle hypodensities, but generally become conspicuous days later when significant edema develops. Hemorrhagic contusions often increase in size within the first 48 h, and nonhemorrhagic contusions can develop delayed hemorrhage. As hemorrhage and edema resolve over several weeks, contusions become less conspicuous but may leave a region of hypodense encephalomalacia. On MRI, nonhemorrhagic contusions are T1 hypointense and T2 hyperintense, usually with reduced diffusion. Acute hemorrhagic contusions will appear T1 isointense and T2 hypointense with a surrounding halo of edema, which often increases during the first week. T2*-weighted imaging better shows small hemorrhages as dark lesions. Contusions follow evolution of intra-axial hematomas and marginal enhancement can also be seen. Lesions can exhibit persistent high T1 and T2 signal for up to a year with a peripheral rim of low signal caused by hemosiderin and ferritin. Encephalomalacia with surrounding gliosis, best seen on FLAIR images as peripheral CSF-like intensity with subjacent hyperintensity, is the hallmark of contusions in the chronic stage.

Pertinent Clinical Information

Cortical contusions are the most common parenchymal brain injuries, identified in 5–10% of patients with moderate to severe head trauma. They tend to be more severe when associated with skull fractures and less severe in patients presenting with a lucid interval after injury. Contusions without significant mass effect typically result in better outcomes than diffuse axonal injury; however, they are associated with a high risk of post-traumatic epilepsy.

Differential Diagnosis

Diffuse Axonal Injury (114)
- typically at the corticomedullary junction, corpus callosum, dorsolateral brainstem

Hypertensive Hemorrhage (177)
- characteristically centered in the putamen, thalamus, pons, or dentate nucleus

Amyloid Hemorrhage (178)
- occurs in elderly patients
- usually large hemorrhages with relatively small mass effect

Traumatic Subarachnoid Hemorrhage
- frequently in association with cortical contusions, may be indistinguishable early on
- follows cortical sulci rather than being located at the crowns of gyri

Cortical Vein Thrombosis (181)
- edema or hemorrhage usually subcortical
- thrombosed cortical vein (cord sign) or dural venous thrombosis may be seen

Infarct with Hemorrhagic Transformation
- shows a vascular distribution

Background

Cortical contusions are bruises of the brain's surface and are characterized histologically by necrosis and hemorrhage of the cortex and leptomeninges. Bleeding into the Virchow–Robin spaces produces linear hemorrhages oriented perpendicular to the pial surfaces of the gyri, which may extend to the cortical surface and into the CSF. Contusions result from either a forceful impact or translational movement between the brain and the overlying skull or skull base and therefore involve the superficial gray matter while relatively sparing the adjacent white matter. Injury patterns vary depending upon whether the patient's head is stationary or moving at the moment of impact, and the terms "coup" and "contrecoup" are traditionally used to describe contusions. Coup injuries commonly occur when the head is stationary and are found at the site of cranial impact. Contrecoup injuries typically occur when the head is accelerating and impacts against an unyielding surface, and are found on the side of the brain opposite the site of impact, with the inferior frontal lobes and temporal poles being particularly vulnerable. Additionally, contusions are also common along the inferior surfaces of the frontal and temporal lobes, presumably due to translational movement of the brain across the rough bony contours of the anterior and middle cranial fossae. Rarely, closed head injuries may result in so-called intermediary hemorrhages of the basal ganglia and thalami, which are presumed to be due to shearing of the perforating vessels supplying these structures.

REFERENCES

1. Hardman JM, Manoukian A. Pathology of head trauma. *Neuroimag Clin N Am* 2002;**12**:175–87.
2. Provenzale J. CT and MR imaging of acute cranial trauma. *Emerg Radiol* 2007;**14**:1–12.
3. Young RJ, Destian S. Imaging of traumatic intracranial hemorrhage. *Neuroimag Clin N Am* 2002;**12**:189–204.
4. Kim JJ, Gean AD. Imaging for the diagnosis and management of traumatic brain injury. *Neurotherapeutics* 2011;**8**:39–53.

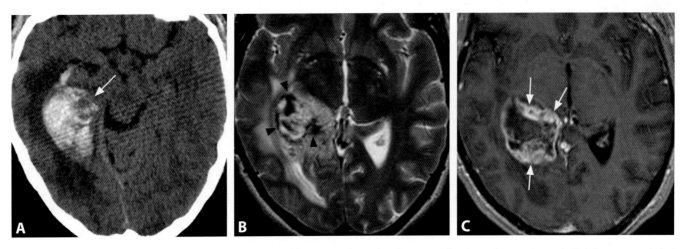

Figure 1. Unenhanced CT image (A) shows a right temporal hematoma (arrow) with surrounding hypodense edema. A slightly more cephalad T2WI (B) reveals heterogeneous signal within the lesion with irregular and discontinuous hemosiderin ring (arrowheads). Corresponding post-contrast T1WI (C) shows irregular and in places nodular (arrows) peripheral enhancement of the lesion.

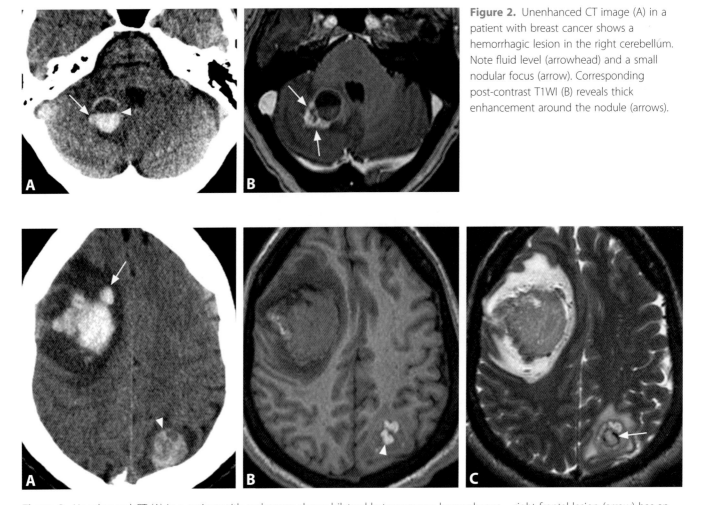

Figure 2. Unenhanced CT image (A) in a patient with breast cancer shows a hemorrhagic lesion in the right cerebellum. Note fluid level (arrowhead) and a small nodular focus (arrow). Corresponding post-contrast T1WI (B) reveals thick enhancement around the nodule (arrows).

Figure 3. Unenhanced CT (A) in a patient with melanoma shows bilateral heterogenous hemorrhages – right frontal lesion (arrow) has an irregular, lobulated contour; left parietal hematoma (arrowhead) is slightly darker and likely to be older. Corresponding pre-contrast T1WI (B) and T2WI (C) show iso- to slightly hyperintense signal in the frontal lesion, indicating more acute hemorrhage. The left parietal lesion contains predominantly central T1 hyperintense areas (arrowhead) suggesting subacute clot (methemoglobin), and concentric internal ring of low T2 signal (arrow) suggesting repeated hemorrhages (hemosiderin).

Hemorrhagic Neoplasms

BENJAMIN HUANG

Specific Imaging Findings

Tumoral intracranial hemorrhages can be difficult to distinguish from more common spontaneous hemorrhages, primarily due to hypertension, amyloid angiopathy, vascular malformations, or venous thrombosis. Features of an acute hemorrhage which favor the presence of an underlying tumor include a complex and heterogeneous appearance, the presence of a nonhemorrhagic mass within or adjacent to the hematoma, multiplicity (suggesting hemorrhagic metastases), and areas of nodular post-contrast enhancement. On CT neoplastic hemorrhages will be heterogeneously hyperdense acutely, and will occasionally demonstrate fluid levels if hemorrhage extends into a cystic portion of a tumor (fluid levels may notably be also seen with amyloid bleeds). The presence of enhancement within or adjacent to a hemorrhage on either CT or MRI is strongly suggestive of an underlying neoplasm, but contrast enhancement may be absent, particularly if the tumor is small and/or compressed or replaced by the hematoma. Evolution of blood products' signal characteristics on MRI tends to be delayed in neoplastic hemorrhages compared to the other etiologies. In the subacute stage, the T1 hyperintensity due to the presence of methemoglobin tends to be centrally located, just the opposite from nontumoral bleeds in which increased signal begins at the periphery and progresses inward. In addition, while edema surrounding other hemorrhages usually begins resolving within a week, edema will persist in the presence of a neoplasm. Lack of a complete hemosiderin ring around the periphery of a resolving hematoma after a few weeks is suggestive of tumor, but this is an inconsistent finding.

Pertinent Clinical Information

The frequency of spontaneous hemorrhage in intracranial neoplasms is roughly 2–3%, and approximately 7% of all non-traumatic intracranial hemorrhages are tumor related. These hemorrhages present most frequently in the sixth decade, but they can occur at any age. In roughly half of these patients, hemorrhage may be the initial presentation of the tumors. Symptoms related to tumoral hemorrhages are nonspecific and depend upon the size and location of the lesions. Decreased level of consciousness, hemiparesis, headache, nausea and vomiting, seizures, imbalance, and visual field defects are more commonly encountered. If any uncertainty exists regarding the etiology of an intracranial hemorrhage, follow-up imaging at 3–6 weeks – after the hematoma has largely resolved – should be performed.

Differential Diagnosis

Hypertensive Hemorrhage (177)
- typical locations are putamen, thalamus, pons, and medial cerebellar hemispheres
- homogeneous with predictable evolution of MR signal changes
- minimal to no enhancement

Amyloid Angiopathy (178)
- typically large lobar bleed in senior individuals with minimal mass effect
- evidence of other hemispheric microhemorrhages on T2* MR imaging
- subarachnoid hemorrhage may be present
- minimal to no enhancement

Hemorrhagic Vascular Malformation (182, 183, 193)
- abnormal flow-voids on T2WI in AVMs
- T1 hyperintensity within the edema may be present with cavernomas

Venous Thrombosis (181)
- evidence of intraluminal clot, may be confirmed with MRV or CTV

Hemorrhagic Transformation of Ischemic Infarction
- evidence of infarcted tissue surrounding the hematoma
- shows a vascular distribution

Background

Hemorrhage can arise within both primary and metastatic tumors. Among primary tumors the most likely to hemorrhage is glioblastoma, but oligodendrogliomas, lower-grade astrocytomas (including pilocytic astrocytomas), ependymomas, choroid plexus papillomas, schwannomas, and meningiomas may also present with hemorrhage. Metastases with the greatest propensity to hemorrhage include primarily melanoma, followed by renal cell carcinoma and choriocarcinoma, but virtually any type of metastasis can exhibit hemorrhage. A number of factors contribute to the development of intratumoral bleeding including the rate of neoplastic growth, tumor vascularity, presence of vascular invasion, tissue infarction and necrosis, and fibrinolysis. Signal heterogeneity and delayed temporal evolution of tumoral hemorrhage have been attributed to continued oozing of fresh blood from the neoplasm, relatively oxygen-poor intratumoral environment, and the rapid absorption of hemoglobin breakdown products within the tumor.

REFERENCES
1. Destian S, Sze G, Krol G, et al. MR imaging of hemorrhagic intracranial neoplasms. AJR 1989;152:137–44.
2. Scrader B, Barth H, Lang EW, et al. Spontaneous intracranial haematomas caused by neoplasms. Acta Neurochir (Wien) 2000;142:979–85.
3. Fischbein NJ, Wijman CA. Nontraumatic intracranial hemorrhage. Neuroimaging Clin N Am 2010;20:469–92.
4. White JB, Piepgras DG, Scheithauer BW, et al. Rate of spontaneous hemorrhage in histologically proven cases of pilocytic astrocytoma. J Neurosurg 2008;108:223–6.

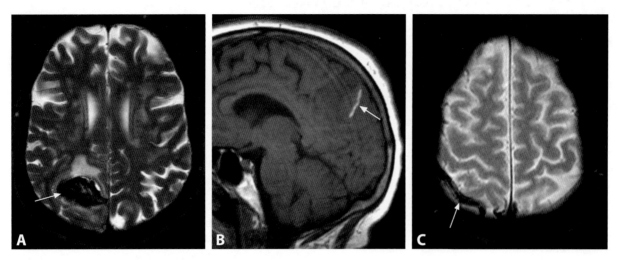

Figure 1. Axial T2WI (A) shows acute (dark due to deoxyhemoglobin) hematoma (arrow) in the right parietal region in a non-arterial distribution. Sagittal T1WI (B) demonstrates a linear hyperintensity (arrow) due to subacute clot. Axial T2*WI image (C) shows a sulcal dark cord (arrow) along the right parietal convexity.

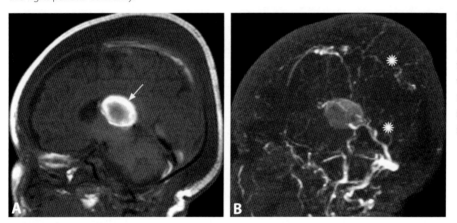

Figure 2. Sagittal T1WI without contrast (A) in a baby shows oval hyperintensity of early subacute blood (methemoglobin) in a thalamus (arrow). Lateral MIP image from MR venogram without contrast shows absence of normal flow-related signal in the major structures of superficial and deep venous systems (*).

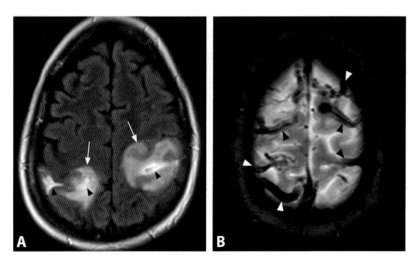

Figure 3. Axial FLAIR image (A) shows bilateral fronto-parietal hemorrhages (arrowheads) with surrounding edema (arrows). Axial T2*WI at a more cephalad level (B) shows bilateral dark superficial structures (arrows head) corresponding to cortical veins along the convexity.

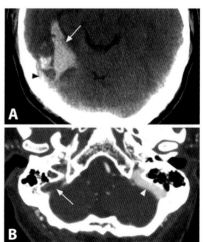

Figure 4. Non-enhanced CT (A) shows parenchymal hemorrhage (arrow) and hyperdensity (arrowhead) in the transverse sinus location. CTA image (B) reveals no enhancement of the right sigmoid sinus (arrow). Normal left sigmoid sinus (arrowhead).

CASE 181

Hemorrhagic Venous Thrombosis

MAURICIO CASTILLO AND BENJAMIN HUANG

Specific Imaging Findings

The thrombosed cortical vein may be hyperdense on non-contrast CT or T1 bright on MRI. The underlying cortex may be edematous and occasionally adjacent subarachnoid hemorrhage is seen. The thrombosed vein is best demonstrated on T2* gradient echo and susceptibility-weighted sequences as an area of signal void. On FLAIR, the thrombus may be hyperintense, as is the underlying swollen cortex. Once hemorrhage occurs, the clot is obviously dense on CT and its MRI signal features vary according to its age. Isolated subarachnoid hemorrhage without parenchymal clots is occasionally seen. A hemorrhage in a non-arterial distribution involving both gray and white matter in a younger patient should raise the suspicion of a thrombosed cortical vein with secondary hemorrhage.

Pertinent Clinical Information

Most patients are adults who present with nonspecific clinical symptoms leading to delays in the appropriate diagnosis. The most common symptom is headache accompanied by signs of increased intracranial pressure. Once an infarct and/or hemorrhage occur, seizures frequently follow. Other symptoms such as altered mental status and paresis may also be present. The main risk factors are hypercoagulable states, pregnancy and malignant tumors. Because of its association with pregnancy, oral contraceptives, and smoking, venous thrombosis is more common in females, particularly younger ones. In children, dehydration due to fever and diarrhea and/or vomiting is the most commonly implicated cause. Patients with the syndrome of intracranial hypotension are also at risk for cortical vein thrombosis.

Differential Diagnosis

Vasculitis (123)
- infarctions and/or cortical subarachnoid hemorrhage may be present
- characteristic scattered leptomeningeal/cortical enhancement in some cases
- vascular studies may be diagnostic

Amyloid Hemorrhage (178)
- large lobar bleeds with minimal associated mass effect
- possible fluid–fluid level
- older patients
- intact venous structures

Hypertensive Hematoma (177)
- typically occurs in characteristic locations
- intact venous structures

Hemorrhagic Neoplasm (180)
- abnormal contrast enhancement frequently present on MRI
- infiltrative edema with primary brain tumors

AVM (182, 193)
- abnormal flow-voids of the nidus and/or enlarged draining veins
- possible calcifications

Cavernoma (183, 193)
- T1 hyperintensity within the edema may be present
- calcifications may be found

Background

For hemorrhage to occur, cortical or deep vein thrombosis must be present. Hemorrhage does not occur if the thrombosis is limited to the superficial venous sinuses. Cortical vein thromboses account for 1% of stroke presentations and about 40% of them will be hemorrhagic. The cause of thrombosis is identified in about 75% of cases (most common: trauma, infection, coagulopathies, pregnancy, contraceptives, cancer, metabolic, collagen-vascular disorders, ulcerative colitis, and drug-induced) and remains unknown in 25% of patients. Clot in the superficial venous sinuses results in symptoms of increased intracranial pressure, but may extend into the adjacent cortical veins producing focal symptoms. Once a cortical vein is occluded by clot, its intrinsic pressure increases leading to breakdown of the blood–brain barrier and vessel wall resulting in cerebral edema and hematoma with or without infarction. Nonhemorrhagic parenchymal abnormalities associated with cerebral venous thrombosis (CVT) have variable appearances on diffusion MR imaging and even large areas with reduced ADC values may be reversible. The treatment of CVT is systemic anticoagulation even if hemorrhage is present. Mortality is over 10%, morbidity rates vary between 40 and 80%, and there is a high rate of recurrence. Endovascular thrombectomy, in conjunction with systemic anticoagulation, is an alternative strategy in patients with deterioration on heparin therapy or in those who are moribund on presentation.

REFERENCES

1. Röttger C, Trittmacher S, Gerriets T, *et al*. Reversible MR imaging abnormalities following cerebral venous thrombosis. *AJNR* 2005; **26**:607–13.
2. Mullins ME, Grant PE, Wang B, *et al*. Parenchymal abnormalities associated with cerebral venous sinus thrombosis: assessment with diffusion-weighted MR imaging. *AJNR* 2004;**25**:1666–75.
3. Chang R, Friedman DP. Isolated cortical venous thrombosis presenting as subarachnoid hemorrhage: a report of three cases. *AJNR* 2004;**25**:1676–9.
4. Linn J, Pfefferkorn T, Ivanicova K, *et al*. Noncontrast CT in deep cerebral venous thrombosis and sinus thrombosis: comparison of its diagnostic value for both entities. *AJNR* 2009;**30**:728–35.
5. Ferro JM, Canhão P, Stam J, *et al*. Prognosis of cerebral vein and dural sinus thrombosis: results of the International Study on Cerebral Vein and Dural Sinus Thrombosis (ISCVT). *Stroke* 2004;**35**:664–70.

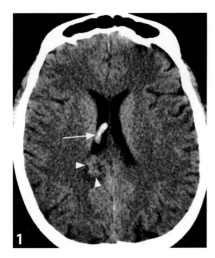

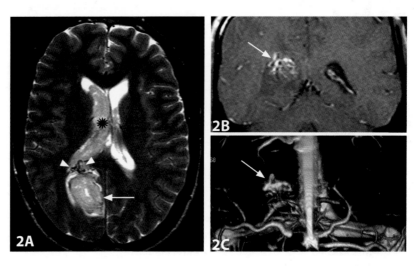

Figure 1. Non-enhanced CT shows intraventricular hemorrhage (arrow) and an adjacent periventricular heterogenous hyperdense lesion (arrowheads).

Figure 2. Axial T2WI (A) shows a parenchymal hematoma (arrow) with intraventricular extension (*) and adjacent abnormal flow-voids (arrowheads). A tangle of abnormal vessels (arrow) is seen on post-contrast images: coronal T1WI with fat-sat (B) and even better on volume rendering of MR venogram (C).

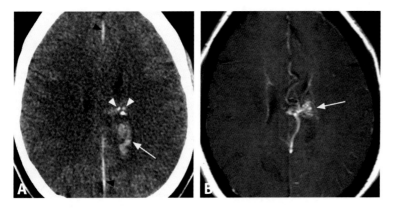

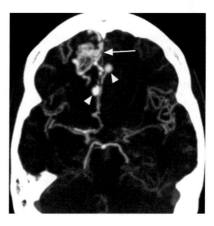

Figure 3. Non-enhanced CT (A) shows a parenchymal bleed (arrow) with subdural extension (black arrowheads) and adjacent punctuate calcifications, which correspond to abnormal vascular structures (arrow) on post-contrast T1WI (B).

Figure 4. Axial CTA MIP image shows a tangle of abnormal vessels (arrow) and aneurysms (arrowheads) on its feeders.

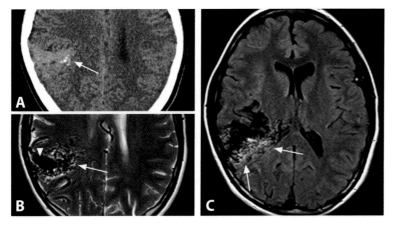

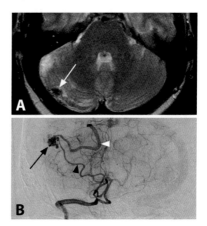

Figure 5. Non-enhanced CT (A) shows a subtle hyperdense abnormality in the right cerebral hemisphere with punctuate calcifications (arrow). Corresponding T2WI (B) reveals multiple abnormal flow-voids (arrow) and a large draining vein (arrowhead). FLAIR at a lower level (C) shows bright perilesional gliosis (arrows).

Figure 6. Axial T2WI (A) shows a focus of right cerebellar flow-voids (arrow). Frontal DSA view of right vertebral artery injection (B) reveals the nidus (arrow), feeding artery (black arrowhead), and draining vein (white arrowhead).

Arteriovenous Malformation

ZORAN RUMBOLDT

Specific Imaging Findings

Cerebral arteriovenous malformations (AVMs) typically present with intracranial, primarily parenchymal, hemorrhage. In most cases a small iso- or slightly hyperdense nodular or tubular defect along the periphery of hemorrhage may be seen on non-enhanced CT, with enhancement on post-contrast images. AVMs without hemorrhage may show irregular hyperdense to calcified areas with contrast enhancement on CT. MRI is the modality of choice for AVM detection, showing the pathognomonic tangle of serpiginous flow-voids, also named "bag of worms", which is best seen on T2-weighted images. The abnormal flow-voids are typically present adjacent to the hematoma in ruptured AVMs. AVM nidus commonly also enhances with contrast. CTA shows enlarged feeding arteries, the nidus, and draining veins. Routine 3D TOF MRA may demonstrate large feeders, while MR venograms better depict the nidus and draining veins. Findings associated with the risk of future hemorrhage include evidence of previous bleed, intranidal aneurysms, venous stenosis, deep venous drainage, and deep nidus location. Secondary effects of brain AVMs that lead to nonhemorrhagic neurologic deficits include edema from venous congestion (due to stenosis and thrombosis), gliosis, arterial steal (with large shunts), and hydrocephalus (from compression).

Pertinent Clinical Information

AVMs usually become evident through intracranial hemorrhage in young adults. Other typical presentations include seizures, progressive neurological deficits, and headaches. The risk of hemorrhage depends on localization and previous bleeding, estimated at 1–4% per year. Therapeutic options comprise microsurgery (primarily for superficially located lesions), radiosurgery, and endovascular embolisation, allowing effective multidisciplinary treatment. It often takes years for complete obliteration following radiosurgery. Spontaneous occlusion occurs in a small percentage of cases. Incidentally diagnosed AVM requires a thorough and individual consideration of treatment indications.

Differential Diagnosis

Developmental Venous Anomaly (DVA) (127)
- characteristic caput medusa appearance without a tangle of serpiginous vessels
- very rare arterialized DVA or DVA with AVM may present with hemorrhage

Moyamoya Disease (122)
- characteristic sulcal hyperintensity on FLAIR and leptomeningeal enhancement
- enlarged perforating vessels but without a nidus of entangled flow-voids

Dural AV Fistula (98)
- hyperintense structures adjacent to dural sinus wall on 3D TOF MRA
- no tangle of serpiginous vessels

Hemorrhagic Neoplasm (180)
- typically prominent surrounding edema
- areas of nodular contrast enhancement are frequently present
- abnormal flow-voids are exceedingly rare

Amyloid Hemorrhage (178)
- lobar location in elderly patients
- usually large hemorrhages with relatively small mass effect
- fluid level may be present in the hemorrhage
- no abnormal flow-voids

Hypertensive Hematoma (177)
- characteristically in putamen, thalamus, pons, and cerebellar white matter
- spot sign with contrast extravasation may be present on CTA
- no abnormal flow-voids

Cortical Contusion (179)
- characteristically superficial in the anterior basal frontal and temporal lobes
- following trauma

Background

Cerebral AVMs are a rare cause of neurologic symptoms with the estimated incidence at about 0.02–0.05% of the population. An AVM is a vascular malformation characterized by arteriovenous shunt through a collection of coiled and tortuous vessels (the nidus) connecting feeding arteries to draining veins, without an intervening capillary bed. The pathogenesis is currently unknown and these malformations were considered congenital in nature. De-novo formation of AVMs is being increasingly reported, especially in young females, indicating that they may arise in early childhood. AVMs are dynamic lesions that may grow and shrink; they also occur as a part of more extensive disease in various rare syndromes. Four-dimensional time-resolved MRA techniques show promising results for non-invasive evaluation, and may eventually obviate the need for diagnostic catheter angiography. Arteriovenous shunt visualization and quantification may be performed with arterial spin-labeling MRI.

REFERENCES

1. Geibprasert S, Pongpech S, Jiarakongmun P, et al. Radiologic assessment of brain arteriovenous malformations: what clinicians need to know. Radiographics 2010;**30**:483–501.

2. Stevens J, Leach JL, Abruzzo T, Jones BV. De novo cerebral arteriovenous malformation: case report and literature review. AJNR 2009;**30**:111–2.

3. Fleetwood IG, Steinberg GK. Arteriovenous malformations. Lancet 2002;**359**:863–73.

4. Wakai S, Nagai M. "Nidus sparing sign" on computerized tomography in intracerebral haemorrhage due to a rupture of arteriovenous malformation. Acta Neurochir (Wien) 1988;**95**:102–8.

5. Yan L, Wang S, Zhuo Y, et al. Unenhanced dynamic MR angiography: high spatial and temporal resolution by using true FISP-based spin tagging with alternating radiofrequency. Radiology 2010;**256**:270–9.

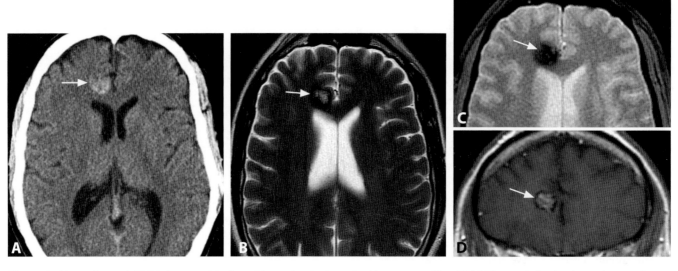

Figure 1. Non-enhanced CT (A) shows a right frontal hyperdensity (arrow) without mass effect. T2WI (B) at a similar level reveals central heterogenous hyperintensity and peripheral dark ring (arrow). Corresponding T2*WI (C) shows signal loss of the lesion (arrow), which appears similar to B (arrow) on coronal T1WI (D).

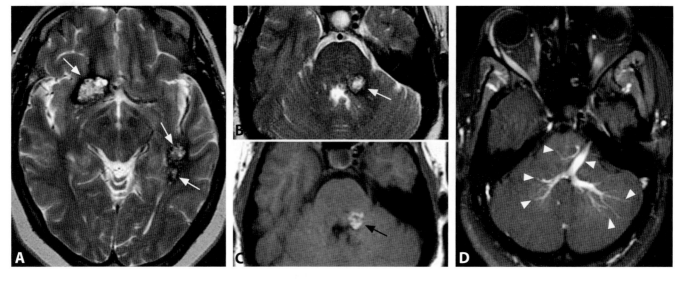

Figure 2. T2WI in another patient shows multiple lesions (arrows). T2WI (B) and T1WI (C) through the pons reveal an additional abnormality (arrows). Corresponding post-contrast T1WI with fat saturation (D) shows a prominent associated DVA (arrowheads).

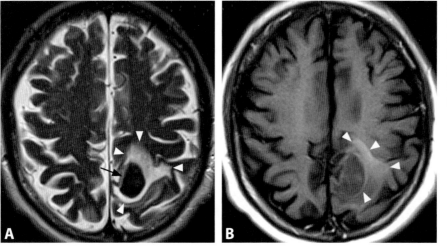

Figure 3. Axial T2WI (A) in a patient with nontraumatic acute cerebral hematoma (arrow) and surrounding edema (arrowheads). Corresponding T1WI without contrast (B) reveals hyperintensity (arrowheads) within the vasogenic edema. This finding is highly suggestive of an underlying cavernoma.

Cavernous Angioma (Cavernoma)

GIULIO ZUCCOLI AND ZORAN RUMBOLDT

Specific Imaging Findings

Cerebral cavernous malformations (CCM, cavernous angiomas/ hemangiomas, cavernomas) show characteristically mild-to-moderate increased density on unenhanced CT reflecting the presence of calcium and blood at various stages of degradation with some cavernomas disclosing clear internal calcifications. MR imaging of CCM demonstrates typical popcorn-like multilobulated lesion with smooth margins and multiple internal septations. There is characteristically high T2 signal centrally, frequently with associated T1 hyperintensities, and a T2 dark peripheral hemosiderin ring. Smaller cavernomas may appear as foci of just low T2 signal. On T2* imaging the characteristic signal loss from hemosiderin due to susceptibility effects reveals cavernomas missed on other sequences. T2* images are very helpful in patients with CCM, as they frequently show multiple lesions, especially in familial cases. Surrounding edema and mass effect may be seen in acute hemorrhage. T1 hyperintensity in the perilesional edema appears to be a characteristic feature of CCMs with a recent bleed. Contrast enhancement is usually absent, while peripheral enhancement may surround an acute hematoma. There is a commonly observed association with a developmental venous anomaly (DVA), which does enhance. CCM are otherwise occult at DSA, CTA, and MRA.

Pertinent Clinical Information

CCM are common vascular malformations of the CNS that may present with seizures, headache, or focal neurological deficits, usually from hemorrhage. They may also be asymptomatic and incidentally discovered. CCM can occur everywhere in the brain, including the extra-axial locations. Compared with adults, pediatric patients with brainstem cavernomas tend to have larger lesions and higher recurrence rate.

Differential Diagnosis

Hemorrhagic and/or Calcified Neoplasms (180, 195)
- small hemorrhagic metastases may be indistinguishable from small CCMs
- absence of surrounding T1 hyperintensity
- hemosiderin rim is usually incomplete
- absence of characteristic "popcorn" appearance
- contrast enhancement and vasogenic edema may be present
- calcifications usually large with bone-like CT density

Amyloid Hemorrhage (CAA) (178)
- almost exclusively in patients over 60 years of age
- absence of "popcorn" appearance
- typically cortico-subcortical microhemorrhages

Hypertensive Hematoma (HCA) (177)
- located in the deep gray and white matter, cerebellum, and pons
- absence of "popcorn" appearance

Cerebral Autosomal Dominant Arteriopathy with Subcortical Infarcts and Leukoencephalopathy (CADASIL) (22)
- bilateral high T2 signal involving the temporal white matter and external capsules
- absence of "popcorn" appearance

Diffuse Axonal Injury (DAI) (114)
- history of trauma, other traumatic injuries
- located at the gray matter–white matter junction, corpus callosum, dorsolateral brainstem

Arteriovenous Malformation (AVM) (182, 193)
- characteristic multiple flow-voids ("bag of worms") on T2WI
- enlarged feeding arteries and draining veins are usually present
- absence of "popcorn" appearance

Background

The prevalence of CCM in the general population is approximately 0.5%. Symptomatic hemorrhage rates range from 0.1% to 2.7% per lesion-year and 0.013–16.5% per patient-year. CCM may be found in association with DVA, superficial siderosis, and hyperkeratotic cutaneous vascular malformation. Three genes associated with CCM have been identified (CCM1–3) and a fourth CCM locus may be present. CCM occur in sporadic or autosomal dominant forms showing incomplete penetrance. Sporadic cases usually present as a single lesion, while familial cases typically show multiple lesions. Number of CCM in familial cases correlates with the patients' age. High-dose whole-brain radiation therapy may induce CCM formation. At least some cavernomas are acquired lesions, as they have been shown to occur de novo adjacent to a pre-existing DVA. CCM are dynamic in nature, and may increase or decrease in size over time. Open surgery or radiosurgery may be performed to eliminate the mass effect and seizure focus.

REFERENCES

1. Yun TJ, Na DG, Kwon BJ, et al. A T1 hyperintense perilesional signal aids in the differentiation of a cavernous angioma from other hemorrhagic masses. AJNR 2008;29:494–500.
2. Washington CW, McCoy KE, Zipfel GJ. Update on the natural history of cavernous malformations and factors predicting aggressive clinical presentation. Neurosurg Focus 2010;29:E7.
3. Rivera PP, Willinsky RA, Porter PJ. Intracranial cavernous malformations. Neuroimaging Clin N Am 2003;13:27–40.
4. Campeau NG, Lane JI. De novo development of a lesion with the appearance of cavernous malformation adjacent to an existing developmental venous anomaly. AJNR 2005;26:156–9.
5. Blitstein MK, Tung GA. MRI of cerebral microhemorrhages. AJR 2007;189:720–5.

Intracranial Calcifications

Cases

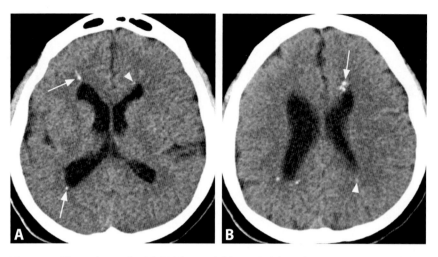

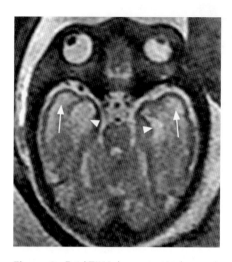

Figure 1. Non-enhanced axial CT (A) in a child reveals bilateral periventricular calcifications, both chunky (arrows) and punctate (arrowhead). A more cephalad image (B) again shows calcifications ranging from very prominent (arrow) to very subtle (arrowhead).

Figure 2. Fetal T2WI shows ventriculomegaly (arrowheads) and hyperintense WM (arrows) in both anterior temporal lobes.

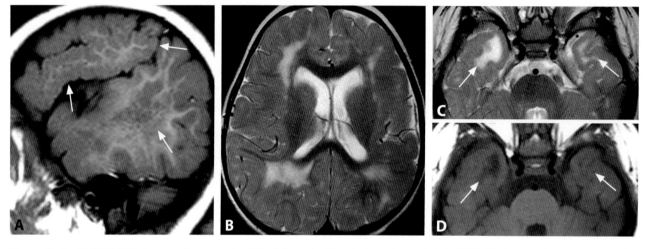

Figure 3. Sagittal T1WI (A) shows polymicrogyria of the left cerebral hemisphere (arrows). Axial T2WI (B) shows polymicrogyria on the left and scattered bilateral deep white matter hyperintensities. A more inferior T2WI (C) reveals bilateral anterior temporal subcortical hyperintensity (arrows), hypointense on T1WI (D).

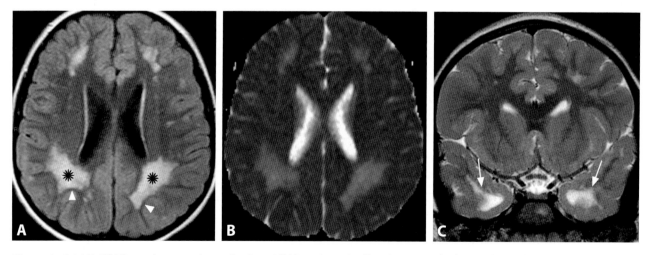

Figure 4. Axial FLAIR (A) reveals a posterior-predominant WM hyperintensity (*) with preserved subcortical (arrowheads) and periventricular WM. ADC (B) shows increased diffusivity of the lesions. Coronal T2WI (C) reveals bilateral anterior temporal subcortical hyperintensity (arrows).

Congenital Cytomegalovirus Infection

ZORAN RUMBOLDT AND CHEN HOFFMAN

Specific Imaging Findings

The most common imaging finding of congenital cytomegalovirus (CMV) infection is intracranial calcifications (in 33–70% of patients), which are typically periventricular thick and chunky, while faint and punctate in other locations. Absence of calcifications does not exclude congenital CMV infection. While calcifications are best seen on CT, MRI is the modality of choice for all other lesions. Neuronal migration abnormalities (in up to 10%) range from lissencephaly to diffuse or focal polymicrogyria. White matter abnormalities (up to 22%) are of low CT attenuation and T1 signal (and high T2 signal over 8–10 months of age), and abnormal anterior temporal white matter, primarily vacuolization and cyst formation, is characteristic. Ventriculomegaly is common (in 10–45%), with or without microcephaly and cerebellar hypoplasia. The most specific findings in children with neurodevelopmental delay are cortical malformations, white matter abnormalities, cerebellar hypoplasia, and temporal lobe lesions. Multifocal predominantly deep parietal white matter lesions in patients with static encephalopathy are indicative of congenital CMV infection. In asymptomatic individuals a posterior-predominant pattern with preserved periventricular and subcortical white matter is characteristically found.

Pertinent Clinical Information

Congenital CMV infection is the most common intrauterine infection, occurring in 0.15–2.0% of all live births. Confirmatory tests are polymerase chain reaction (PCR) in amniotic fluid and virus isolation from urine in the first weeks of life. Neonatal signs of infection include jaundice, hepatosplenomegaly, petechiae, microcephaly, and chorioretinitis. About 90% of affected infants are, however, asymptomatic at birth, and only 10–15% of these will develop persistent problems, primarily sensorineural hearing loss, mental retardation, cerebral palsy, and seizures. Lissencephaly and pachygyria indicate early fetal infection and are associated with a worse outcome. Normal prenatal US examinations appear to predict a normal early outcome in fetuses with congenital CMV infection. Fetal MRI can detect abnormalities when transabdominal US results are normal, but the outcome may not correlate with the abnormal white matter findings. Positive predictive value of both ultrasound and MRI for symptomatic infection is low, in the range of 30%. Treatment with antiviral agents may have a place in neonates with CNS involvement.

Differential Diagnosis

Congenital Toxoplasmosis (185)
- calcifications random in location, typically more prominent and chunky
- no "leukodystrophic" pattern
- frequent ventriculomegaly with posterior prevalence

Aicardi–Goutières Syndrome (186)
- more prominent calcifications in deep gray matter, white matter and cerebellum
- diffuse white matter involvement
- cortex not affected
- clinically progressive

Congenital Muscular Dystrophies (Muscle–Eye–Brain Disease and Fukuyama Type) (92)
- pontine hypoplasia
- cerebellar cysts
- muscle weakness

Megalencephalic Leukoencephalopathy with Subcortical Cysts (23)
- macrocephaly
- cortex is not affected
- clinically progressive

Background

CMV is a ubiquitous virus that usually results in asymptomatic or clinically benign infection. The time of prenatal infection is strongly associated with the level of disability and children infected during the third trimester are rarely affected. The goal of prenatal evaluation is to assess the specific neurotrophic effects of CMV – reduced neuronal proliferation, incomplete migration, and abnormal cortical cell organization. The inflammatory process with infection of astroglia may produce neurotoxic factors leading to focal necroses and calcifications. Congenital CMV infection and periventricular leukomalacia (PVL) affect the white matter in the same developmental period and their pathology is similarly characterized by axonal loss, lack of myelin, and astrogliosis. The introduction of PCR testing of blood stored on Guthrie cards has created the opportunity for correct diagnosis beyond the neonatal period.

REFERENCES

1. Fink KR, Thapa MM, Ishak GE, Pruthi S. Neuroimaging of pediatric central nervous system cytomegalovirus infection. *Radiographics* 2010;**30**:1779–96.
2. van der Knaap MS, Vermeulen G, Barkhof F, *et al.* Pattern of white matter abnormalities at MR imaging: use of polymerase chain reaction testing of Guthrie cards to link pattern with congenital cytomegalovirus infection. *Radiology* 2004;**230**:529–36.
3. Farkas N, Hoffmann C, Ben-Sira L, *et al.* Does normal fetal brain ultrasound predict normal neurodevelopmental outcome in congenital cytomegalovirus infection? *Prenat Diagn* 2011;**31**:360–6.
4. Doneda C, Parazzini C, Righini A, *et al.* Early cerebral lesions in cytomegalovirus infection: prenatal MR imaging. *Radiology* 2010;**255**:613–21.
5. van der Voorn JP, Pouwels PJ, Vermeulen RJ, *et al.* Quantitative MR imaging and spectroscopy in congenital cytomegalovirus infection and periventricular leukomalacia suggests a comparable neuropathological substrate of the cerebral white matter lesions. *Neuropediatrics* 2009;**40**:168–73.

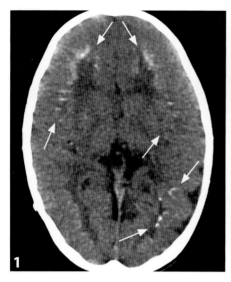

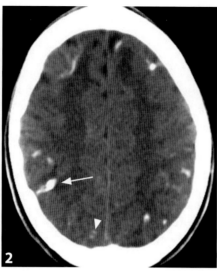

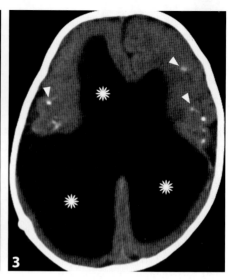

Figure 1. Non-enhanced axial CT image in a young child with seizures reveals numerous bilateral calcifications (arrows), primarily in the white matter.

Figure 2. Axial CT in another patient shows multiple bilateral cortical and subcortical calcifications, ranging from subtle (arrowhead) to chunky (arrow).

Figure 3. CT image in a child with developmental delay and chorioretinitis reveals a very prominent ventriculomegaly (*) and bilateral peripheral calcifications (arrowheads).

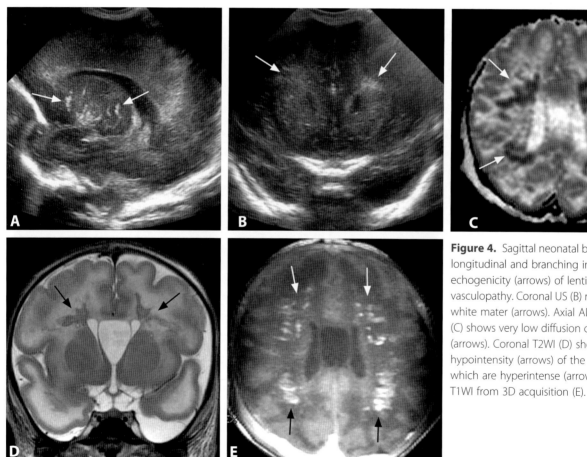

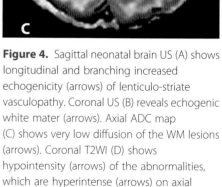

Figure 4. Sagittal neonatal brain US (A) shows longitudinal and branching increased echogenicity (arrows) of lenticulo-striate vasculopathy. Coronal US (B) reveals echogenic white mater (arrows). Axial ADC map (C) shows very low diffusion of the WM lesions (arrows). Coronal T2WI (D) shows hypointensity (arrows) of the abnormalities, which are hyperintense (arrows) on axial T1WI from 3D acquisition (E).

Congenital Toxoplasmosis

CHEN HOFFMAN

Specific Imaging Findings

The involvement of the brain in congenital toxoplasmosis may range from mild to severe. Subtle to coarse and chunky calcifications without periventricular predilection are commonly present and randomly distributed. There is destruction of the brain parenchyma with hydrocephalus and atrophy in severe cases. Ventriculomegaly is due to aqueductal atresia from ependymal involvement and shows a somewhat typical posterior predominance. In addition to calcifications, CT may show focal hypodense areas in the white matter. US demonstrates calcifications and cystic lesions in the periventricular white matter. Lenticulo-striate vasculopathy (LSV) with hyperechogenic linear branching structures corresponding to vasculature is a nonspecific finding, suggesting an infectious process. Ultrasound and CT have comparable sensitivity for intracranial calcifications of congenital toxoplasmosis. MR findings include periventricular foci of bright T1 signal due to calcification and gliosis. T2-weighted images demonstrate cystic white matter lesions and abnormal white matter hyperintensity due to gliosis, while the calcifications are dark. Recent cystic changes may be bright on DWI and show decreased diffusivity from cytotoxic edema. MR spectroscopy is not specific, but may reveal a prominent lactate peak. In contrast to CMV, cortical malformations such as polymicrogyria are infrequent.

Pertinent Clinical Information

Congenital toxoplasmosis is caused by transplacental contamination of the fetus following maternal primary infection. It is substantially less frequent than cytomegalovirus (CMV) infection; however, it is more commonly symptomatic. Education and serological screening of pregnant women are the only currently available strategies for the prevention, diagnosis, and treatment since the infection usually goes unrecognized in pregnant women. Ventriculomegaly associated with multiple calcifications is characteristic of severe fetal toxoplasmosis and carries a poor prognosis, while normal ventricular size on fetal ultrasound is suggestive of a good outcome. The affected neonates are usually normal at birth and become symptomatic after a few days with seizures, chorioretinitis, hydrocephalus, and abnormal CSF. Developmental delay, hematological abnormalities, hepatosplenomegaly, blindness and hearing loss may follow. Although the infection cannot currently be prevented, postnatal therapy can substantially improve outcome, primarily with an alternating pyrimethamine–sulfonamide regimen.

Differential Diagnosis

Congenital CMV Infection (184)
- cortical malformations are much more common
- microcephaly is more common
- chunky calcifications are typically periventricular in location

Meningitis (120)
- calcifications are uncommon
- meningeal contrast enhancement and/or hyperintensity on FLAIR is frequently present

Aicardi–Goutières Syndrome (186)
- more prominent calcifications in the deep gray matter and cerebellum
- diffuse white matter involvement, cortex not affected
- clinically progressive

Congenital HIV
- bilateral symmetric homogenous calcifications primarily involving the basal ganglia and frontal white matter

Cysticercosis (167, 194)
- does not occur in neonates and infants

Background

The infection with protozoan *Toxoplasma gondii* is usually acquired from ingestion of infected, undercooked meat or transmitted from cats. The risk of mother-to-child transmission is lower than 5% in the first trimester, but can reach 90% in the last days of pregnancy. Inversely, however, fetal disease is more severe when contamination occurs early in pregnancy. When maternal infection is suspected, preventive treatment with spiramycin may be started; the treatment is changed to a combination of pyrimethamine–sulfonamide if fetal infection is confirmed. Recent multicenter studies raised questions about the effectiveness of the prenatal treatment on transplacental transmission and on the reduction in the number and severity of fetal sequelae. As soon as the infection is confirmed, children are treated with the pyrimethamine–sulfonamide combination for 3–24 months. Recent studies have shown that postnatal treatment does not prevent ocular lesions: 5% of treated children had choroiditis lesions at birth, 20% at 5 years, and 30% at 8 years of age.

REFERENCES

1. Lago EG, Baldisserotto M, Hoefel Filho JR, *et al*. Agreement between ultrasonography and computed tomography in detecting intracranial calcifications in congenital toxoplasmosis. *Clin Radiol* 2007;**62**:1004–11.
2. Virkola K, Lappalainen M, Valanne L, Koskiniemi M. Radiological signs in newborns exposed to primary *Toxoplasma* infection in utero. *Pediatr Radiol* 1997;**27**:133–8.
3. Malinger G, Werner H, Rodriguez Leonel JC, *et al*. Prenatal brain imaging in congenital toxoplasmosis. *Prenat Diagn* 2011 Jun 27. doi: 10.1002/pd.2795. [Epub ahead of print]
4. Barkovich AJ, Girard N. Fetal brain infections. *Childs Nerv Syst* 2003;**19**:501–7.
5. Kaye A. Toxoplasmosis: diagnosis, treatment, and prevention in congenitally exposed infants. *J Pediatr Health Care* 2011;**25**:355–64.

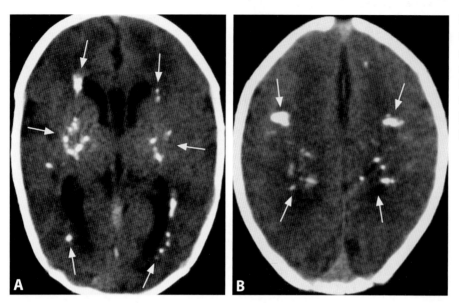

Figure 1. Axial non-enhanced CT images at the level of the lateral ventricles (A) and centrum semiovale (B) in a 6-day-old newborn show extensive calcifications of varying sizes (arrows) involving bilateral basal ganglia and supratentorial white matter. The pathologic process clearly had a prenatal onset in this patient.

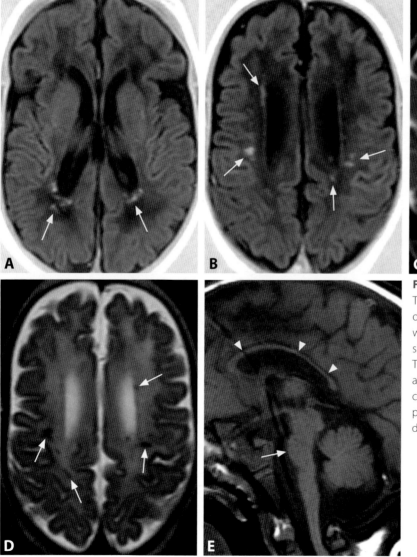
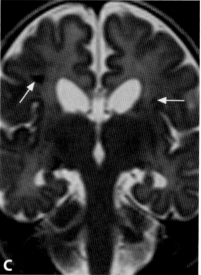

Figure 2. Another patient at 4 months of age. IR T1WI (A, B) and T2WI (C, D) show diffuse prominence of CSF spaces consistent with cerebral atrophy. The white matter is abnormal, with high T2 and low T1 signal. Calcifications show up as T2 hypointense and T1 hyperintense spots (arrows). The cerebellum appears spared. Sagittal T1WI (E) shows thin corpus callosum (arrowheads) and brainstem, especially the pontine protuberance (arrow), due to Wallerian degeneration.

Aicardi–Goutières Syndrome

ANDREA ROSSI

Specific Imaging Findings

The cardinal features of Aicardi-Goutières syndrome (AGS) on brain imaging consist of intracranial calcification, leukodystrophy, and cerebral atrophy. CT scan may be normal in the earliest stages of the disease, but almost invariably shows extensive calcifications involving the basal ganglia, thalami, periventricular white matter, and cerebellum. Calcifications are not always recognized on MRI; when seen, they appear as T2 hypointense, T1 hyperintense spots that stand out against the background of diffusely dysmyelinated white matter, and are better depicted on susceptibility-weighted (T2*) sequences. The abnormal signal (mild T1 hypointensity and moderate to marked T2 hyperintensity) in bilateral supratentorial white matter ranges from just periventricular involvement in milder cases to a striking fronto-temporal leukodystrophy with temporal cystic lesions in the most severely affected patients. Abnormal white matter shows two patterns of distribution: diffuse or anteroposterior gradient, each present in about half of the patients. Infra-tentorially, the pyramidal tracts within the medulla oblongata may be involved while the cerebellum is spared. Cortical atrophy can already be present at the onset and progresses over time; the corpus callosum may be markedly atrophic.

Pertinent Clinical Information

Affected patients present during early infancy with a rapidly progressive picture characterized by feeding difficulties, delayed psychomotor development, progressive microcephaly, irritability, truncal hypotonia with limb spasticity and dystonic ocular and buccolingual movements, convulsions, opisthotonus, and blindness. Demise usually occurs within a few months or years in these severe forms, although patients with apparently static or slowly progressive disease, sometimes presenting after several months of normal development, have also been reported. Thrombocytopenia, hepatosplenomegaly, elevated hepatic transaminases, and intermittent fevers may erroneously suggest an infective process. CSF pleocytosis with an increased lymphocyte count and intrathecal interferon-α (IFN-α) synthesis is found in the majority of patients. However, the levels of white cells and IFN-α in the CSF of affected patients fall to normal over the first few years of life, and the white cell count may be normal despite elevated IFN-α. Cerebrovascular stenoses and stroke have also been described in patients with AGS.

Differential Diagnosis

Congenital Cytomegalovirus (184)
- calcifications are mostly periventricular
- white matter abnormalities more focal, typically periventricular and deep parietal
- subcortical temporal pole cavitations
- cortical abnormalities (polymicrogyria) often present
- clinically stable

Congenital Toxoplasmosis (185)
- calcifications random in location
- no "leukodystrophic" pattern
- frequent ventriculomegaly with posterior prevalence

Baraitser–Reardon syndrome
- white matter extensively atrophic, but not with abnormal signal
- CSF lymphocytosis is absent

Background

AGS is a rare, genetically determined encephalopathy with clinical and imaging features closely mimicking the sequelae of congenital infection, and may therefore be misdiagnosed as such. AGS is caused by mutations (usually recessive) in any of the genes encoding the exonuclease TREX1 on chromosome 3p21 (AGS 1), the three nonallelic components of the RNASEH2 endonuclease complex (AGS 2–4), and the *SAMHD1* gene on chromosome 20 (AGS 5). AGS is an inflammatory encephalopathy associated with increased intrathecal production of IFN-α, and this is in common with the pathogenesis of both congenital infections and systemic lupus erythematosus (SLE), where an IFN-α mediated immune response is triggered by viral and host nucleic acids, respectively. The phenotypic overlap of AGS with congenital infection and SLE is probably explained by the putative role of the causative AGS genes, which are implicated in the removal of nucleic acids produced during apoptosis. Failure of this removal results in activation of the immune system, leading to inflammation and white matter dysmyelination. Mutations in *TREX1* may also be found with SLE.

REFERENCES

1. Uggetti C, La Piana R, Orcesi S, *et al.* Aicardi–Goutieres syndrome: neuroradiologic findings and follow-up. *AJNR* 2009;**30**:1971–6.
2. Crow YJ, Rehwinkel J. Aicardi–Goutières syndrome and related phenotypes: linking nucleic acid metabolism with autoimmunity. *Hum Mol Genet* 2009;**18**:R130–6.
3. Rice GI, Bond J, Asipu A, *et al.* Mutations involved in Aicardi–Goutières syndrome implicate SAMHD1 as regulator of the innate immune response. *Nat Genet* 2009;**41**:829–32.
4. Abdel-Salam GM, Zaki MS, Lebon P, Meguid NA. Aicardi–Goutières syndrome: clinical and neuroradiological findings of 10 new cases. *Acta Paediatr* 2004;**93**:929–36.
5. Orcesi S, Pessagno A, Biancheri R, *et al.* Aicardi–Goutières syndrome presenting atypically as a sub-acute leukoencephalopathy. *Eur J Paediatr Neurol* 2008;**12**:408–11.

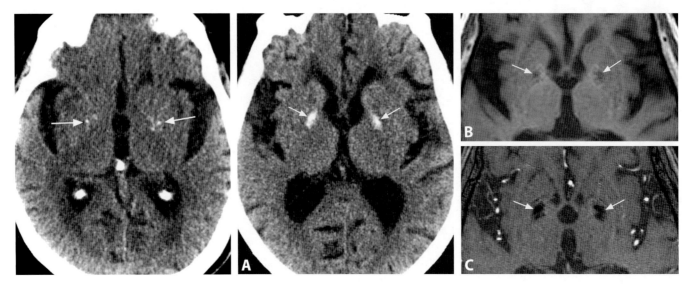

Figure 1. Axial unenhanced CT image through the basal ganglia demonstrates bilateral scattered and punctuate calcifications (arrows), confined to the globi pallidi.

Figure 2. Axial un-enhanced CT image (A) shows more confluent calcifications (arrows) in bilateral globi pallidi. Corresponding T1WI (B) demonstrates decreased signal in the region of calcifications (arrows). Source image from a gradient echo 3D TOF MRA (C) reveals increased size of hypointensities (arrows) due to magnetic susceptibility.

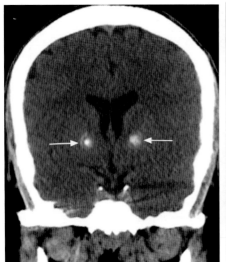

Figure 3. Non-enhanced CT image reconstructed in the coronal plane shows bilateral dense calcifications (arrows) within the globi pallidi.

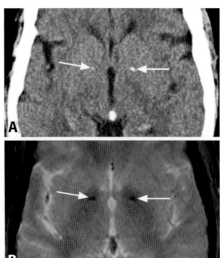

Figure 4. Axial non-enhanced CT image (A) shows subtle punctate calcifications (arrows) in bilateral globi pallidi. Corresponding T2*WI (B) demonstrates a slightly more prominent decreased signal in the region of calcifications (arrows).

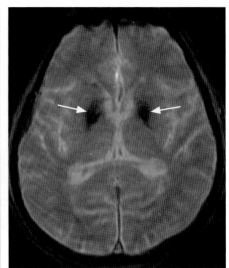

Figure 5. Axial T2*WI in a different patient reveals prominent bilateral hypointensities (arrows) conforming to the globus pallidus, consistent with calcification.

Physiologic Basal Ganglia Calcifications

BENJAMIN HUANG

Specific Imaging Findings

Physiologic parenchymal calcifications are generally confined to the globi pallidi, but can be seen elsewhere in the basal ganglia, and in the cerebellar dentate nuclei. They are typically punctate or smudgy and almost always bilateral. Occasionally they can be quite prominent. T1 and T2 signal intensities vary depending on the concentration of calcium salts within the tissues. T2*-weighted sequences demonstrate blooming with signal loss due to increased magnetic susceptibility.

Pertinent Clinical Information

Basal ganglia calcifications are an incidental finding in roughly 1% of head CTs. They generally occur over the age of 30 and their prevalence increases with age. The median age at which physiologic basal calcification is seen is in the 60s. They usually have no clinical significance. However, if they are observed in patients with extrapyramidal signs or under the age of 30, clinical evaluation to rule out an underlying endocrine process affecting calcium and phosphate metabolism should be undertaken.

Differential Diagnosis

Fahr Disease
- also involves cerebral white matter and cerebellum

Hyperparathyroidism, Hypoparathyroidism (188)
- may involve thalamus, white matter, cerebellum, and dura
- abnormal serum PTH levels

Aicardi–Goutières Syndrome (186)
- also thalamic, periventricular and cerebellar calcifications
- leukodystrophy with abnormal white matter signal
- cerebral atrophy
- presents in infancy

Radiation/Chemotherapy-Induced Leukoencephalopathy (26, 191)
- CT hypodense and T2 hyperintense white matter
- typically in young children
- calcifications are primarily in the white matter

Congenital HIV Infection
- also frontal white matter and cerebellar calcifications

Background

Macroscopic basal ganglia calcifications are seen in roughly 3.4% of autopsies, and microscopic calcifications isolated to the basal ganglia may be present in up to 70% of cases. The physiology of these calcifications is unknown. It has been suggested that they are the result of colloid deposition in and around the finer cerebral blood vessels with subsequent calcification. The increased density may in part be due to the presence of admixed metals such as iron.

REFERENCES
1. Cohen CR, Duchesneau PM, Weinstein MA. Calcification of the basal ganglia as visualized by computed tomography. *Radiology* 1980;**134**:97–9.
2. Makariou E, Patsalides AD. Intracranial calcifications. *Applied Radiol* 2009;**38**:48–60.

Brain Imaging with MRI and CT, ed. Zoran Rumboldt *et al.* Published by Cambridge University Press. © Cambridge University Press 2012.

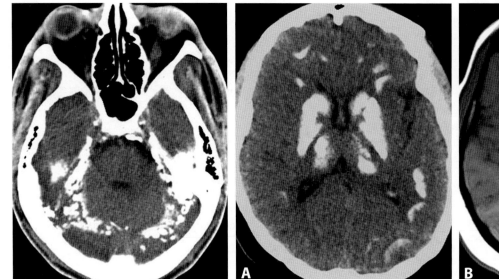

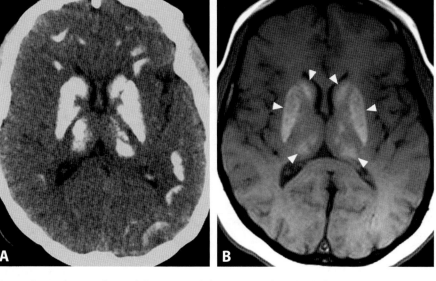

Figure 1. Axial non-enhanced CT image demonstrates typical dense, nodular calcifications along the tentorium in a patient with end-stage renal disease. No parenchymal calcifications are evident.

Figure 2. Axial non-enhanced CT image (A) shows parenchymal calcifications in another patient. Dense calcifications are present in the bilateral basal ganglia, thalami and subcortical regions. Matching T1WI without contrast (B) reveals hyperintensities in the deep gray matter structures (arrowheads) corresponding to calcifications.

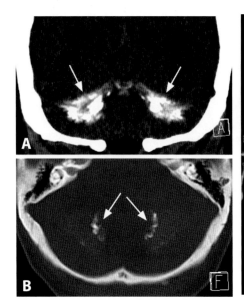

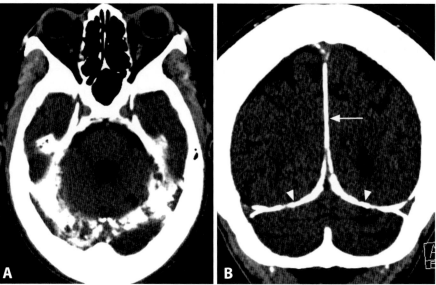

Figure 3. Non-enhanced CT in the coronal plane (A) shows prominent bilateral cerebellar calcifications (arrows). Axial CT image with bone algorithm and window (B) reveals that the densest of these calcifications (arrows) reflect the shape of the dentate nuclei.

Figure 4. Axial non-enhanced CT image (A) in a different patient shows dense calcifications along the tentorium cerebelli. CT image in the coronal plane (B) demonstrates thick calcifications along the tentorium (arrowheads) and falx cerebri (arrow).

Hyperparathyroidism

BENJAMIN HUANG

Specific Imaging Findings

Intracranial calcifications from hyperparathyroidism are typically nodular and symmetric on CT, most commonly seen along dural surfaces, particularly the tentorium and falx. Parenchymal calcifications in the deep gray matter, subcortical regions, and cerebellar folia are frequently dense and bulky. Both parenchymal and dural calcifications can occur in isolation. Extracranial calcifications may be observed in corneas, sclerae, and salivary glands. The calcifications are of variable MR signal intensities, with parenchymal calcifications being frequently T1 hyperintense. T2*-weighted sequences demonstrate signal loss with blooming due to magnetic susceptibility.

Pertinent Clinical Information

Neurologic presentations are related to hypercalcemia and include weakness, fatigue, lethargy, depression, or cognitive impairment. Intracranial calcifications are primarily reported with secondary or tertiary hyperparathyroidism.

Differential Diagnosis

Physiologic Basal Ganglia Calcifications (187)
- typically localized to globus pallidus
- no dural involvement

Fahr Disease
- no dural involvement
- periventricular white matter may be affected

Hypoparathyroidism
- no dural involvement

Aicardi–Goutières Syndrome (186)
- also periventricular calcifications

- no dural involvement
- leukodystrophy with abnormal white matter and atrophy
- presents in infancy

Radiation/Chemotherapy-Induced Leukoencephalopathy (26, 190)
- CT hypodense and T2 hyperintense white matter
- calcifications primarily in the white matter

Background

Parathyroid hormone (PTH) is secreted in response to decreased calcium levels and exerts three main effects: (1) increased tubular resorption of calcium by the kidneys; (2) stimulation of osteoclast resorption to release calcium from bone; and (3) increased calcium absorption by the bowel, by stimulating production of 1,25-dihydroxyvitamin D in the kidneys. Most patients with primary hyperparathyroidism are asymptomatic and diagnosed based on incidental hypercalcemia. In secondary hyperparathyroidism, increased PTH is a response to lowered calcium levels caused by kidney, liver, or bowel disease, or vitamin D deficiency. In tertiary hyperparathyroidism, autonomous secretion of PTH occurs in longstanding secondary hyperparathyroidism, usually due to kidney disease. The mechanism by which hyperparathyroidism causes tissue calcification is not entirely clear.

REFERENCES

1. Dorenbeck U, Leingartner T, Bretschneider T, et al. Tentorial and dural calcification with tertiary hyperparathyroidism: a rare entity in chronic renal failure. *Eur Radiol* 2002;**12**:S11–3.
2. Henkelman RM, Watts JF, Kucharczyk W. High signal intensity in MR images of calcified brain tissue. *Radiology* 1991;**179**:199–206.

Brain Imaging with MRI and CT, ed. Zoran Rumboldt *et al.* Published by Cambridge University Press. © Cambridge University Press 2012.

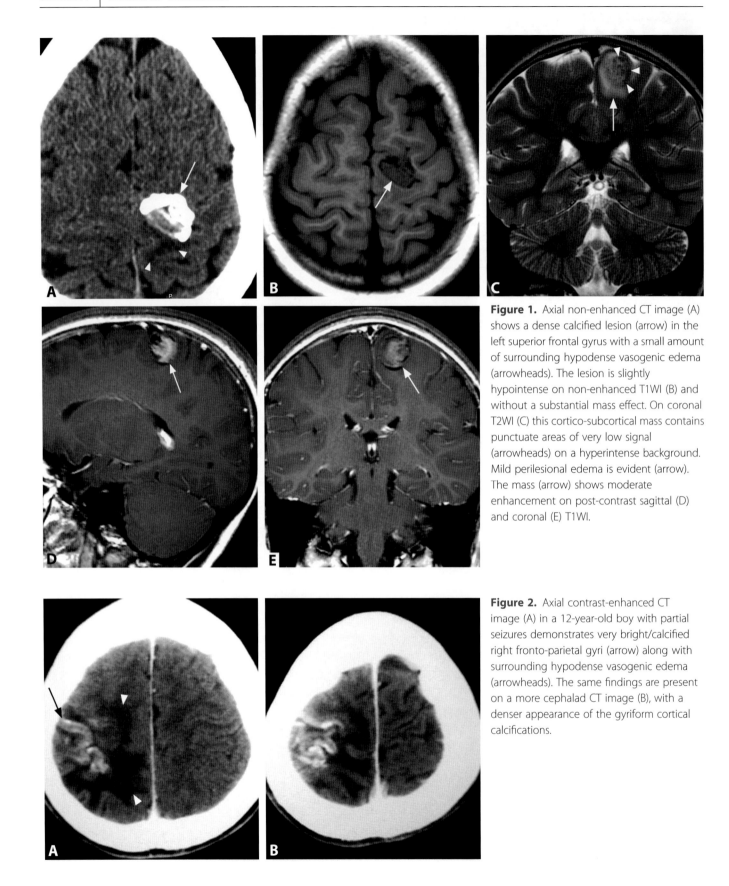

Figure 1. Axial non-enhanced CT image (A) shows a dense calcified lesion (arrow) in the left superior frontal gyrus with a small amount of surrounding hypodense vasogenic edema (arrowheads). The lesion is slightly hypointense on non-enhanced T1WI (B) and without a substantial mass effect. On coronal T2WI (C) this cortico-subcortical mass contains punctuate areas of very low signal (arrowheads) on a hyperintense background. Mild perilesional edema is evident (arrow). The mass (arrow) shows moderate enhancement on post-contrast sagittal (D) and coronal (E) T1WI.

Figure 2. Axial contrast-enhanced CT image (A) in a 12-year-old boy with partial seizures demonstrates very bright/calcified right fronto-parietal gyri (arrow) along with surrounding hypodense vasogenic edema (arrowheads). The same findings are present on a more cephalad CT image (B), with a denser appearance of the gyriform cortical calcifications.

Meningioangiomatosis

GIOVANNI MORANA

Specific Imaging Findings

On non-enhanced CT scans, meningioangiomatosis (MA) may appear as a nodular calcification, as a thickened gyriform mass with or without surrounding hypodense edema, or as hypodense lesion with central calcification. On MRI it is of either low T1 signal, or shows a mixed signal on both T1- and T2-weighted images, depending primarily on the amount of calcific deposition. A pattern of gyriform hyperintensity has been recently reported as a characteristic feature on FLAIR. Contrast enhancement is usually very prominent and may show a gyriform distribution. Surrounding vasogenic edema involving the adjacent white matter is quite common, and the lesion may cause mass effect. Advanced imaging techniques such as MRS may be degraded by contamination artifacts due to calcific deposition; nevertheless, increase in the choline peak with loss of the n-acetyl aspartate peak have been described. Imaging findings are often nonspecific and do not allow for a definite diagnosis.

Pertinent Clinical Information

MA usually affects children and young adults, with a male predominance; it may occur sporadically (most of reported cases) or in association with NF2 (approximately 20%), when it is often multifocal. Sporadic and NF2-associated forms are histologically similar but clinically different. The sporadic type typically presents with partial seizures that are difficult to control, whereas lesions associated with NF2 are often asymptomatic and discovered incidentally. The genetic basis of the sporadic form is not well clarified. Regarding seizures, the outcome after surgery is variable because the epileptogenic activity may arise from the lesion itself, from the perilesional cortex, and/or from a remote cortical site, thus explaining persistent seizure after removal of the meningiomatosis alone.

Differential Diagnosis

Sturge–Weber Syndrome Type III (without facial nevus) (86)
- progressive cortical atrophy, no mass effect, no perifocal edema
- progressive involution of leptomeningeal vessels due to spontaneous thrombosis

Primary Brain Tumors (Oligodendroglioma, Ganglioglioma) (161, 166, 196, 197)
- cortical thickening and gyriform enhancing pattern are uncommon
- may be indistinguishable

Atypical or Malignant Meningioma (138, 203)
- usually a broad dural base
- more common in adult population

Intra-axial Schwannoma
- extremely rare
- subtle calcifications

Granulomatous Disease (TB, Fungal Infections, Sarcoidosis) (118, 160)
- rim enhancement more common
- often multiple lesions
- calcifications, when present, are usually more subtle

Background

MA is a rare benign lesion characterized by a plaque-like or gyriform, variably calcified, cerebral hemispheric mass, with focal leptomeningeal thickening, most often involving the temporal and/or frontal lobes. Histologically, there is cortical meningovascular proliferation with perivascular spindled cells and leptomeningeal calcification interwoven with bands of fibrous connective tissue. Individual cases may be classified into those with predominantly cellular and those with predominantly vascular lesions. The pathogenesis remains unclear, and it has been debated whether the biological nature is that of a hamartoma or a neoplasm. A non-neoplastic, hamartomatous etiology is favored based on its typically benign clinical course and lack of significant proliferative activity in most cases. MA has rarely been reported to coexist with meningiomas and any variant of meningioma might be present in this lesion. Meningioangiomatosis-associated meningiomas seem to occur frequently in young patients, whereas conventional meningiomas occur most commonly in middle-aged or elderly patients.

REFERENCES

1. Yao Z, Wang Y, Zee C, et al. Computed tomography and magnetic resonance appearance of sporadic meningioangiomatosis correlated with pathological findings. *J Comput Assist Tomogr* 2009; **33**:799–804.

2. Rokes C, Ketonen LM, Fuller GN, et al. Imaging and spectroscopic findings in meningioangiomatosis. *Pediatr Blood Cancer* 2009; **53**:672–4.

3. Aizpuru RN, Quencer RM, Norenberg M, et al. Meningioangiomatosis: clinical, radiologic, and histopathologic correlation. *Radiology* 1991;**179**:819–21.

4. Wiebe S, Munoz DG, Smith S, Lee DH. Meningioangiomatosis. A comprehensive analysis of clinical and laboratory features. *Brain* 1999;**122**:709–26.

5. Deb P, Gupta A, Sharma MC, et al. Meningioangiomatosis with meningioma: an uncommon association of a rare entity – report of a case and review of the literature. *Childs Nerv Syst* 2006; **22**:78–83.

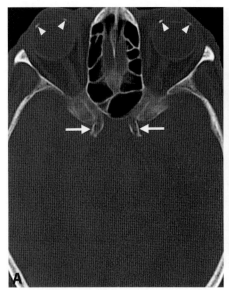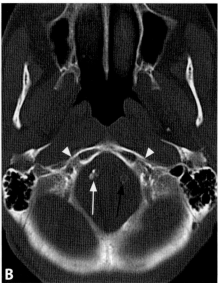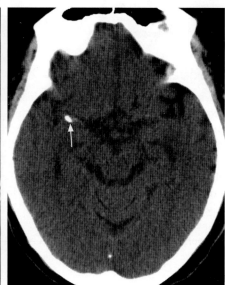

Figure 1. Un-enhanced axial CT image with bone algorithm and window at the level of the orbits (A) shows bilateral tubular calcifications (arrows) at the location of supraclinoid internal carotid arteries. Note also limbus calcifications (arrowheads) in both globes. CT image (B) at the level of the hypoglossal foramina (arrowheads) demonstrates bilateral intradural calcifications. On the right, the calcifications appear more plaque-like (white arrow). On the left, they are more ring-like (black arrow).

Figure 2. Axial un-enhanced CT image with soft tissue algorithm and window shows a very bright linear lesion (arrow) consistent with calcium at the location of the middle cerebral artery in the right sylvian fissure.

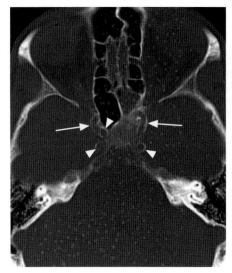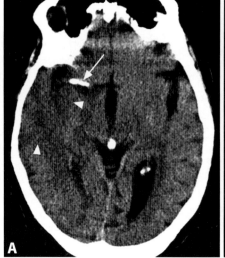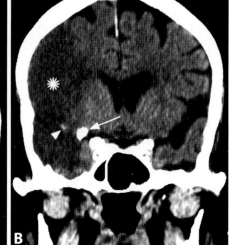

Figure 3. Axial non-enhanced CT image with bone algorithm and window shows bilateral tubular (arrow) and ring-like (arrowheads) calcifications delineating the entire course of the cavernous internal carotid arteries.

Figure 4. Non-enhanced axial CT image with soft tissue algorithm and window (A) shows a linear calcification (arrow) in the location of the right middle cerebral artery. Note also a subtle hypodensity with mild mass effect involving the right insula and temporal lobe (arrowheads). Follow-up coronal CT image (B) reveals a large infarct (*) along with a dense right middle cerebral artery (arrowhead). Again seen is the more proximal calcification (arrow), which is much brighter and bulkier.

Vascular Wall Calcification

BENJAMIN HUANG

Specific Imaging Findings

Wall calcifications are most commonly seen on unenhanced CT along the internal carotid arteries (carotid siphon), the vertebral arteries, middle cerebral arteries, and basilar artery. They range from fine and barely perceptible to chunky ones, several millimeters in thickness. When viewed in cross-section, mural calcifications appear ring-like, curvilinear, or stippled; when the affected artery is viewed longitudinally, they appear tubular, stippled and discontinuous, or plaque-like. Associated luminal narrowing may or may not be present. They are difficult to see on routine MRI, but very thick ones appear as a hypointense vessel rim.

Pertinent Clinical Information

Intracranial arterial calcifications are extremely common and often incidental on head CT, but are exceedingly uncommon under the age of 20. Their prevalence is roughly 50% at 41–60 and 90% at 61–80 years of age. In younger patients they may indicate an underlying metabolic disorder.

Differential Diagnosis

Calcified Aneurysms (144, 192)
- affected segment is dilated
- confirmed with CTA or MRA
- atherosclerotic calcifications can be mistaken for small aneurysms on CTA but distinguished with unenhanced CT

Dense Vessel Sign in Early Infarction (111)
- the vessel is mildly hyperdense, not calcified
- may coexist

Calcified Vascular Malformations (182, 183, 193)
- patchy calcifications common in cavernomas and AVMs
- typically peripherally located

Background

Calcifications within the arterial walls are a presumed sequela of advanced arteriosclerotic disease. Histologically, mineral deposits are found primarily in lesions containing prominent fibrous connective tissue layers, and it has been proposed that these deposits replace the accumulated remnants of dead cells and extracellular lipid within atherosclerotic plaques. The severity of intracranial carotid artery calcification appears to correlate with arteriosclerotic changes on catheter angiograms; however, intracranial vascular calcifications have not been found to predict or correlate with future stroke risk.

REFERENCES

1. de Weert TT, Cakir H, Rozie S, et al. Intracranial internal carotid artery calcifications: association with vascular risk factors and ischemic cerebrovascular disease. AJNR 2009;**30**:177–84.
2. Taoka T, Iwasaki S, Nakagawa H, et al. Evaluation of arteriosclerotic changes in the intracranial carotid artery using the calcium score obtained on plain cranial computed tomography scan: correlation with angiographic changes and clinical outcome. J Comput Assist Tomogr 2006;**30**:624–8.

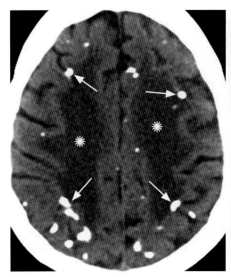

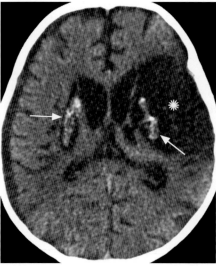

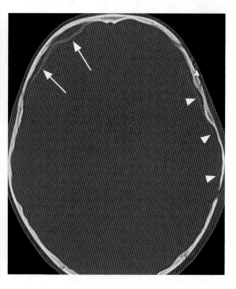

Figure 1. Axial unenhanced CT in a patient who had undergone whole-brain irradiation several years ago shows multiple calcifications (arrows), predominantly subcortical at the gray–white matter junction. Note diffuse white matter hypodensity (*).

Figure 2. Axial unenhanced CT image obtained several months after ischemic infarctions in a young child shows encephalomalacia (*) and calcifications in both basal ganglia (arrows). Also a small right-sided extra-axial collection.

Figure 3. Bone algorithm and window CT many months after surgery complicated by extra-axial hemorrhage reveals a smooth rind of calcification covering hematoma remnants (arrows) and subtle dural calcifications deep to the craniotomy (arrowheads).

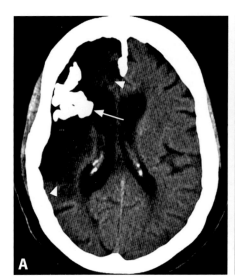

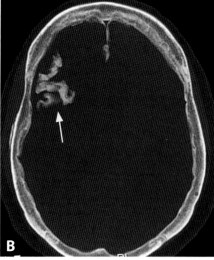

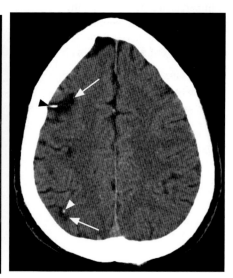

Figure 4. Non-enhanced axial CT image shows a large area of hypodense encephalomalacia in the anterior right cerebral hemisphere (arrowheads). Within the encephalomalacia there is an irregular bone-like structure (arrow). Corresponding CT image with bone algorithm and window (B) reveals that this bright structure (arrow) corresponds to a very dense somewhat gyriform calcification.

Figure 5. Non-enhanced axial CT image in another patient shows two small hypodense areas (arrows) in the right cerebral hemisphere. There are associated dystrophic calcifications (arrowheads).

Dystrophic Calcifications

BENJAMIN HUANG

Specific Imaging Findings

Dystrophic calcifications within previously damaged CNS tissue are best seen as very bright lesions on non-enhanced CT images. They occur in a wide range of diseases, more commonly in young children. Underlying areas of encephalomalacia are usually a consequence of ischemic injury, infections, trauma, and iatrogenic causes. Dural calcification is commonly associated with chronic subdural hematomas. Dystrophic calcification with mineralizing microangiopathy occurs in children treated with whole-brain radiation. The calcifications are characteristically bilateral and most commonly found in a cerebral subcortical location at the gray–white matter junction, followed by the basal ganglia and cerebellar dentate nuclei. Associated leukoencephalopathy with diffusely hypodense/T2 hyperintense white matter is usually present. The findings are more severe in younger children, particularly if they received radiation therapy under 3 years of age.

Pertinent Clinical Information

Dystrophic calcifications are usually not a major clinical concern as they occur in a previously already-injured tissue. The incidence of mineralizing microangiopathy has substantially decreased with improved treatment regimens for pediatric malignancies.

Differential Diagnosis

Physiologic Basal Ganglia Calcifications (187)
- typically localized to globus pallidus
- no underlying encephalomalacia

Hyperparathyroidism (188)
- no underlying encephalomalacia or leukoencephalopathy

Aicardi–Goutières Syndrome (186)
- scattered basal ganglia, thalamic, periventricular and cerebellar calcifications
- leukodystrophy with abnormal white matter signal and cerebral atrophy
- presents in infancy

Meningioangiomatosis (189)
- focal gyriform cortical calcifications, adjacent edema may be present

Sturge–Weber Syndrome (86)
- gyriform cortical calcifications with associated cerebral hemiatrophy
- additional typical findings are usually present

Meningioma (138, 203)
- typically focal extra-axial mass with contrast enhancement of the non-calcified portion

Background

Dystrophic calcification refers to heterotopic formation of calcium in soft tissue. They can occur in injured tissue wherein deposits of devitalized cells, blood cells, and lipids may act as a nidus for calcification. In the presence of infection, bacteria may also serve as a nidus.

REFERENCES

1. Lewis E, Lee YY. Computed tomography findings of severe mineralizing microangiopathy in the brain. *J Comput Tomogr* 1986;**10**:357–64.

2. Yu YL, Chiu EK, Woo E, *et al.* Dystrophic intracranial calcification: CT evidence of "cerebral steal" from arteriovenous malformation. *Neuroradiology* 1987;**29**:519–22.

Brain Imaging with MRI and CT, ed. Zoran Rumboldt *et al.* Published by Cambridge University Press. © Cambridge University Press 2012.

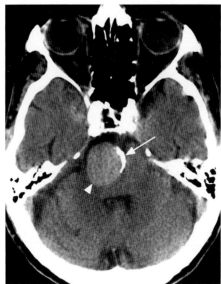

Figure 1. Axial non-enhanced CT image shows an oval hyperdense mass (arrowhead) in the prepontine cistern compressing the pons. The lesion contains peripheral shell-like calcification (arrow).

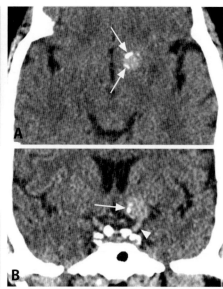

Figure 2. Non-enhanced axial CT (A) shows a hyperdense round lesion with peripheral calcifications (arrows) at the anterior commissure level. Reformatted coronal image (B) reveals the lesion (arrow) is an ICA (arrowhead) aneurysm.

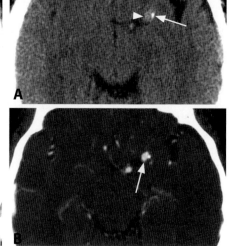

Figure 3. Non-enhanced CT (A) shows an oval hyperdensity (arrowhead) with marginal calcification (arrow) in the right sylvian fissure region. Source CTA image (B) shows dense enhancement of this MCA aneurysm (arrow).

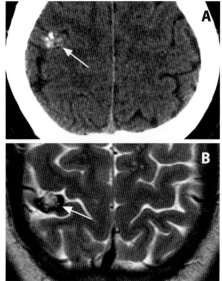

Figure 1. Non-enhanced axial CT image (A) shows speckled calcifications (arrow) in the right postcentral gyrus. T2WI (B) reveals that the lesion is a typical cavernoma (arrow) with "popcorn" hyperintensities and a dark hemosiderin rim.

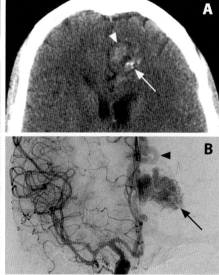

Figure 2. Non-enhanced axial CT (A) shows calcifications (arrow) within a heterogenous left frontal mass (arrowhead). Frontal DSA image of a right ICA injection (B) reveals left frontal AVM nidus (arrow) and a draining vein (arrowhead).

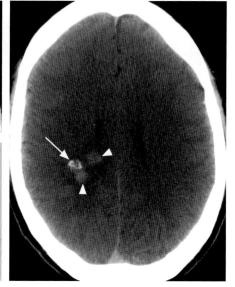

Figure 3. Axial non-enhanced CT image demonstrates an oval calcified lesion (arrow) and adjacent round hyperdensities (arrowheads) in the right centrum semiovale. The findings correspond to an AVM with draining veins.

CASE 192 — Calcified Aneurysms

ZORAN RUMBOLDT

Also 144

CASE 193 — Vascular Malformations

ZORAN RUMBOLDT

Also 182 & 183

CASE 192 — Calcified Aneurysms

ZORAN RUMBOLDT

Also 144

CASE 193 — Vascular Malformations

ZORAN RUMBOLDT

Also 182 & 183

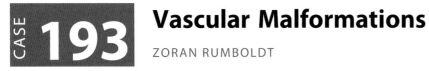

THE

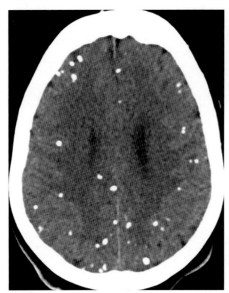

Figure 1. Axial non-enhanced CT image in a patient with epilepsy shows diffuse nodular parenchymal calcifications, predominantly in a cortico-subcortical location at the gray–white matter junction.

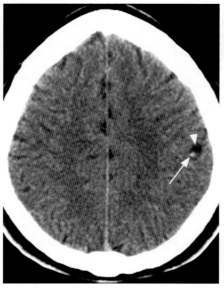

Figure 2. Axial non-enhanced CT image in another patient with neurocysticercosis demonstrates a characteristic peripheral cyst (arrowhead) with a tiny focal calcification (arrow).

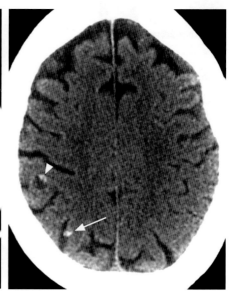

Figure 3. Non-enhanced CT reveals a small cortico-subcortical cyst with wall calcification (arrowhead) and an additional cortical calcification (arrow) in the right hemisphere.

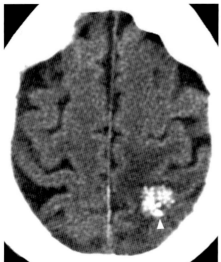

Figure 1. Axial non-enhanced CT image demonstrates a left parietal calcified lesion (arrowhead) and surrounding white matter hypodensity. Previously irradiated colon adenocarcinoma metastasis.

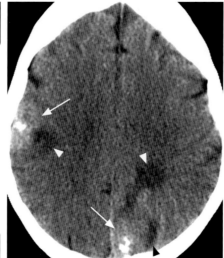

Figure 2. Non-enhanced CT shows partially calcified right frontal and left parietal lesions (arrows) at the gray–white matter junction with vasogenic edema (arrowheads). Lung cancer metastases.

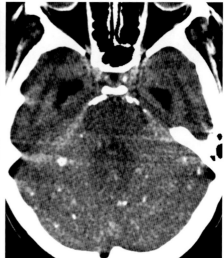

Figure 3. Non-enhanced CT in a patient with metastatic breast cancer shows multiple calcifications ranging from small to barely perceptible throughout the cerebellar hemispheres.

Cysticercosis

MATTHEW OMOJOLA

Also 167

Calcified Metastases

BENJAMIN HUANG

Also 155 & 180

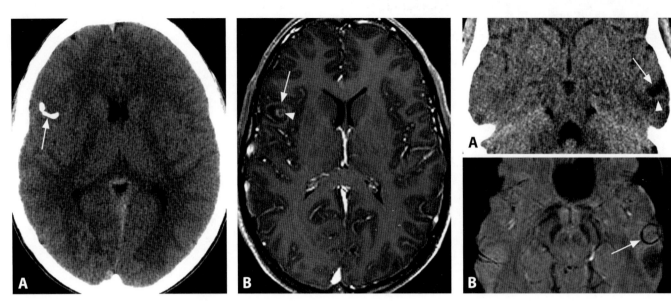

Figure 1. Axial non-enhanced CT image (A) in a 29-year-old patient with epilepsy shows a curvilinear calcification (arrow) in the left frontal lobe without a clear associated abnormality. Axial post-contrast T1WI (B) demonstrates a corresponding rim-enhancing oval hypointense cortical lesion (arrow). The lesion contains internal nodular enhancement (arrowhead), while the calcification is not appreciated. Right frontal ganglioglioma.

Figure 2. Non-enhanced CT (A) shows a peripheral hypodense oval lesion (arrow) in the left temporal lobe with a subtle peripheral calcification (arrowhead), which is better appreciated as a dark ring (arrow) on SWI (B).

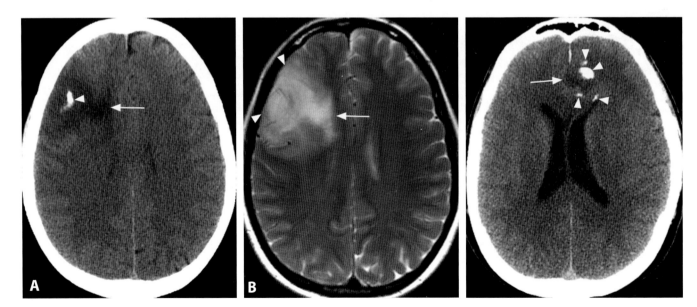

Figure 1. Axial non-enhanced CT image (A) in a 41-year-old patient with new onset seizures shows a right frontal intra-axial hypodense lesion (arrow), which contains central chunky calcification (arrowhead). Corresponding T2WI (B) reveals hyperintense signal of the lesion (arrow), which exhibits mild mass effect and infiltrative edema with involvement of the cortical gray matter (arrowheads). Oligodendroglioma.

Figure 2. Non-enhanced CT image in another patient with oligodendroglioma reveals a hypodense paramedian frontal lesion (arrow) with central and peripheral dense calcifications (arrowheads).

Ganglioglioma

MAURICIO CASTILLO

Also 166

Oligodendroglioma

ZORAN RUMBOLDT

Also 161

Brain Imaging with MRI and CT, ed. Zoran Rumboldt *et al.* Published by Cambridge University Press. © Cambridge University Press 2012.

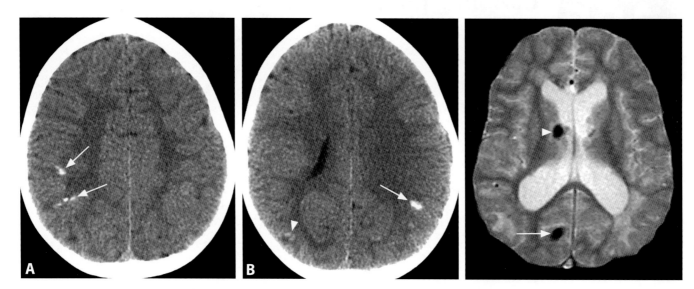

Figure 1. Axial non-enhanced CT image (A) in a patient with epilepsy shows cortico-subcortical calcifications (arrows) in the right cerebral hemisphere. CT image at a slightly lower level (B) shows a peripheral calcification (arrow) in the left hemisphere. An additional subtle calcification (arrowhead) is present in a cortico-subcortical location on the right. The findings are consistent with cortical tubers in tuberous sclerosis.

Figure 2. Axial T2*WI shows a focal cortico-subcortical area of signal loss (arrow) in the right occipital lobe. There is also a subependymal lesion of similar appearance (arrowhead).

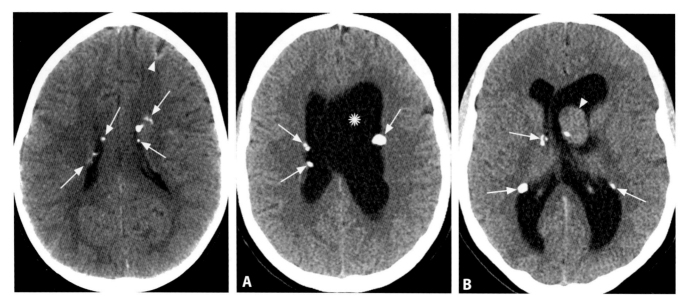

Figure 3. Axial non-enhanced CT image shows multiple calcifications along the walls of the lateral ventricles (arrows). There is also a subtle peripheral calcification (arrowhead).

Figure 4. Axial non-enhanced CT image (A) demonstrates calcified nodules along the lateral ventricular walls (arrows), as well as ventriculomegaly (*). A more caudal CT image (B) reveals additional subependymal nodules (arrows). There is also a soft tissue mass (arrowhead) arising in the region of the left foramen of Monro and engulfing one of the calcifications. Subependymal giant cell astrocytoma causing obstructive hydrocephalus.

Cortical Tubers in Tuberous Sclerosis

ZORAN RUMBOLDT

Also 107

Subependymal Nodules in Tuberous Sclerosis

ZORAN RUMBOLDT

Also 107

403

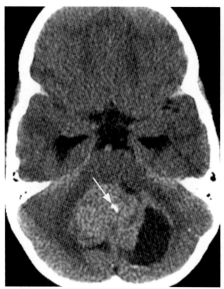

Figure 1. Axial non-enhanced CT image in a 9-year-old child shows a heterogenous posterior fossa mass that is centered at the fourth ventricle and contains calcifications (arrow). Dilated temporal horns indicate hydrocephalus.

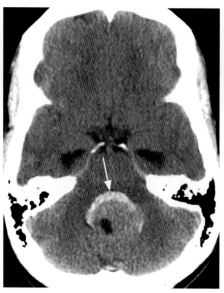

Figure 2. Non-enhanced axial CT image in a different young patient demonstrates a heterogenous mass within the fourth ventricle containing prominent peripheral calcifications (arrow). Ependymoma.

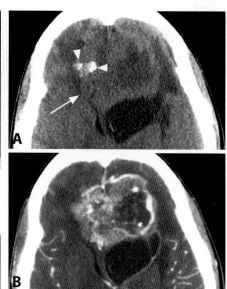

Figure 3. Non-enhanced CT (A) shows a frontal paraventricular mass (arrow) with internal calcifications (arrowheads). Post-contrast image (B) reveals marked heterogenous enhancement of this anaplastic ependymoma.

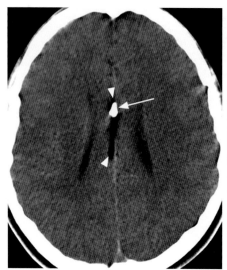

Figure 1. Axial non-enhanced CT image shows a midline curvilinear pericallosal lesion of very low attenuation (arrowheads) with a focus of calcification (arrow).

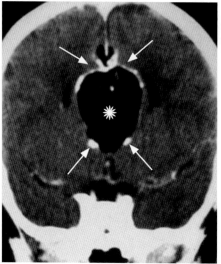

Figure 2. Coronal contrast-enhanced CT image demonstrates a large hypodense mass (*) with scattered peripheral calcifications (arrows).

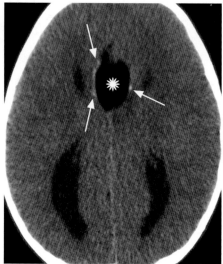

Figure 3. Axial non-enhanced CT image shows an anterior tubulonodular interhemispheric lipoma (*) with faint peripheral calcifications (arrows).

Ependymoma

ZORAN RUMBOLDT

Also 172

Lipoma With Calcification

BENJAMIN HUANG

Also 76

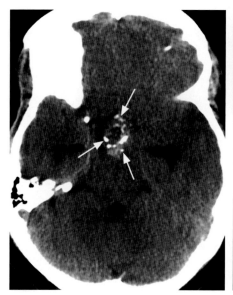

Figure 1. Axial non-enhanced CT image in a 10-year-old child shows a heterogenous suprasellar mass with scattered calcifications (arrows). Dilated temporal horns indicate hydrocephalus.

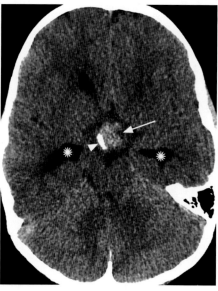

Figure 2. Axial non-enhanced CT image in another patient reveals a hyperdense suprasellar mass (arrow) with peripheral calcification (arrowhead). Note dilated temporal horns (*).

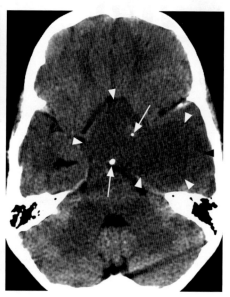

Figure 3. Non-enhanced CT shows a large hypodense suprasellar and left middle cranial fossa mass (arrowheads). Internal foci of calcification (arrows) are seen in this craniopharyngioma.

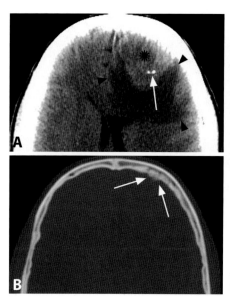

Figure 1. Non-enhanced CT (A) shows a left frontal mass (*) with a wide dural base and calcifications (arrow). Note surrounding vasogenic edema (arrowheads) and mass effect. Bone algorithm and window (B) reveals associated hyperostotic reaction (arrows).

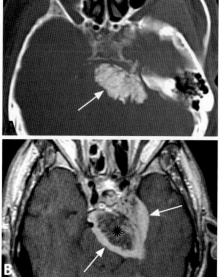

Figure 2. Axial bone algorithm and window CT (A) shows a densely calcifed mass (arrow) adjacent to the petrous bone and clivus. Post-contrast T1WI (B) shows the full size of the meningioma (arrows) with typical dense enhancement around the calcified portion (*).

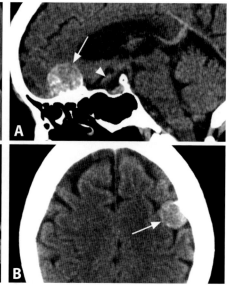

Figure 3. Non-enhanced reformatted sagittal CT image (A) shows a hyperdense partly calcified mass (arrow) with the base along the anterior cranial fossa, and intact optic chiasm (arrowhead). Axial image (B) reveals an additional left frontal meningioma (arrow).

Also 44

CASE

203

Meningioma

ALESSANDRO CIANFONI

Also 47, 138, 149

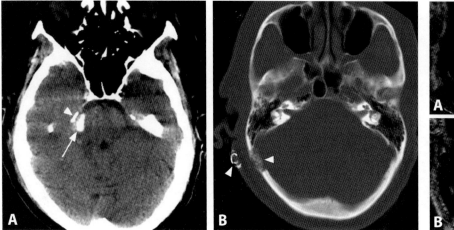

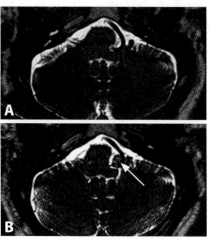

Figure 1. Non-enhanced CT image (A) shows a densely calcified lesion (arrow) in the location of the right trigeminal nerve, medial to the tentorium (arrowhead). A previous CT with bone window and algorithm demonstrates status post right retromastoid craniotomy (arrowheads) – typical approach for microvascular decompression.

Figure 2. Axial high-resolution 3D T2WIs before (A) and after neurovascular surgery (B) show a new mass (arrow) next to the vertebral artery.

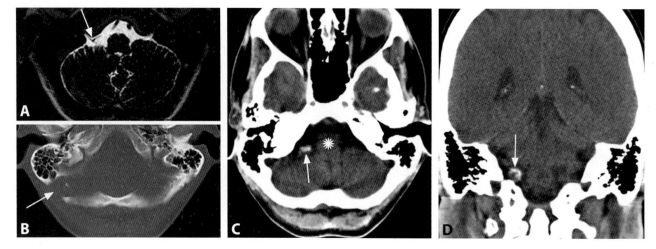

Figure 3. Axial high-resolution 3D T2WI (A) shows a possible neurovascular conflict between right PICA and IX–X exiting nerve complex (arrow). Follow-up CT (B) shows retromastoid postoperative defect (arrow). A calcified mass (arrow) to the right of the medulla oblongata (*), in the location of the preoperative conflict is seen on other axial (C) and coronal (D) CT images.

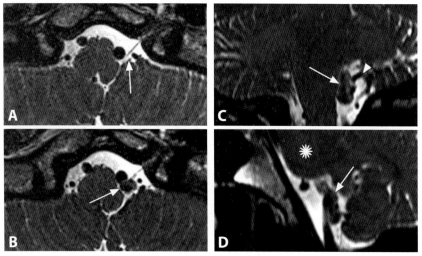

Figure 4. Preoperative axial high-resolution 3D T2WI (A) shows close proximity of the left vertebral artery and PICA to the IX–X nerve complex (arrow). Postoperative follow-up image after recurrence of symptoms (B) reveals a new heterogeneously hypointense mass (arrow) in the same area. Coronal (C) and sagittal (D) reconstructed images show the extent of the lesion (arrow) adjacent to PICA (arrowhead). Normal pons (*).

Specific Imaging Findings

Teflon granuloma is seen as a focal calcification on CT images and tends to be hypointense on all MRI sequences. They may range from a few millimeters to a few centimeters in size and frequently enhance on post-contrast MR images. The typical location is in the cerebellopontine angle at the site of previous neurosurgical vascular decompression procedure. Granulomas are most commonly seen following surgery for intractable trigeminal neuralgia, characteristically at the root entry zone (REZ) of the nerve within the first few millimeters from the brainstem. The lesions are best depicted on high-resolution 3D MR images, either T2-weighted (such as CISS, DRIVE, FIESTA) or post-contrast T1-weighted, as elongated oval to round heterogenous structures, characteristically located between the vessel and the nerve or brainstem.

Pertinent Clinical Information

Microvascular decompression (MVD) is commonly performed for medically refractory trigeminal neuralgia (tic douloureux) and hemifacial spasm. A piece of polytetrafluoroethylene (PTFE, Teflon) is usually placed between the nerve (or pons) and the blood vessel compressing the nerve. Deleterious effects of this procedure are rare; however, cases of enlarging enhancing masses that were mistaken for neoplasms have been described. More commonly the patients present with recurrence of the initial symptomatology, usually within a few years, frequently accompanied by new facial numbness. Teflon granuloma is found on surgical re-exploration, sometimes with prominent adhesions. Polyvinyl alcohol foam (Ivalon sponge) has also been used for MVD and may also lead to granulomatous reaction and scar formation. Cases of foreign-body granuloma occurring after craniotomy with dura-cranioplasty and other materials have also been described.

Differential Diagnosis

Meningioma (138, 203)
- typically dural-based homogenously enhancing mass

Schwannoma (141)
- calcifications are rare
- may be indistinguishable from granuloma
- usually no history of MVD

Aneurysm (144, 192)
- presence of flow-void and vascular enhancement
- contiguous with the vessel lumen on high-resolution 3D MRI

Granulomatous Diseases (TB, Sarcoidosis) (118, 160)
- dural and leptomeningeal thickening and enhancement is rarely limited to a single small area

Background

Recurrent trigeminal neuralgia after MVD may be due to insufficient decompression, dislocation of the implant, or the development of granuloma. The Teflon felt used in MVD procedures is not absolutely inert and an inflammatory giant-cell foreign body reaction can be induced when it contacts the tentorium and/or dura. It has therefore been suggested that it should be kept away from the tentorium and dura intraoperatively, and placed completely within the CSF cisterns. Small bleeding into the felt at surgery might also trigger inflammatory reaction and formation of dense fibrous tissue. Histopathological examination reveals foreign body granuloma with multinuclear giant cells, collagen-rich hyalinized scar tissue, focal hemosiderin depositions, and microcalcifications. These lesions also show increased FDG uptake on PET/CT scans (such as with vocal cord injections) and may be confused with malignant neoplasms. Teflon-induced granuloma occurs in a small percentage of patients undergoing MVD and may be treated by nerve preserving surgical removal and placement of a new Teflon felt.

REFERENCES

1. Chen J, Lee S, Lui T, et al. Teflon granuloma after microvascular decompression for trigeminal neuralgia. Surg Neurol 2000;53:281–7.
2. Capelle HH, Brandis A, Tschan CA, Krauss JK. Treatment of recurrent trigeminal neuralgia due to Teflon granuloma. J Headache Pain 2010;11:339–44.
3. Megerian CA, Busaba NY, McKenna MJ, Ojemann RG. Teflon granuloma presenting as an enlarging, gadolinium enhancing, posterior fossa mass with progressive hearing loss following microvascular decompression. Am J Otol 1995;16:783–6.
4. Harrigal C, Branstetter BF 4th, Snyderman CH, Maroon J. Teflon granuloma in the nasopharynx: a potentially false-positive PET/CT finding. AJNR 2005;26:417–20.
5. Barker FG 2nd, Jannetta PJ, Bissonette DJ, et al. The long-term outcome of microvascular decompression for trigeminal neuralgia. N Engl J Med 1996;334:1077–83.

INDEX